HUMAN IMMUNODEFICIENCY VIRUS AND THE LUNG

LUNG BIOLOGY IN HEALTH AND DISEASE

Executive Editor

Claude Lenfant
Director, National Heart, Lung and Blood Institute
National Institutes of Health
Bethesda, Maryland

1. Immunologic and Infectious Reactions in the Lung, *edited by Charles H. Kirkpatrick and Herbert Y. Reynolds*
2. The Biochemical Basis of Pulmonary Function, *edited by Ronald G. Crystal*
3. Bioengineering Aspects of the Lung, *edited by John B. West*
4. Metabolic Functions of the Lung, *edited by Y. S. Bakhle and John R. Vane*
5. Respiratory Defense Mechanisms (in two parts), *edited by Joseph D. Brain, Donald F. Proctor, and Lynne M. Reid*
6. Development of the Lung, *edited by W. Alan Hodson*
7. Lung Water and Solute Exchange, *edited by Norman C. Staub*
8. Extrapulmonary Manifestations of Respiratory Disease, *edited by Eugene Debs Robin*
9. Chronic Obstructive Pulmonary Disease, *edited by Thomas L. Petty*
10. Pathogenesis and Therapy of Lung Cancer, *edited by Curtis C. Harris*
11. Genetic Determinants of Pulmonary Disease, *edited by Stephen D. Litwin*
12. The Lung in the Transition Between Health and Disease, *edited by Peter T. Macklem and Solbert Permutt*
13. Evolution of Respiratory Processes: A Comparative Approach, *edited by Stephen C. Wood and Claude Lenfant*
14. Pulmonary Vascular Diseases, *edited by Kenneth M. Moser*
15. Physiology and Pharmacology of the Airways, *edited by Jay A. Nadel*
16. Diagnostic Techniques in Pulmonary Disease (in two parts), *edited by Marvin A. Sackner*
17. Regulation of Breathing (in two parts), *edited by Thomas F. Hornbein*
18. Occupational Lung Diseases: Research Approaches and Methods, *edited by Hans Weill and Margaret Turner-Warwick*
19. Immunopharmacology of the Lung, *edited by Harold H. Newball*
20. Sarcoidosis and Other Granulomatous Diseases of the Lung, *edited by Barry L. Fanburg*

21. Sleep and Breathing, *edited by Nicholas A. Saunders and Colin E. Sullivan*
22. *Pneumocystis carinii* Pneumonia: Pathogenesis, Diagnosis, and Treatment, *edited by Lowell S. Young*
23. Pulmonary Nuclear Medicine: Techniques in Diagnosis of Lung Disease, *edited by Harold L. Atkins*
24. Acute Respiratory Failure, *edited by Warren M. Zapol and Konrad J. Falke*
25. Gas Mixing and Distribution in the Lung, *edited by Ludwig A. Engel and Manuel Paiva*
26. High-Frequency Ventilation in Intensive Care and During Surgery, *edited by Graziano Carlon and William S. Howland*
27. Pulmonary Development: Transition from Intrauterine to Extrauterine Life, *edited by George H. Nelson*
28. Chronic Obstructive Pulmonary Disease: Second Edition, Revised and Expanded, *edited by Thomas L. Petty*
29. The Thorax (in two parts), *edited by Charis Roussos and Peter T. Macklem*
30. The Pleura in Health and Disease, *edited by Jacques Chrétien, Jean Bignon, and Albert Hirsch*
31. Drug Therapy for Asthma: Research and Clinical Practice, *edited by John W. Jenne and Shirley Murphy*
32. Pulmonary Endothelium in Health and Disease, *edited by Una S. Ryan*
33. The Airways: Neural Control in Health and Disease, *edited by Michael A. Kaliner and Peter J. Barnes*
34. Pathophysiology and Treatment of Inhalation Injuries, *edited by Jacob Loke*
35. Respiratory Function of the Upper Airway, *edited by Oommen P. Mathew and Giuseppe Sant'Ambrogio*
36. Chronic Obstructive Pulmonary Disease: A Behavioral Perspective, *edited by A. John McSweeny and Igor Grant*
37. Biology of Lung Cancer: Diagnosis and Treatment, *edited by Steven T. Rosen, James L. Mulshine, Frank Cuttitta, and Paul G. Abrams*
38. Pulmonary Vascular Physiology and Pathophysiology, *edited by E. Kenneth Weir and John T. Reeves*
39. Comparative Pulmonary Physiology: Current Concepts, *edited by Stephen C. Wood*
40. Respiratory Physiology: An Analytical Approach, *edited by H. K. Chang and Manuel Paiva*
41. Lung Cell Biology, *edited by Donald Massaro*
42. Heart–Lung Interactions in Health and Disease, *edited by Steven M. Scharf and Sharon S. Cassidy*
43. Clinical Epidemiology of Chronic Obstructive Pulmonary Disease, *edited by Michael J. Hensley and Nicholas A. Saunders*
44. Surgical Pathology of Lung Neoplasms, *edited by Alberto M. Marchevsky*
45. The Lung in Rheumatic Diseases, *edited by Grant W. Cannon and Guy A. Zimmerman*

46. Diagnostic Imaging of the Lung, *edited by Charles E. Putman*
47. Models of Lung Disease: Microscopy and Structural Methods, *edited by Joan Gil*
48. Electron Microscopy of the Lung, *edited by Dean E. Schraufnagel*
49. Asthma: Its Pathology and Treatment, *edited by Michael A. Kaliner, Peter J. Barnes, and Carl G. A. Persson*
50. Acute Respiratory Failure: Second Edition, *edited by Warren M. Zapol and Francois Lemaire*
51. Lung Disease in the Tropics, *edited by Om P. Sharma*
52. Exercise: Pulmonary Physiology and Pathophysiology, *edited by Brian J. Whipp and Karlman Wasserman*
53. Developmental Neurobiology of Breathing, *edited by Gabriel G. Haddad and Jay P. Farber*
54. Mediators of Pulmonary Inflammation, *edited by Michael A. Bray and Wayne H. Anderson*
55. The Airway Epithelium, *edited by Stephen G. Farmer and Douglas Hay*
56. Physiological Adaptations in Vertebrates: Respiration, Circulation, and Metabolism, *edited by Stephen C. Wood, Roy E. Weber, Alan R. Hargens, and Ronald W. Millard*
57. The Bronchial Circulation, *edited by John Butler*
58. Lung Cancer Differentiation: Implications for Diagnosis and Treatment, *edited by Samuel D. Bernal and Paul J. Hesketh*
59. Pulmonary Complications of Systemic Disease, *edited by John F. Murray*
60. Lung Vascular Injury: Molecular and Cellular Response, *edited by Arnold Johnson and Thomas J. Ferro*
61. Cytokines of the Lung, *edited by Jason Kelley*
62. The Mast Cell in Health and Disease, *edited by Michael A. Kaliner and Dean D. Metcalfe*
63. Pulmonary Disease in the Elderly Patient, *edited by Donald A. Mahler*
64. Cystic Fibrosis, *edited by Pamela B. Davis*
65. Signal Transduction in Lung Cells, *edited by Jerome S. Brody, David M. Center, and Vsevolod A. Tkachuk*
66. Tuberculosis: A Comprehensive International Approach, *edited by Lee B. Reichman and Earl S. Hershfield*
67. Pharmacology of the Respiratory Tract: Experimental and Clinical Research, *edited by K. Fan Chung and Peter J. Barnes*
68. Prevention of Respiratory Diseases, *edited by Albert Hirsch, Marcel Goldberg, Jean-Pierre Martin, and Roland Masse*
69. *Pneumocystis carinii* Pneumonia: Second Edition, Revised and Expanded, *edited by Peter D. Walzer*
70. Fluid and Solute Transport in the Airspaces of the Lungs, *edited by Richard M. Effros and H. K. Chang*
71. Sleep and Breathing: Second Edition, Revised and Expanded, *edited by Nicholas A. Saunders and Colin E. Sullivan*
72. Airway Secretion: Physiological Bases for the Control of Mucous Hypersecretion, *edited by Tamotsu Takishima and Sanae Shimura*

73. Sarcoidosis and Other Granulomatous Disorders, *edited by D. Geraint James*
74. Epidemiology of Lung Cancer, *edited by Jonathan M. Samet*
75. Pulmonary Embolism, *edited by Mario Morpurgo*
76. Sports and Exercise Medicine, *edited by Stephen C. Wood and Robert C. Roach*
77. Endotoxin and the Lungs, *edited by Kenneth L. Brigham*
78. The Mesothelial Cell and Mesothelioma, *edited by Marie-Claude Jaurand and Jean Bignon*
79. Regulation of Breathing: Second Edition, Revised and Expanded, *edited by Jerome A. Dempsey and Allan I. Pack*
80. Pulmonary Fibrosis, *edited by Sem Hin Phan and Roger S. Thrall*
81. Long-Term Oxygen Therapy: Scientific Basis and Clinical Application, *edited by Walter J. O'Donohue, Jr.*
82. Ventral Brainstem Mechanisms and Control of Respiration and Blood Pressure, *edited by C. Ovid Trouth, Richard M. Millis, Heidrun F. Kiwull-Schöne, and Marianne E. Schläfke*
83. A History of Breathing Physiology, *edited by Donald F. Proctor*
84. Surfactant Therapy for Lung Disease, *edited by Bengt Robertson and H. William Taeusch*
85. The Thorax: Second Edition, Revised and Expanded (in three parts), *edited by Charis Roussos*
86. Severe Asthma: Pathogenesis and Clinical Management, *edited by Stanley J. Szefler and Donald Y. M. Leung*
87. *Mycobacterium avium*–Complex Infection: Progress in Research and Treatment, *edited by Joyce A. Korvick and Constance A. Benson*
88. Alpha 1–Antitrypsin Deficiency: Biology • Pathogenesis • Clinical Manifestations • Therapy, *edited by Ronald G. Crystal*
89. Adhesion Molecules and the Lung, *edited by Peter A. Ward and Joseph C. Fantone*
90. Respiratory Sensation, *edited by Lewis Adams and Abraham Guz*
91. Pulmonary Rehabilitation, *edited by Alfred P. Fishman*
92. Acute Respiratory Failure in Chronic Obstructive Pulmonary Disease, *edited by Jean-Philippe Derenne, William A. Whitelaw, and Thomas Similowski*
93. Environmental Impact on the Airways: From Injury to Repair, *edited by Jacques Chrétien and Daniel Dusser*
94. Inhalation Aerosols: Physical and Biological Basis for Therapy, *edited by Anthony J. Hickey*
95. Tissue Oxygen Deprivation: From Molecular to Integrated Function, *edited by Gabriel G. Haddad and George Lister*
96. The Genetics of Asthma, *edited by Stephen B. Liggett and Deborah A. Meyers*
97. Inhaled Glucocorticoids in Asthma: Mechanisms and Clinical Actions, *edited by Robert P. Schleimer, William W. Busse, and Paul M. O'Byrne*
98. Nitric Oxide and the Lung, *edited by Warren M. Zapol and Kenneth D. Bloch*

99. Primary Pulmonary Hypertension, *edited by Lewis J. Rubin and Stuart Rich*
100. Lung Growth and Development, *edited by John A. McDonald*
101. Parasitic Lung Diseases, *edited by Adel A. F. Mahmoud*
102. Lung Macrophages and Dendritic Cells in Health and Disease, *edited by Mary F. Lipscomb and Stephen W. Russell*
103. Pulmonary and Cardiac Imaging, *edited by Caroline Chiles and Charles E. Putman*
104. Gene Therapy for Diseases of the Lung, *edited by Kenneth L. Brigham*
105. Oxygen, Gene Expression, and Cellular Function, *edited by Linda Biadasz Clerch and Donald J. Massaro*
106. $Beta_2$-Agonists in Asthma Treatment, *edited by Romain Pauwels and Paul M. O'Byrne*
107. Inhalation Delivery of Therapeutic Peptides and Proteins, *edited by Akwete Lex Adjei and Pramod K. Gupta*
108. Asthma in the Elderly, *edited by Robert A. Barbee and John W. Bloom*
109. Treatment of the Hospitalized Cystic Fibrosis Patient, *edited by David M. Orenstein and Robert C. Stern*
110. Asthma and Immunological Diseases in Pregnancy and Early Infancy, *edited by Michael Schatz, Robert S. Zeiger, and Henry N. Claman*
111. Dyspnea, *edited by Donald A. Mahler*
112. Proinflammatory and Antiinflammatory Peptides, *edited by Sami I. Said*
113. Self-Management of Asthma, *edited by Harry Kotses and Andrew Harver*
114. Eicosanoids, Aspirin, and Asthma, *edited by Andrew Szczeklik, Ryszard J. Gryglewski, and John R. Vane*
115. Fatal Asthma, *edited by Albert L. Sheffer*
116. Pulmonary Edema, *edited by Michael A. Matthay and David H. Ingbar*
117. Inflammatory Mechanisms in Asthma, *edited by Stephen T. Holgate and William W. Busse*
118. Physiological Basis of Ventilatory Support, *edited by John J. Marini and Arthur S. Slutsky*
119. Human Immunodeficiency Virus and the Lung, *edited by Mark J. Rosen and James M. Beck*
120. Five-Lipoxygenase Products in Asthma, *edited by Jeffrey M. Drazen, Sven-Erik Dahlén, and Tak H. Lee*

ADDITIONAL VOLUMES IN PREPARATION

Complexity in Structure and Function of the Lung, *edited by Michael P. Hlastala and H. Thomas Robertson*

Biology of Lung Cancer, *edited by Madeleine A. Kane and Paul A. Bunn, Jr.*

The Lung at Depth, *edited by Claes Lundgren and John N. Miller*

Lung Tumors, *edited by Christian Brambilla and Elisabeth Brambilla*

Diagnostic Pulmonary Pathology, *edited by Philip Cagle*

Immunotherapy of Asthma, *edited by Jean Bousquet and Hans Yssel*

Rhinitis, *edited by Robert M. Maclerio, Stephen R. Durham, and Niels Mygind*

Interleukin-5: From Molecule to Drug Target for Asthma, *edited by Colin Sanderson*

Viral Infections of the Lung, *edited by Raphael Dolin and Peter F. Wright*

Pediatric Asthma, *edited by Shirley J. Murphy, H. William Kelly, and Bennie C. McWilliams*

LAM and Other Diseases Characterized by Smooth Muscle Proliferation, *edited by Joel Moss*

GERD and Airway Disease, *edited by Mark R. Stein*

Control of Breathing in Health and Disease, *edited by Murray D. Altose and Yoshikazu Kawakami*

Neurobiology of Sleep and Circadian Rhythms, *edited by Fred Turek and Phyllis Zee*

Multimodality Treatment of Lung Cancer, *edited by Arthur T. Skarin*

Cytokines in Pulmonary Infectious Disease, *edited by Steven Nelson and Thomas Martin*

Air Pollutants and the Respiratory Tract, *edited by David L. Swift*

Exercise-Induced Asthma, *edited by E. Regis McFadden Jr.*

The opinions expressed in these volumes do not necessarily represent the views of the National Institutes of Health.

HUMAN IMMUNODEFICIENCY VIRUS AND THE LUNG

Edited by

Mark J. Rosen

Albert Einstein College of Medicine and
Beth Israel Medical Center
New York, New York

James M. Beck

University of Michigan Medical School and
Veterans Affairs Medical Center
Ann Arbor, Michigan

MARCEL DEKKER

MARCEL DEKKER, INC. NEW YORK • BASEL • HONG KONG

Library of Congress Cataloging-in-Publication Data

Human immunodeficiency virus and the lung/edited by Mark J. Rosen, James M. Beck.
p. cm.—(Lung biology in health and disease; v. 119)
Includes bibliographical references and index.
ISBN: 0-8247-9883-X
1. Respiratory infections. 2. Lungs—Diseases. 3. AIDS (Disease)—Complications. I. Rosen, Mark J. II. Beck, James M. III. Series.
[DNLM: 1. HIV Infections—complications. 2. Lung Diseases—complications. WC 503.5 H918 1998]
RC740.H86 1998
616.2'407—dc21
DNLM/DLC
for Library of Congress 98-7847
CIP

This book is printed on acid-free paper.

Headquarters
Marcel Dekker, Inc.
270 Madison Avenue, New York, NY 10016
tel: 212-696-9000; fax: 212-685-4540

Eastern Hemisphere Distribution
Marcel Dekker AG
Hutgasse 4, Postfach 812, CH-4001 Basel, Switzerland
tel: 44-61-261-8482; fax: 44-61-261-8896

World Wide Web
http://www.dekker.com

The publisher offers discounts on this book when ordered in bulk quantities. For more information, write to Special Sales/Professional Marketing at the headquarters address above.

Current printing (last digit)
10 9 8 7 6 5 4 3 2 1

PRINTED IN THE UNITED STATES OF AMERICA

INTRODUCTION

Since its inception in 1976, the first year of publication, the Lung Biology in Health and Disease series has had two specific, but interrelated, purposes: to inform and to challenge.

The first goal has largely been advanced by the definite arrival of pulmonary medicine as a medical specialty that now has joined forces with critical care medicine. The second goal has been driven by a continuous flow of discoveries in the area of lung biology and medicine. Thus, it should not be surprising that this series of monographs has devoted much attention to the relationship between the lung and HIV infection and other associated infections.

As early as 1984, the series presented Volume 22, titled Pneumocystis carinii *Pneumonia: Pathogenesis, Diagnosis, and Treatment*, edited by Lowell S. Young. Although *Pneumocystis* infections in some forms of immunodeficiency had been described in 1957 by Gajducek, interest in this relatively rare condition faded until the fundamental description of a "new acquired cellular immunodeficiency" by M.S. Gottlied et al. in 1981. This was only three years before Lowell Young's publication in the series. By then, AIDS and its cause, HIV, had appeared!

The years that followed led to an ever-increasing amount of knowledge about AIDS and its pulmonary involvement and complications. And so, in 1992, the topic received prominent attention in Volume 59, *Pulmonary Complications of Systemic Disease*, edited by John F. Murray. But what we knew then was so extensive that a single chapter was not enough to meet the purposes of the series of monographs. Thus, Volume 69, Pneumocystis carinii *Pneumonia: Second Edition, Revised and Expanded*, edited by Peter D. Walzer, went to press in 1993.

More knowledge has been acquired and major discoveries have been made—much to the benefit of the growing number of patients, whose life expectancy keeps on increasing. Although the disease is not conquered, what we know today is a triumph of basic research and clinical investigations, including drug discovery.

Unfortunately, there is a trade-off! At the beginning of the AIDS epidemic, *Pneumocystis carinii* pneumonia and Kaposi's sarcoma were the major threats to the lungs of AIDS patients. Since, we have found that the prolonged survival of these patients has resulted in the development of a greater number of associated lung complications, with ever greater severity.

This book is a major treatise on Human Immunodeficiency Virus and the Lung. It truly exemplifies the purpose of the series as a whole: to inform and to challenge . . . and there is a good reason for it. The editors and the authors are physicians and investigators who are on the front line of the care of AIDS patients, and they are at the cutting edge of research on this disease. As the Executive Editor of this series of monographs, I want to express my gratitude to all of them for their contributions.

Claude Lenfant, M.D.
Bethesda, Maryland

PREFACE

The first cases of the acquired immunodeficiency syndrome (AIDS) were reported on June 4, 1981, when the Centers for Disease Control (CDC) described five gay men in Los Angeles who had *Pneumocystis carinii* pneumonia. Although *P. carinii* infection was known to occur only in severely immunocompromised hosts, these men had no recognized cause of immunosuppression. Since that initial report, an explosion of information has been obtained concerning the biology of the human immunodeficiency virus (HIV) and its attendant immunological effects.

From that initial report until the present day, pulmonary complications have figured prominently in AIDS-related morbidity and mortality. In 1983, the Division of Lung Diseases of the National Heart, Lung and Blood Institute (NHLBI), National Institutes of Health, sponsored a workshop on the pulmonary complications of AIDS. This meeting brought together clinicians from centers with vast experience in the diagnosis and treatment of patients with AIDS to share their data. The result was a report that detailed the types and relative incidence of pulmonary disorders, recommended algorithms for diagnosis and treatment, and suggested avenues for further research (1). In 1987, the NHLBI and the National Institute of Allergy and Infectious Diseases jointly initiated the Pulmonary Complications of HIV Infections Study, a multicenter, prospective effort designed to describe the lung diseases associated with all stages of HIV infection. This study's contributions to the literature was a small part of an enormous international effort to describe the mechanisms and clinical features of HIV infection as it relates to pulmonary disease.

Throughout the epidemic, the NHLBI has supported basic and clinical investigations of HIV-related disease, and the current volume represents another in the NHLBI's efforts to disseminate, in a timely manner, information about HIV's effects in the lung. As editors for this volume, we realize that the brisk pace of investigation in this field produces new information on a monthly, if not daily, basis. Therefore, we attempted to include the most comprehensive and current information available, emphasizing that which is unlikely to change by the time the book is published. We are privileged to include as authors some of the investigators whose work established the scientific basis of HIV infection of the lung, collaborators in the Pulmonary Complications of HIV Infections Study, and clinical leaders with great experience in diagnosing and treating patients with HIV-related lung diseases.

The volume begins with an overview of the pulmonary complications of HIV infection, stressing epidemiological approaches and intensive care. We then follow with a section describing the basic biology of HIV infection in the lung, including HIV's effects on lung immune cells. In this way, we hope to provide both clinically and research-oriented readers with a sound scientific foundation for the clinical chapters that follow. Next, diagnosis of pulmonary disorders in HIV-infected individuals is covered, including invasive and noninvasive testing as well as screening. A comprehensive review of infectious causes of pulmonary disease during HIV infection follows, considering each etiological entity individually. In the reviews of noninfectious pulmonary disorders, we consider the neoplastic, inflammatory, and immunological complications of HIV infection. Finally, infection control for the pulmonary specialist is reviewed.

As we complete this volume, recent advances in antiretroviral therapy for HIV infection have created tremendous optimism that HIV infection will eventually become a chronic, manageable disease. Based on the devastating pulmonary effects of HIV infection that we have diagnosed and treated for many years, this enthusiasm is welcome. However, many HIV-infected individuals will not be able to tolerate this therapy. Furthermore, societal inequities in availability and delivery of health care result in persistent barriers that block access to these medications for many patients. On a global scale, limited health care resources mean that HIV will continue to have a devastating effect. Even here, however, there is some cause for optimism. For example, public health measures, such as condom distribution in Thailand, have reduced the spread of HIV infection in that country, and directly observed therapy of tuberculosis in the United States reversed the steady increases of that infection. However, it is likely that both clinicians and basic scientists will be dealing with the pulmonary complications of HIV infection for many years to come. We hope that this volume will provide a comprehensive compendium of these complications, and will synthesize disparate information into an accessible format.

Mark J. Rosen
James M. Beck

Reference

1. Murray JF, Felton CP, Garay SM, Gottlieb MS, Hopewell PC, Stover DE, Teirstein AS. Pulmonary complications of the acquired immunodeficiency syndrome. Report of a National Heart, Lung and Blood Institute workshop. N Engl J Med 1984; 310:1682–1688.

CONTRIBUTORS

Frank L. Acerra, D.O. Fellow, Pulmonary and Critical Care Medicine, Beth Israel Medical Center, New York, New York

Carlo Agostini, M.D. Deputy, Department of Clinical and Experimental Medicine, Padua University School of Medicine, Padua, Italy

Thomas L. Benfield, M.D. Research Fellow, Department of Infectious Diseases, Hvidovre University Hospital, Hvidovre, Denmark

Juan Carlos Celedón, M.D., F.A.C.P., F.C.C.P. Research Fellow, Department of Medicine, Harvard Medical School, and Channing Laboratory, Brigham and Women's Hospital, Boston, Massachusetts

Scott F. Davies, M.D. Professor of Medicine, University of Minnesota Medical School, and Division Director, Pulmonary and Critical Care Medicine, Department of Internal Medicine, Hennepin County Medical Center, Minneapolis, Minnesota

Vera A. De Palo, M.D. Assistant Professor of Medicine, Pulmonary and Critical Care Medicine, Brown University School of Medicine, Providence, Rhode Island

Don C. Des Jarlais, Ph.D. Professor of Epidemiology and Social Medicine, Albert Einstein College of Medicine and Director of Research, Chemical Dependency Institute, Beth Israel Medical Center, New York, New York

Samuel R. Friedman, Ph.D. Senior Research Fellow, Institute for AIDS Research, National Development and Research Institutes, Inc., New York, New York

Jeffrey Glassroth, M.D. Thomas J. Vischer Professor and Chairman, Department of Medicine, MCP-Hahnemann Medical School, Philadelphia, Pennsylvania

Robert E. Hirschtick, M.D. Assistant Professor of Medicine, Section of Infectious Diseases, Northwestern University Medical School, Chicago, Illinois

Jeffrey I. Kuritzky, M.D. Department of Pulmonary and Critical Care Medicine, Beth Israel Medical Center, New York, New York

Paul A. Kvale, M.D. Professor of Medicine, Case Western Reserve University School of Medicine, and Henry Ford Hospital, Cleveland, Ohio

Jens D. Lundgren, M.D., D.M.Sc. Consultant and Assistant Professor, Department of Infectious Diseases, University of Copenhagen, and Hvidovre University Hospital, Hvidovre, Denmark

Bonita T. Mangura, M.D. Associate Professor of Clinical Medicine, Department of Medicine, University of Medicine and Dentistry of New Jersey–New Jersey Medical School, and New Jersey Medical School National Tuberculosis Center, Newark, New Jersey

Frederick P. Ognibene, M.D. Senior Investigator, Department of Critical Care Medicine, Warren G. Magnuson Clinical Center, National Institutes of Health, Bethesda, Maryland

Court Pedersen, M.D., Ph.D. Head, Department of Infectious Diseases C, Odense University Hospital, Odense, Denmark

Beth G. Raucher, M.D. Associate Professor of Clinical Medicine, Albert Einstein College of Medicine, and Hospital Epidemiologist, Department of Infection Control, Beth Israel Medical Center, New York, New York

Lee B. Reichman, M.D., M.P.H. Professor of Medicine, Preventive Medicine and Community Health, Department of Medicine, University of Medicine and Dentistry of New Jersey–New Jersey Medical School, and Executive Director, New Jersey Medical School National Tuberculosis Center, Newark, New Jersey

Elizabeth A. Rich, M.D. Associate Professor, Department of Medicine, Case Western Reserve University, and University Hospitals of Cleveland, Cleveland, Ohio

Mark J. Rosen, M.D. Professor of Medicine, Albert Einstein College of Medicine, and Chief, Pulmonary and Critical Care Medicine, Beth Israel Medical Center, New York, New York

Steve H. Salzman, M.D. Albert Einstein College of Medicine, and Director, Pulmonary Diagnostic Laboratory, Department of Pulmonary and Critical Care Medicine, Beth Israel Medical Center, New York, New York

George A. Sarosi, M.D. Chief, Medical Service, and Professor of Medicine, Department of Veterans Affairs, Roudebush VA Medical Center, Indiana University School of Medicine, Indianapolis, Indiana

Roslyn F. Schneider, M.D. Assistant Professor, Department of Medicine, Albert Einstein College of Medicine, and Beth Israel Medical Center, New York, New York

Gianpietro Semenzato, M.D. Associate Professor of Medicine, Department of Clinical and Experimental Medicine, Padua University School of Medicine, Padua, Italy

John D. Stansell, M.D. Associate Professor, Department of Medicine, University of California at San Francisco, San Francisco, California

William D. Travis, M.D. Professor, Department of Pulmonary and Mediastinal Pathology, Armed Forces Institute of Pathology, Washington, D.C.

Homer L. Twigg III, M.D. Associate Professor, Division of Pulmonary and Critical Care, Department of Medicine, Indiana University Medical Center, Indianapolis, Indiana

Deborah M. Ushkow, M.D. Department of Pulmonary and Critical Care Medicine, Beth Israel Medical Center, New York, New York

Jeanne Marie Wallace, M.D. Associate Professor, Department of Medicine, Olive View–UCLA Medical Center at Los Angeles, Sylmar, California

Dorothy A. White, M.D. Attending Physician, Department of Medicine, Memorial Sloan–Kettering Cancer Center, New York, New York

Emanuel I. Wurm, D.O. Fellow, Pulmonary and Critical Care Medicine, Beth Israel Medical Center, New York, New York

CONTENTS

Part One

OVERVIEW OF HIV INFECTION

1

Overview of Respiratory Disease in HIV Infection

MARK J. ROSEN

Albert Einstein College of Medicine and
Beth Israel Medical Center
New York, New York

I. Introduction

The acquired immunodeficiency syndrome (AIDS) epidemic is now well into its second decade, and is arguably the most important global health problem of the 20th century. By July 1996, almost 550,000 cases of AIDS were reported in the United States, and over 340,000 persons had died of the disease (1). Approximately 50,000 Americans with AIDS die each year, and AIDS is the leading cause of death in the age group 25–44 years (2,3). The annual US death rate in persons with AIDS increased steadily until 1994, but declined for the first time during 1996 (2). However, the prevalence of AIDS in the population continues to increase, with an estimated 225,000 persons as of June 1996. The number of persons with human immunodeficiency virus (HIV) infection in the United States is difficult to determine, but is estimated at 650,000–950,000 (2). The worldwide effect of the AIDS epidemic is devastating: some sub-Saharan countries could lose a quarter of their adult population, and an estimated 10 million Asians may die of AIDS-related illnesses before the year 2015.

Since the beginning of the epidemic, lung diseases were among the most important causes of illness and death. The first cases of AIDS were described in homosexual men in Los Angeles who had *Pneumocystis carinii* pneumonia (PCP), without a known reason for immunodeficiency (4). In the early 1980s, AIDS was known as "GRID," or "gay-related immune deficiency," and PCP was considered the predominant opportunistic infection and pulmonary disorder. In October 1983, the National Heart, Lung and Blood Institute-sponsored Workshop on Pulmonary Complications of HIV Infection reported that 41% of the 1067 patients diagnosed with AIDS in the participating institutions had "serious" pulmonary disorders, and PCP accounted for 85% of cases (5). As the epidemic progressed, it became apparent that AIDS was not just a disease of gay men, and that other lung diseases were important, not only in those with full-blown AIDS, but also in HIV-infected persons with less severe immune compromise. Also, the types of lung diseases that people with HIV infection develop changed over the years, as the demographics of HIV-infected populations shifted and prophylaxis against *P. carinii* became widely used.

II. Definition of AIDS

To track the epidemic, the Centers for Disease Control (CDC) established a case definition of AIDS in 1983 (6). AIDS was defined by the presence of specific opportunistic infections and neoplasms that occurred with advanced immunosuppression, and PCP was the most common AIDS-defining disorder. Because the purpose of surveillance is to describe the affected populations to anticipate trends and guide public health planning and responses, the case definition was revised in 1987 and in 1992 to reflect the new understanding of AIDS-related disorders (7,8). Since 1993, recurrent pneumonia, pulmonary tuberculosis, and carcinoma of the cervix are AIDS-defining disorders in HIV-infected persons. Advanced immunosuppression, defined as a $CD4^+$ lymphocyte count of fewer than 200/μl, or less than 20% of total lymphocytes, was also included in the case definition, even without opportunistic infections or neoplasms. The expanded definition of AIDS led to a 111% increase in reported cases from 1992 to 1993 (Fig. 1), and new case reports increased disproportionally in women, racial and ethnic minorities, and injection drug users (9).

The revised case definition reflects the recognition that PCP is not the predominant pulmonary disorder in HIV-infected persons. This perception came from early reports that only considered patients who met the older definitions for AIDS, almost all of whom had advanced immunosuppression, and it did not consider people who did not meet the criteria for AIDS. Our appreciation of a wider spectrum of disease increased with observations in patients with less severe immunosuppression.

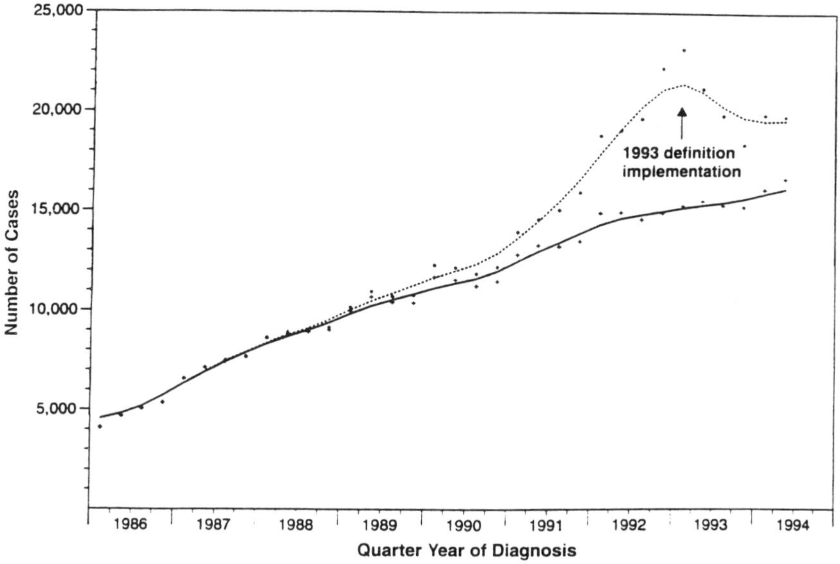

Figure 1 AIDS incidence and estimated AIDS–opportunistic illness incidence, adjusted for delays in reporting, by quarter year of diagnosis, January 1986 through June 1994, United States. (From Ref. 55.)

III. Risk Factors for Specific Pulmonary Diseases

Table 1 lists the major infectious, neoplastic, inflammatory, and other diseases that occur in patients with HIV infection. The full spectrum of pulmonary disorders that are associated with HIV infection range from abnormalities in pulmonary function, unaccompanied by respiratory symptoms, to fatal opportunistic infections. The risk for developing each of these disorders is strongly influenced by the severity of immunosuppression, the patient's demographic characteristics and place of current or prior residence, and whether they are using prophylaxis against common HIV-associated infections. Genetic factors are undoubtedly important, but less precisely defined.

A. Influence of Immune Function

The severity and type of immunosuppression has a major influence on the risk of developing different pulmonary disorders. Because immune competence is difficult to quantify, the $CD4^+$ lymphocyte count is used most often as a surrogate marker for severity of immunosuppression and as a predictor of the probability of developing specific diseases (10). Until re-

Table 1 Pulmonary Complications of HIV Infection

Bacteria	
	Streptococcus pneumoniae
	Hemophilus influenzae
	Staphylococcus aureus
	Moraxella catarrhalis
	Pseudomonas aeruginosa
	Rhodococcus equii
	Nocardia asteroides
	Mycobacterium tuberculosis
	M. avium–intracellulare
	Other nontuberculous mycobacteria
Protozoa	
	Pneumocystis carinii (fungus?)
	Strongyloides stercoralis
	Toxoplasma gondii
Viruses	
	Cytomegalovirus
	Adenovirus
	Herpes simplex
Fungi	
	Aspergillus fumigatus
	Cryptococcus neoformans
	Blastomyces dermatitides
	Coccidioides immitis
	Histoplasma capsulatum
Malignancies	
	Kaposi's sarcoma
	Non-Hodgkin's lymphoma
	Carcinoma of the lung
Other pulmonary disorders	
	Lymphocytic interstitial pneumonitis
	Nonspecific interstitial pneumonitis
	Bronchiolitis obliterans-organizing pneumonia
	Primary pulmonary hypertension

cently, the $CD4^+$ lymphocyte count was also used to predict the likelihood of progression of HIV disease (11). However, measurement of HIV-1 RNA in the plasma has replaced $CD4^+$ lymphocyte counts as the strongest predictor of progression of disease and response to antiretroviral therapy (12–14).

Following infection with HIV, most persons develop a progressive decline in immune function over years, although some "nonprogressors" remain well, with stable $CD4^+$ counts for at least 10 years (15,16). Early in the course of HIV infection, when the immune system is not severely compromised, respiratory disorders tend to be similar to those that affect the general population; opportunistic infections occur only with severe immunodeficiency. Recent studies confirmed the relation of immune function to the risk of common problems such as upper respiratory infection, bacterial pneumonia, and pulmonary tuberculosis. In the Pulmonary Complications of HIV Infection Study, 1353 subjects were followed prospectively in six U.S. cities to determine the prevalence, incidence, and types of lung diseases that occur in persons in selected HIV transmission categories (17). To describe the types of disorders that occur in early HIV infection, patients with an AIDS-defining diagnosis (1987 case definition) were excluded from enrollment. After 18 months of follow-up, the most frequent respiratory diagnoses in the HIV-seropositive subjects were upper respiratory infection (33.4%), acute bronchitis (16%), and acute sinusitis (5.3%). Although these disorders were also common in a control group of HIV-seronegative gay men and injection drug users, the incidences of acute bronchitis and sinusitis were significantly higher in the HIV-infected subjects. Surprisingly, upper respiratory infections (defined as a mild, self-limited illnesses with coryza, and sometimes, sore throat and cough), occurred less frequently in subjects with a baseline $CD4^+$ cell count of fewer than 250/μl, compared with those with higher lymphocyte counts. The reason for this is unknown, but it is possible that patients with severe immunosuppression may have a less vigorous immune response and milder symptoms with this self-limited illness. In the same study, bacterial pneumonia and PCP occurred more frequently in subjects with baseline $CD4^+$ lymphocyte counts of few than 250/μl than in those with higher counts.

The association between reduction in the $CD4^+$ lymphocyte count and the risk of developing specific diseases was explored in a survey of the medical records of more than 18,000 HIV-infected subjects who received care in more than 100 sites in ten U.S. cities (Table 2; 18). Common disorders, such as sinusitis, bronchitis, and pharyngitis, occurred at all strata of $CD4^+$ cell counts. With lower counts, different pulmonary infections occurred with increasing frequency: 80% of cases of bacterial pneumonia, and pulmonary tuberculosis occurred with $CD4^+$ cell counts of fewer than 400/μl, recurrent pneumonia and nontuberculous pulmonary mycobacterioses at $CD4^+$ counts fewer than 300/μl, and PCP, Kaposi's sarcoma, and disseminated *Mycobacterium tuberculosis* at $CD4^+$ of fewer than 200/μl. More than 80% of cases of disseminated nontuberculous mycobacterioses, including *M. avium–intracellulare*, disseminated fungal infections, central nervous system toxoplasmosis, and cytomegalovirus disease occurred in

Table 2 Selected Disease Conditions Listed by $CD4^+$ Below Which 80% of HIV-Infected Patients Were Diagnosed (Number of Cases, Percent Reported During Follow-up)

Disease	Patients (*n*)	(%)
$CD4^+ < 100/\mu l$		
Disseminated *M. avium* complex	1144	(6.5)
Cytomegalovirus disease	513	(2.9)
Extrapulmonary cryptococcosis	280	(1.6)
Disseminated histoplasmosis	57	(0.3)
Pulmonary candidiasis	35	(0.2)
Disseminated coccidioidomycosis	14	(0.1)
$CD4^+$ 100–199/μl		
P. carinii pneumonia	1097	(7.3)
Kaposi's sarcoma	695	(4.0)
Bacterial sepsis	557	(3.1)
Disseminated *M. tuberculosis*	153	(0.9)
$CD4^+$ 200–299/μl		
Pulmonary *Mycobacterium* (excludes tuberculosis)	464	(2.6)
Recurrent pneumonia	375	(2.1)
$CD4^+$ 300–399/μl		
Pneumonia (one episode)	1418	(8.4)
Pulmonary *M. tuberculosis*	149	(0.8)
Cardiomyopathy	158	(0.9)
$CD4^+ > 500/\mu l$		
Infectious sinusitis/mastoiditis/otitis	2350	(14.2)
Bronchitis	2037	(12.2)
Pharyngitis	1613	(9.5)
Lung Cancer	17	(0.1)

Source: Ref. 18.

patients with the most severe immunosuppression ($CD4^+$ counts of fewer than 100/μl).

Therefore, common respiratory problems such as sinusitis and bronchitis may occur at any $CD4^+$ count, and bacterial pneumonia and tuberculosis often occur before AIDS-defining opportunistic infections and neoplasms. Declining immune function increases the risk for all HIV-associated respiratory disease, except perhaps for mild upper respiratory tract infections.

B. Demographic Factors

In the United States, the demographic characteristics of persons with HIV infection have a major influence on the incidence of specific pulmonary disorders, and demographic trends during the AIDS epidemic are accompanied by a changing spectrum of disease. Persons who acquired HIV infection through injection drug use and heterosexual contact represent an increasing proportion of new cases of AIDS. From 1981 to 1987, 64% of cases of AIDS were in gay men, compared with 45% of new cases from 1993 to 1995 (19). In the early years of the epidemic, most patients with AIDS were white. Now, the majority are black and Hispanic (2,20).

The increased number of injection drug users in the HIV-infected population is paralleled by the recognition of bacterial pneumonia and pulmonary tuberculosis as important HIV-associated infections. The CDC surveillance data in the 1980s showed that mortality rates for "pneumonia" doubled among persons aged 25–44 years in cities with a high prevalence of injection drug use and AIDS (21). Selwyn et al. found that the incidence of bacterial pneumonia was five times greater in HIV-infected than in non–HIV-infected injection drug users, and that bacterial infections accounted for substantial mortality (22,23). In the Pulmonary Complications of HIV Infection Study cohort, bacterial pneumonia occurred more frequently than PCP, and the risk of developing bacterial pneumonia was significantly higher in injection drug users than in others (17).

Race and ethnicity may also influence the risk of developing bacterial pneumonia and tuberculosis, but these associations are confounded by differences in access to health care, the higher prevalence of tuberculosis in minority communities, and disproportionally high numbers of injection drug users who are black or Hispanic (24–26). Nevertheless, the risk of tuberculosis is higher in blacks and Hispanics than in whites, whereas whites have a higher risk of HIV-associated malignancies and cytomegalovirus disease (25–27).

C. Residence

A person's place of residence strongly influences the risk of developing specific infections. The high incidence of PCP in the United States and Europe contrasts sharply with many nations in Africa, where it is much less common (28,29). It is still unknown whether genetic or environmental factors account for the lower incidence of PCP in Africa. In the United States, the incidence of HIV-associated tuberculosis is highest in the Northeast (17,25). The geographic distribution of endemic fungi is a strong determinant of risk of those infections; disseminated histoplasmosis and coccidioidomycosis are common in patients with AIDS who live in endemic areas (30,31). These infections may also occur as reactivation disease after HIV-infected persons move to other areas and develop immunocompromise. For example, cases of disseminated histoplasmosis were reported in New York in patients with AIDS who had relocated from Puerto Rico years before (32).

D. Use of Prophylaxis

Antipneumocystis prophylaxis probably had the most profound effect on the changing spectrum of HIV-associated pulmonary diseases by reducing the incidence and mortality rate of that infection. From 1987 to 1992, the percentage of HIV-related deaths from PCP fell from 32.5% to 13.8%, whereas the percentage of deaths of nontuberculous mycobacteriosis, cytomegalovirus disease, bacterial infections, non-Hodgkin's lymphoma, and tuberculosis increased (Fig. 2; 33). The prognosis for survival after developing immunosuppression or an AIDS-defining diagnosis also improved, largely attributable to antipneumocystis prophylaxis (34). However, longevity may be accompanied by progressive immunosuppression and susceptibility to other potentially fatal infections and neoplasms. In an analysis of 844 gay men enrolled in the Multicenter AIDS Cohort Study, the 138 who received prophylaxis for PCP before their AIDS diagnosis had a lower incidence of PCP and lower mean $CD4^+$ count at the time of the AIDS diagnosis than the 73 who did not (35). However, they had a higher incidence of *M.* avium disease (33.4 vs. 24.8%), wasting syndrome (18.4 vs. 6.4%), and esophageal candidiasis (21.3 vs. 12.8%). The PCP prophylaxis also appeared to delay the time to the first AIDS-related illness by 6–12 months.

The incidence of new cases of tuberculosis in the United States began to decline in 1992, despite the increasing numbers of patients with AIDS (36). Expanded use of antituberculous prophylaxis in high-risk groups undoubtedly played a role in this phenomenon, along with earlier and more effective treatment of active cases by improved methods to identify the organism, broader use of drug susceptibility testing, and enhanced adherence through directly observed therapy. Transmission of tuberculosis in congregative settings, such as hospitals and correction facilities, was probably also reduced by implementing infection-control guidelines.

IV. Respiratory Symptoms

Persons with HIV infection who have diagnosed pulmonary disorders usually have respiratory symptoms, which may include dyspnea, cough, sputum production, and wheezing. The specific disorders that cause these symptoms are discussed in other sections of this text. However, HIV-infected persons with no defined pulmonary diagnosis may also have similar symptoms.

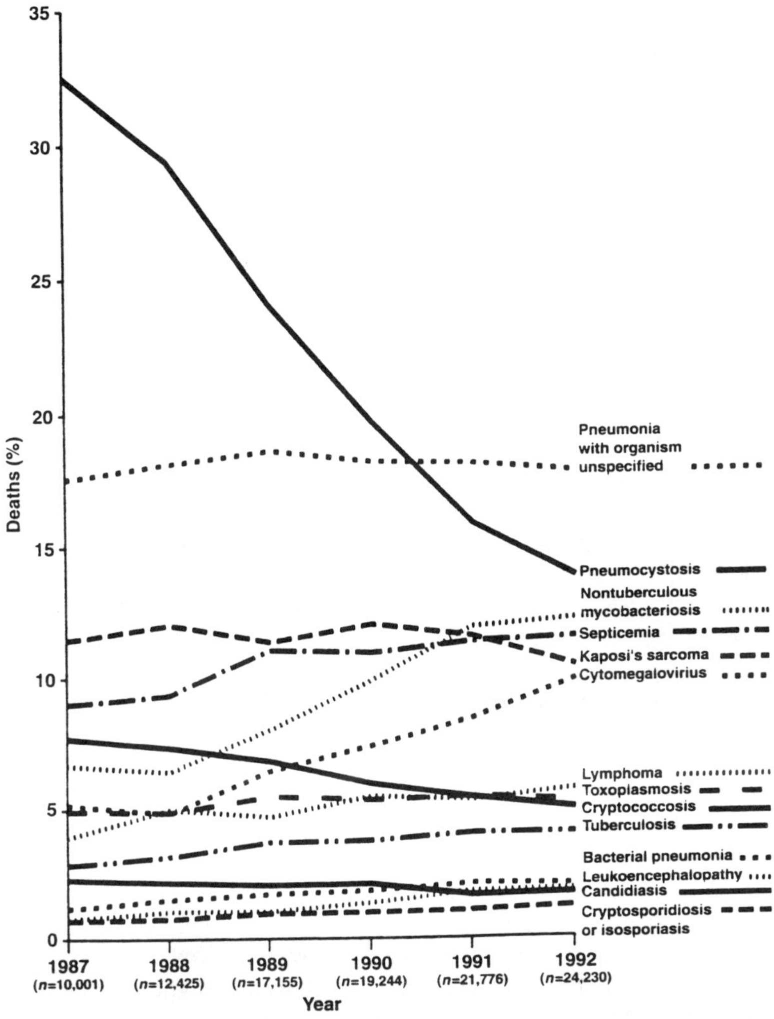

Figure 2 Trends in the prevalence of infectious diseases and cancers reported among persons dying of HIV infection in the United States from 1987 to 1992. (From Ref. 33.)

In the evaluation of a symptomatic patient, disorders seen in the general population should be considered, including asthma and chronic bronchitis. Even in the absence of these conditions, pulmonary symptoms may be still be more common in HIV-infected persons than in the general population. At the time of enrollment in the Pulmonary Complications of HIV Infection Study, the 1171 evaluable HIV-seropositive subjects reported dyspnea and productive cough in 15% of cases, respectively (17). Moderate to severe dyspnea was reported more frequently in the HIV-seropositive subjects than in the seronegative control group. Both dyspnea and cough were more prevalent in injection drug users than others, and were strongly associated with cigarette smoking.

For unknown reasons, patients with advanced HIV infection may also have chronic bronchitis and bronchiectasis, even if they do not smoke (37,38). These patients usually have $CD4^+$ counts of fewer than 100/μl. Standard antimicrobial agents are usually effective, but symptoms are likely to recur, especially when *Pseudomonas aeruginosa* is isolated from the sputum (38). The role and efficacy of bronchodilators and anti-inflammatory agents in HIV-associated airway disease have not been studied systematically.

V. Spectrum of Pulmonary Disorders

Early investigations of the types of pulmonary disorders that occur in patients with HIV infection were limited by analysis of data at single sites, and by restricting the scope of analysis to patients who had CDC-defined AIDS (39). This approach systematically underestimated the incidence and importance of pulmonary disorders that occur earlier in the course of HIV infection. Despite the declining incidence of PCP owing to prophylaxis, it remains an important pathogen. Most patients who develop PCP do not take prophylaxis at all, or do not take it regularly. Even patients who adhere to their regimen may develop PCP, and the risk of prophylaxis failure increases with declining $CD4^+$ cell counts (40).

The types and frequencies of lower respiratory tract disorders diagnosed in the first 18 months of follow-up in the Pulmonary Complications of HIV Infection Study are listed in Table 3 (17). Bacterial pneumonia was the most common serious lower respiratory tract disorder. After follow-up of up to 64 months, bacterial pneumonia still had a higher incidence than PCP (5.5 and 5.1 episodes per 100 person-years, respectively; 41). The risk of developing bacterial pneumonia increases as the $CD4^+$ lymphocyte count declines, but it usually occurs before an AIDS diagnosis (41,42). Injection drug users are at higher risk than other groups, and neutropenia and drug smoking are independent risk factors (43,44). Bacterial pneumonia may also accelerate the course of HIV disease because it causes a transient increase in plasma HIV RNA and is an independent predictor of mortality (41,45).

Prophylaxis with trimethoprim–sulfamethoxazole appears to reduce the risk of developing bacterial pneumonia. (41,46) *Streptococcus, Haemo-*

Table 3 The 18-Month Incidence Rates of Lower Respiratory Disorders in 1116 HIV-Seropositive Persons

Disorder	Patients (*n*)	(%)
Bacterial pneumonia	53	(4.8)
P. carinii	43	(3.9)
Nontuberculous mycobacteria	12	(1.1)
M. tuberculosis	10	(0.9)
Nonspecific pneumonitis	8	(0.7)
C. neoformans	5	(0.5)
Cytomegalovirus	3	(0.3)
Carcinoma	3	(0.3)
Kaposi's sarcoma	2	(0.2)
Congestive heart failure	2	(0.2)
Herpes simplex	1	(0.1)
T. gondii	1	(0.1)
H. capsulatum	1	(0.1)
Lung abscess	1	(0.1)
Pulmonary embolism	1	(0.1)
Pneumothorax	1	(0.1)

Source: Ref. 17.

philus, and *Staphylococcus aureus* are still the most common pathogens, but disturbing patterns of antimicrobial resistance are emerging, and new etiologies of pneumonia are recognized more commonly, especially in patients with advanced HIV disease (47–50). For example, pneumonia caused by *Pseudomonas aeruginosa*, which was rarely diagnosed in the 1980s, is emerging as a common pathogen in patients with advanced immunosuppression, and especially following another opportunistic infection, or when the $CD4^+$ cell count is fewer than 50/μl (51–53). Although many patients have histories of recent hospitalization, this infection usually presents as a community-acquired pneumonia, and it is not necessarily associated with neutropenia or the use of corticosteroids. Cavitation is common, and the infection is often recurrent or chronic.

Patients with severe immunosuppression are predisposed to the development of disseminated fungal infections, often with prominent pulmonary involvement (54). In endemic areas, histoplasmosis, blastomycosis, and coccidioidomycosis are important causes of mortality in HIV-infected persons. *Cryptococcus neoformans* and *Aspergillus fumigatus* are ubiquitous pathogens that are potentially life-threatening in persons with advanced HIV disease.

Noninfectious disorders may also involve the lung, including neoplasms (especially Kaposi's sarcoma), nonspecific and lymphocytic interstitial pneumonitis, primary pulmonary hypertension, and bronchiolitis obliterans-organizing pneumonia. These disorders may vary in severity from asymptomatic to life-threatening.

References

1. Centers for Disease Control and Prevention (CDC). HIV/AIDS surveillance report, 1996; 8:1–33.
2. Centers for Disease Control and Prevention. Update: trends in AIDS incidence, deaths and prevalence—United States, 1996. MMWR 1997; 46:165–173.
3. Selik RM, Chu SY, Buehler JW. HIV infection as leading cause of death among young adults in US cities and states. JAMA 1993; 269:2991–2994.
4. Centers for Disease Control: *Pneumocystis pneumonia*—Los Angeles. MMWR 1980; 30:250–254.
5. Murray J, Felton CP, Garay SM, Gottlieb MS, Hopewell PC, Stover DE, Geirstein AS. Pulmonary complications of the acquired immunodeficiency syndrome: report of National Heart, Lung and Blood Institute Workshop. N Engl J Med 1984; 310:1682–1688.
6. Centers for Disease Control and Prevention. Update on acquired immune deficiency syndrome (AIDS)—United States. MMWR 1982; 31:507–513.
7. Centers for Disease Control and Prevention. Revision of the CDC surveillance case definition for acquired immunodeficiency syndrome. MMWR 1987; 36(suppl 1S):3–13.
8. Centers for Disease Control and Prevention. 1993 revised classification system for HIV infection and expanded surveillance case definitions for AIDS among adolescents and adults. MMWR 1992; 41 (RR-17):1–19.
9. Centers for Disease Control and Prevention. Update: trends in AIDS diagnosis and reporting under the expanded surveillance definition for adolescents and adults—United States, 1993. MMWR 1994; 43:826–831.
10. Fauci AS (moderator). Immunopathogenic mechanisms in human immunodeficiency virus (HIV) infection. Ann Intern Med 1991; 114:678–693.
11. Choi S, Lagakos SW, Schooley RT, Volberding PA. $CD4^+$ lymphocytes are an incomplete surrogate marker for clinical progression in persons with asymptomatic HIV infection taking zidovudine. Ann Intern Med 1993; 118:674–680.
12. Mellors JW, Kinsley LA, Rinaldo CR, Todd JA, Hoo BS, Kokka RP, Gupta P. Quantitation of HIV-1 RNA in plasma predicts outcome after seroconversion. Ann Inten Med 1995; 122:573–579.
13. O'Brien TR, Blattner WA, Waters D, Eyster ME, Helgartner MW, Cohen AR, Luban N, Hatzakis A, Aledort LM, Rosenberg PS, Miley WJ, Krover BL, Goedert JJ, for the Multicenter Hemophilia Cohort Study. Serum HIV-1 RNA levels and time to development of AIDS in the Multicenter Hemophilia Cohort Study. JAMA 1996; 276:105–110.
14. O'Brien WA, Hartigan PM, Martin D, Esinhart J, Hill A, Benoit S, Rubin M, Simberkoff MS, Hamilton JD, Veterans Affairs Cooperatine Study Group on

AIDS. Changes in plasma HIV-1 RNA and CD4+ lymphocyte counts and the risk of progression to AIDS: Veterans Affairs Cooperative Study Group on AIDS. N Engl J Med 1996; 334:426–431.

15. Buchbinder SP, Katz MH, Hessol NA, O'Malley PM, Holmberg SD. Long-term HIV infection without immunologic progression. AIDS 1994; 8:1123–1128.
16. Pantaleo G, Menzo S, Vaccarezza M, Graziosi C, Cohen OJ, Demarest JF, Montegiori D, Orenstein JM, Fox C, Schrager LK, Margolick JB, Buchbinder S, Georgi JV, Fanci AS. Studies in subjects with long-term nonprogressive human immunodeficiency virus infection. N Engl J Med 1995; 332:209–216.
17. Wallace JM, Rao AV, Glassroth J, Hausen NI, Rosen MJ, Arakaki C, Kvale PA, Reichman LB, Hopewell PC and the Pulm Comps of HIV Infection Study Group. Respiratory illness in persons with human immunodeficiency virus infection. Am Rev Respir Dis 1993; 148:1523–1529.
18. Hanson DL, Chu SY, Farizo KM, Ward JW, and the Adult and Adolescent Spectrum of HIV Disease Study Group. Distribution of CD4+ lymphocytes at diagnosis of acquired immunodeficiency syndrome-defining and other human immunodeficiency virus-related illnesses. Arch Intern Med 1995; 155:1537–1542.
19. Centers for Disease Control and Prevention. First 500,000 AIDS cases—United States, 1995. MMWR 1995; 44:849–853.
20. Centers for Disease Control and Prevention. AIDS among racial ethnic minorities—United States, 1993. MMWR 1994; 43:644–647, 653–655.
21. Centers for Disease Control. Increase in pneumonia mortality among young adults and the HIV epidemic—New York City, United States. MMWR 1988; 37:593–596,
22. Selwyn PA, Feingold AR, Hartel, et al. Increased risk of bacterial pneumonia in HIV-infected intravenous drug users without AIDS. AIDS 1988; 2:267–272.
23. Selwyn PA, Alcabes P, Hartel D, Buono D, Schoenbaum EE, Klein RS, Davenny K, Friedland GH. Clinical manifestations and predictors of disease progression in drug users with human immunodeficiency virus infection. N Engl J Med 1992; 327:1697–1703.
24. Chaisson RE, Keruly JC. Moore RD. Race, sex, drug use, and progression of human immunodeficiency virus disease. N Engl J Med 1995; 333:751–756.
25. Chan ISF, Neaton JD, Saravolatz LD, Crane LR, Osterberger, Community Programs for Clinical Research on AIDS. Frequencies of opportunistic diseases prior to death among HIV-infected persons. AIDS 1995; 9:1145–1151.
26. Hu DJ, Fleming PL, Castro KG, Jones JL, bush TJ, Hanson D, Chu SY, Kaplan J, Ward JW. How important is race/ethnicity as an indicator of risk for specific AIDS-defining conditions? J Acquir Immune Defic. Syndr 1995; 10:374–380.
27. Gallant JE, Moore RD, Richman DD, Keruly J, Chaisson RE. Risk factors for Kaposi's sarcoma in patients with advanced human immunodeficiency virus disease treated with zidovudine. Arch Intern Med 1994; 154:566–572.
28. Batungwanayo J, Taelman H, Lucas S, Bogaerts J, Alard D, Kagame A, Blanche P, Clerinx J, Van De Perre P, Allen S, Aris E, MToni IM, Cegielski JP, Lallinger

G, Mbaga I, Murray JF. Pulmonary disease associated with human immunodeficiency virus in Kigali, Rwanda: a fiberoptic bronchoscopic study of 111 cases of undetermined etiology. Am Rev Respir Crit Care Med 1994; 149:1591–1596.
29. Daley CL, Mugusi F, Chen LL, Schmidt DM, Small PM, Bearer E. Pulmonary complications of HIV infection in Dar es Salaam, Tanzania: role of bronchoscopy and bronchoalveolar lavage. Am J Respir Crit Care Med 1996; 154:105–110.
30. Wheat LJ, Connoly-Stringfield PA, Baker RL, Curfman MF, Eads ME, Israel KS, Norris SA, Webb DH, Jeckel ML. Disseminated histoplasmosis in the acquired immune deficiency syndrome. Clinical findings, diagnosis and treatment and review of the literature. Medicine 1990; 69:361–374.
31. Jones JL, Fleming PL, Ciesielski CA, Hu DJ, Kaplan JE, Ward JW. Coccidioidomycosis in patients infected with AIDS in the United States. J Infect Dis 1995; 171:961–966.
32. Salzman S, Smith RL, Aranda CP. Histoplasmosis in patients at risk for the acquired immunodeficiency syndrome in a nonendemic setting. Chest 1988; 93:916–921.
33. Selik RM, Chu SY, Ward JW. Trends in infectious diseases and cancers among persons dying of HIV infection in the United States from 1987 to 1992. Ann Intern Med 1995; 123:933–936.
34. Enger C, Graham N, Peng Y, Climiel JS, Kingley LA, Detels R, Muñoz A.. Survival from early, intermediate and late stages of HIV infection. JAMA 1996; 275:1329–1334.
35. Hoover DR, Saah AJ, Bacellar H, Phair J, Detels R, Anderson R, Kaslow RA for the Multicenter AIDS Cohort Study. Clinical manifestations of AIDS in the era of *Pneumocystis* prophylaxis. N Engl J Med 1993; 329:1922–1926.
36. Centers for Disease Control and Prevention. Tuberculosis morbidity—United States. MMWR 1996; 45:365–370.
37. Wallace JM, Hansen N, Lavange L, Glassroth J, Brody BL, Rosen MJ, Kvale PA, Mangura BT, Reichman LB, Hopewell PC and the Pulmonary Complications of HIV Infection Study Group. Respiratory disease trends in the pulmonary complications of HIV infection study cohort. Am J Respir Crit Care Med 1997; 155:72–80.
38. Verghese A, Al-Samman M, Nabhan D, Naylor AD, Rivera M. Bacterial bronchitis and bronchiectasis in human immunodeficiency virus infection. Arch Intern Med 154:2086–2091, 1994.
39. Murray JF, Garay SM, Hopewell PC, Mills J, Snider GL, Stover DE. Pulmonary complications of the acquired immunodeficiency syndrome: an update. Am Rev Respir Dis 1987; 135:504–509.
40. Saah AJ, Hoover DR, Peng Y, Phair JP, Vascher B, Kingsley LA, Schrager LK, for the Multicenter AIDs Cohort Study. Predictors of failure of *Pneumocystis carinii* prophylaxis. JAMA 1995; 273:1197–1202.
41. Hirschtick RE, Glassroth J, Jordan MC, Wilcosky TC, Wallace JM, Kvale PA, Markowitz N, Rosen MJ, Mangura BT, Hopewell PC and the Pulm Comp of HIV Infection Study Group. Bacterial pneumonia in patients infected with human immunodeficiency virus. N Engl J Med 1995; 333:845–851.

42. Falco V, de Sevilla TF, Alegre J, Barbé J, Ferrer A, Ocaña I, Ribera E, Martinez-Vasquez JM. Bacterial pneumonia in HIV-infected patients: a prospective study of 68 episodes. Eur Respir J 1994; 7:235–239.
43. Moore RD, Keruly JC, Chaisson RE. Neutropenia and bacterial infection in acquired immunodeficiency syndrome. Arch Intern Med 1995; 155:1965–1970.
44. Caiaffa WT, Vlahov D, Graham NMH, Astembarski J, Solomon L, Nelson KE, Munoz A. Drug smoking, *Pneumocystis carinii* pneumonia, and immunosuppression increase risk of bacterial pneumonia in human immunodeficiency virus-seropositive injection drug users. Am J Respir Crit Care Med 1994; 150:1493–1498.
45. Bush CE, Donovan RM, Markowitz NP, Kvale P, Saravolatz LD. A study of HIV RNA viral load in AIDS patients with bacterial pneumonia. J AIDS 1996; 13:23–26.
46. Hardy WD, Feinberg J, Finkelstein DM, Power ME, Weili H, Kaczka C, Frame PE, Homes M, Waskin H, Fass RJ, Powderly WG, Steigbigel RT, Zuger A, Holzman RS. A controlled trial of trimethoprim–sulfamethoxazole or aerosolized pentamidine for secondary prophylaxis of *Pneumocystis carinii* pneumonia in patients with the acquired immunodeficiency syndrome. N Engl J Med 1992; 327:1842–1848.
47. Blatt SP, Dolan MJ, Hendrix CW, Melcher GP. Legionnaires' disease in human immunodeficiency virus-infected patients: eight cases and review. Clin Infect Dis 1994; 18:227–232.
48. Donisi A, Suardi MG, Casari S, Longo M, Cadeo GP, Carosi G. *Rhodococcus equi* infection in HIV-infected patients. AIDS 1996; 10:359–362.
49. Uttamchandani RB, Daikos GL, Reyes RR, Fischl MA, Dickinson GM, Yamaguchi E, Kramer MR. Nocardiosis in 30 patients with advanced immunodeficiency virus: clinical features and outcome. Clin Infect Dis 1994; 18:348–353.
50. Burack JH, Hahn JA, Saint-Maurice D, Jacobson MA. Microbiology of community-acquired bacterial pneumonia in persons with and at risk for human immunodeficiency virus type 1 infection. Arch Intern Med 1994; 154:2589–2596.
51. Baron AD, Hollander H. *Pseudomonas aeruginosa* bronchopulmonary infection in late human immunodeficiency virus infection. Am Rev Respir Dis 1993; 148:992–996.
52. Dropulic LK, Leslie JM, Eldred LJ, Zenilman J, Sears CL. Clinical manifestations and risk factors of *Pseudomonas aeruginosa* infection in patients with AIDS. J Infect Dis 1995, 171:930–937.
53. Schuster MG, Norris AH. Community-acquired *Pseudomonas aeruginosa* pneumonia in patients with HIV infection. AIDS 1994; 8:1437–1441.
54. Sarosi GA, Ampel N, Cohn DL, et al. Fungal infection in HIV-infected persons. Am J Respir Crit Care Med 1995, 152:816–822.
55. Centers for Disease Control and Prevention. HIV/AIDS surveillance report. 1994; 6(2):1.

2

HIV Infection in Europe

An Overview of Epidemiology and Pulmonary Complications

COURT PEDERSEN

Odense University Hospital
Odense, Denmark

THOMAS L. BENFIELD

Hvidovre University Hospital
Hvidovre, Denmark

JENS D. LUNDGREN

University of Copenhagen and
Hvidovre University Hospital
Hvidovre, Denmark

I. Introduction

The first AIDS cases in Europe occurred simultaneously with the start of the epidemic in the epicenters in the United States and predominantly affected homosexual men. Subsequently, the epidemic in Europe spread to the intravenous drug-using community. The estimated total number of human immunodeficiency virus (HIV)-infected persons in Europe is now 500,000, and a total of 170,000 patients have developed the acquired immunodeficiency syndrome (AIDS). The HIV pandemic is primarily caused by HIV-1 with HIV-2 accounting for less than 1% of HIV infections. Most cases of HIV-2 infection have been described in persons from West African countries.

The epidemiology of the HIV epidemic in Europe has many similarities to the situation in North America, as has the epidemiology of HIV-related disorders, including pulmonary complications. However, in certain areas there are important differences. In this chapter we discuss the epidemiology of HIV and AIDS in Europe, as well as how patients are treated in different regions of Europe. Thereafter, the epidemiology of the main pulmonary pathogens affecting European HIV-infected patients will be reviewed.

II. Data Sources

The data discussed in the following have been derived from several sources, in particular the European Centre for the Epidemiological Monitoring of AIDS (ECEMA, Saint-Maurice, France) and two large cohort studies (entitled the AIDS In Europe and the EuroSIDA studies). The ECEMA generates data from national health authorities reporting on the number and characteristics of patients with AIDS (1), comparable with the function of the Centers for Disease Control and Prevention (CDC) in the United States. The data are presented quarterly in a report entitled *HIV/AIDS Surveillance in Europe*. Because of reported delays, the center also presents adjusted data, using a method that assumes constant patterns of reporting.

The AIDS In Europe study collected data from patient records of 6578 patients from 17 European countries, with AIDS diagnoses between 1979 and December 31, 1989 (2). The EuroSIDA study is an ongoing cohort study that prospectively follows more than 4000 unselected patients from 16 European countries with CD4 cell counts of fewer than 500/μl (3). In contrast with the two cohort studies, ECEMA reports only on patient characteristics (including diseases) at the time of the AIDS diagnosis. Because of differences in inclusion criteria, the EuroSIDA study—as opposed with the AIDS in Europe study—provides the incidence data of individual HIV-related disorders in non-AIDS patients, whereas both studies provide incidence data of HIV-related disorders after the AIDS diagnosis. In addition, data has been collected from single-center published reports, and from a consecutive cohort of HIV-infected patients requiring bronchoscopy for diagnostic evaluation at the Hvidovre Hospital in Copenhagen, Denmark.

In several analyses, western Europe is divided in regions (Fig. 1): northern (Denmark [DK], Ireland [IR], Finland [SF], northern Germany [D], The Netherlands [NL], Norway [N], Sweden [S], and the United Kingdom [UK]); central (Belgium [B], France [F], southern Germany [D], Hungary [HU], Luxembourg [LUX], and Switzerland [CH]); south (southeast: Greece [GR], Israel, Italy [I]; southwest: Portugal [P] and Spain [S]).

III. Use of Prophylaxis in European HIV-Infected Persons

Most centers in Europe started to use trimethoprim–sulfamethoxazole (TMP–SMX) in 1986–1987 to prevent the recurrence of *Pneumocystis carinii* pneumonia (PCP) in patients who had recovered from an episode of PCP

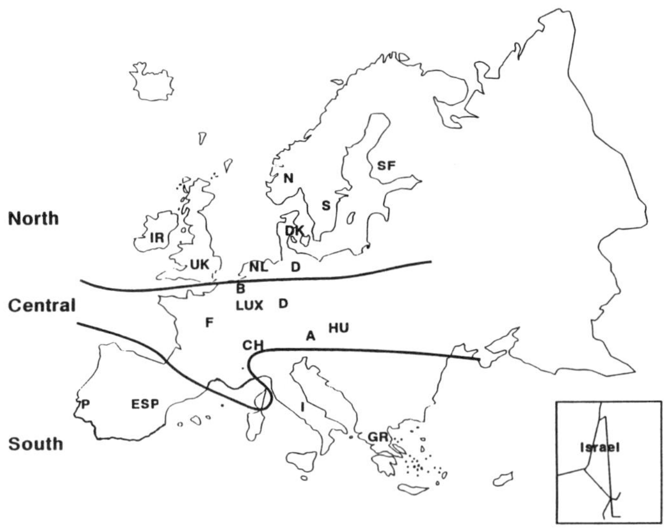

Figure 1 Europe divided into geographic regions (north, central, south). (From Refs. 2 and 3.)

(4). Secondary prophylaxis is now considered standard care. Primary prophylaxis was introduced considerably later. Only 4% of AIDS patients diagnosed before 1987 received treatment that could be considered to be primary PCP prophylaxis, most of whom received it as therapy for other opportunistic infections (e.g., cerebral toxoplasmosis). This percentage increased to 18% among patients diagnosed in 1989, but only 1.4% received primary prophylaxis before they were diagnosed with AIDS (4). Subsequently, the identification of HIV-infected persons at particular risk (namely, those with a CD4 cell count of fewer than 200/μl) was followed by guidelines for primary PCP prophylaxis (5). The situation has changed considerably. At the time of enrollment in the EuroSIDA study (mid-1994), 89% of the patients considered at risk of PCP were receiving some type of primary prophylaxis. The proportion of patients receiving primary prophylaxis was higher among those with a CD4 cell count of fewer than 100/μl as compared with those with a CD4 cell count between 100 and 200/μl (3) (Fig. 2), indicating that both patients and treating physicians appreciate that the risk of contracting PCP correlates with the CD4 cell count as it drops below 200/μl (4,6,7). Trimethoprim–sulfamethoxazole is the predominant primary prophylaxis, followed by aerosolized pentamidine and dapsone (3).

Some countries recommend preventive therapy for tuberculin skin test-positive HIV-infected individuals (8). In Italy and Spain, preventive therapy

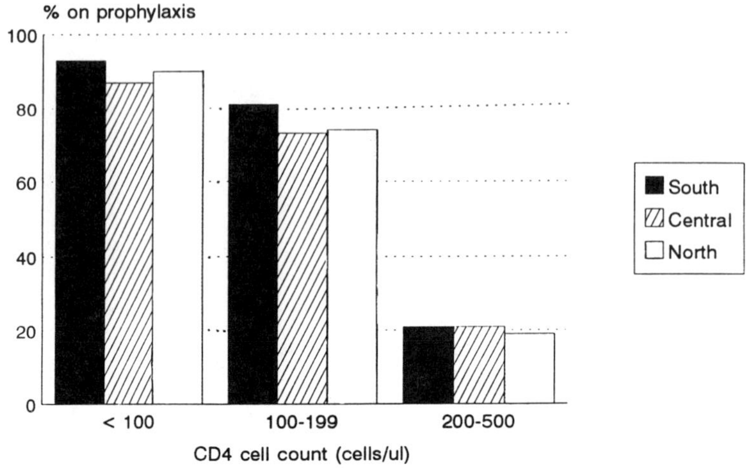

Figure 2 PCP prophylaxis used in HIV-infected patients in Europe for different CD4 cell count strata. (From Ref. 3.)

is also recommended for HIV-infected patients with cutaneous anergy (8–10). Most countries with low incidence rates of tuberculosis (TB) have no national recommendations on skin testing and preventive therapy.

In Europe, primary prophylaxis against atypical mycobacterioses has been introduced on only a very limited scale (3).

IV. HIV and AIDS Epidemiology in Europe

Surveillance of AIDS is conducted by 45 countries in the World Health Organization (WHO) European Region. It is estimated almost all AIDS cases in Europe are reported. National estimates of underreporting vary among countries, less than 5% in Scandinavia, 6% in Switzerland, 13% in United Kingdoms, 15% in Germany, and 10–20% in southern Europe. In eastern Europe estimates of underreporting varies considerably, from 0% in Croatia to 25% in Poland (1). Until 1993 the AIDS case definitions used for surveillance were identical with the definitions prepared by the CDC in the United States in 1982, 1985, and 1987. The European case definition for adults and adolescents was revised in 1993 (11), adding pulmonary tuberculosis, recurrent bacterial pneumonia, and invasive cervical cancer to the list of AIDS-defining diseases. This definition differs from the CDC's revised definition by not including low CD4 cell counts as an AIDS-defining criterion. The case definition used for children in Europe is essentially the same as that used in the United States (12).

By March 1996, a cumulative total of 161,764 adult AIDS cases and 6,297 pediatric cases (younger than 13 years) had been reported. After adjustments for reporting delays, it is estimated that the total number of adult cases is 172,854 and the number of pediatric cases 6,532 (1). The AIDS incidence is much higher in western Europe than in eastern Europe (13; Table 1), reflecting that the epidemic is at its beginning in most parts of eastern Europe. From 1994 to 1995 the number of newly diagnosed cases increased by 23% in eastern Europe (2), with rapidly rising incidences in Poland and in the Federal Republic of Yugoslavia. In western Europe, the highest numbers of cases have been reported from France, Spain, and Italy, each, with more than 35,000 cases (see Table 1).

The highest annual incidence rates in 1995 were observed in Spain (183 cases per million populations), Italy (103 cases per million), France (89 cases per million), Switzerland (85 cases per million), and Portugal (77

Table 1 AIDS Cases in Selected European Countries Adjusted for Reporting Delays[a]

	Year of diagnosis			
Country	1993	1994	1995	Cumulative
All Europe	**22,743**	**26,181**	**26,256**	**179,445**
Belgium	248 (24.7)	253 (25.1)	251 (24.8)	2,247
Bulgaria	6 (0.7)	10 (1.1)	1 (0.1)	39
Croatia	10 (2.2)	17 (3.8)	15 (3.3)	98
Denmark	239 (46.3)	239 (46.2)	219 (42.3)	1,892
France	5468 (92.6)	5760 (97.1)	5329 (89.4)	43,062
Germany	1815 (22.4)	1841 (22.7)	1715 (21.0)	15,612
Greece	161 (15.5)	225 (21.6)	230 (22.0)	1,477
Ireland	70 (19.9)	68 (19.2)	39 (11.0)	538
Italy	4881 (84.2)	5619 (98.3)	5914 (103.4)	35,120
Netherlands	462 (30.2)	463 (30.1)	513 (33.1)	4,128
Norway	63 (14.7)	73 (16.9)	70 (16.1)	521
Poland	68 (1.8)	96 (2.5)	129 (3.4)	466
Portugal	515 (52.3)	642 (65.3)	754 (76.8)	3,600
Romania	435 (18.9)	491 (21.4)	662 (29.0)	3,989
Russian Federation	13 (0.1)	27 (0.2)	35 (0.2)	224
Spain	5261 (133.1)	7217 (182.4)	7259 (183.2)	42,281
Sweden	181 (20.8)	185 (21.2)	194 (22.1)	1,402
Ukraine	12 (0.2)	16 (0.3)	45 (0.9)	93
United Kingdom	1717 (29.6)	785 (30.7)	1721 (29.5)	13,335
Yugoslavia, F.R.	71 (6.7)	86 (8.0)	109 (10.0)	573

[a]Numbers of patients with rates (cases per million population) in parentheses.
Source: Ref. 13.

cases per million). Since 1988 the annual rates have increased in all countries in western Europe, but with impressive geographic differences. Table 2 shows annual rates in 1990 and 1995 for some of the countries, emphasizing that the AIDS epidemic has spread more extensively in southern Europe than in northern Europe (11,13,14). Within the last 5 years the annual AIDS rates appear to have stabilized in northern Europe, whereas they are still increasing in southern Europe.

The male/female ratio of all AIDS cases is 4.7, but has steadily declined to 3.8 in 1995. Most cases have been reported among homosexual men (36.7%) and among intravenous drug users (39.3%), whereas 13.9% of cases were heterosexual contacts. Most women with AIDS diagnosed in 1995 were injection drug users (46%) or had been infected through heterosexual contact (43%).

During the epidemic there has been a shift in the various transmission categories' relative contribution to new AIDS cases (14; Fig. 3). The proportion of cases attributed to homosexual transmission decreased from 63% in 1985 to 28% in 1995, whereas the proportion of cases attributed to injection drug use increased from 16 to 43% in the same period. The proportion of cases attributed to transmission through treatment of coagulation disorders or through blood transfusions decreased from 7.2% to 1%.

Table 2 Annual AIDS Incidence Rates in Some European Countries: Rates for 1995 Are Also Shown for the Main HIV Transmission Categories

	Incidence rates (cases per million population)				
		1995[a]			
Country	1990	All	Ho	IVDU	Het
South					
Greece	14	22	12	0.5	3
Italy	55	103	13	61	16
Portugal	25	77	10	41	19
Spain	96	183	24	115	27
Central					
Belgium	21	25	11	2	11
France	74	89	35	22	21
Switzerland	86	85	27	32	22
North					
Denmark	38	42	24	6	10
Sweden	15	22	11	3	7
United Kingdom	22	30	18	2	7

[a]Ho, homosexual men; IVDU, intravenous drug users; Het, heterosexual contacts.
Source: Ref. 1.

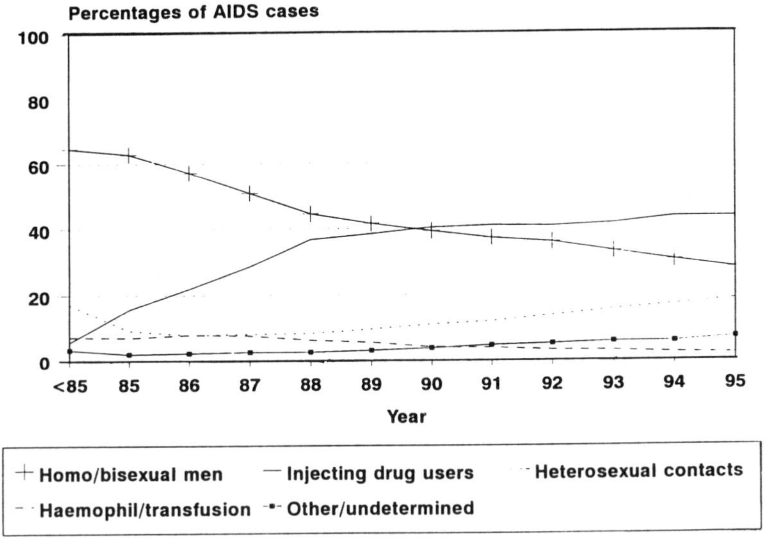

Figure 3 Adult AIDS cases by transmission group and year of diagnosis. (From Ref. 13.)

In 1995, heterosexual transmission accounted for 19% of notified cases, compared with only 9% in 1985. The proportion of heterosexuals among cases reported before 1985 was relatively high, probably owing to cases among immigrants from Central Africa.

There are pronounced differences within Europe relative to incidences of AIDS in the main HIV transmission categories (1). The incidence rates of injection drug users with AIDS are much higher in most parts of southern Europe than in central and northern Europe, an exception being Greece, which has a distribution of AIDS cases more like northern Europe (see Table 2). As an example of the differences, the ratio of injection drug users to homosexual men among AIDS cases who had been reported in 1995 was 4.8 in Spain, 4.7 in Italy, 1.1 in Switzerland, 0.6 in France, 0.25 in Denmark, and 0.1 in the United Kingdom (1). The differences in AIDS rates for injection drug users largely explain the differences in total AIDS rates within Europe, because the rates for homosexual men and heterosexuals with AIDS are not that different.

Although surveillance data from European countries provide a reliable picture of the AIDS epidemic, data concerning HIV seroprevalence and seroincidence are less accurate. Estimates are based on national HIV surveillance systems—screening of blood donors and pregnant women—and surveys undertaken on various other populations. Among pregnant women, the highest prevalence is among women in urban areas in central and southern Europe (1:7000–4:1000 pregnant women), whereas the prevalence is much lower in northern Europe (1,15). The number of HIV-positive blood donations is fewer than 3:100,000 in most countries (15). From national estimates of HIV seroprevalence (1), it has been estimated that the cumulative number of adults with HIV infection in Europe by January 1, 1994 was between 500,000 and 600,000. Injection drug users account for an estimated 41% of the cases, homosexual contact 28%, heterosexual contact 17%, and 14% infected either through blood or blood products or with unknown mode of transmission. The estimates of HIV prevalence must be interpreted cautiously, and especially in the eastern part of Europe, where the epidemic is new, it is very difficult to predict the future incidence rates of HIV infection.

So far, HIV infection has remained at a low endemic level, but there are indications that the situation is vulnerable. Surveillance data from the southern part of Ukraine have shown that the HIV prevalence among injection drug users has increased more than ten-fold in less than 1 year, from close to zero to 30.7% in Odessa and to 17.7% in Mykolayiv (16). An explosive rise in the incidence rate of syphilis has been observed in the Russian Federation (170 cases per 100,000 populations)—Ukraine, Belarus, and the Republic of Moldova (17). These data give rise to concern, suggesting that preventive measures should be initiated immediately to prevent epidemic spread of HIV infection.

A. AIDS-Defining Diseases

Among 6578 adult AIDS cases diagnosed between 1979 and 1989 (3), the most common AIDS-defining diseases were *Pneumocystis carinii* pneumonia, Kaposi's sarcoma, esophageal candidiasis, extrapulmonary tuberculosis, and cerebral toxoplasmosis. This pattern has changed owing to the introduction of the new AIDS definition in 1993, changes in demographics among AIDS patients, and therapeutic changes. The most common AIDS-defining diseases, based on surveillance data from January 1994 to March 1996 (1) are shown in Table 3.

It must be remembered that surveillance data give an incomplete picture of disease patterns. Diseases occurring after an AIDS diagnosis are not reported to national surveillance systems. A complete picture of disease patterns can be obtained only through prospective studies of well-defined HIV-infected populations. In a Danish study of Kaposi's sarcoma among 520 AIDS cases in homosexual men diagnosed from 1979 to 1990, data showed that the proportion of men who had Kaposi's sarcoma as an AIDS-defining illness decreased steadily from 31 to 13%, suggesting a

Table 3 AIDS-Defining Diseases in 43,685 Adults and 425 Children with an AIDS Diagnosis in Europe from January 1994 to March 1996

	Frequency of disease (%)	
Disease[a]	Adults	Children
Pneumocystis carinii pneumonia	22.0	22
Esophageal candidiasis	17.0	13
Pulmonary tuberculosis	10.7	
Extrapulmonary tuberculosis	9.4	
Cerebral toxoplasmosis	8.9	
Kaposi's sarcoma	8.1	
HIV wasting syndrome	7.6	12
Cytomegalovirus disease	6.1	8
HIV encephalopathy	5.6	20
Malignant lymphoma	3.5	
Recurrent pneumonia	3.1	
Disseminated infection with atypical mycobacteria	2.8	
Cryptosporidiosis	2.8	4
Cryptococcosis	2.7	
Progressive multifocal leukoencephalopathy	2.5	
Lymphoid interstitial pneumonia		15
Multiple or recurrent bacterial infections		20

[a]Only diseases occurring in more than 2% of cases are included.
Source: Ref. 1.

decline in the incidence of Kaposi's sarcoma (18). However, complete follow-up of the patients from time of AIDS diagnosis to death showed constant rates of Kaposi's sarcoma, the explanation being that Kaposi's sarcoma occurred at a later stage of HIV infection among more recent AIDS cases. This finding of an apparent discrepancy between surveillance data and prospective follow-up studies has subsequently been confirmed in a larger European study (19). Surveillance data may also underestimate the incidences and may fail to detect changes in the incidences of diseases such as infection with atypical mycobacteria and cytomegalovirus (CMV), which mainly occur with severe immune suppression.

V. The Spectrum of Pulmonary Disorders

A. Experience from a Single Center

We evaluated the results of 515 diagnostic bronchoscopies including bronchoalveolar lavage (BAL) in consecutive HIV-infected patients with pulmonary disease from 1989 to 1996 (Table 4). Only the first bronchoscopy for each episode of pneumonia was included. The bronchoscopy service supports a middle-sized HIV clinic in Copenhagen, Denmark, with approximately 700–800 unselected HIV-infected patients. Bronchoscopy is the primary choice for diagnostic workup if tracheal suction is noninformative.

Most of the bronchoscopies (58%) were done in patients with a CD4 cell count of fewer than 50/μl, as expected based on the opportunistic nature of the possible pathogens (20). *Pneumocystis carinii* pneumonia was the leading pathogen identified among patients with CD4 counts of fewer than 200/μl, whereas bacterial pneumonia was more frequently diagnosed in patients with CD4 counts of 200 μl, or more. Three percent of the patients had tuberculosis, and CMV was cultured in 36% of the patients (see later discussion for possible implications thereof). The distribution of pathogens is comparable with that found in bronchoscopy series from the United States (21,22).

The number of patients who underwent bronchoscopy per year decreased from 102 in 1990 to 59 in 1995. This was primarily due to a gradual decline in the number of PCP cases (in 1990: 46 cases; in 1995 24 cases), whereas the percentage of patients with PCP for each calender year remained constant (range: 32–45%).

B. *Pneumocystis carinii* Pneumonia

Pneumonia caused by *P. carinii* was the leading cause of AIDS-related disease among patients with HIV infection in Europe in the 1980s. Thirty-nine percent of cases had PCP at the time of their AIDS diagnosis, and

Table 4 Diagnostic Result of 515 Bronchoscopies Performed on 396 HIV-Infected Patients with Pulmonary Symptoms, Associated with the Department of Infectious Diseases, Hvidovre Hospital, Copenhagen, Denmark (1989–1995)[a]

CD4 cell count	PCP	Bacterial pneumonia	Tuberculosis	CMV culture[b]	Total
< 50	48	14	2	43	58
50–99	37	22	3	33	11
100–199	28	19	5	25	11
> 200	22	28	2	22	11
Unknown	28	23	3	26	8
Total	40	18	3	36	100

[a]Percentage of patients with various diagnoses in different CD4 cell count strata at the time of the bronchoscopy is presented.

[b]Result of CMV culture from bronchoalveolar lavage fluid available in 420 of 515 bronchoscopies.

additionally 11% developed PCP thereafter (4). Because primary prophylaxis against PCP was rarely used in this time period, these figures provide a reliable picture of the susceptibility of this population to PCP.

The occurrence of PCP showed marked regional differences. A total of 50.2% of patients from northern Europe has developed PCP at the time of their AIDS diagnosis, compared with 36% in patients from central Europe, and 30% in patients from southern Europe (Fig. 4). Incidences of first-episode PCP after the time of the AIDS diagnosis showed similar regional differences (see Fig. 4). These findings could not be explained by differences in diagnostic strategies, differences in degree of immunosuppression, or other independent risk factors (4), indicating that patients in southern Europe may be less exposed to *P. carinii*.

In northern Europe, the proportion of AIDS patients with PCP in the 1980s approximate data from North America (23) from the same time period. However, in African HIV-infected patients, PCP is rarely detected, despite careful diagnostic workup (24–26), although it is a significant differential diagnosis in selected patients (27). Identification of a possible reservoir for human pathogenic *P. carinii*, outside the human organism, remains to be identified. If such a reservoir exists, it may help in explaining the global variation in the occurrence of PCP.

The epidemiology of PCP in European HIV-infected patients has changed markedly in recent years, parallel with the widespread introduc-

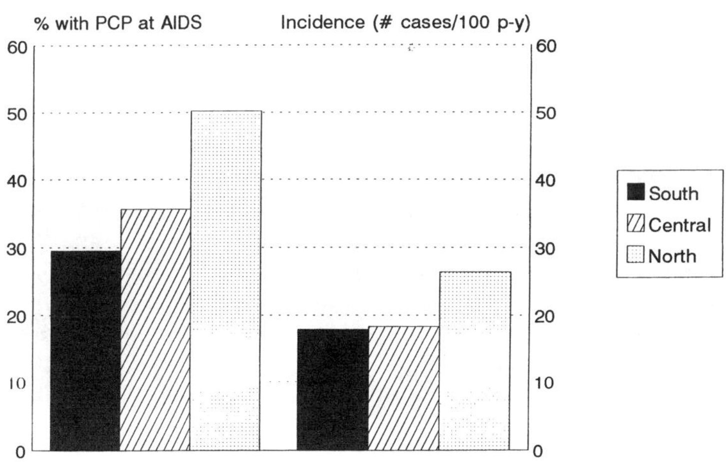

Figure 4 Regional differences in occurrence of PCP: Proportion of patients with PCP at the diagnosis of AIDS (left three columns, $p < 0.0001$). Incidence of PCP after the AIDS diagnosis (right three columns, $p < 0.0001$). (From Ref. 4.)

tion of primary prophylaxis in at-risk patients (see foregoing). Whereas 30–50% of patients had PCP at the time of the AIDS diagnosis in the 1980s, only 10–20% of the patients who developed AIDS, after inclusion in the EuroSIDA cohort in 1994, had PCP as their AIDS-defining illness. This corresponds to figures from other observational studies from United States and Europe of patients who receive primary PCP prophylaxis (4,28–30; Table 5). Furthermore, the incidence of PCP diminished to approximately one-third (7.4 cases per 100-person years of follow-up) in patients with similar degrees of immunosuppression, compared with the AIDS patients from the 1980s (see Fig. 4). Similar incidence rates were observed in HIV-infected patients from Baltimore, Maryland. This cohort of patients had CD4 cell counts of fewer than 300/μl, and most received PCP prophylaxis. Here the incidence of PCP was 8.9 cases per 100 person-years (7). The MACS studies reported incidence rates of PCP in patients on PCP prophylaxis and CD4 cell counts of fewer than 200/μl of 5.3 cases per 100 person-years (30).

In the EuroSIDA study, there was no regional difference in the occurrence of PCP among patients with a diagnosis of AIDS, from 1994 to 1996, probably because the incidence of PCP in a given population is now determined to a larger degree by the use of effective PCP prophylaxis than by exposure to the microorganism.

Although PCP has become less prevalent in European HIV clinics in recent years, it remains one of the leading causes of AIDS-related illness. In the EuroSIDA patient population referred to earlier, PCP remains the second most frequent cause of AIDS-related illness, and only esophageal candidiasis was diagnosed more often in these patients. However, AIDS surveillance data suggest that PCP remains the leading cause of AIDS illness in Europe (see Table 3). This apparent discrepancy is most likely explained by the fact that the HIV diagnosis is established about the same time as the AIDS diagnosis in a fraction of the patients, and that these patients are not represented in a cohort study such as EuroSIDA. In newly HIV-diagnosed AIDS patients, the risk of having PCP as initial AIDS-defining illness is similar to that observed among AIDS patients in the 1980s. In a study of all Danish AIDS patients reported in 1992 and 1993, 15% of the patients had a diagnosis of HIV infection less than 4 months before the development of AIDS (31). Among these patients, 49% had PCP as their AIDS-defining illness, whereas only 17% of the patients with previously established HIV infection had PCP. Thus, PCP remains the most significant cause of AIDS in Europe.

There are several possible explanations why primary prophylaxis does not provide complete protection against PCP. The primary choice of treatment, trimethoprim–sulfamethoxazole, is almost 100% effective when taken

Table 5 Influence of Primary *Pneumocystis carinii* Prophylaxis, When Initiated Before the AIDS Diagnosis, on the Rate of PCP as AIDS-Defining Event[a]

Region studied	Ref.	Prior prophylaxis: With PCP (%)	Prior prophylaxis: Total number of patients	No prior prophylaxis: With PCP (%)	No prior prophylaxis: Total number of patients
United States	28	17	138	47	706
Europe	4	25	72	40	4953
Denmark	29	20	46	54	633

Source: Data from Refs. 4, 28, and 29.

regularly. However, half of the patients discontinue therapy because of side effects (32,33). The second choice, inhaled pentamidine, is better tolerated, but less effective than trimethoprim–sulfamethoxazole (32,33). Some centers prefer dapsone as a second choice, but a similar proportion of patients to those receiving trimethoprim–sulfamethoxazole discontinue dapsone owing to side effects (32). Besides tolerance and efficacy, patient compliance is an important determinant of the outcome of PCP prophylaxis. A case–control study from Switzerland reported a 35-fold increased risk of developing PCP for patients taking prophylaxis irregularly, compared with patients taking it regularly (34).

Survival from an episode of PCP and also the long-term survival after successful treatment of the pneumonia have improved in the 1980s in Europe. The acute mortality was 18% in those diagnosed before 1988, compared with 11% of those diagnosed in 1988–1989 (35). The median survival time for patients whose disease was diagnosed before 1987 was only 13 months compared with 18 months for those diagnosed in 1987–1989 (35; Fig. 5). The improvement in sudden mortality may relate to earlier diagnosis of PCP after the onset of symptoms (36,37), and the introduction of adjunctive glucocorticoid therapy (38). The most likely explanations for improvement in long-term prognosis include the introduction of secondary prophylaxis and antiretroviral therapy (35).

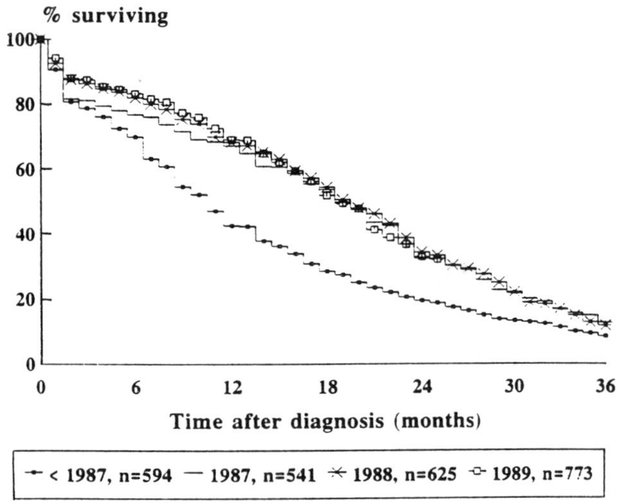

Figure 5 Changes in survival over time from an episode of *Pneumocystis carinii* pneumonia at the time of the AIDS diagnosis among 2,533 patients diagnosed with AIDS between 1979 and December 31, 1989. (From Ref. 35.)

Subsequently, more effective antiretroviral drugs and combinations thereof have been introduced (39–41), but this will probably not lead to further improvement in long-term survival after a diagnosis of PCP. PCP is a late-stage disease, which occurs in severely immunocompromised patients not responding to antiretroviral and prophylactic treatment.

In the years to come, there is a realistic hope for further improvement in the effect of the antiretroviral drug regimens. As a result, the risk per year of developing opportunistic infections (including PCP) will be lowered. However, as long as HIV-infected patients develop severe immunosuppression, PCP will be one of the leading serious HIV-associated diseases. There is an urgent need for new and less toxic prophylactic regimens, especially for patients intolerant to trimethoprim–sulfamethoxazole.

C. Tuberculosis

Since the mid-1980s, it has become increasingly clear that HIV infection has had a major effect on the epidemiology of tuberculosis (TB; 42).

Extrapulmonary tuberculosis has been considered an AIDS-defining illness since 1987, and knowledge of the epidemiology of extrapulmonary TB, therefore, may be derived from AIDS surveillance data and from prospective studies of AIDS patients. Results from the AIDS in Europe study showed that among cases diagnosed between 1979 and 1989, 8.7% had extrapulmonary TB at time of AIDS diagnosis (43). The incidence of extrapulmonary TB after the AIDS diagnosis was 1.9/100 persons-years. In a multivariate analysis, only geographic regions were significantly associated with the risk of developing extrapulmonary TB after AIDS, with an increasing risk from northern Europe to central and southern Europe. Reanalysis of these data, dividing southern Europe in a western (Portugal, Spain) and an eastern part (remaining countries) emphasizes the great diversity in incidences of HIV-related TB within Europe. Extrapulmonary TB was significantly more common in the southwestern part than in other parts of Europe (Table 6). Rates in the eastern part of southern Europe were much like the rates in northern Europe.

In 1993 pulmonary TB was included in the AIDS definition. European surveillance data for 1994 show that among 19,778 AIDS cases, 3,805 (19%) were diagnosed with TB (1; Table 7). Of these cases, 44.5% were reported with extrapulmonary TB alone, 49.1% with pulmonary TB alone, and 6.4% with both. The proportion of patients with a diagnosis of TB was highest in Portugal and Spain, reaching astounding 51 and 42%. In a prospective study of HIV-infected persons with relatively well-preserved immune function (median CD4 cell counts of 467/μl) from Spain, the annual rate of TB was 9.1 cases per 100 person-years (10). The prevalence of HIV

Table 6 Extrapulmonary Tuberculosis (ETB) in European AIDS Patients Stratified by Region

Region	Percentage with ETB at AIDS	Incidence of ETB after AIDS (cases per 100 person-years)
North	2.0	0.7
Central	5.9	2.0
Southeast	4.7	2.6
Southwest	35.2	7.8

Source: Adapted from Ref. 43.

in patients with tuberculosis has been estimated to be between 10 and 30% in Spain (1), which is much higher than in other western industrialized country. For comparison, the percentage of reported TB cases with an AIDS match in the United States in 1990 was 9.5% (44), with the highest rates in New York City (23%), Puerto Rico (19%), and Florida (17%). Besides the association with country, an increased risk of TB was significantly associated with a younger age, injection drug use, and the heterosexual HIV transmission category. The higher risk of TB in the heterosexual transmission category compared with homosexual men is probably caused by heterosexual cases among immigrants from countries with high prevalence of infection with *M. tuberculosis*.

Surveillance data give a minimum estimate of the proportion of patients who will develop TB, for cases diagnosed after AIDS are not reported.

Table 7 Proportion of AIDS Cases Reported in 1994 with Diagnosed Tuberculosis

Country	Number of AIDS cases	%TB
Austria	147	12.9
Belgium	209	16.7
Denmark	232	7.3
France	4831	10.7
Germany	1305	6.5
Greece	121	12.4
Italy	5079	7.4
Portugal	452	51.1
Spain	5618	42.4
Switzerland	424	6.6
United Kingdom	1360	7.3

Source: Ref. 1.

Preliminary data from the EuroSIDA study indicate that the incidence rate of TB among HIV-infected patients with CD4 cell counts of fewer than 200/μl is about 30 cases per 100 person-years in southwestern Europe, compared with rates of fewer than 2.5 cases per 100 person-years in other parts of Europe.

As might be expected, the incidence rates of HIV-associated TB are highest in countries with the highest TB incidence rates in the general population (Table 8; 1), suggesting that the prevalence of latent infection with *M. tuberculosis* in the population has a major influence on the rates among persons infected with HIV. However, the epidemiological pattern cannot be explained simply by reactivation of latent *M. tuberculosis* infection in immunocompromised individuals. The association with younger age strongly suggests that a significant proportion of HIV-related TB cases in Europe, as in the United States (45,46), are caused by more recent infection. A study from Spain has demonstrated that HIV-infected injection drug users with TB are more likely to generate microepidemics of TB than HIV-seronegative TB patients (7.9 vs. 3.8% TB cases among contacts), probably reflecting that the living conditions of abusers of injected drugs may favor contact transmission of *M. tuberculosis* (47). Furthermore, those latently infected are at increased risk for developing active TB and thus becoming infectious themselves.

In a European study of TB and mortality (48), survival was reduced by 34% in AIDS patients who developed tuberculosis, after adjustment for other factors having a significant influence on survival. This may seem surprising because TB is considered a curable disease in patients with HIV

Table 8 Incidence Rates (Cases per 100,000 Population) of TB and AIDS-Associated TB in Some European Countries

Country	AIDS-associated TB in 1994	TB in 1993
Austria	0.3	16.1
Belgium	0.4	14.9
Denmark	0.3	7.9
France	1.1	16.6
Germany	0.2	17.5
Greece	0.1	8.8
Italy	0.7	7.2
Portugal	3.4	55.6
Spain	8.2	24.1
Switzerland	0.6	13.3
United Kingdom	0.2	11.3

Source: Ref. 1.

infection. However, early death before the treatment is effective and lack of compliance may have contributed to the increased mortality observed among TB patients. It is possible that other factors, such as malnutrition or severe immune suppression, that are not reflected by CD4 cell counts, may contribute to shortened survival.

Coinciding with the increase in TB incidence in the United States in the late 1980s and early 1990s, outbreaks of multidrug-resistant TB occurred in hospitals and institutions (49–51). In Europe multidrug-resistant TB is uncommon, but within the past 4 years, several hospital outbreaks have been reported from Spain (52–53), Italy (54), and the United Kingdom (55).

The triad *M. tuberculosis*, HIV and injection drug use has created a background for an epidemic spread of TB among at-risk individuals. At the moment Spain and Portugal face the greatest problem, having outstandingly high TB rates. However, rates are not negligible in other parts of Europe. There is an urgent need for programs to prevent further development of TB in HIV-infected individuals, and to prevent nosocomial outbreaks of multidrug-resistant TB. Source control through rapid identification and effective treatment, including direct observed therapy, should be the primary goal. Other measures should include preventive therapy with isoniazid and isolation of sputum-positive individuals who are in settings where transmission may occur, such as hospitals, prisons, and institutions for users of injection drugs.

D. Bacterial Pneumonia

The development of pneumonia caused by encapsulated bacteria, in particular *Streptococcus pneumoniae* and *Haemophilus influenzae*, occurs more frequently in HIV-infected patients when compared with the background population, in studies from both Europe (56,57) and the United States (58–64). Several studies have found a four- to fivefold increased risk for contracting bacterial pneumonia for HIV-infected injection drug users, compared with non-HIV–infected injection drug users. However, the risk of developing pneumonia with the encapsulated bacteria may increase 13- to 16-fold for HIV-infected injection drug users (56). In addition, the rate of *S. pneumoniae* bacteremia is also substantially higher in AIDS patients than in community-based studies within the same age range (9.4 vs. 0.07 cases per 1000 patient-years, respectively; 65). The risk of developing bacterial pneumonia increases markedly for patients with low CD4 cell counts (56,61,62,64; in one study 37% per 100 cells per microliter; 56), which probably relates to a HIV-induced B-lymphocyte dysfunction (56). Injection drug users are at increased risk compared with homosexual men (56,64). The incidence of bacterial pneumonia in injection drug users with a CD4 cell count of fewer than 200/μl may be as high as 21 cases per 100 person-years (56). In the patient series presented in Table 4, many cases of bacterial pneumonia were diagnosed without use of bronchoscopy and, therefore, were not included in the table.

Once an episode of bacterial pneumonia has emerged, HIV-infected patients are at particular risk of recurrence of the pneumonia. A study of injection drug users from Italy found a 13-fold increased risk of recurrence for HIV-infected patients, compared with non-HIV–infected persons (56).

Besides the encapsulated bacteria, HIV-infected patients may develop bacterial pneumonia caused by *Staphylococcus aureaus* (56,64,67), *Pseudomonas aeruginosa* (68), *Rhodococcus equi* (69), and *Nocardia* spp. (70). Finally, outbreaks of other causes in the community (e.g., *Clamydia pneumoniae*, *Mycoplasma pneumoniae*, or *Legionella* spp.) may also result in increased pulmonary morbidity in HIV-infected persons (56).

E. Viral Pneumonia

Cytomegalovirus (CMV) can be cultured from bronchoalveolar lavage (BAL) fluid from about one-third of HIV-infected persons presenting with pulmonary symptoms, and with increased frequency the lower the CD4 cell count is (Table 4).

CMV as a cause of pulmonary symptoms in AIDS patients has been questioned. Most series have studied CMV as a possible copathogen in cases of PCP. Several larger studies have failed to show any difference in survival for patients from whom both *P. carinii* and CMV (by culture) were identified in BAL fluid, when compared with patients in whom only *P. carinii* was identified (71–74). Thus, CMV does not appear to be an important pathogen for causing pneumonia in HIV-infected patients, whereas the virus is a well-recognized cause of pneumonia in other immunocompromised patients (75).

However, a few cases of isolated CMV infection in the lung with related pneumonia symptoms have been reported, especially in patients who already have established extrapulmonary CMV infection and a CD4 cell count of fewer than 50/μl (76–78). Viral burden within the lung may correlate with disease presentation and outcome in HIV-infected patients (76), whereas in transplant patients, the severity of disease is thought to be primarily related to the degree of inflammation (79). Furthermore, the causative nature of the CMV in pneumonia in HIV-infected persons is suggested by clinical response to anti-CMV therapy in some of the patients (76–78). Culture of CMV from the BAL fluid is a marker for increased risk of contracting extrapulmonary CMV infection. In the patient series presented in Table 4, patients with CMV culture-positive BAL fluid had an 8.7-fold increased risk of developing CMV retinitis during a median of 14 months of follow-up after the bronchoscopy (80).

Finally, the detection of CMV in BAL fluid tends—although not significantly—to predict short-term survival for PCP patients receiving steroids as comedication (81). It remains controversial whether this reflects increased risk of developing herpetic infections; some studies have suggested increased risk of contracting herpetic infection after use of steroids (36,82–84), whereas others have not been able to demonstrate such an association (85–88).

F. Other Pulmonary Complications

Fungal infections (*Aspergillus* spp. and *Candida* spp.), nonspecific interstitial pneumonitis (NIP), and lymphoid interstitial pneumonitis (LIP), are observed in European AIDS patients. The fungal infections are rare, whereas NIP is a significant differential diagnosis in adult patients, and LIP is the leading cause of pediatric AIDS-related illness. Kaposi's sarcoma (KS) is almost exclusively seen in patients with already diagnosed cutanous, oral, or pharyngeal Kaposi's sarcoma. The AIDS in Europe study estimates that 35% of patients also have pulmonary KS, 2 years after the first manifestation of this disorder. Malignant lymphoma located within the lung is rarely detected (personal communication).

VI. Conclusions

The epidemiology of HIV and AIDS in Europe has changed markedly since the beginning of the epidemic. Initially, AIDS cases were primarily observed among homosexual men in northern Europe. However, the HIV infection is now spreading rapidly in injection drug users, especially in southern Europe. Pulmonary complications vary for different regions of Europe. In the 1980s, PCP was by far the most frequent form of pneumonia, especially in northern Europe. However, because of widespread introduction of primary prophylaxis against PCP, its occurrence has diminished considerably in recent years. However, PCP remains the leading cause of AIDS-related illness, partly because the current available prophylactic regimens are not 100% effective, and partly because not all at-risk individuals are identified before they develop PCP. Tuberculosis is a major problem, especially in Spain and Portugal, with incidence rates of more than 30 cases per 100 person-years in patients with CD4 cell counts of fewer than 200/μl. Bacterial pneumonia is a significant cause of morbidity, especially in injection drug users. Surveillance data and large prospectively followed cohorts are important complementary methods to identify patient groups especially susceptible to different causes of pulmonary complications and to detect the ever-changing epidemiology thereof.

References

1. European Centre for the Epidemiological Monitoring of AIDS. HIV/AIDS surveillance in Europe. 1994–1996. St. Maurice, France, 1996.
2. Lundgren JD, Pedersen C, Clumeck N, Gatell JM, Johnson AM, Ledergerber B, Vella S, Phillips AN, Nielsen JO. Survival differences in European AIDS patients 1979–1989. AIDS in Europe Study Group. Br Med J 1994; 308:1068–1073.
3. Lundgren JD, Phillips AN, Vella S, Katlama C, Ledergerber B, Johnson AM, Reiss P, Gatell J, Clumeck N, Dietrich M, Benfield TL, Nielsen JO, Pedersen C. Regional differences in use of antiretrovirals and primary prophylaxis in 3122 European HIV-infected patients. EuroSIDA Study Group. J AIDS 1997; 16:93–99.
4. Lundgren JD, Barton SE, Lazzarin A, Danner S, Geobel FD, Pehrson P, Mulcahy F, Kosmidis J, Pedersen C, Phillips AN. Factors associated with the occurrence of *Pneumocystis carinii* pneumonia in 5025 European AIDS patients. AIDS in Europe Study Group. Clin Infect Dis 1995; 21:106–113.
5. Masur H. Prevention and treatment of *Pneumocystis* pneumonia. N Engl J Med 1992; 327:1853–1860.
6. Phair J, Munoz A, Detels R, Kaslow R, Rinaldo C, Saah A, and the Multicenter AIDS Cohort Study Group. The risk of *Pneumocystis carinii* pneumonia among men infected with human immunodeficiency virus type 1. N Engl J Med 1990; 322:161–165.
7. Moore RD, Chaisson RE. Natural history of opportunistic disease in an HIV-infected urban clinical cohort. Ann Intern Med 1996; 124:633–642.
8. European Centre for the Epidemiological Monitoring of AIDS. HIV testing and surveillance among tuberculosis patients and tuberculosis prevention in HIV-infected persons in Europe. HIV/AIDS Surveillance Eur (quarterly report). St. Maurice, France; 1995: 46.
9. Guelar A, Gatell JM, Verdejo J, Podzamczer D, Lozano L, Aznar E, Miro JM, Mallolas J, Zamora L, Gonzales J, Soriano E. A prospective study of the risk of tuberculosis among HIV-infected patients. AIDS 1993; 7:1345–1349.
10. Moreno S, Baraia-Etxaburu J, Bouza E, Parras F, Perez-Tascon M, Miralles P, Vicente T, Alberdi JC, Cosin J, Lopez-Gay D. Risk for developing tuberculosis among anergic patients infected with HIV. Ann Intern Med 1993; 119:194–198.
11. Ancelle-Park R. Expanded European AIDS case definition. Lancet 1993; 341:441.
12. European Centre for the Epidemiological Monitoring of AIDS. European case definition for AIDS—surveillance in children—revision 1995. HIV/AIDS Surveillance Eur (quarterly report). St. Maurice, France; 1995; 48:46–53.
13. European Centre for the Epidemiological Monitoring of AIDS. HIV/AIDS Surveillance Eur (quarterly report). St. Maurice, France; 1995: 49.
14. European Centre for the Epidemiological Monitoring of AIDS. HIV/AIDS Sur-

veillance in the European Community and COST countries, quarterly report. 1996; 34. St. Maurice, France.
15. European Centre for the Epidemiological Monitoring of AIDS. HIV/AIDS Surveillance in the European Community and COST countries, quarterly report. 1995; 33, St. Maurice, France, 1996.
16. Kobyshcha Y, Shcherbinskaya A, Khodakevich L, Andruschak L, Kruglov Y. HIV infection among drug users in Ukraine—beginning of the epidemic. XI International Conference on AIDS, Vancouver. 1996; Abstract Tu.C.204.
17. Gromyko A. Epidemiological trends of AIDS and other sexually transmitted diseases in the eastern part of Europe. XI International Conference on AIDS, Vancouver. 1996; Abstract Tu.C.205.
18. Lundgren JD, Melbye M, Pedersen C, Rosenberg PS, Gerstoft J. Changing pattern of Kaposi's sarcoma in Danish acquired immunodeficiency syndrome patients with complete follow-up. Am J Epidemiol 1995; 141:652–658.
19. Hermans P, Lundgren J, Sommereijns B, Pedersen C, Vella S, Katlama C, Luthy R, Pinching AJ, Gerstoft J, Pherson P, Clumeck N, for the AIDS in Europe Study Group. Epidemiology of AIDS-related Kaposi's sarcoma in Europe over 10 years. AIDS 1996; 10:911–917.
20. Masur H, Ognibene FP, Yarchoan R, Shelhamer JH, BF, Travis W, Suffredini AF, Deyton L, Kovacs JA, Falloon J, Davey R, Polis M, Metcalf J, Baseler M, Wesley R, Gill VJ, Fauci AS, Lane HC. CD4 counts as predictors of opportunistic pneumonias in human immunodeficiency virus (HIV) infection. Ann Intern Med 1989; 111:223–231.
21. Murray JF, Felton CP, Garay SM, Gottlibe MS, Hopewell PC, Stover DE, Tierstein AS. Pulmonary complications of the acquired immunodeficiency syndrome. N Engl J Med 1984; 310:1682–1688.
22. Murray JF, Mills J. Pulmonary complications of human immunodeficiency virus: Part I. Am Rev Respir Dis 1990; 141:1356–1372.
23. Jones JL, Hanson DL, Chu SY, Fleming PL, Hu DJ, Ward JW. Surveillance of AIDS-defining conditions in the United States. AIDS 1994; 8:1489–1493.
24. Daley CL, Mugusi F, Chen LL, Schmidt DM, Small PM, Bearer E, Aris E, Mtoni IM, Cegielski JP, Lalinger G, Mbaga I, Murray JF. Pulmonary complications of HIV infection in Dar es Salaam, Tanzania: role of bronchoscopy and bronchoalveolar lavage. Am J Respir Crit Care Med 1996; 154:105–110.
25. Elvin KM, Lumbwe CM, Luo NP, Bjørkman A, Kallenius G, Linder E. *Pneumocystis carinii* is not a major cause of pneumonia in HIV infected patients in Lusaka, Zambia, Trans R Soc Trop Med Hyg 1989; 83:553–555.
26. Serwadda D, Goodgame R, Lucas S, Kocjan G. Absence of pneumocystosis in Ugandan AIDS patients. AIDS 1989; 3:47–48.
27. Malin AS, Gwanzura LKZ, Klein S, Robertson VJ, Musvaire P, Mason PR. *Pneumocystis carinii* pneumonia in Zimbabwe, Lancet 1995; 346:1258–1261.
28. Hoover DR, Saah AJ, Bacellar H, et al. Clinical manifestations of AIDS in the era of pneumocystis prophylaxis. N Engl J Med 1993; 329:1922–1926.
29. Lundgren JD, Bentsen KD, Pedersen C, Gerstoft J, Seefelt-Nielsen T, Nielsen TL, Jensen GF, AIDS in Denmark (I). Opportunistic infections and malignancies. Ugesk Laeger 1995; 157:1347–1351.

30. Munoz A, Schrager LK, Bacellar H, Speizer I, Vermund SH, Detels R, Saah AJ, Kingsley LA, Seminara D, Phair JP. Trends in the incidence and outcomes defining acquired immunodeficiency syndrome (AIDS) in the multicenter AIDS cohort study: 1985–1991. Am J Epidemiol 1993; 137:423–438.
31. Smith E, Orholm MK. Danish AIDS patients 1988–1993: a recent decline in *Pneumocystis carinii* pneumonia as AIDS-defining disease related to the period of known HIV positivity. Scand J Infect Dis 1994; 26: 517–522.
32. Bozzette SA, Finkelstein DM, Spector SA, Frame P, Powderly WG, He W, Phillips L, Craven D, Horst C, Feinberg J. A randomised trial of three antipneumocystis agents in patients with advanced human immunodeficiency virus infection. N Engl J Med 1995; 332:693-699.
33. Schneider MME, Hoepelman AIM, Schattenkerk JKME, Nielsen TL, Graaf Y, Frissen JPHJ, Ende IME, Kolsters AFP, Borleffs JCC. A controlled trial of aerosolized pentamidine or trimethoprim–sulfamethoxazole as primary prophylaxis against *Pneumocystis carinii* pneumonia in patients with human immunodeficiency virus infection. N Engl J Med 1992; 327:1836–1841.
34. Flepp M, Ledergerber B, Schenker C, Egger M, Gebhardt M, Lüthy R. *Pneumocystis carinii* pneumonia as first AIDS defining disease in the era of primary prophylaxis—why does it still occur [abstr]? XI International Conference on AIDS, Vancouver, July 1996.
35. Lundgren JD, Barton SE, Katlama C, Ledergerber B, Gonzales-Lahoz J, Pinching AJ, Proenca R, Hemmer R, Pedersen C, Phillips AN. Changes in survival over time after a first episode of *Pneumocystis carinii* pneumonia for 2533 European patients with acquired immunodeficiency syndrome. AIDS in Europe Study Group. Arch Intern Med 1995; 155:822–828.
36. Caumes E, Roudier C, Rogeaux O, Bricaire F, Gentilini M. Effect of corticosteroids on the incidence of adverse cutanous reactions to trimethoprim–sulfamethoxazole during treatment of AIDS-associated *Pneumocystis carinii* pneumonia. Clin Infec Dis 1994; 18:319–323.
37. Bennett CL, Adams J, Bennett RL, Rodrique D, George L, Cassileth B, Gilman SC. The learning curve for AIDS-related *Pneumocystis carinii* pneumonia: experience from 3,981 cases in Veterans Affairs Hospitals 1987–1991. J AIDS 1995; 8:373–378.
38. The NIH-UC Expert Panel. Consensus statement on the use of corticosteroids as adjunctive therapy for pneumocystis pneumonia in the acquired immunodeficiency syndrome. N Engl J Med 1990; 323:1500–1504.
39. Danner SA, Carr A, Leonard JM, Lehman LM, Guidol F, Gonzales J, Aguado AG, De Lomas JG, Delgado R, Borleffs JCC, Hsu A, Joaquin VM, Boucher CAB, Cooper DA. A short-term study of the safety, pharmacokinetics, and efficacy of ritonavir, an inhibitor of HIV-1 protease. European–Australian Collaborative Ritonavir Study Group. N Engl J Med 1995; 333:1528–1533.
40. Bartlett JA, Benoit SL, Johnson VA, Quinn JB, Sepulveda GE, Ehmann WC, Tsoukas C, Fallon MA, Self PL, Rubin M. Lamivudine plus zidovudine compared with zalcitabine plus zidovudine in patients with HIV infection. Ann Intern Med 1996; 124:161–172.
41. D'Auila RT, Hughes MD, Johnson VA, Fischl MA, Sommadossi J-P, Liou S-H,

Timpone J, Myers M, Basgoz N, Niu M, Hirsch MS. Nevirapine, zidovudine, and didanosine compared with zidovudine and didanosine in patients with HIV-1 infection. Ann Intern Med 1996; 124:1019–1030.

42. Shafer RW, Edlin BR. Tuberculosis in patients infected with human immunodeficiency virus: perspective on the past decade. Clin Infect Dis 1996; 22:683–704.
43. Sudre P, Hirschel BJ, Gatell JM, Schwander S, Vella S, Katlama C, Ledergerber B, Monforte A, Goebel F, Pehrson P, Pedersen C, Lundgren JD, and the AIDS in Europe Study Group. Tuberculosis among European patients with AIDS. Tuberc Lung 1996; 77:322–328.
44. Burwen DR, Bloch AB, Griffin LD, Ciesielski CA, Stern HA, Onarato IM. National trends in the concurrence of tuberculosis and acquired immunodeficiency syndrome. Arch Intern Med 1995; 155:1281–1286.
45. Small PM, Hopewell PC, Singh SP, Paz A, Parsonnet J, Ruston DC, Schecter GF, Daley CL, Schoolnik GK. The epidemiology of tuberculosis in San Francisco. N Engl J Med 1994; 330:1703–1709.
46. Alland D, Kalkut GE, Moss AR, McAdam RA, Hahn JA, Bosworth W, Drucker E, Bloom BR. Transmission of tuberculosis in New York City. N Engl J Med 1994; 330:1710–1716.
47. Cayla JA, de Olalla PG, Galdos-Tanguis H, Vidal R, Lopez-Colomes JL, Gatell JM, Jansa JM. The influence of intravenous drug use and HIV infection in the transmission of tuberculosis. AIDS 1996; 10:95–100.
48. Perneger TV, Sudre P, Lundgren JD, Hirschel B, for the AIDS in Europe Study Group. Does the onset of tuberculosis in AIDS predict shorter survival? Results of a cohort study in 17 European countries over 13 years. Br Med J 1995; 311:1468–1471.
49. Fischl M, Uttamchandani RB, Daikos GL, Pobelete RB, Moreno JN, Reyes RR, Boota AM, Thompson LM, Cleary TJ, Lai S. An outbreak of tuberculosis caused by multiple-drug-resistant tubercle bacilli among patients with HIV infection. Ann Intern Med 1992; 117:177–183.
50. Pearson ML, Jereb JA, Friden TR, Crawford JT, Davis BJ, Dooley SW, Jarvis WR. Nosocomial transmission of multidrug-resistant *Mycobacterium tuberculosis*. Ann Intern Med 1992; 117:191–196.
51. Daley CL, Small PM, Schecter GF, Schoolnik GK, McAdam RA, Jacobs WR, Hopewell PC. An outbreak of tuberculosis with accelerated progression among persons infected with the human immunodeficiency virus. N Engl J Med 1992; 326:231–235.
52. Centers for Disease Control and Prevention. Multidrug-resistant tuberculosis outbreak on an HIV ward—Madrid, Spain 1991–1995. MMWR 1996; 45:330–333.
53. Mellado M, Fontelos P, Cilleruelo M, Garcia M, Barreiro G, Jurado M, Ortega A, Villota J. Nosocomial outbreak of multidrug resistant tuberculosis in HIV infected children. XI International Conference on AIDS, Vancouver, 1996; abstract Mo.B. 1310.
54. Caggese L, Volonterio A, Orcese C, Penati V, Astolfi A, Rastrelli M. Human tuberculosis and multidrug-resistance: clinicoepidemiological remarks following

a nosocomial outbreak. XI International Conference on AIDS, Vancouver, 1996; abstract Mo.C.1660.
55. Easterbrook P, Bell A, Hannan M, Hayward A, Troop M, Shave A, Nelson M, Hawkins D, Gazzard BG, Azadian B, Lau YK. Nosocomial outbreak of multidrug resistant tuberculosis in a London HIV unit: outbreak investigation and clinical follow-up. XI International Conference on AIDS, Vancouver, 1996; abstract We.B.305.
56. Bocchini A, Smacchia C, DiFine M, Schiesari A, Ballalini P, Arlotti M, Gabrielli C, Castellani G, Genova M, Pantani P, Lepri AC, Rezza G. Community-acquired pneumonia in a cohort of former injecting drug users with and without human immunodeficiency virus infection: incidence, etiologies, and clinical aspects. Clin Infect Dis 1996; 23:107–113.
57. Mientjes GH, van Ameijden EJ, van den Hoek JAR, Coutinho RA. Increasing morbidity without rise in non-AIDS mortality among HIV-infected intravenous drug users in Amsterdam. AIDS 1992; 6:207-212.
58. Polsky B, Gold JWM, Whimbey E, Dryjanski J, Brown AE, Schiffman G, Armstrong D. Bacterial pneumonia in patients with the acquired immunodeficiency syndrome. Ann Intern Med 1986; 104:38–41.
59. Stoneburner RL, Des Jarlais DC, Benezra D, Gorelkin L, Sotheran JL, Friedman S, Schultz S, Marmor M, Mildvan D, Maslansky R. A larger spectrum of severe HIV-1–related disease in intravenous drug users in New York City. Science 1988; 242:916–919.
60. Selwyn PA, Feingold AR, Hartel D, Schoenbaum EE, Alderman MH, Klein RS, Friedland GH. Increased risk of bacterial pneumonia in HIV-infected intravenous drug users without AIDS. AIDS 1988; 2:267–272.
61. Wallace JM, Rao AV, Glassroth J, Hansen NI, Rosen MJ, Arakaki C, Kvale PA, Reichman LB, Hopewell PC. Respiratory illness in persons with human immunodeficiency virus infection. Am Rev Respir Dis 1993; 148:1523–1529.
62. Caiaffa WT, Vlahov D, Graham NMH, Astemborski J, Solomon L, Nelson KE, Munoz A. Drug smoking, *Pneumocystis carinii* pneumonia, and immunosuppression increase risk of bacterial pneumonia in human immunodeficiency virus-seropositive injection drug users. Am J Respir Crit Care Med 1994; 150:1493–1498.
63. Schlamm HT, Yancovitz SR. *Haemophilus influenzae* pneumonia in young adults with AIDS, ARC, or risk of AIDS. Am J Med 1989; 86:11–14.
64. Hirschtick RE, Glassroth J, Jordan MC, Wilcosky TC, Wallace JM, Kvale PA, Markowitz N, Rosen MJ, Mangura BT, Hopewell PC. Bacterial pneumonia in persons infected with the human immunodeficiency virus. N Engl J Med 1995; 333:845–851.
65. Janoff EN, Breiman RF, Daley CL, Hopewell PC. Pneumococcal disease during HIV infection. Ann Intern Med 1992; 117:314–324.
66. Toews GB. Predisposition to respiratory disease: immunologic and nonimmunologic factors. In: Shelhamer JH, moderator. Respiratory Disease in the Immunosuppressed Patient. Ann Intern Med 1992; 117:415–431.
67. Levine SJ, White DA, Fels AOS. The incidence and significance of *Staphylococ-*

cus aureus in respiratory cultures from patients infected with the human immunodeficiency virus. Am Rev Respir Dis 1990; 141:89–93.
68. Schuster MG, Norris AH. Community-acquired *Pseudomonas aeruginosa* pneumonia in patients with HIV infection. AIDS 1994; 8:1437–1441.
69. Vestbo J, Lundgren JD, Gaub J, Røder B, Gutschik E. Severe *Rhodococcus equi* pneumonia: case report and literature review. Eur J Clin Microbiol Infect Dis 1991; 10:762–768.
70. Rodriguez JL, Barrio JL, Pitchenik AE. Pulmonary nocardiosis in the acquired immunodeficiency syndrome. Chest 1986; 90:912–914.
71. Millar AB, Patou G, Miller RF, Grundy JE, Katz DR, Weller IV, Semple SJ. Cytomegalovirus in the lungs of patients with AIDS. Am Rev Respir Dis 1990; 141:1474–1477.
72. Broaddus VC, Leoung G, Feigal DW. Morbidity and mortality of patients with AIDS and first-episode *Pneumocystis carinii* pneumonia unaffected by concomitant pulmonary cytomegalovirus infection. Am Rev Respir Dis 1991; 144:6–9.
73. Mils PR, Baughman RP, Linnemann CC. Cytomegalovirus in the bronchoalveolar lavage fluid of patients with AIDS. Chest 1990; 97:1072–1076.
74. Bower MB, Barton SE, Nelson MR, Bobby J, Smith D, Youle M, Gazzard BG. The significance of the detection of cytomegalovirus in the bronchoalveolar lavage fluid in AIDS patients with pneumonia. AIDS 1990; 4:317–320.
75. van den Berg AP, van den Bij W, van Son WJ, Anema J, van der Giessen M, Schirm J, Tegzess AM, The TH. Cytomegalovirus antigenemia as a useful marker of symptomatic cytomegalovirus infection after renal transplantation—a report of 130 consecutive patients. Transplantation 1989; 48:991–995.
76. Rodriguez-Barradas MC, Stool E, Musher DM, Gathe J, Goldstein J, Genta RM, Yoffe B. Diagnosing and treating cytomegalovirus pneumonia in patients with AIDS. Clin Infect Dis 1996; 23:76–81.
77. Lundgren JD, Vestbo J, Junge J, mathiesen LR. CMV pneumonia and response to ganciclovir treatment in an AIDS patient. Respir Med 1991; 85:437–439.
78. Vasudevan VP, Mascarenhas DAN, Klapper P, Lomvardias S. Cytomegalovirus necrotizing bronchiolitis with HIV infection. Chest 1990; 97:483–484.
79. Grundy JE, Shanley JD, Griffiths PD. Is cytomegalovirus interstitial pneumonitis in transplant recipients an immunopathological condition? Lancet 1987; 2:996–999.
80. Hansen KK, Vestbo J, Benfield TL, Lundgren JD, Mathiesen LR. Rapid detection of cytomegalovirus in bronchoalveolar lavage fluid and serum samples: correlation to virus isolation and clinical outcome in patients with HIV infection. Inf Dis 1997; 24:878–883.
81. Jensen A-MB, Lundgren JD, Benfield T, Nielsen TL, Vestbo J. Does cytomegalovirus predict a poor prognosis in *Pneumocystis carinii* pneumonia treated with corticosteroids? Chest 1995; 108:411–414.
82. Nelson MR, Erskine D, Hawkins DA, Gazzard BG. Treatment with corticosteroids—a risk factor for the development of clinical cytomegalovirus disease in AIDS. AIDS 1993; 7:375–378.
83. Bozzette SA, Sattler FR, Chiu J, Wu AW, Gluckstein D, Kemper C, Bartok A,

Niosi J, Abramson I, Coffman J, Hughlett C, Loya R, Cassens B, Akil B, Meng T-C, Boylen CT, Nielsen D, Richman DD, Tilles JG, Leedom J, McCutchan JA. A controlled trial of early adjunctive treatment with corticosteroids for *Pneumocystis carinii* pneumonia in the acquired immunodeficiency syndrome. N Engl J Med 1990; 323:1451–1457.

84. Elliott AM, Halwiindi B, Bagshawe A, Hayes RJ, Luo N, Pobee JO, McAdam KP. Use of prednisolone in the treatment of HIV-positive tuberculosis patients. Q J Med 1992; 85:855–860.
85. Gagnon S, Boota AM, Fischl MA, Baier H, Kirksey OW, Voie LL. Corticosteroids as adjunctive therapy for severe *Pneumocystis carinii* pneumonia in the acquired immunodeficiency syndrome. N Engl J Med 1990; 323:1444–1450.
86. Lambertus MW, Goetz MB, Murthy AR, Mathiesen GE. Complications of corticosteroid therapy in patients with the acquired immunodeficiency syndrome and *Pneumocystis carinii* pneumonia. Chest 1990; 98:38–43.
87. LaRocco A Jr, Amundson DE, Wallace MR, Malone JL, Oldfeild EC III. Corticosteroids for *Pneumocystis carinii* pneumonia with acute respiratory failure. Chest 1992; 102:892–895.
88. Montaner JS, Lawson LM, Levitt N, Belzberg A, Schechter MT, Ruedy J. Corticosteroids prevent early deterioration in patients with moderately severe *Pneumocystis carinii* pneumonia and the acquired immunodeficiency syndrome. Ann Intern Med 1990; 113:14–20.

3

HIV and Injecting Drug Users

DON C. DES JARLAIS

Albert Einstein College of Medicine
and Beth Israel Medical Center
New York, New York

SAMUEL R. FRIEDMAN

National Development and Research Institutes, Inc.
New York, New York

I. Introduction

Human immunodeficiency virus (HIV) infection has been reported among injecting drug users (IDUs) in 80 countries throughout the world (1). In many areas, HIV has spread extremely rapidly among IDUs, with the HIV-seroprevalence rate (the percent of IDUs infected with HIV) increasing from less than 10 to 40% or higher within a period of 1–2 years (2). Two factors have been associated with extremely rapid transmission of HIV among IDUs: (1) lack of awareness of HIV or acquired immunodeficiency syndrome (AIDS) as a local threat; and (2) mechanisms for rapid, efficient mixing within the local IDU population. Without an awareness of AIDS as a local threat, injecting drug users are likely to use each other's equipment very frequently. Indeed, before an awareness of HIV–AIDS developed, providing previously used equipment to another IDU was likely to be seen as an act of solidarity among IDUs, or as a service for which one could legitimately charge a small fee.

"Shooting galleries" (places where IDUs can rent injection equipment, which is then returned to the gallery owner for rental to other IDUs) and "dealer's works" (injection equipment kept by a drug seller, which can be lent to successive drug purchasers) are examples of situations that provide rapid, efficient mixing within an IDU population. The "mixing" (or "sharing" of injection equipment) is rapid in that many IDUs may use the gallery or the dealer's injection equipment within very short time periods. Several studies have indicated that the infectiousness of HIV is many times greater in that period after initial infection compared with the long "latency" period between initial infection and the development of severe immunosuppression (3,4). Thus, rapid mixing can lead to highly infectious IDUs transmitting HIV to very large numbers of other drug injectors.

Efficient mixing refers to the sharing of drug injection equipment with few restrictions on who shares with whom. Thus efficient mixing serves to spread HIV across potential social boundaries, such as friendship groups, which otherwise might have served to limit transmission. Shooting galleries and dealer's works situations tend to arise where there are legal restrictions on sale and possession of drug injection equipment. These restrictions can both make it difficult to purchase sterile injection equipment, and make it difficult for IDUs to carry their own equipment with them for fear of being arrested (5,6).

In some European countries, such as Spain and Italy, injecting drug use has long been the most common risk factor for HIV infection and AIDS. In the United States, injecting drug use has been associated with approximately one-third of the cumulative cases of AIDS (7). Over half of the US heterosexual transmission cases have involved transmission from an IDU, and over half of the perinatal transmission cases have occurred in women who injected drugs themselves or were the sexual partners of IDUs. In the most recent estimate of new HIV infections in the United States, approximately half of all new infections in the country are occurring among the IDUs (8).

II. Outcomes of HIV Infection Among Injecting Drug Users

In sharp contrast to HIV infection among homo- or bisexual men, HIV infection among IDUs leads to a wider variety of illnesses than the original opportunistic infections that were used to define AIDS. Table 1 lists some of the illnesses in which HIV infection is associated with increased morbidity or increased mortality among injecting drug users. The 1987 and 1993 revisions of the Centers for Disease Control (CDC) surveillance definition for AIDS were based partly on the studies of the wider spectrum of HIV-related illnesses among IDUs. Before these revisions, many IDUs were dying of HIV-related illnesses, without ever being classified as having AIDS (9).

Table 1 "Nonopportunistic" Infections Associated with HIV Immunosuppression Among Injecting Drug Users

Disease	Comments	Ref.
Bacterial pneumonia	Higher incidence, higher morbidity, more severe course	66, 67
Endocarditis	Higher incidence, higher morbidity, more severe course	9,67
Tuberculosis	Higher incidence, higher morbidity, and reactivation of preexisting infection, multi-drug resistant	9,67
Pelvic inflammatory disease	Possible more severe course	68
Cervical cancer	Interaction with human papillomavirus (HPV) infection	69

The mechanisms through which HIV infection leads to this wider spectrum of illnesses have not yet been identified. Tuberculosis (TB) infection is controlled primarily through cell-mediated immunity, so that one would expect HIV infection to lead to increased reactivation of latent TB infection and increased susceptibility to such infection. HIV infection can also affect humoral immune functioning (10), so that resistance to many infectious agents may be compromised. The lifestyle of many IDUs may also put them at greater risk for exposure to a wide variety of pathogens and reduce immune functioning through mechanism such as poor nutrition.

Whether continued use of psychoactive drugs influences the course of HIV infection among IDUs has been an important question since AIDS was first noticed among them. A wide variety of psychoactive substances have at least some in vitro effects on components of the immune system. There have been a few studies suggesting more rapid CD4 cell count decline or more rapid development of AIDS among IDUs who continue to inject at high levels (11,12). Studies comparing progression of HIV infection among IDUs and among men infected through male-with-male sex, however, have generally shown no differences in the rate of CD4 cell count loss or development of AIDS (13).

At present, it does not appear that continued use of psychoactive drugs per se has any strong effect on the course of HIV infection among IDUs. Immune system activation, however, may increase replication of HIV (14), so that very high frequencies of nonsterile injections, or development of other infections, such as pneumonia, may increase progression of HIV infection. Developing other infections, such as pneumonia, may be a consequence of a high-frequency drug-use lifestyle.

A high-frequency drug-use lifestyle may also interfere with adherence to medical treatment regimens. IDUs in drug abuse treatment programs have often shown very good adherence to medical regimens, particularly tuberculosis screening and directly observed tuberculosis treatment (15).

Some psychoactive drugs may also interact with medications needed by HIV-infected persons. The interaction between methadone and rifampin is the best known. In this particular case, IDUs receiving methadone maintenance treatment, and who need to take rifampin, should have their methadone dosage adjusted upward to provide proper methadone medication (see Chap. 13).

III. HIV and AIDS Prevention for Injecting Drug Users

A. Early Studies

The common stereotype that IDUs are not at all concerned about health led to initial expectations that they would not change their behavior because of AIDS. In sharp contrast with these expectations, reductions in risk behavior were observed among IDU participants in a wide variety of early prevention programs, including outreach distribution of bleach (16,17), "education only" (18,19), drug abuse treatment (20,21), syringe exchange (22,23), increased over-the-counter sales of injection equipment (24,25), and HIV counseling and testing (26,27).

Also, importantly, there is evidence that IDUs will reduce HIV risk behavior in the absence of any specific prevention program. IDUs in New York City reported risk reduction before the implementation of any formal HIV prevention programs (28,29). They had learned about AIDS through the mass media and the oral communication networks within the drug-injecting population (28), and the illicit market in sterile injection equipment had expanded to provide additional equipment (30).

Rather than having to overcome indifference to AIDS among IDUs, the scientific problem became one of understanding and quantifying the change processes. The differences in research design and measurement instruments in these early studies have generally precluded any comparisons of the differential effectiveness of the different HIV prevention programs. It was also difficult to determine how a specific prevention program might be contributing to behavior change processes, and the effects of the behavior change on the rate of new HIV infections among IDUs and their sexual partners.

B. Large-Scale Comparative Studies

Then in late 1980s, two large-scale multisite studies were undertaken that used standardized methods and thus permitted cross-site comparisons. The World Health Organization (WHO) Multisite Study of HIV and Injecting Drug Use (31) was conducted in 11 different cities (Athens, Bangkok, Berlin, Glasgow, London, Madrid, New York, Rio de Janeiro, Rome, Santos, and Toronto). In each city, samples of IDUs were recruited from both drug-abuse treatment programs and nontreatment sites. A standardized interview covering demographic information, drug use history, HIV infection, and sexual risk behavior was administered by a trained interviewer. Blood or saliva samples, or both, were obtained for anti-HIV testing.

The biggest difference among the sites was the seroprevalence at the beginning of the study, ranging from a low of under 1% (Athens, Greece) to a high of approximately 60% (Santos, Brazil). The WHO study found a number of strong similarities across the different sites. A variety of different HIV prevention programs had been implemented for IDUs in each of the cities. Most IDUs from all sites reported having changed their behavior in response to concerns about AIDS. There was only modest variation in the frequencies of risk behaviors across the different sites.

The HIV seroprevalence had stabilized in the different of the cities; however, there was still substantial risk behavior among the IDUs in all of the cities. HIV incidence was estimated using reports of previous negative HIV tests (32). Estimated HIV incidence closely paralleled HIV seroprevalence: All cities with low seroprevalence had low seroincidence, whereas all cities with high seroprevalence had moderate to high rates of seroincidence.

The best explanation for the differences in seroprevalence and seroincidence among the cities was not the implementation of specific HIV prevention programs across the cities nor differential responses to HIV prevention programs by IDUs in the different cities. Rather, the most important factor relating to the large differences in seroprevalence was the HIV seroprevalence level at the time when large-scale HIV prevention programs were first implemented in each of the cities.

The National AIDS Demonstration Research/AIDS Targeted Outreach Model (NADR/ATOM) program was begun in the United States in 1987, and eventually included 41 projects in nearly 50 different cities (33). In all of the cities, the NADR/ATOM project involved street outreach to IDUs not in treatment programs. The eligibility requirements for subjects to be enrolled in the research component of the NADR/ATOM projects required that the person must have injected illicit drugs in the previous 6 months and must not have been in drug-abuse treatment in the proceeding 1 month. Approximately 40% of the more than 30,000 subjects enrolled in the NADR/ATOM projects reported that they had never been in drug-abuse treatment.

Many of the NADR/ATOM projects used experimental designs to test psychological theories of health behavior change. All subjects were provided with a "standard" intervention to reduce HIV risk behavior, which included information about HIV and AIDS, a baseline risk assessment, and the option of HIV counseling and testing. Some of these subjects were then randomly assigned to an "enhanced" condition, which typically involved several additional hours of counseling, education, and skill-training, that incorporated components of the psychological theories of health behavior. Subjects were followed at 6-month intervals to assess changes in HIV risk behaviors and the incidence of new HIV infections.

The NADR/ATOM projects provided a wealth of data about HIV risk behaviors among IDUs not in drug treatment programs. Relative to changes in HIV risk behaviors, there were two strong and very consistent findings. First, almost all of the NADR/ATOM projects showed substantial reductions in injection risk behavior from the baseline assessment to the follow-up interviews, with the percentage of IDUs reporting that they did not "always use a sterile needle" declining from 64 to 41%, while those reporting ever sharing needles declined from 54 to 23% (34).

The second consistent finding was that almost none of the different projects showed significant differences in risk reduction between the standard intervention and the enhanced interview. The general lack of differences between the standard and the enhanced interventions should not be interpreted as meaning that the psychological theories of health behavior are not relevant to HIV risk reduction among IDUs. Rather, these results suggest two other possible explanations. First, after the provision of basic information about AIDS (as in the standard intervention), 2–6 hr of additional education and counseling does little to further "strengthen" anti-AIDS attitudes, perceptions, and intentions.

A second explanation is that risk reduction among IDUs—again, after basic HIV and AIDS education—is primarily a function of social processes, rather than the characteristics of individual IDUs. Thus, information about HIV and AIDS, new attitudes toward risk behaviors, and skills in practicing new behaviors would have been transmitted among active IDUs, influencing persons who had not participated in the enhanced conditions.

IV. HIV Incidence as an Outcome of Prevention Programs

Almost all studies of HIV prevention programs for IDUs have found pre- to postintervention changes in risk behaviors. There are now enough data on HIV incidence among IDUs to draw some conclusions about the relations between risk reduction and the incidence of new HIV infections among IDUs.

The NADR/ATOM studies included follow-up of the participants with repeated HIV counseling and testing to detect new HIV infections. Table 2 presents data on new HIV infections among participants in the NADR/ATOM projects for which these outcome data are available (35). (The cities are not identified individually, because researchers in those cities are preparing individual research reports.)

There are two clear findings from the NADR/ATOM HIV incidence (new infection) studies. First, as in the WHO study, the new infection rates are substantially lower in the cities where the initial (background) HIV seroprevalence rates were low. Second, both background HIV seroprevalence and the new infection rates are generally much lower in areas that permit over-the-counter sales of sterile injection equipment (i.e., do not have prescription requirements for the sale of injection equipment).

The higher new infection rates in areas with higher HIV seroprevalence are easily understood in epidemiological terms. An uninfected person who engages in risk behavior (sharing of drug injection equipment or unprotected sexual intercourse) is more likely to encounter an HIV-infected risk partner. Indeed, even within the low-seroprevalence cities, in the NADR/ATOM seroincidence data, there was a direct relation between higher background seroprevalence and higher incidence (35).

The overall incidence rate was also much lower in areas with legal over-the-counter sales of injection equipment (0.79 per hundred person-years at risk) than in areas that had prescription requirements for sale of injection equipment (1.99 per hundred person-years at risk) (6). Current HIV seroprevalence is the product of past seroincidence (plus changes in the composition of the IDU population), and the presence of over-the-counter sales was also strongly linked with current seroprevalence (so strongly that multivariate analyses were not possible).

However, given the difficulties in establishing factors accounting for current HIV seroprevalence in U.S. cities where over-the-counter sales of injection equipment are legal, one must be cautious in drawing conclusions about causal relations between such sales and lower rates of HIV incidence. The data in Table 2, however, strongly suggest that over-the-counter sales may be one factor in facilitating safer injection among injecting drug users. Studies from France (24,36), Glasgow, Scotland (25), and Connecticut (37)—where the prescription requirement was recently repealed—all show HIV risk reduction associated with over-the-counter sales, supporting the interpretation of a causal role for over-the-counter sales in reducing HIV transmission among IDUs.

Table 2 HIV Seroprevalence and HIV Seroconversions per 100 Person-Years at Risk, Among Injecting Drug Users in 14 Localities[a], by Legal Status of Over-the-Counter Syringe Sales

			Person-years seroconversions per 100		
No. HIV	No. HIV+	%HIV+	Seroconversions	At risk[b]	Person-years at risk
Localities where over-the-counter sales are illegal					
A. 288	311	51.9	4	49.3	8.11
B. 1088	908	45.5	6	146.1	4.10
C. 855	589	40.8	3	81.9	3.66
D. 669	194	22.5	17	262.8	6.47
E. 1222	76	5.9	2	956.1	0.21
F. 787	14	1.7	0	109.0	0.00
Localities where over-the-counter sales are legal					
G. 1760	138	7.3	7	184.0	3.80
H. 652	43	6.2	5	187.0	2.67
I. 1968	61	3.0	8	732.5	1.09
J. 651	17	2.5	0	225.3	0.00
K. 2099	31	1.5	2	765.1	0.26
L. 891	13	1.4	3	983.4	0.31
M. 372	4	1.1	0	18.0	0.00
N. 514	5	1.0	0	53.7	0.00

[a]The principal investigators of specific sites are preparing detailed analyses of their data on seroconversion rates. Data are publicly available (with locality identifiers removed) through Nova Research Company, Bethesda, Maryland.
[b]Numbers presented for person-years at risk by locality do not add up to those for the summary table owing to rounding error.

In addition to the NADR/ATOM outreach bleach-distribution program data, presented in Table 2, one such program deserves additional consideration. The NADR program in Chicago not only had one of the strongest theoretical bases, but also the Chicago research group was able to collect 4 years of HIV incidence data in the cohort of IDUs who participated in the program. There was a dramatic drop in injection risk behavior over the 4-year period, from 95% of the subjects reporting recent injection risk behavior at the start of the project, to only 15% reporting injection risk behavior in the fourth year. HIV incidence in the cohort fell from approximately 9 per 100 person-years at risk during the first year of the cohort follow-up to approximately 2 per 100 person-years at risk for the rest of the follow-up period. Most importantly, there was a strong relation between self-reported injection risk behavior and actual HIV seroconversion: all of the subjects who became infected with HIV were from among those who reported current injection risk behavior. All subjects who reported that they stopped injection risk behavior avoided HIV infection (17). The study did not include a comparison group, so that caution is needed in making causal inferences. Nevertheless, the dramatic drop in reported injection risk behavior and the strong association between HIV incidence and reported injection risk behavior suggests that this project did lead to a substantial reduction in HIV transmission among IDUs in the study.

Many of the NADR/ATOM programs distributed small bottles of bleach to IDUs for disinfection of used injection equipment. Bleach is a relatively strong viricide, but there is some doubt about whether the bleach disinfection as practiced by IDUs in the field actually protects against HIV infection. Two recent studies from Baltimore (38) and New York City (39) have failed to show any relation between self-reported use of bleach to disinfect injection equipment and protection from infection with HIV. (A third study from Miami, however, did find a significant protective effect against HIV incidence (McCoy CB, personal communication). There are numerous difficulties in attempting to find such a relation. Reporting on the frequency and circumstances of using bleach may not be very accurate. Drug users may not know how to "properly" use bleach to disinfect injection equipment (the current recommendation is for 30 sec of contact time of full-strength [not diluted] bleach in the needle and syringe). Even if the drug injectors know how to properly use bleach, they may not be using it properly under field conditions (40).

Thus, the effectiveness of the outreach bleach-distribution programs in lowering rates of new HIV infections among injecting drug users may be a result of participants obtaining more sterile injection equipment (from pharmacies or on the illicit market), rather than resulting from the actual use of bleach to disinfect used injection equipment.

Table 3 presents HIV incidence data among participants in syringe-exchange programs. First, as with the outreach bleach-distribution programs, HIV incidence is quite low in areas with low background HIV prevalence. HIV incidence is, among other factors, related to the probability of a seronegative IDU sharing equipment with a seropositive IDU. Because of this, it may be that almost any HIV prevention program will appear to be effective in a low-seroprevalence area. Conversely, the presence of syringe-exchange programs (or other reliable access to sterile injection equipment) may itself be an important reason why HIV seroprevalence and HIV incidence has remained low in many populations of injecting drug users.

The IDUs from the Montreal exchange have an HIV incidence rate notably above that of the other cities in Table 3. The Montreal program appears to attract a subgroup of injecting drug users with extremely high initial risk levels (41,42), including high rates of cocaine injection and high

Table 3 Recent Studies of HIV Incidence Among Syringe-Exchange Participants

City	HIV Prevalence[a]	Measured HIV seroconversions[b]	Estimated HIV seroconversions[c]	Ref.
Lund	Low	0		70
Glasgow	Low		0–1 (2)	31
Sydney	Low		0–1 (2)	31
Toronto	Low		102 (1)	31
England and Wales (except London)	Low		0–1 (1)	1
Kathmandu	Low	0		71
Tacoma, WA	Low	< 1		72
Portland, OR	Low	< 1		73
Montreal	Moderate	13		42
London	Moderate		1–2 (3)	1
Amsterdam	High	4		
Chicago, IL	High	0		74
New York, NY	Very high	2		75
New Haven, CT	Very high		0 (4)	76

[a]Low = 0–5%
Moderate = 6–20%
High = 21–40%
Very high = 41+%
[b]Cohort study or repeated testing of participants in per 100 person-years at risk
[c]Estimated from: (1) stable, very low < 2% seroprevalence in area; (2) self-reports of previous seronegative test and a current HIV blood or saliva test; (3) stable or declining seroprevalence; (4) from HIV testing of syringes collected at exchange per 100 person-years at risk.

levels of unprotected commercial sex work. Still, additional data are needed to fully explain the Montreal incidence rate, and new studies are presently being initiated in Montreal (Hankins C, personal communication).

The HIV incidence data from the three US high-HIV seroprevalence cities (New Haven, Chicago, and New York) with syringe-exchange programs are based on relatively small sample sizes of person-years at risk. Nevertheless, these results must be considered extremely encouraging in reducing HIV transmission in high-seroprevalence areas. The data from New Haven are generally consistent with the previously developed mathematical model to assess the effectiveness of the New Haven syringe-exchange program (43).

A recent study on incident hepatitis B and hepatitis C infection among IDUs in Tacoma, WA, may contain the strongest evidence for the effectiveness of syringe-exchange programs on reducing transmission of blood-borne viruses (44,45). Tacoma, Pierce County is one of the four counties in the US Centers for Disease Control Hepatitis Surveillance System, and thus has among the best data on hepatitis incidence in the United States. A case–control design was used. Cases of hepatitis B and hepatitis C among IDUs were identified through the surveillance reporting system. Controls were identified among IDUs attending the drug treatment and HIV-counseling clinics in the county. (Sera is collected at both clinics, and could thus be tested to identify IDUs who were seronegative for hepatitis.) Demographic data, drug-injection history data, and whether the subject had ever used the local syringe-exchange program were abstracted from the clinics' records.

Multiple logistic regression analyses were used to identify statistically independent factors differentiating the incident IDU hepatitis cases from the controls. Failure to use the local syringe exchange was strongly associated with both incident hepatitis B and incident hepatitis C. After statistical control for age, gender, race–ethnicity, and duration of injection, the odds ratio for acute infection with hepatitis B among IDUs who had never used the exchange compared with any use of the exchange was over 5 for hepatitis C, the adjusted odds ratio also was over 5 for "never" versus "ever" using the exchange. One of the possible reasons for the strength of these associations is that the local syringe-exchange program is the primary HIV prevention program in the area. Although pharmacies in the area are legally permitted to sell injection equipment without a prescription, many pharmacists choose not to sell to persons suspected of being IDUs.

The HIV seroincidence data in Table 3 and the hepatitis data from the Tacoma study are far from constituting "experimental proof" of the effectiveness of syringe-exchange programs in reducing transmission of blood-borne viruses. Nevertheless, these data clearly indicate that IDUs will use syringe-exchange programs to successfully protect themselves against infection with blood-borne viruses.

V. Integrating Multiple Prevention Programs

While assisting drug injectors to practice safer injection and providing drug-abuse treatment to reduce drug injection per se are often perceived as contradictory strategies, in practice, they have been complementary strategies. One of the most important lessons of the early outreach programs was that the process of teaching drug injectors how to practice safer injection uncovered previously hidden demand for entry into drug-abuse treatment. This unexpected demand for drug-abuse treatment led to a program in which New Jersey outreach workers distributed vouchers that could be redeemed for no-cost detoxification treatment (18). Over 95% of the vouchers were redeemed by drug users entering treatment, many of whom had never before been in drug-abuse treatment.

The NADR/ATOM projects also uncovered previously hidden demand for treatment, and they were able to successfully refer many persons into treatment (46). The limiting factor in the ability of these programs to place drug users into treatment was usually the lack of available treatment capacity in the different cities.

There are also examples of syringe-exchange programs that have become important sources of referral to drug-misuse treatment programs. For example, the New Haven program reports 33% of the first 569 participants were referred to drug treatment (43). The Tacoma syringe-exchange program has become the leading source of referrals to the local drug treatment program (47). The "harm reduction" philosophy used in many outreach bleach-distribution programs and in most syringe-exchange programs emphasizes reducing drug injection as a preferred method for reducing the risk of HIV infection, as soon as the individual drug user believes that he or she is ready for such treatment. The "user-friendly" staff attitude that has been adopted in most syringe exchanges also emphasizes providing a variety of services to IDUs, including referrals to other health and social services, particularly to drug-abuse treatment. The capacity of outreach bleach-distribution programs and syringe-exchange programs to make effective referrals to drug treatment programs may depend primarily upon the availability of treatment in the local area, and whether the programs can afford the appropriate staff to make and follow through on referrals.

Although much progress has been made in providing referrals from outreach bleach-distribution programs to drug-abuse treatment programs, HIV prevention efforts in the United States are still hampered by a lack of "referrals" from drug-abuse treatment programs to bleach-distribution and syringe-exchange programs. Even though drug-abuse treatment programs lead to substantial and well-documented reductions in illicit drug use (48), it would be unrealistic to expect that all IDUs who enter treatment programs will abstain from further illicit drug injection. Indeed, most are likely to fail to complete treatment or to use illicit drugs while in treatment. Some US drug treatment programs currently include information about the locations and hours of operation of local bleach-distribution and syringe-exchange programs as part of the "AIDS education" provided to all entrants into treatment. (Many European drug treatment programs actually provide syringe-exchange services on site.) In general, however, US drug treatment programs have not yet developed strategies for reducing the likelihood that persons who relapse back to drug injection will not become infected with HIV through sharing of drug injection equipment.

VI. Current Problematic Issues in Preventing HIV Infection Among Injecting Drug Users

Much has been learned in the last decade of research on prevention of HIV infection among IDUs. Most importantly, all studies to date have shown that the large majority of injecting drug users will modify their behavior to reduce the chances of becoming infected with HIV. The theoretical bases for HIV prevention efforts have expanded from "factual education" to psychological and social-change theories. Prevention programs are increasingly providing the means for behavior change (for safer injection and, less frequently, for reducing drug injection).

Despite the progress in terms of research findings, increasing sophistication of prevention programs, and actual reduction in HIV transmission, there still are several problem areas related to prevention of new HIV infections among IDUs in some industrialized countries—the United States in particular—and in many developing countries.

A. Provision of Prevention Services

The biggest single problem may simply be the scarcity of HIV prevention services for IDUs in the nation. In the United States, the Presidential Commission on the HIV Epidemic recommended in 1988 that drug-abuse treatment be provided to all persons who desire it. The US National Commission on AIDS made the same recommendation in 1991 (49). The National Commission on AIDS also recommended the removal of "legal barriers to the purchase and possession" of sterile injection equipment. Although there has been some expansion of syringe-exchange services in the United States in the last several years, the commissions' recommendations would appear as valid today as when they were initially made.

In many developing countries, drug addiction is not seen as a health problem, and there are few resources to provide either HIV prevention or drug-abuse treatment for IDUs.

B. Sexual Transmission of HIV

Although there is highly consistent evidence that IDUs will make large changes in their injection risk behavior in response to concerns about AIDS, changes in sexual behavior appear to be much more modest. All studies that have compared changes in injection risk behavior with changes in sexual risk behavior found greater changes in injection risk behavior (50). In general, IDUs appear more likely to make risk-reduction efforts (reduced numbers of partners, increased use of condoms) for "casual" sexual relationships rather than in "primary" sexual relationships (51).

The reasons for the difficulties in changing the sexual behavior of IDUs have not been fully clarified, but the problem appears in many different cultural settings, including IDUs in Asia, Europe, and South America, as well as in the United States (52). To place the problem in perspective, however, IDUs have undoubtedly changed their sexual risk behavior more than noninjecting heterosexuals in the United States as a whole (53).

One factor that appears to be important in increasing condom use among IDUs is an altruistic desire to avoid transmitting HIV to a noninjecting sexual partner. In both Bangkok (54) and New York City (51), IDUs who know (or have reason to suspect) that they are HIV-positive are particularly likely to use condoms in relationships with sexual partners who do not inject illicit drugs. Most programs that have urged IDUs to use condoms thus far have focused on the self-protective effects of condom usage. Appealing to altruistic feelings of protecting others from HIV infection may be an untapped source of motivation for increasing condom use.

Heterosexual transmission from IDUs to their sexual partners who do not inject drugs has occurred in the United States since the first heterosexual IDUs were infected with HIV. The use of crack cocaine is often associated with high frequencies of unsafe sexual behaviors. In cities such as New York and Miami, where there are large numbers of HIV-infected IDUs who also use crack cocaine, the use of crack without injection drug use has itself become an important risk factor for infection with HIV (55). While intervening in the nexus of injection drug use–crack use–unsafe sex will be quite difficult, one strategy that might be used is to provide prompt treatment for genital ulcerative sexually transmitted diseases such as syphilis. The presence of these ulcerative sexually transmitted diseases appears to greatly increase the likelihood of HIV transmission (56).

Also, additional strategies are needed for increasing safer sex among IDUs who engage in male-with-male sexual activities. IDUs who also engage in male-with-male sex can act as a bridge population between non–drug-injecting men who engage in male-with-male sex and the larger IDU population. In many areas of the United States, HIV seroprevalence among men who engage in male-with-male sex is substantially higher than among exclusively heterosexual IDUs (7). There are indications of "slippage" back to high-risk sexual behavior among men-who-have-sex-with-men in San Francisco (57,58) and Amsterdam (59). If slippage back to unsafe sex should occur among men-who-have-sex-with-men in the United States as a whole, this could lead to more HIV infection among IDU men who engage in male-with-male sex, followed by more transmission from these men to other IDUs.

C. The Role of Voluntary HIV Counseling and Testing

Voluntary HIV counseling and testing receives more federal funding than any other type of prevention activity. The use of voluntary HIV counseling and testing as an HIV prevention strategy has recently been reviewed by the Centers for Disease Control and Prevention (60). HIV counseling and testing can be considered as a standard part of health care. Anyone at any risk of being infected with HIV should have the right to learn his or her HIV status. HIV counseling and testing may also be an important gateway for engaging HIV-infected persons into full treatment for HIV infection, which would both improve the quality and length of their own lives and reduce the chances that they will transmit HIV to others. This requires, however, that counseling and testing services reach persons who are likely to be infected with HIV. Unfortunately, the present alternative-site counseling and testing system in the United States generally does not reach persons at high risk for HIV infection. Injecting drug users, in particular, are not likely to use the present HIV-counseling and testing sites.

It is also unclear how counseling and testing affects the risk behavior of persons who receive these services. Although there are studies showing reductions in risk behavior among persons who have been counseled and tested (61), there are also concerns about (1) the stress associated with learning that one is infected with HIV; and (2) the possibility that some persons who test negative might see this result as an indication that they will not become infected, despite their risk behavior.

The role of voluntary counseling and testing is undergoing some revision in HIV prevention. Rather than being seen as a method of "primary" prevention, voluntary counseling and testing is now being viewed as a method for engaging HIV-infected persons, providing them with access to medical treatment, and facilitating behavior change so that they do not transmit HIV to others.

D. HIV Prevention in High-Seroprevalence Areas

Current prevention programs for IDUs in low-seroprevalence areas appear capable of achieving control over HIV transmission (44). These programs cannot prevent all new HIV infections, but it does appear that they can maintain low seroprevalence indefinitely. In these low–HIV-seroprevalence areas, almost all of the remaining risk behavior among IDUs occurs among persons who are HIV-seronegative and, therefore, without transmission of the virus. In high–HIV-seroprevalence areas, however, even moderate levels of injection risk behavior are likely to involve persons of different HIV serostatus and thus lead to transmission of the virus. Recent analyses conducted by Holmberg of the CDC (8) suggest that transmission of HIV among IDUs in high-seroprevalence areas may account for the plurality of new HIV infections in the United States.

A new generation of HIV prevention programs may thus be needed for IDUs in high–HIV-seroprevalence areas. In addition to more intensive programs focusing on safer injection, there is a need for programs to reduce the numbers of persons injecting illicit drugs in high-seroprevalence areas. Massive expansion of drug-abuse treatment could lead to large reductions in the numbers of persons who are injecting illicit drugs. Programs to reduce initiation into drug injection would also be very useful for high-seroprevalence areas, as these would also lead to a reduction over time in the numbers of injecting drug users (2).

VII. Harm Reduction

The worldwide epidemic of HIV infection among IDUs has led to important conceptual developments on injecting drug use as a health problem. HIV and AIDS have dramatically increased the adverse health consequences of injecting drug use, and thus have led to seeing psychoactive drug use as more of a health problem and not just a criminal justice problem. At the same time, HIV infection can be prevented without requiring the cessation of injecting drug use. This potential separation of a severe adverse potential consequence of drug use from the drug use itself has encouraged analysis of other areas in which adverse consequences of drug use might be reduced without requiring its cessation.

The ability of many injecting drug users to modify their behavior to reduce the chances of HIV infection has also led to consideration of drug addicts as both concerned about their health and as capable of acting on that concern (without denying the compulsive nature of drug dependence).

These ideas have formed much of the basis for what has been termed the "harm-reduction" perspective on psychoactive drug use (62–65). This perspective emphasizes the pragmatic need to reduce harmful consequences of psychoactive drug use while acknowledging that eliminating psychoactive drug use and misuse is not likely to be feasible in the foreseeable future. One of the major strengths of the harm-reduction perspective is its applicability to both licit (alcohol and nicotine) as well as illicit psychoactive drugs.

Acknowledgments

Sections of this chapter were originally prepared as reports to the United Kingdom Department of Health and for the United States Congress Office of Technology Assessment.

References

1. Stimson GV. The health and social costs of drug injecting: the challenge to developing countries. Presented at the Sixth International Conference on the Reduction of Drug-Related Harm, Florence, Italy, March 26–30, 1995.
2. Des Jarlais DC, Friedman SR, Choopanya K, Vanichseni S, Ward TP. International epidemiology of HIV and AIDS among injecting drug users. AIDS 1992; 6:1053–1068.
3. Jacquez J, Koopman J, Simon C, Longini I. Role of the primary infection in epidemic HIV infection of gay cohorts. J Acquir Immune Defic Syndr 1994; 7:1169–1184.
4. Salzberg A, Dolins S, Salzberg C. HIV transmission among IV drug abusers in NYC. JAMA 1989; 162:1329–1331.
5. Des Jarlais DC, Friedman SR. The AIDS epidemic and legal access to sterile equipment for injecting illicit drugs. Ann Am Acad Polit Soc Sci 1992; 521:42–65.
6. Friedman SR, Jose B, Neaigus A, Des Jarlais DC. Over-the-counter syringe sales and HIV among drug injectors in the United States. Presented at the Second National Conference on Human Retroviruses and Related Infections. Washington, D.C. Jan. 29–Feb. 2, 1995.

7. Centers for Disease Control and Prevention. HIV/AIDS surveillance report. Atlanta, GA: Centers for Disease Control, 1994.
8. Holmberg SD. Emerging epidemiological patterns in the USA. Presented at the 6th Annual Meeting of the National Cooperative Vaccine Development Group for AIDS, Alexandria, VA, November 1993.
9. Stoneburner RL, Des Jarlais DC, Benezra D, Singh T, Sotheran JL, Friedman SR, Schultz S, Marmor M, Mildvan D, Maslansky R. A larger spectrum of severe HIV-1-related disease in intravenous drug users in New York City. Science 1988; 242:916–919.
10. Zolla-Pazner S, Des Jarlais DC, Friedman SR, Spira TJ, Marmor M, Holzman R, Mildvan D, Yancovitz S, Mathur-Wagh U, Garber J, El-Sadr W, Cohen H, Smith D, Kalyanaraman VS, Kaplan JE, Fishbein DB. Non-random development of immunologic abnormalities after infection with human immunodeficiency virus: implications for immunologic classification of the disease. Proc Natl Acad Sci USA 1987; 84:5404–5408.
11. Des Jarlais DC, Friedman SR, et al. Development of AIDS, HIV seroconversion, and potential co-factors for T4 cell loss in a cohort of intravenous drug users. AIDS 1987; 1:105–112.
12. Weber R, Ledergerber G, Opravil M, Lüthy R. Cessation of intravenous drug use reduces progression of HIV infection in HIV-positive drug users. Sixth International Conference on AIDS, San Francisco. 1990. Abstract TH.C.36.
13. Margolick JB, Munoz A, Vlahov D, Astemborski, Solomon L. Direct comparison of the relationship between clinical outcome and change in $CD4^+$ lymphocytes in human immunodeficiency virus-positive homosexual men and injecting drug users. Arch Intern Med 1994; 154:868–875.
14. Zagury D, Bernard J, Leonard R, Cheynier R, Feldman M, Sarin PS, Gallo RC. Long-term cultures of HTLV-III-infected T cells: a model of cytopathology of T-cell depletion in AIDS. Science 1986; 231:850–853.
15. Altrac D, Dansky SF. Tuberculosis treatment through directly observed therapy in a large multisite Methadone Maintenance Treatment Program: addressing the public health needs of a high-risk population. J Public Health Manage Pract. In press.
16. Thompson PI, Jones TS, Cahill K, Medina V. Promoting HIV prevention outreach activities via community-based organizations. Presented at the Sixth International Conference on AIDS, San Francisco, CA. June 1990. Abstract FD797.
17. Wiebel W, Jimenez A, Johnson W, Ouellet L, Murray J, O'Brien M. Positive effect on HIV seroconversion of street outreach intervention with IDU in Chicago, 1988–1992. Presented at the Ninth International Conference on AIDS, Berlin, 1993. Abstract WS-C15-2.
18. Jackson J, Rotkiewicz L. A coupon program: AIDS education and drug treatment. Presented at the Third International Conference on AIDS, Washington, DC, 1987. Abstract TH.5.2.
19. Ostrow DG. AIDS prevention through effective education. Daedalus 1989; 118:229–254.
20. Blix O, Gronbladh L. AIDS and IV heroin addicts: the preventive effect of

methadone maintenance in Sweden. Poster presented at the Fourth International Conference on AIDS, Stockholm, Sweden, 1988.
21. Hartel D, Selwyn PA, Schoenbaum EE, Klein RS, Friedland GH. Methadone maintenance treatment (MMTP) and reduced risk of AIDS and AIDS-specific mortality in intravenous drug users (IVDUs). Poster presented at the Fourth International Conference on AIDS, Stockholm, Sweden, June 1988.
22. Buning EC, Hargers C, Verster AD, van Santen GW, Coutinho RA. The evaluation of the needle/syringe exchange in Amsterdam. Presented at the Fourth International Conference on AIDS, Stockholm, Sweden, June 1988. Abstr 8513.
23. Hart GJ, Carvell ALM, Woodward N, Johnson AM, Williams P, Parry J. Evaluation of needle exchange in central London: behaviour change and anti-HIV status over one year. AIDS 1989; 3:261–265.
24. Espinoza P, Bouchard I, Ballian P, Polo DeVoto J. Has the open sale of syringes modified the syringe exchanging habits of drug addicts. Presented at the Fourth International Conference on AIDS, Stockholm, Sweden, June 12–16, 1990. Abstract 8522.
25. Goldberg D, Watson H, Stuart F, Miller M, Gruer L, Follett E. Pharmacy supply of needles and syringes: the effect on spread of HIV intravenous drug misusers. Presented at the Fourth International Conference on AIDS, Stockholm, Sweden, June 1988. Abstract 8521.
26. Cartter ML, Petersen LR, Savage RB, Donagher J. Providing HIV counseling and testing services in methadone maintenance programs. AIDS 1990; 4:463–465.
27. Higgins DL, Galavotti C, Johnson R, O'Reilly KR, Rugg DL. The effect of HIV antibody counseling and testing on risk behaviors: are the studies consistent? Presented at the Sixth International Conference on AIDS, San Francisco, June 1990.
28. Friedman SR, Des Jarlais DC, Sotheran JL, Garber J, Cohen H, Smith D. AIDS and self-organization among intravenous drug users. Int J Addict 1987; 22:201–219.
29. Selwyn PA, Feiner C, Cox CP, Lipshutz C, Cohen R. Knowledge about AIDS and high-risk behavior among intravenous drug abusers in New York City. AIDS 1987; 1:247–254.
30. Des Jarlais DC, Hopkins W. "Free" needles for intravenous drug users at risk for AIDS: current developments in New York City (letter). N Engl J Med 1985; 313:1476.
31. World Health Organization, Program on Substance Abuse. Multi-centre study on drug injecting and risk of HIV infection. A Report Prepared on Behalf of the International Collaborative Group, 1994.
32. Des Jarlais DC, Marmor M, Paone D, Titus S, Shi Q, Perlis T, Jose B, Friedman SR. HIV incidence among injecting drug users in New York City syringe-exchange programmes. Lancet 1996; 348:987–991.
33. Brown BS, Beschner GM. Introduction: at risk for AIDS—injection drug users and their sexual partners. In: Brown BS, Beschner GM, eds. Handbook on Risk of AIDS. Westport, CT: Greenwood Press. 1993:xxxi-xl.

34. Stephens RC, Simpson DD, Coyle SL, McCoy CB, and the National AIDS Research Consortium. Comparative effectiveness of NADR interventions. In: Brown BS, Beschner GM, eds. Handbook on Risk of AIDS Westport, CT: Greenwood Press. 1993:519–556.
35. Friedman SR, Jose B, Deren S, Des Jarlais DC, Neaigus A, National AIDS Research Consortium. Risk factors for HIV seroconversion among out-of-treatment drug injectors in high- and low-seroprevalence cities. Am J Epidemiol 1995; 142(8):864–874.
36. Ingold FR, Ingold S. The effects of the liberalization of syringe sales on the behaviour of intravenous drug users in France. Bull Narc 1989; 41:67–81.
37. Valleroy L, Groseclose S. Legislative changes: the Connecticut experience. Presentation given at the National Academy of Sciences Workshop on Needle Exchange and Bleach Distribution Programs, Baltimore, MD, 1993.
38. Vlahov D, Asemborski J, Solomon L, Nelson KE. Field effectiveness of needle disinfection among injecting drug users. J Acquir Immune Defic Syndr 1994; 7:760–766.
39. Titus S, Marmor M, Des Jarlais DC, Kim M, Wolfe H, Beatrice S. Bleach use and HIV seroconversion among New York City injection drug users. J Acquir Immune Defic Syndr 1994; 7:700–704.
40. Gleghorn AA, Doherty MC, Vlahov D, Celentano DD, Jones TS. Inadequate bleach contact times during syringe cleaning among injection drug users. J Acquir Immune Defic Syndr 1994; 7:767–772.
41. Bruneau J, Lamothe F, Lachance N, Soto J, Vincelette J. HIV prevalence and incidence in a cohort of IDUs in Montreal, according to their needle exchange attendance. Presented at the Tenth International Conference on AIDS, Yokohama, Japan, 1994. Abstr PD0496.
42. Hankins C, Gendron S, Tran T. Montreal needle exchange attenders versus non-attenders: what's the difference? Presented at the Tenth International Conference on AIDS, Yokohama, Japan, 1994. Abstr PC0464.
43. O'Keefe E, Kaplan E, Khoshnood K. Preliminary report: City of New Haven Needle Exchange Program. New Haven, CT: New Haven Health Department, 1991 July.
44. Des Jarlais DC, Goldberg D, Tunving K, Wodak A, Hagan H, Friedman SR. Characteristics of prevented HIV epidemics. Presented at the Ninth International Conference on AIDS, Berlin, Germany, 1993. Abstract WS-C15-6.
45. Hagan H, Des Jarlais DC, Friedman SR, Purchase D, Alter M. Reduced risk of hepatitis B and hepatitis C among injecting drug users participating in the Tacoma syringe-exchange program. Am J Public Health 1995; 85(11):1531–1537.
46. Ashery RS, Davis H, Davis WH, Ross RI. Entry into treatment of IDUs based on the association of outreach workers with treatment programs. In: Brown BS, Beschner GM, eds., Handbook on Risk of AIDS. Westport, CT: Greenwood Press. 1993:386–395.
47. Hagan H, Des Jarlais DC, Friedman SR, Purchase D. Risk for human immunodeficiency virus and hepatitis B virus in users of the Tacoma syringe exchange program. In: Proceedings: Workshop on Needle Exchange and Bleach Distribution Programs Washington, DC: National Academy Press, 1994:24–34.

48. Hubbard RL, Marsden ME, Rachal JV, Harwood HJ, Cavanaugh ER, Ginzburg HM. Drug Abuse Treatment: a National Study of Effectiveness. Chapel Hill, NC: University of North Carolina Press, 1989.
49. National Commission on AIDS. Report: the twin epidemics of substance use and HIV. Washington, DC: US Government Printing Office, July 1991.
50. Friedman SR, Des Jarlais DC, Ward TP, Jose B, Neaigus A, Goldstein M. Drug injectors and heterosexual AIDS. In: Sherr L, ed. AIDS and the Heterosexual Population Chur, Switzerland: Harwood Academic Publishers, 1993:41–65.
51. Friedman SR, Jose B, Neaigus A, Goldstein M, Curtis R, Ildefonso G, Mota P, Des Jarlais DC. Consistent condom use in relationships between seropositive injecting drug users and sex partners who do not inject drugs. AIDS 1994; 8:357–361.
52. Ball A, Des Jarlais DC, Donoghoe M, et al. Multi-Centre Study on Drug Injecting and Risk of HIV Infection. Geneva: World Health Organization, Programme on Substance Abuse, 1994.
53. Laumann EO, Gagnon JH, Michael RT, Michaels S. The Social Organization of Sexuality: Sexual Practices in the United States. Chicago: University of Chicago Press, 1994.
54. Vanichseni S, Des Jarlais DC, Choopanya K, Friedmann P, Wenston J, Sonchai W, Sotheran JL, Raktham S, Carballo M, Friedman SR. Condom use with primary partners among injecting drug users in Bangkok, Thailand and New York City, USA. AIDS 1993; 7:887–891.
55. Edlin BR, Irwin KL, Faruque S, et al. Intersecting epidemics: crack cocaine use and HIV infection among inner-city young adults. N Engl J Med. 1994; 331:1422–1427.
56. Chiasson MA, Stoneburner RL, Hildebrandt DS, Ewing WE, Telzak EE, Jaffe HW. Heterosexual transmission of HIV-1 associated with the use of smokable freebase cocaine (crack). AIDS 1991; 5:1121–1126.
57. Ekstrand ML, Coates TJ. Maintenance of safer sexual behaviors and predictors of risky sex: the San Francisco Men's Health Study. Am J Public Health 1990; 80:973–977.
58. Stall R, Ekstrand ML, Pollack L, McKusick L, Coates TJ. Relapse from safer sex: the next challenge for AIDS prevention efforts. J Acquir Immune Defic Syndr 1990; 3:1181–1187.
59. de Wit JFB, de Vroome EMM, Sandfort TGM, van Griensven GJP, Coutinho RA, Tielman RAP. Safe sexual practices not reliably maintained by homosexual men. Am J of Public Health 1992; 82:615–616.
60. Centers for Disease Control and Prevention. External Review of CDC's HIV Prevention Strategies by the CDC Advisory Committee on the Prevention of HIV Infection. Atlanta, GA: Centers for Disease Control, 1994.
61. Higgins DL, Galavotti C, O'Reilly KR, Schnell DJ, Moore M, Rugg DL, Johnson R. Evidence for the effects of HIV antibody counseling and testing on risk behaviors. JAMA 1991; 266:2419–2429.
62. Brettle RP. HIV and harm reduction in injection drug users. AIDS 1991; 5:125–136.

63. Des Jarlais DC. Harm reduction—a framework for incorporating science into drug policy [editorial]. Am J Public Health 1995; 85:10–12.
64. Des Jarlais DC, Friedman SR, Ward TP. Harm reduction: a public health response to the AIDS epidemic among injecting drug users. Annu Rev Public Health 1993; 14:413–450.
65. Heather N, Wodak A, Nadelmann E, O'Hare P, eds. Psychoactive Drugs and Harm Reduction: From Faith to Science. London: Whurr Publishers, 1993.
66. Selwyn PA, Feingold AR, Hartel D, et al. Increased risk of bacterial pneumonia in HIV-infected intravenous drug users without AIDS. AIDS 1988; 2:267–272.
67. Nelson KE, Vlahov D, Cohn S, Lindsay A, Solomon L, Anthony JC. Diabetes is protective against HIV infections in IV drug users. Paper presented at the Sixth International Conference on AIDS, San Francisco, CA, 1990.
68. Minkoff HL, DeHovitz JA. Care of women infected with the human immunodeficiency virus. JAMA 1991; 266:2253–2258.
69. Vermund S.H, Kelley KF, Klein RS, et al. High risk of human papillomavirus infection and cervical squamous intraepithelial lesions among women with symptomatic human immunodeficiency virus infection. Am J Obstet Gynecol 1991; 165:392–400.
70. Ljungberg B, Christensson B, Tunving K, Anderson B, Landvall B, Lundberg M, Zall-Friberg AC. HIV prevention among injecting drug users: three years of experience from a syringe exchange program in Sweden. J Acquir Immune Defic Syndr 1991; 4:890–895.
71. Maharjan,SH, Peak A, Rana S, Crofts N. Declining risk for HIV among IDUs in Kathmandu: impact of a harm reduction programme. Paper presented at the Tenth International Conference on AIDS, Yokohama, Japan, 1994.
72. Hagan H, Des Jarlais DC, Purchase D, Reid TR, Friedman SR, Bell TA. The incidence of HBV infection and syringe exchange programs [letter]. JAMA 1991; 266:1646–1647.
73. Oliver K, Maynard H, Friedman SR, Des Jarlais DC. Behavioral and community impact of the Portland Syringe Exchange Program. In: Proceedings of the Workshop on Needle Exchange and Bleach Distribution Programs. Washington, DC: National Academy Press, 1994:35–39.
74. O'Brien M, Murray JR, Rahemian A, Wiebel W. Three topics from the Chicago Needle Exchange Cohort Study: seroconversion; the behavior of HIV-positive NX users; and the need for additional prevention around non-needle injection risks. Paper presented at the Annual North American Syringe Exchange Conference, Santa Cruz, CA, 1994.
75. Paone D, Des Jarlais DC, Caloir S, Friedmann PB, Ness I, Friedman SR. New York City syringe exchange: an overview. In: Proceedings of the Workshop on Needle Exchange and Bleach Distribution Programs. Washington, DC: National Academy Press, 1994:47–59.
76. Kaplan E, Heimer R. What happened to HIV transmission among HIV drug injectors in New Haven? Chance: New Direct Stat Comput 1993; 6:9–14.

4

Intensive Care for Patients with HIV Infection

VERA A. DE PALO

Brown University School of Medicine
Providence, Rhode Island

I. Introduction

Patients who develop a life-threatening illness must decide with their physicians whether aggressive forms of treatment, such as mechanical ventilation, are appropriate, and the expected outcome of these therapies are an important consideration. Despite the optimism engendered by new treatments that forestall the progression of human immunodeficiency virus (HIV) disease, prevent opportunistic infection, and prolong survival, the death rate remains high, and no cure for HIV infection or its consequences yet exists. Knowledge of the outcome of intensive care in patients with HIV-related illnesses is crucial in deciding if these treatments are appropriate and in the patient's best interests.

II. Respiratory Failure in *Pneumocystis carinii* Pneumonia

Because *P. carinii* pneumonia (PCP) was considered the predominant pulmonary disorder in HIV infection, most investigations of intensive care in acquired immunodeficiency syndrome (AIDS) focused on patients with that infection. These reports deal with PCP and respiratory failure, usually defined as the need for intubation and mechanical ventilation. In these studies, survival is usually defined as discharge from the hospital. As changes in therapy modified the prognosis, three "eras" of critical care for patients with PCP and respiratory failure were identified (1). The first era comprised the experience through 1986, when outcomes were uniformly dismal. From 1986 through 1993, the prognosis seemed to improve, but after 1993, survival of patients with PCP and respiratory failure was again reported to be unlikely. Table 1 summarizes the reports on mortality following intubation and mechanical ventilation for PCP.

A. Early Experience

Intensive care for patients with PCP in the early years of the AIDS epidemic carried a dismal prognosis. The first description of the outcome of

Table 1 Outcome of Mechanical Ventilation in Patients with *Pneumocystis carinii* Pneumonia and AIDS

Ref.	Study period	Mortality (%)
2	10/80–7/83	88/102 (86)[a]
4	1/82–6/85	21/25 (84)
5	3/81–12/85	39/45 (87)
7	1/85–6/86	41/45 (91)
8	Pre-1988	45/58 (78)
10	Pre-1986	18/22 (82)
11	1/84–9/88	32/37 (87)
16	1/82–12/86	11/19 (58)
17	1/81–3/87	5/6 (83)
		7/18 (39)[b]
19	7/81–3/87	15/24 (63)
30	1/86–12/88	21/35 (60)
31	12/84–6/88	15/32 (46)
33	1/87–12/90	40/75 (53)
35	4/87–3/91	24/27 (89)
44	1/85–4/89	15/17 (88)
45	4/85–12/87	7/12 (58)
36	1/87–1/92	27/33 (82)
37	11/91–11/92	13/16 (81)
40	11/88–3/94	5/7 (71)
62	1/90–9/94	36/41 (88)

[a]"Nearly all of these patients" were reported to have PCP.
[b]Received high-dose corticosteroid therapy at the onset of respiratory failure.

mechanical ventilation in patients with AIDS was included in the 1984 National Institutes of Health Workshop on the Pulmonary Complications of HIV Infection (2). Six centers in the United States reported that 102 patients with AIDS received mechanical ventilation, "nearly all" for PCP, and 88 (86%) died.

Some of these patients were described in greater detail in reports from centers in New York and San Francisco. At Memorial Sloan-Kettering Hospital in New York, all 22 patients with AIDS who required mechanical ventilation died (3). At Mount Sinai Hospital, New York, only 4 of 31 patients (13%) who required mechanical ventilation survived to be discharged from the hospital, and all 4 survivors (diagnosed with PCP) had complicated and prolonged hospitalizations (4). Three required mechanical ventilation for more than 30 days, and 3 survivors died within 9 months of hospital discharge. However, 1 lived for more than 2 years. Of the 31 patients, 6 had respiratory failure owing to causes other than PCP, including pulmonary lymphoma, Kaposi's sarcoma, septic shock, invasive endobronchial aspergillosis, and disseminated *Mycobacterium avium-intracellulare* infection. In 1985, Wachter et al. reported on 86 intensive care unit (ICU) admissions for 82 patients with AIDS at San Francisco General Hospital (5): 49 required mechanical ventilation for respiratory failure; 45 had PCP and 4 owing to other causes. Only 6 (13%) survived, all with PCP, and 5 of them died within a year of hospital discharge. Nine patients were admitted with PCP who did not require mechanical ventilation; 4 survived to discharge, but died within 1 year.

After 1986, other studies confirmed the poor outcome of respiratory failure in AIDS. In Miami, 23 of the 31 patients with AIDS admitted to the ICU had respiratory failure, 70% caused by PCP, and almost all of them died (6). Similar dismal outcomes were described at other centers in New York (7-9) and the United Kingdom (10,11).

B. Altered ICU Utilization Patterns

Knowledge of these outcome data led to the belief that endotracheal intubation and mechanical ventilation were unlikely to improve the prognosis of respiratory failure caused by PCP. Although the absolute number of patients admitted to San Francisco General Hospital with AIDS continued to rise through 1985, the number of ICU admissions for AIDS patients decreased dramatically because of changes in physicians' and patients' attitudes (5). Awareness of a poor prognosis made physicians less likely to recommend aggressive interventions; surveys of medical housestaff showed that the greater the physician's experience in caring for patients with AIDS, the more accurately he was able to estimate ICU prognosis for these patients (12). Other data from San Francisco indicated that patients preferences contributed to the decline in ICU admissions. Although patients with AIDS tended to overestimate the likelihood of survival after respiratory failure, 45% said they would decline mechanical ventilation, suggesting that many patients chose not to be admitted to the ICU (13). Patients with HIV infection are often keen to participate in decisions about their care (14,15). Furthermore, the national survey of medical residents indicated that physicians with greater experience in caring for AIDS patients were more willing to discuss ethical issues concerning health care decisions early on in their patient's illness (12).

C. New Successes in ICU Treatment of Respiratory Failure

After 1986, reports from several institutions began to dispel the notion of a bleak prognosis for respiratory failure in AIDS (16–21). The reasons for this were not explored systematically, but several factors undoubtedly contributed to reports of improved outcomes. The first is reporting bias, because centers that achieved improved survival statistics would be more likely to try to report their data, and journals would be more likely to publish this new information. Also, there was probably a shift in selection of patients who received ICU care. Early in the epidemic, patients with AIDS and critical illnesses were usually treated very aggressively, because their likely outcomes were unknown. With more experience, patients with obviously poor prognoses were less likely to be offered or to agree to mechanical ventilation. Finally, adjunctive steroids were introduced as part of the treatment of severe PCP in the late 1980s, with a corresponding improvement in survival.

At the New York Veterans Administration Medical Center, 8 of 19 patients (42%) who received mechanical ventilation during a first episode of PCP survived (16). However, 7 of the 8 survivors were admitted immediately after diagnostic fiberoptic bronchoscopy, suggesting that the procedure was largely responsible for the need for mechanical ventilation. In Vancouver, British Columbia, Montaner et al. described a striking reduction in mortality in patients who received ventilatory support for PCP, attributed to the use of adjunctive high-dose corticosteroid therapy and early diagnosis (17). Five of the six patients (84%) who did not receive corticosteroids died, compared with 7 of the 18 patients (39%) who also received intravenous hydrocortisone. Data derived from patients in Copenhagen who required mechanical ventilation with a first episode of PCP found survival rates to be over 50%, and the long-term prognosis to be no different than that for patients no requiring mechanical ventilation (22,23).

The influence of clinical experience on outcomes of patients with PCP was studied by Bennett et al. using a modified version of the Uniform

Hospital Discharge Data Set from 15 hospitals in metropolitan areas of California (24,25). The data were organized into a group of seven hospitals with a high degree of familiarity with AIDS, and another group of eight with a low degree of familiarity. Intensive care utilization was similar in both groups, but the hospitals with low AIDS experience had higher hospital mortality rates. After adjusting for severity of illness, a two-stage multivariate regression analysis showed that patients with PCP were 3.6 times as likely to die in a hospitals with low AIDS familiarity, as in a hospitals with high AIDS experience. These data were confirmed by a population-based AIDS surveillance data analysis from Massachusetts (26). Not only was there a higher risk of mortality at hospitals with less AIDS experience, but also a significantly higher frequency of ICU use.

Given these observations, some suggested that regionalization of care to centers with a high level of experience caring for patients with AIDS would lead to improved outcomes, but others pointed out that this would take patients away from their primary care providers and social support (27). This strategy would also negatively impinge on many teaching hospitals, who might find it difficult to attract house staff if the proportion of medical admissions who had HIV infection increased (27–29).

To find out whether the outcome of intensive care for patients with AIDS had really improved, a longitudinal examination of patients with PCP and respiratory failure was undertaken at San Francisco General Hospital (30). Patients were divided into two eras. Era I described 42 patients admitted to the ICU between 1981 and 1985; 36 patients (86%) died and 2 (5%) received corticosteroids. Between 1986 and 1988 (era II), patients, 26 of the 35 patients (74%) were treated with adjunctive steroids, and 21 (60%) died. In a stepwise logistic regression model, corticosteroid use was not independently associated with improved survival; the only variables were intensive care in the later era and a higher serum albumin level at the time of admission. The authors concluded that their data supported an optimistic short-term prognosis for severe PCP and ICU treatment. Others expressed similar optimism in reports of survival, in the range of 50%, among patients with PCP who required mechanical ventilation (31–33).

D. The "Third Era" of Outcomes

After the reports of improved outcomes associated with the use of adjunctive corticosteroid therapy, we are now in a third era of outcomes, with higher mortality rates reported after 1993 (1). The apparent decline in survival is best explained by shifts in characteristics of patients who receive intensive care toward those who are expected to have a worse prognosis. In San Francisco General Hospital, mortality increased from 61% in the period from 1986 through 1988, to 76% in the next 2 years (34). In the latter period, more patients were injection drug users, and there were more episodes of recurrent PCP. Mortality was strongly associated with a CD4 lymphocyte count of fewer than 50/mm^3 (94%), and with the development of a pneumothorax (no survivors).

Recent patients who required mechanical ventilation are also more likely to represent failures of prophylaxis, antipneumocystis treatment, and adjunctive corticosteroids. These patients would be expected to have a poor prognosis. In Vancouver, the proportion of patients who received mechanical ventilation for PCP decreased from 1981 through 1991, but mortality rates increased from 50% in 1981–1987, to 89% in 1987–1991 (35). Simultaneously, corticosteroid use before intubation increased from "almost never" to 50%. In another retrospective analysis, Staikowsky et al. found an overall mortality rate of 82% among patients who required mechanical ventilation for the treatment of PCP between 1987 and 1992 (36). Only 1 of the 22 patients (5%) who started mechanical ventilation after 5 days of treatment with trimethoprim–sulfamethoxazole and corticosteroids survived, compared with 5 of the 14 (36%) who received a shorter course of therapy. Similarly, 13 of 16 (81%) patients who required mechanical ventilation for PCP at Beth Israel Hospital in New York from July 1991 to June 1992 died, despite the routine use of adjunctive corticosteroids (37). Taken together, these studies show that when respiratory failure follows several days of appropriate therapy for PCP, the probability of survival is only 10–20%. Patients who require intubation before receiving antipneumocystis treatment have a better outlook.

The outcome of respiratory failure in PCP is also inversely related to the length of stay in the ICU, but data on the duration of mechanical ventilation for PCP that is associated with no survival is scarce. In the multicenter trial of corticosteroids for PCP, survival after 2 weeks of mechanical ventilation was unprecedented (38). However, the number of patients in the analysis was too small to support a conclusion that ventilatory support for more than 2 weeks is futile.

The prospects for long-term survival following PCP and respiratory failure are more hopeful than earlier in the epidemic, when patients who lived until hospital discharge rarely lived longer than 1 year (4,5). Friedman et al. studied 73 patients with 75 episodes of PCP who received positive-pressure ventilation in the ICU from 1987 through 1990 (33). Among the 34 survivors, 20 (74%) survived for 1 year. In a follow-up study from the same center, which included more patients, the survival rate was 80% at 1 year, 49% at 2 years, 18% at 3 years, and 6% at 4 years (39). Prolonged survival is probably related to the selection of patients for mechanical ventilation who have a better prognosis, and to improvements in prophylaxis and treatment of subsequent infections. With newer antiretroviral treatments, it is possible that the long-term prognosis may improve further.

III. Intensive Care for Causes Other Than PCP

Admission rates to ICUs for other diagnoses are not adequately studied. Information on intensive care in patients with HIV infection who do not have PCP is scant, and it is difficult to make generalizable conclusions on the data that exist. First, most studies consider only patients with AIDS; only a few consider HIV-infected persons without an AIDS-defining disorder who receive intensive care. These studies were conducted over more than 10 years, and all but one come from single centers (40). Depending on local patient populations and physicians' practice patterns, inferences about the types of critical illnesses and their outcomes may show strong bias. For example, in an analysis of 120 consecutive patients with AIDS admitted to an ICU in Paris, the overall mortality was only 28% (41). However, the unit's admission policy excludes patients with dementia or severe wasting, and admits all patients with a significant pneumothorax. Thus, patients with a poor prognosis are systematically excluded, whereas some with a good prognosis (who would not be admitted to another center's ICU) are included.

Despite problems with the available data, some conclusions may be drawn. Although PCP is probably the single most common diagnosis leading to ICU admission, it still accounts for the minority of ICU admissions of persons with HIV infection. There is a diverse range of diseases that prompt admission to ICUs, and outcomes for patients who do not have respiratory failure is significantly better than for those who do. In the study of patients with AIDS, by Lazard et al., half the patients were admitted with acute respiratory failure, and half of them had PCP (41). The 39 patients who required mechanical ventilation had a 61% mortality, compared with only 9% mortality in the 81 who did not. At Beth Israel Medical Center, New York, 32 of the 65 adults (49%) with HIV infection or AIDS admitted to the ICU from 1991 to 1992 survived to be discharged from the hospital (37). The principal reasons for admission included respiratory failure, sepsis syndrome, neurological diseases, cardiac disease, hypotension, and drug overdose. Although respiratory failure from PCP was the most common reason for admission to the ICU, it accounted for only a third of total admissions. Twenty percent of the admissions for respiratory failure were for causes other than PCP, and 37% survived. However, patients admitted for other reasons enjoyed a 67% survival rate. Similarly, 88 of the 161 patients (55%) with HIV infection admitted to Yale–New Haven

Hospital's medical ICU between 1986 and 1991 had primary disorders other than pneumonia and sepsis (42). The overall mortality rate was 44.1%, but 85.7% of patients with CD4 lymphocyte counts of $200/mm^3$, or fewer, who had pneumonia or sepsis died. In a multicenter prospective study of 1130 persons with HIV infection (but not AIDS) at the time of enrollment, there were 68 ICU admissions after 4298 patient-years of follow-up, and PCP accounted for only 16% (Table 2; 40). The overall hospital mortality was 40%, but 67% of patients with respiratory failure died, compared with 25% of the others.

IV. Predictors of ICU Survival

Some investigators attempted to predict ICU survival based on laboratory tests and scoring systems, but the data are conflicting on the reliability of prognostic variables, and no measurements are sufficiently predictive to make firm conclusions on whether intensive care will be effective for an individual patient. In various studies of patients with PCP, a worse prognosis was associated with age older than 45 years, PaO_2 less than 50 mmHg, $P(A\text{-}a)O_2$ greater than 50 mmHg, lactate dehydrogenase (LDH) levels higher than 800 IU/L, metabolic acidosis, and higher APACHE score (11,42–45). Poor nutritional status also appears to predict a worse prognosis (5,37).

It is clear that neither HIV infection nor AIDS alone is associated with a significantly worse outcome of intensive care interventions than in other patients. In the study by Lazard et al., patients with AIDS had a higher mortality rate than others admitted to the ICU (28 vs. 20%), despite similar severity of illness scores and lengths of stay (41). However, a multivariate analysis identified three factors that predicted death independently: a Simplified Acute Physiology score I (SAPS I) higher than 10, an serum albumin level lower than 30 g/L, and CDC-defined AIDS (1987 definition) for more than 1 year. Nevertheless, 82% of ICU survivors were alive at 1 month, 53% at 6 months, and 39% at 1 year.

These and other studies suggest that, in patients with HIV infection, the short-term prognosis depends primarily on the nature and severity of the acute illness and the physiological reserve of the patient, rather than measurements such as the CD4 lymphocyte count (40). Long-term survival is related to the severity of the underlying HIV disease. Because the outcome of intensive care does not depend directly on the patient's HIV status, then serostatus and CD4 lymphocyte counts should not be overriding considerations in deciding whether to offer or withhold intensive care. Rather, these decisions should be made using the same criteria as for all patients, namely, the likelihood of benefit and the patient's wishes.

Table 2 Admissions to Intensive Care Units: Principal Diagnosis and Mortality

	Admissions	Mortality (%)
Total	68	25 (40)
Pulmonary	24	16 (67)
Pneumocystis carinii pneumonia[a]	11	6 (55)
Other lung disease	13	10 (77)
Bacterial pneumonia	4	2 (50)
Pulmonary edema (renal failure)	2	1 (50)
Pulmonary tuberculosis	1	1 (100)
ARDS	1	1 (100)
Kaposi's sarcoma	1	1 (100)
Pulmonary fibrosis	1	1 (100)
Pneumothorax	1	1 (100)
Cytomegalovirus pneumonia	1	1 (100)
Metastatic adenocarcinoma	1	1 (100)
Gastrointestinal	14	4 (29)
Cardiovascular	9	1 (13)
Sepsis syndrome	6	3 (50)
Neurological	5	1 (20)
Procedure	4	0 (0)
Metabolic	3	0 (0)
Trauma	2	0 (0)
Drug overdose	1	0 (0)
Unknown	1	0 (0)

[a]One patient had coinfection with *P. carinii*, *Legionella pneumophilia*, and *Aspergillus fumigatus*
Source: Ref. 40.

V. Surgical Intensive Care

Patients with AIDS or HIV infection may be admitted to the ICU after surgery. In addition to open lung biopsy, brain biopsy, and other diagnostic procedures, patients with HIV infection may have the same indications for surgery as the rest of the population. In a retrospective review, the postoperative complication rate in HIV-infected patients was not increased compared with HIV-seronegative controls (46). In another, 52 patients with HIV infection in a surgical ICU were compared with 350 who were not infected (47). The groups had similar APACHE II scores, and all had conditions not directly related to HIV infection. After adjustment for age, there were no differences in mortality or length of stay. These data suggest that HIV-infected persons do not have an increased risk of posteroperative complications compared with others, and that decisions concerning whether surgery should be performed should be based on the same criteria as those for other patients.

VI. The Economics of Intensive Care for HIV-Infected Patients

There is national debate on the allocation of health care resources that often centers on critically ill patients with terminal illness. Many patients with AIDS are in this category. Assessment of costs and outcomes is inevitable with all interventions. Similar questions are asked about intensive care in patients with AIDS as new therapies for HIV-associated disorders are introduced, and outcomes of critical illness change (34,48–51). In San Francisco, the cost of each hospitalization for PCP and respiratory failure treated with mechanical ventilation was estimated at 35,000 dollars and ICU admission and subsequent hospitalization cost an average of 174,781 dollars per year of life saved (34,49). Analysis of the economics of ICU and hospital care, spanning the length of the AIDS epidemic revealed that care cost 305,795 dollars per year of life saved in era I (1981 through 1985), 94,528 dollars during era II (1986 through 1988), and 215,233 dollars in era III (1989 through 1991). It is impossible to predict the effect of improving antiretroviral therapies and prophylaxis on costs associated with intensive care in AIDS. In parallel with the epidemiology of AIDS, patients will almost surely be more likely to be injection drug users, and perhaps more likely to have failed antiretroviral therapy, with an associated poor short-term prognosis. On the other hand, survival after intensive care treatment may improve owing to new therapies.

VII. Ethical and Moral Considerations

The decision to provide intensive care to patients with AIDS or any other terminal illness is often difficult, involving the patient's or surrogate's wishes, the physician's experience, and the expected outcome if ICU interventions are provided. Armed with sound medical knowledge and accurate data, patients and physicians are better equipped to choose or refuse more aggressive and life-sustaining therapies (52,53). In cases for whom these interventions offer no reasonable prospect of survival, the physician has no ethical, medical, or legal obligation to provide a futile therapy, even if requested by the patient or his surrogate (54–56). However, decisions of futility may still be debatable, as futility involves value judgment, as well as scientific knowledge (57).

The patient's capacity to make decisions concerning their care must also be considered, for some patients with AIDS are rendered incompetent by AIDS-related dementia, infections, or neoplasms of the brain, or by metabolic encephalopathy. It is the consensus of medical, ethical, and legal opinions that the care of the incompetent patient should be guided by the patient's previously stated wishes. Often, when a patient's wishes are unknown, families may be asked to act as surrogates. This may not be appropriate for some patients, as many gay men with AIDS prefer their lovers or partners to make health care decisions, instead of their biological families (57). This emphasizes the importance of health care proxies, durable power of attorney, and discussions with patients about their health care wishes early in their illness.

Moral and ethical issues are also raised when considering allocation of intensive care resources to patients with such a grave prognosis (58). In the event of scarce bed availability, assignment of individual patients should occur according to standard triage guidelines (57). Limiting resources to treat patients with AIDS based on economic considerations would be difficult to justify, unless resources for patients with other diseases, but similar prognoses, were also restricted (59). Similarly, the argument that intensive care resources should be limited to patients with HIV infection because their condition is in some way self-inflicted is indefensible, unless we limit treatment of persons with diseases attributed to other "unhealthful" behaviors, such as dietary indulgences, tobacco smoking, or in an extreme example, to police officers or firefighters who willfully engage in risky behaviors that can cause injury and disease (60).

Currently, a competent patient has the right to choose intensive care therapy, even if its benefits are few and its burdens, including its financial costs, are many (61). With finite resources, and a potential for increased ICU utilization by persons with HIV infection, guidelines for the intensive care of AIDS patients may be proposed. However, any policy that limits the access of patients with AIDS to intensive care must also limit care for other patient populations with similar prognoses, to meet the goal of using fixed resources to provide adequate health care to all.

References

1. Wachter RM, Luce JM. Respiratory failure from severe *Pneumocystis carinii* pneumonia: entering the third era. Chest 1994; 106:1313–1315.
2. Murray JF, Felton CP, Garay SM, et al. Pulmonary complications of the acquired immunodeficiency syndrome. Report of National Heart, Lung and Blood Institute Workshop. N Engl J Med 1984; 310:1682–1688.

3. Stover DE, White DA, Romano PA, et al: Spectrum of pulmonary disease associated with the acquired immunodeficiency syndrome. Am J Med 1985; 78:429–437.
4. Rosen MJ, Cucco RA, Teirstein AS. Outcome of intensive care in patients with the acquired immunodeficiency syndrome. J Intensive Care Med 1986; 1:55–60.
5. Wachter RM, Luce JM, Turner J, Volberding P, Hopewell PC. Intensive care of patients with the acquired immunodeficiency syndrome: outcome and changing patterns of utilization. Am Rev Respir Dis 1986; 134:891–896.
6. Schein RMH, Fischl MA, Pitchenik AE, Sprung CL. ICU survival of patients with the acquired immunodeficiency syndrome. Crit Care Med 1986; 14:1026–1027.
7. Baggott LA, Baggott BB. *Pneumocystis carinii* pneumonia (PCP) in AIDS patients in intensive care. Chest 1987; 92(suppl):132.
8. DeVita MA, Greenbaum DM. The critically ill patient with the acquired immunodeficiency syndrome. In: Shoemaker WC, Ayres S, Grenvik A, Holbrook PR, Thompson WL, eds. Textbook of Critical Care Medicine. Philadelphia: WB Saunders, 1989:862–869.
9. Smith RL, Levine SM, Lewis ML. Prognosis of patients with AIDS requiring intensive care. Chest 1989; 96:857–861.
10. Deam R, Kimberley APS, Anderson M, Soni N. AIDS in ICUs: outcome. Anaesthesia 1988; 43:150–151.
11. deRuiter A, Webb A, Mindel A, Scaravilli F, Michaels L, Miller RF. Intensive care for advanced HIV disease. Genitourin Med 1992; 68:154–158.
12. Wachter RM, Cooke M, Hopewell PC, Luce JM. Attitudes of medical residents regarding intensive care for patients with the acquired immunodeficiency syndrome. Arch Intern Med 1988; 148:149–152.
13. Steinbrook R, Lo B, Moulton J, Saika G, Hollander H, Volberding PA. Preferences of homosexual men with AIDS for life-sustaining treatment. N Engl J Med 1986; 314:457–460.
14. Wachter RM. AIDS, activism and the politics of health. N Engl J Med 1992; 326:128–133.
15. Wachter RM, Luce JM, Hearst N, Lo B. Decisions about resuscitation: inequities among patients with different diseases but similar prognoses. Ann Intern Med 1989; 111:525–532.
16. El-Sadr W, Simberkoff MS. Survival and prognostic factors in severe *Pneumocystis carinii* pneumonia following mechanical ventilation. Am Rev Respir Dis 1988; 137:1264–1267.
17. Montaner JSG, Russell JA, Lawson L, Ruedy J. Acute respiratory failure secondary to *Pneumocystis carinii* pneumonia in the acquired immunodeficiency syndrome: a potential role for systemic corticosteroids. Chest 1989; 95:881–884.
18. Luce JM, Wachter RM, Hopewell PC. Intensive care of patients with acquired immunodeficiency syndrome: time for a reassessment? Am Rev Respir Dis 1988; 137:1261–1263.
19. Rogers PL, Lane HC, Henderson DK, Parillo J, Masur H. Admission of AIDS patients to a medical intensive care unit: causes and outcome. Crit Care Med 1989; 17:113–117.

20. Friedman Y, Franklin C. Admission of AIDS patients to a medical intensive care unit: causes and outcomes. Crit Care Med 1990; 18:346–347.
21. Tucker KJ, Anton B, Tucker HJ. The effect of human immunodeficiency virus infection on the distribution and outcome of pneumonia in intensive care units. West J Med 1992; 157:637–640.
22. Pedersen C, Lundgren JD, Nielsen T, Andersen WH. The outcome of *Pneumocystis carinii* pneumonia in Danish patients with AIDS. Scand J Infect Dis 1989; 21:375–380.
23. Nielsen TL, Guldager H, Pedersen C, Mathiesen L, Nielsen JO. The outcome of mechanical ventilation in patients with an AIDS-associated primary episode of *Pneumocystis carinii* pneumonia. Scand J Infect Dis 1991; 23:37–41.
24. Bennett CL, Garfinkle JB, Draper D, Rogers W, Mathews WC, Knouse DE. The relation between hospital experience and in-hospital mortality for patients with AIDS-related PCP. JAMA 1989; 261:2975–2979.
25. Bennett CL, Gertler P, Guze PA, Garfinkle JB, Knouse DE, Greenfield S. The relation between resource use and in-hospital mortality for patients with acquired immunodeficiency syndrome-related *Pneumocystis carinii* pneumonia. Arch Intern Med 1990; 150:1447–1452.
26. Stone VE, Seage GR, Hertz T, Epstein AM. The relation between hospital experience and mortality for patients with AIDS. JAMA 1992; 268:2655–2661.
27. Shapiro MF, Greenfield S. Experience and outcome in AIDS. JAMA 1992; 288:2698–2699.
28. Wachter RM. The impact of the acquired immunodeficiency syndrome on medical residency training. N Engl J Med 1986; 314:177–180.
29. Hayward RA, Kravitz RL, Shapiro MF. Program directors' attitudes toward residents' care of patients who have AIDS. J Gen Intern Med 1991; 6:18–26.
30. Wachter RM, Russi MB, Bloch DA, Hopewell PC, Luce JM. *Pneumocystis carinii* pneumonia and respiratory failure in AIDS: improved outcomes and increased use of intensive care units. Am Rev Respir Dis 1991; 143:251–256.
31. Efferen LS, Nadarajah D, Palat DS. Survival following mechanical ventilation of *Pneumocystis carinii* pneumonia in patients with the acquired immunodeficiency syndrome. Am J Med 1989; 87:401–404.
32. Friedman Y, Franklin C, Rackow EC, Weil MH. Improved survival in patients with AIDS, *Pneumocystis carinii* pneumonia, and severe respiratory failure. Chest 1989; 96:862–866.
33. Friedman Y, Franklin C, Freels, Weil MH. Long-term survival of patients with AIDS, *Pneumocystis carinii* pneumonia and respiratory failure. JAMA 1991; 266:89–92.
34. Wachter RM, Luce JM, Safrin S, Berrios DC, Charlebois E, Scitovsky AA. Cost and outcome of intensive care for patients with AIDS, *Pneumocystis carinii* pneumonia and severe respiratory failure. JAMA 1995; 273:230–235.
35. Hawley PH, Ronco JJ, Guillemi SA, et al. Decreasing frequency but worsening mortality of acute respiratory failure secondary to AIDS-related *Pneumocystis carinii* pneumonia. Chest 1994; 106:1456–1459.
36. Staikowsky F, Lafon B, Guidet B, Denis M, Mayaud C, Offenstadt G. Mechani-

cal ventilation for *Pneumocystis carinii* pneumonia in patients with the acquired immunodeficiency syndrome: is the prognosis really improved? Chest 1993; 104:756–62.
37. De Palo VA, Millstein BH, Mayo PH, Salzman SH, Rosen MJ. Outcome of intensive care in patients with HIV infection. Chest 1995; 107:506–510.
38. Bozzette SA, Feigal D, Chiu J, et al. Length of stay and survival after intensive care for severe *Pneumocystis carinii* pneumonia: a prospective study. Chest 1992; 101:1404–1407.
39. Franklin C, Friedman Y, Wong T, Hu T. Improving long-term prognosis for survivors of mechanical ventilation in patients with AIDS with PCP and acute respiratory failure: five-year follow-up of intensive care unit discharges. Arch Intern Med 1995; 155:91–95.
40. Rosen MJ, Clayton K, Schneider RF, et al. Intensive care of patients with HIV infection: utilization, critical illnesses and outcomes. Am J Respir Crit Care Med 1997; 155:67–71.
41. Lazard T, Retel O, Guidet B, Maury E, Valleron A-J, Offenstadt G. AIDS in a medical intensive care unit. Immediate prognosis and long-term survival. JAMA 1996; 276:1240–1245.
42. Brown MC, Crede WB. Predictive ability of Acute Physiology and Chronic Health Evaluation II scoring applied to human immunodeficiency virus-positive patients. Crit Care Med 1995; 23:848–853.
43. Antinori A, Maiuro G, Fallavicini F, et al. Prognostic factors of early fatal outcome and long-term survival in patients with *Pneumocystis carinii* pneumonia and acquired immunodeficiency syndrome. Eur J Epidemiol 1993; 9:189–199.
44. Peruzzi WT, Skoutelis A, Shapiro BA, et al. Intensive care unit patients with acquired immunodeficiency syndrome and *Pneumocystis carinii* pneumonia: suggested predictors of hospital outcome. Crit Care Med 1991; 19:892–900.
45. Benson CA, Spear J, Hines D, Pottage JC, Kessler HA, Trenholme GM. Combined APACHE II score and serum lactate dehydrogenase as predictors of in-hospital mortality caused by first episode *Pneumocystis carinii* pneumonia in patients with acquired immunodeficiency syndrome. Am Rev Respir Dis 1991; 144:319–323.
46. Ayers J, Howton MJ, Layon AJ. Postoperative complications in patients with human immunodeficiency virus disease: clinical data and a literature review. Chest 1993; 103:1800–1807.
47. Bhagwanjee S, Muckart DJJ, Jeena PM, Moodley P. Does HIV status influence the outcome of patients admitted to a surgical intensive care unit? A prospective double blind study. Br Med J 1997; 314:1077–1084.
48. Wachter RM, Luce JM. Intensive care for patients with *Pneumocystis carinii* pneumonia and respiratory failure: are we prepared for our new success? [editorial]. Chest 1989; 96:714–715.
49. Scitovsky AA, Cline M, Lee P. Medical care costs of patients with AIDS in San Francisco. JAMA 1986; 526:3103–3106.
50. Singer P, Askanazi J, Akiva L, Bursztein S, Kvetan V. Reassessing intensive care for patients with the acquired immunodeficiency syndrome. Heart Lung 1990; 19:387–394.

51. Curtis JR, Greenberg DL, Hudson LD, Fisher LD, Krone MR, Collier AC. Changing use of intensive care for HIV-infected patients with *Pneumocystis carinii* pneumonia. Am J Respir Crit Care Med 1994; 150:1305–1310.
52. Brown J, Sprung CL. Ethical considerations in the treatment of patients in the intensive care unit. Crit Care Clin North Am 1993; 9:115–123.
53. Nerlich S. The option of intensive care for the patient with AIDS. Aust Crit Care 1993; 6:8–10.
54. Steinbrook R, Lo B, Tirpak J, Dilley JW, Volberding P. Ethical dilemmas in caring for patients with the acquired immunodeficiency syndrome. Ann Intern Med 1985; 103:787–790.
55. Lo B, Jonsen AR. Clinical decisions to limit treatment. Ann Intern Med 1980; 93:764–768.
56. Szafelarski NL. Respiratory failure in the patient with AIDS: is critical care warranted? AACN Clin Issues Crit Care Nurs 1990; 1:215–224.
57. Lo B, Raffin TA, Cohen NH, Wachter RM, Luce JM, Hopewell PC. Ethical dilemmas about intensive care for patients with AIDS. Rev Infect Dis 1987; 9:1163–1167.
58. Banks RA, Lindley, Pozniak AL. AIDS: a problem for intensive care. Intensive Care Med 1985; 11:169–171.
59. Englehardt HT, Rie MA. Intensive care units, scarce resources, and conflicting principles of justice. JAMA 1986; 255:1159–1164.
60. Terry PB, Fessler HE. [Editorial]. Should intensive care be limited for patients with self-induced disease? Am J Med Sci 1994; 307:374–377.
61. Luce JM, Wachter RM. Intensive care for patients with the acquired immunodeficiency syndrome. Intensive Care Med 1989; 15:481–482.
62. El-Solh AA, Stubeusz DL, Grant GB, Brant BJB. Outcome of AIDS patients requiring mechanical ventilation predicted by recursive partitioning. Chest 1996; 109:1584–1590.

Part Two

EFFECTS OF HIV ON THE LUNG

5

HIV Biology and Infection of Lung Cells

ELIZABETH A. RICH

Case Western Reserve University and
University Hospitals of Cleveland
Cleveland, Ohio

I. Introduction

In human immunodeficiency virus (HIV)-infected persons, the lung is often beset by a wide variety of infectious or noninfectious complications as discussed in several chapters in this book. The high prevalence of pulmonary problems that accompany HIV disease suggests a certain constancy of viral effects on the lung. Yet, the sheer diversity of pulmonary disorders also raises the likelihood that HIV interacts in complex ways with multiple cell types. The infectious disorders can most clearly be attributed to effects of HIV on immune effector cells in the lung, whereas the noninfectious complications, such as nonspecific interstitial pneumonitis, emphysema, and pulmonary hypertension, may be a consequence of effects of HIV on pulmonary parenchymal cells.

Major insights into pathogenesis of HIV disease have been made by studying HIV infection of blood and lymph node cells. The source of HIV in these compartments is predominantly the CD4 T lymphocyte; the HIV load is astonishingly higher in lymph node cells than in the blood. Viral load increases with disease progression, yet evidence of active viral replication is observed even during asymptomatic stages of disease. Although several direct and indirect mechanisms of depletion of CD4 T cells have been examined, recent studies showing remarkably high rates of viral turnover indicate that the major mechanism of CD4 depletion in HIV disease is probably through direct cell destruction and not through impaired production. Another major concept that has emerged from studies of HIV infection of blood and lymph node cells is that the phenotype and biology of HIV may vary during the course of disease and depend on the cell type infected. Such viral heterogeneity has important implications for development of therapeutic strategies and also demonstrates that the pathogenesis of disease may be organ-specific. Finally, one of the clearest hallmarks of HIV pathogenesis is that the infected host cell must be activated for replication of the virus to occur.

Because an understanding of HIV infection of lung cells requires knowledge of the virus, this chapter first summarizes current concepts of HIV biology. Next, the lessons learned about pathogenesis of HIV disease, as gleaned from studies of infection of cells with this virus, will be discussed in general and as it specifically pertains to the lung. These concepts include the following: cellular targets of the virus; relation between viral load and disease progression; mechanisms of CD4 depletion; viral determinants of infection; and role of cellular activation in replication of HIV.

II. HIV Biology

A. Classification of HIV

Human immunodeficiency virus is a member of the *Retroviridae* family of viruses. The three exogenous viral subfamilies of this family include the oncoviruses, spumaviruses, and lentiviruses. HTLV-1 and HTLV-2 are the members of the oncovirus subgroup that infect humans and, as the name oncovirus implies, these viruses cause transformation of cells. HTLV-1, but apparently not HTLV-2, causes disease manifested as leukemia. Spumaviruses cause foamy degeneration in the cytoplasm of infected cells, but do not cause any known disease. In contrast to oncoviruses and spumaviruses, lentiviruses are cytopathic to cells and, as their name suggests, cause slow disease progression. Lentiviruses that infect nonhuman primates include the visna virus that causes encephalitis and pneumonitis in sheep; caprine arthritis virus, which causes chronic arthritis in goats; equine infectious anemia virus in horses; and simian immunodeficiency virus (SIV) of monkeys. HIV is a lentivirus that infects humans only. HIV-1 is the major cause of the acquired immunodeficiency syndrome (AIDS). HIV-2 is another strain of lentivirus that is more closely related to SIV than to HIV-1. HIV-2 is found primarily in West African patients and also causes AIDS, but may be less pathogenic than HIV-1. HIV, as used in this chapter, will refer to studies of the pathogenesis of HIV-1.

B. Structure and Life Cycle of HIV

The HIV is a spherical structure comprised principally of a viral coat, called the envelope, and a core that contains the genetic RNA material (Fig. 1a). The envelope is a lipid bilayer derived from the host cell membrane and is studded with external viral glycoproteins, called gp120, attached to transmembrane proteins known as gp41. The gp120 protein binds to its receptor CD4 on host cells, whereupon fusion with the cell membrane by gp41 results in entry of the virus (see Fig. 1b).

Within the envelope and surrounding the core is the viral protein p17 (see Fig. 1a). The major core protein is p24, which encompasses several viral enzymes, including reverse transcriptase, integrase, and protease, and two strands of RNA that, in turn, are encircled by the p7 nucleocapsid protein. The p24 core protein is a common measure of extent of HIV replication in the plasma of HIV-infected patients and in experimental systems in vitro. The first major step after entry of HIV into host cells is reverse transcription of RNA into DNA, catalyzed by viral reverse transcriptase (see Fig. 1b). Viral DNA then enters the cell nucleus and is integrated into host chromosomal DNA by viral integrase.

For HIV to complete its life cycle and make new virions, integrated DNA must be transcribed back into RNA (reviewed in Refs. 1 and 2). This process of converting latent DNA provirus into RNA is extremely complex. Unlike many other retroviruses, HIV has several regulatory genes that interact in complex and still incompletely understood ways to accomplish the transcriptional and viral packaging processes. These genes include *tat*, *nef*, and *rev*. Before transcription can occur, however, the infected host cell itself must be activated. Numerous stimuli may activate the cell, including antigens, mitogens, and cytokines (discussed later in this chapter). With exposure to such stimuli, cell proteins, in particular those from the NF-κB/Rel protein family, become activated and bind to specific enhancer sites in the viral long-terminal repeat (LTR; located on both ends of the viral genome; 3). This binding step of cellular proteins to the HIV promoter (in the LTR) initiates viral transcription through activation of still another host cell protein, RNA polymerase II, which is required for completion of transcription. Thus, latent HV DNA is transcribed into RNA only after cellular activation and through use of cellular proteins. This concept is of fundamental importance for understanding the mechanisms of activation of HIV replication, in general, and in the lung specifically.

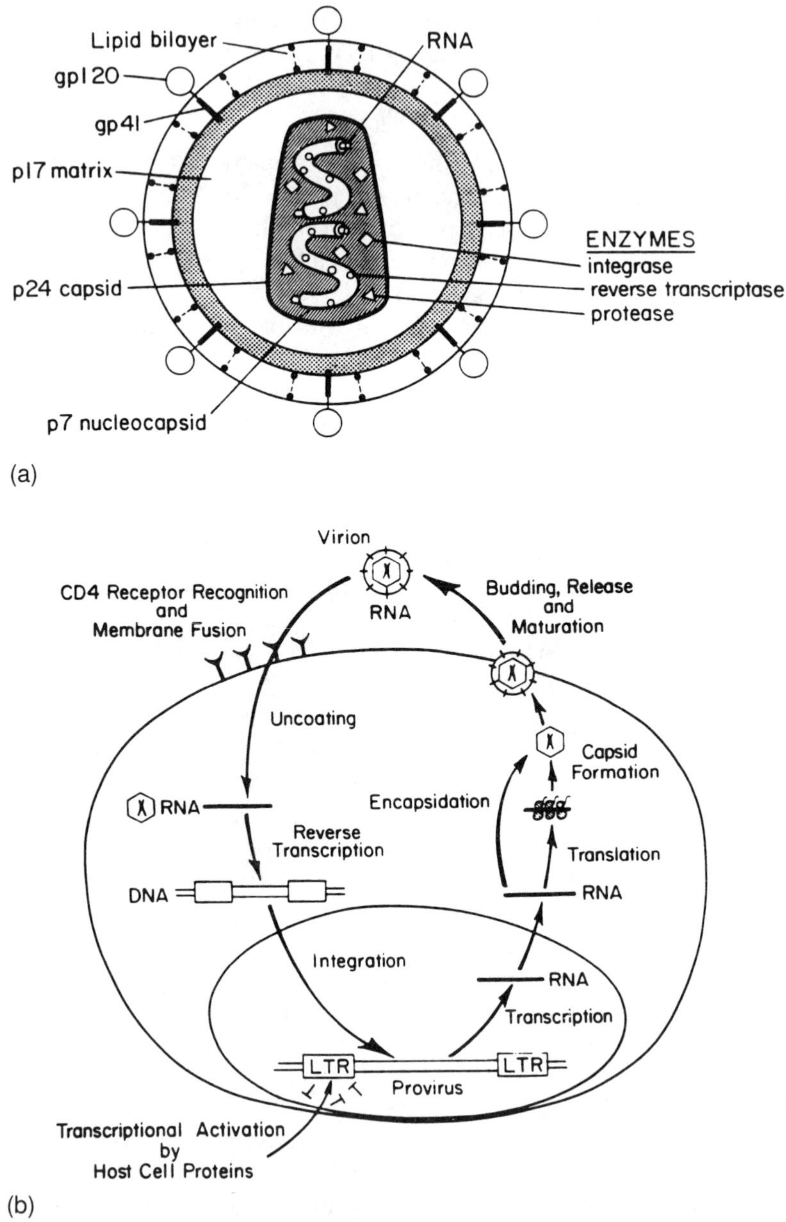

Figure 1 Structure of HIV: HIV comprises an envelope and a core. The envelope is a lipid bilayer containing the viral proteins gp120 and gp41. The core contains the viral proteins p17 (outer core) and p24 (inner core). The cone-shaped p24 structure con-

After cellular activation, the viral regulatory genes are transcribed first, and these short RNAs leave the nucleus. The *tat* gene, in particular, functions to accelerate transcription of HIV DNA (3). The *nef* gene is also expressed early, and although it has both positive and negative influences on transcription in vitro, in vivo it must be expressed to develop AIDS (4,5). The *rev* gene product switches the transcriptional process to the longer RNAs that code for the structural proteins of HIV, including those of the envelope (gp120 and gp41 from the *env* gene), and core (p24, p7, and p6 from the *gag* gene), as well as the viral enzymes (reverse transcriptase, integrase, protease, and ribonuclease from the *pol* gene; 6). Also present in the longer RNAs are the *vif*, *vpr*, and *vpu* regulatory genes, the functions of which are still being discerned, but which may be involved in viral assembly after transcription, and in viral infectivity. The precursor protein products of all these genes, as well as complete copies of viral RNA, accumulate in the cytoplasm and then move to the cell surface. Viral particles bud off from the cell membrane, acquiring their envelope lipid bilayer. Viral protease becomes active during this last stage, cutting up the precursor proteins to complete the assembly of core proteins and enzymes.

III. HIV Infection of Cells: Lessons in Pathogenesis

A. Cellular Targets of HIV

General

As early as 1984, 3 years after the first patient with AIDS was described, Klatzman et al. (7) and Popovic et al. (8) demonstrated that HIV is selectively tropic for $CD4^+$ helper T lymphocytes from the blood. Several studies have since shown that blood monocytes from HIV-infected persons also may

---

tains two strands of viral RNA surrounded by the nucleocapsid protein p7. Viral enzymes, including reverse transcriptase, integrase, and protease, are also contained within the core. The HIV replication cycle: Viral gp120 binds to cellular CD4 receptors, and the virus gains entry into the cell by directly fusing with the cell membrane. Virus is uncoated in the cell cytoplasm and is reverse transcribed into DNA. After transport to the nucleus, the viral genome is integrated into host cell chromosomal DNA where it may remain stable for long periods. The stably integrated provirus is transcribed back into RNA through complex mechanisms, first requiring stimulation of the cell, which activates cellular proteins, such as NF-κB that then enhance transcription after binding to the viral promoter (in the LTR). Transcription of provirus results in mRNA that is translated to regulatory and then structural proteins and enzymes. Transcripts are packaged into virion particles. Budding from the cell wall where the viral envelope is formed leads to release of progeny virions capable of initiating a new cycle of infection.

harbor HIV and can be infected in vitro (9–15). Because monocytes are less susceptible to the cytopathic effects of HIV, demonstration that HIV can infect monocytes led to the widespread opinion that monocytes, or their derived tissue macrophages, may be the major reservoir of HIV. Indeed, as will be discussed later, tissue macrophages may be a major reservoir at sites such as the lung and brain. In the blood, however, studies using a variety of techniques, including viral cultures, gene amplification by the polymerase chain reaction (PCR), and in situ hybridization, reveal that the major cell that harbors HIV in infected individuals is the CD4 T lymphocyte and not blood monocytes (16–18). Nevertheless, the load of HIV; even in blood CD4 T cells from HIV-infected subjects, is surprisingly low for the degree of immunodeficiency (ranging from approximately 1:100 to 1:1000 cells; reviewed in Refs. 19 and 20).

Dendritic cells are potent antigen-presenting cells for T-cell activation that constitute less than 1% of circulating leukocytes, but are abundant in the T-cell–dependent areas of lymph nodes (21). Blood dendritic cells support HIV replication when infected in vitro, but although controversial, most purified blood dendritic cells do not appear to be productively infected in vivo (reviewed in Ref. 22). Remarkably, however, during antigen-stimulated responses with cluster formation by T cells, blood dendritic cells exposed to HIV in vitro can efficiently transmit HIV to T cells (23). Subsequent productive infection of the T cells results in death by apoptosis (24).

In lymph nodes, as in the blood, HIV infection of follicular dendritic cells is infrequent when compared with T cells (25–27). However, high levels of HIV particles are observed extracellularly attached to follicular dendritic cells in germinal centers (19,27–29). Furthermore, CD4 T lymphocytes from lymph nodes (and other lymphoid tissue) of infected patients harbor significantly higher levels of HIV than do CD4 T lymphocytes from the blood of the same patients (28,29).

Thus, in the blood and in lymph nodes CD4 T lymphocytes are the predominant cell type infected. The load of HIV, however, is significantly higher in T cells from lymph nodes than in those from blood, indicating distinct immunopathogenetic processes in these two compartments. It has been hypothesized that the viral particles associated with (but not infecting) follicular dendritic cells of lymphoid tissue are trapped there as would be any other virus or particle as part of the normal immune responses (19,20). Trapped virus may, in turn, be aggressively transmitted to T cells that have been recruited to lymphoid tissue to mount an immune response against HIV.

Cellular Targets of HIV in the Lung

It is imperative that a full delineation of the extent of HIV infection of lung cells be determined because this information is vital to understanding the pathogenesis of the pulmonary complications of HIV disease. The lung is not a lymphoid organ and would not be expected to show the same findings of high HIV loads as such organs. The lung is beset, however, by infectious and noninfectious complications during HIV disease. It is likely that understanding the distinctive features of viral interactions with lung cells may help elucidate how such common and heterogeneous problems occur; thus, ultimately, how such complications might be prevented or treated.

The search for evidence of HIV infection of lung cells has been directed at several compartments, including lung tissue, bronchoalveolar lavage (BAL) fluid, bronchoalveolar cells, alveolar lymphocytes, alveolar macrophages, and fibroblasts. HIV infection of lung dendritic cells has not been reported. The methods used for detection of HIV have included immunohistochemistry for expression of HIV antigens, viral culture (to detect any capacity for viral transmission), in situ hybridization for HIV mRNA, and PCR for HIV DNA. Table 1 shows a compilation of studies that have focused on infection of lung cells with HIV and is organized according to in which compartment of the lung HIV was being measured. With rare exceptions (30), all of the studies described were performed on HIV-infected individuals undergoing diagnostic studies for clinical purposes, indicating that many of the individuals had some kind of concurrent pulmonary problem (such as opportunistic or nonopportunistic infection of the lung or airways, or LIP). Therefore, these studies should generally be viewed as reflecting HIV infection of lung cells during active pulmonary complications. The following six subsections describe the general conclusions that may be drawn from the numerous studies cited in Table 1.

Lung Tissue

Surprisingly little is known about HIV infection of lung cells as can be determined by examination of tissue. Chayt and co-workers, in 1986, reported the results of lung biopsies from 11 HIV-infected patients (31). In situ hybridization to detect viral mRNA was performed. In 10 patients, either no HIV was found (7 of 10 subjects) or levels were very low (3 of 10 subjects, 0.002% of cells). These patients had a variety of concurrent opportunistic and other infections. In the 1 patient with lymphocytic interstitial pneumonitis (LIP), HIV expression was significantly higher (0.1% of alveolar cells) than in the 3 subjects with infectious complications, suggesting activation of viral expression in LIP. The cell type expressing HIV

Table 1 HIV Infection of Lung Cells

Compartment	Methods of identification	HIV detected no. subjects +/total (% + subjects)	Refs.
Lung	In situ hybridization for HIV mRNA	3/10 with OI (30%) (0.002% of cells +)	31
		1/1 with LIP (100%) (0.1% of cells +)	
		1/1 (100%) (grossly +)	32
BAL fluid (cell-free)	p 24 antigen	0/8 (0%)	33
		1/15 (7%)	34
	Viral culture	0/24 (0%)	35
BAL fluid	p 24 antigen	2/2 (100%)	36
		1/10 (10%)	37
		11/26 (42%)	43
	Viral culture (basal growth HIV)	10/10 (100%)	37
BAC	Viral culture	2/23 (9%)	35
		37/63 (59%)	38
		2/6 Early HIV (33%)	30
		3/7 Late HIV (43%)	
	DNA–PCR	12/14 (86%) (3–90 copies per 10^5 cells)	39
		(297 copies per 10^6 cells)	40
		3/6 early HIV (50%)	30
		7/8 late HIV (88%)	
Alveolar lymphocytes	HIV antigen	0/9 (0%)	47
		8/10 (80%)	43
	Viral culture	26/32 (81%)	44
	DNA–PCR	8/8 (100%)	33
		40/63 (64%)	38
		1746 ± 8717 copies per 10^6 cells	40
		4/4 (100%) (9–162 copies per 10^5 CD8 cells)	48a

Alveolar macrophages	HIV antigen	9/9 (100%)	47
		2/2 (100%)	32
		0/15 (0%)	34
	In situ hybridization for HIV mRNA	0/15 (0%)	34
		2/4 (50%)	43
	Viral culture (basal growth HIV)	0/4 (0%)	43
		6/18 (33%)	44
	Viral culture	15/39 (38%)	43
		0/6 early HIV (0%); 6/8 late HIV (75%)	30
		21/44 (47%)	46
		3/3 (100%)	32
	DNA-PCR	8/14 (57%) (35 ± 22 copies per 10^5 cells)	39
		8/8 (100%)	33
		42/63 (67%)	38
		1478 ± 6320 copies per 10^6 cells or 0.01–1% of total cells	40
		7/7 (100%)	35
		2/6 early HIV (33%)	30
		5/8 late HIV (64%)	
Fibroblasts	HIV antigen	4/4 (100%)	32
	In situ hybridization for HIV mRNA viral culture	1/1 (100%)	
		4/4 (100%)	
	DNA-PCR	4/4 (100%)	

mRNA could not be determined in this study. Plata et al. performed in situ hybridization on lung tissue from one patient with AIDS (32). In this subject, HIV mRNA expression was high and appeared to be expressed by alveolar macrophages and lung fibroblasts.

These two studies showed that HIV is present in lung cells, but, according to the larger study by Chayt et al., the frequency of cells expressing active viral mRNA is extremely low, and viral mRNA is not expressed in the lungs of all subjects. Expression of latent HIV (presence of viral DNA) has not been studied in lung tissue, and more sensitive measures of active viral expression such as reverse transcription (RT)-PCR have not been applied to lung tissue in HIV disease. Therefore, conclusions cannot yet be drawn about infection of lung interstitial cells, either in late stages of disease or during evolution of pulmonary complications of HIV disease. It may never be possible to study lung tissue in early stages of disease because lung biopsy on asymptomatic subjects cannot be justified under most instances. Future studies should, however, focus on HIV load (latent vs. active viral expression) and cell type infected in lung tissues, as can be obtained from patients at late stages of disease undergoing diagnostic lung biopsy, or from autopsy samples.

Bronchoalveolar Lavage Fluid

Bronchoalveolar lavage has revolutionized our understanding of the pathogenesis of a variety of pulmonary diseases, including sarcoidosis, idiopathic pulmonary fibrosis, and asthma. The cellular and acellular constituents of the lower respiratory tract can be sampled in a relatively noninvasive manner. The major drawback is that the cellular activities may not always reflect interstitial activities of immune effector cells; and parenchymal cells, such as epithelial, endothelial, and fibroblasts, cannot be assessed.

From the studies listed in Table 1 it can be concluded that cell-free lavage fluid does not contain free virus (33–35). When bronchoalveolar cells are included in BAL fluid, however, HIV can be detected by viral culture in the BAL material and most AIDS patients undergoing clinical diagnostic lavage (37).

Bronchoalveolar Cells

There are several studies of HIV infection of unseparated bronchoalveolar cells obtained by BAL, as shown in Table 1 (30,35,38–40). In viral cultures that can determine capacity for transmission of HIV, bronchoalveolar cells are positive in 9–59% of HIV-infected subjects (excluding asymptomatic subjects with early HIV disease). By PCR for HIV DNA, 50–86% of individuals studied (excluding asymptomatic subjects with early HIV disease) show evidence of harboring HIV in bronchoalveolar cells.

In summary, for unseparated bronchoalveolar cells, transmissable HIV is generally detectable in fewer than half of the subjects, whereas latent HIV, as determined by DNA PCR, is present in bronchoalveolar cells from more than half of subjects. Therefore, the proportion of subjects in whom HIV DNA is present in bronchoalveolar cells is higher than those in whom the cells readily transmit HIV in coculture.

Alveolar Lymphocytes

Several studies of HIV-infected individuals demonstrate an increase in the number of alveolar lymphocytes that are highly enriched for CD8 cells. A few studies (see Table 1) examined HIV load in nonadherent bronchoalveolar cells that are enriched for lymphocytes. In most of these studies, alveolar lymphocytes were not highly purified and, indeed, it is quite difficult to purify these cells because they are so few in comparison with alveolar macrophages, even in HIV disease. Semenzato et al., however, recently reported that highly purified alveolar CD8 T lymphocytes from HIV-infected patients harbor HIV (48b). Overall, HIV DNA is present in alveolar lymphocytes from 64 to 100% of HIV-infected patients undergoing diagnostic lavage (33,38,40). Detection of HIV antigen is highly variable (43,47). Viral cultures from most subjects were positive in one study (44). Therefore, from extant studies, it appears that alveolar lymphocytes from most AIDS patients are infected with HIV.

Because most alveolar lymphocytes in HIV disease are CD8 T cells, which generally are not infectable with HIV, the high level of proviral expression in the studies noted may reflect an unusual propensity for HIV infection of CD8 cells in the lung, contamination of nonadherent cells with HIV-positive alveolar macrophages, or a huge level of virus in the few CD4 T cells that might be present. Studies need to be performed to clarify the load and frequency of HIV-infected alveolar T cells and the subpopulation infected. Even more importantly, the relation between HIV infection of alveolar lymphocytes, function of these cells, and clinical disease needs to be explored in both cross-sectional and longitudinal studies.

Alveolar Macrophages

Alveolar macrophages (AM) are the predominant cell type lining the alveolar wall and, therefore, are contained within the bronchoalveolar cell population retrieved by BAL, in both health (approximately 90% of the cells) and HIV disease (70–90%, depending on stage of disease and concurrent other infections). Macrophages have generally been considered to be the major reservoir of HIV in tissues because these cells are relatively resistant to the cytopathic effects of HIV. Mononuclear (MN) phagocytes express CD4 on their surface, such that HIV would have a way of entering the cell.

Harbison demonstrated that soluble CD4 inhibits productive infection of HIV in alveolar macrophages (41). Furthermore, in other lentiviral infections of animals, such as sheep, tissue macrophages carry extraordinarily high levels of these viruses (42).

Salahuddin and co-workers were the first to specifically assess whether purified alveolar macrophages from BAL fluid of infected subjects carry HIV (43). In two patients, HIV was present, as detected by basal culture (but not by coculture) of alveolar macrophages (see Table 1). Alveolar macrophages from healthy subjects were also infectable with HIV in vitro, as shown by detection of HIV p24 antigen in culture supernatants. Thus, alveolar macrophages are infectable in vitro and in vivo with HIV.

Subsequent studies have confirmed that alveolar macrophages from AIDS patients can be infected with HIV (30,32–34,38–40,43,44,46,47). Alveolar macrophages from early-stage HIV disease (CD4 cell levels of more than 400/μl) are rarely infected with HIV, as determined by viral cultures and DNA PCR (30). Alveolar macrophages from 33 to 75% of HIV-infected subjects, generally with late-stage disease, are positive for HIV by viral cocultures. Alveolar macrophages from 47 to 100% of HIV-infected individuals are positive for HIV DNA by PCR. Thus, most, but not all, patients with later-stage HIV disease carry proviral HIV in their alveolar macrophages, and approximately half carry virus in alveolar macrophages that is transmissable to lymphocytes in vitro. HIV infection of alveolar macrophages and unseparated bronchoalveolar cells was comparable in one study, suggesting that the major cell type infected in alveolar spaces is macrophages (30).

Only one study has specifically examined whether the HIV in alveolar macrophages is predominantly latent or if the virus is active replicating. Lebargy et al. compared expression of HIV DNA by PCR with assays that indicate active viral expression, including in situ hybridization and viral antigen expression in alveolar macrophages from HIV-infected subjects (34). Alveolar macrophages from all the subjects were positive for HIV DNA, but in none of the subjects was HIV antigen or mRNA expressed. Therefore, it appears from this study by Lebargy that HIV in alveolar macrophages during symptomatic HIV disease is predominantly latent and not undergoing active replication. Other studies, however, show that viral antigen is being expressed by alveolar macrophages from most subjects with AIDS who have been studied (32,47).

It is not yet possible to resolve these conflicting data on the latency of HIV in alveolar macrophages during HIV disease. Possible explanations for failure to find evidence of active viral replication, even in AIDS patients with opportunistic infection, include insensitivity of assays used for evidence of active HIV expression (RT-PCR should be able to resolve the issue); influx of blood cells that are not yet showing evidence of viral replication at the site of lung disease; and cytotoxic death in vivo of alveolar macrophages carrying actively replicating virus, such that little active viral expression could be detected ex vivo. Longitudinal studies of evidence of latent versus active viral infection of alveolar macrophages (and lymphocytes) in HIV-infected subjects before and during development of lung symptomatology and other opportunistic infections could shed light on the role of HIV infection and growth in lung cells in the pathogenesis of lung disease associated with HIV infection. If HIV is truly latent in these cells, then one can speculate that mechanisms of suppression of viral growth in the lung are efficient and dominant over the factors that might activate viral replication.

Lung Fibroblasts and Cells of the Alveolocapillary Membrane

It is difficult to attribute all of the known pulmonary pathology associated with HIV disease to infection of T cells and macrophages, because pathological changes may occur relatively early in the course before viral burden in these lung cells is high. These inexplicable pathological and functional entities associated with HIV disease include emphysema, pulmonary hypertension, nonspecific interstitial pneumonitis, low diffusion capacity, and unexplained dyspnea (48b,49). One explanation for the development of these pulmonary disorders that appear to be unrelated to immunodeficiency is that nonlymphoid or nonmacrophage-derived cells such as mesenchymal or ectodermal cells are infected with HIV. Alternatively, such parenchymal cells may be damaged by inflammatory responses induced by products of HIV or by HIV infection of immune effector cells. There is an increase in alveolocapillary permeability in HIV-infected patients, without active opportunistic infection, but with a cytotoxic T-lymphocytic alveolitis suggesting T-cell–induced injury to the alveolocapillary membrane (50).

There is precedence for HIV infection of mesenchymal and ectodermal cells derived from nonpulmonary tissues in vivo, including skin fibroblasts, brain endothelial cells, intestinal epithelial cells, and others (reviewed in Ref. 51). Such infection is generally quite low grade, but may have important biological sequelae. Contact between monocytes and endothelial cells increases HIV replication (52) and endothelial cell permeability (53). Such interactions in vivo could lead to influx of cells from the blood to the tissues or may cause tissue damage. HIV can also be transmitted from monocytes to epithelial cells (54).

There is only one study of HIV infection of lung parenchymal cells in vivo: Plata et al. found that fibroblasts in the lungs of HIV-infected individuals express HIV antigen and HIV mRNA and contain provirus (see Table 1; 32). Three other studies have documented that lung-derived fibroblasts can be productively infected with HIV in vitro (55–57): epithelial cells derived from the lung can be infected in vitro (55). There are as yet no reports of HIV infection in vivo of epithelial or endothelial cells of the alveolocapillary membrane. Nevertheless, whether such cells are infected directly or damaged indirectly during HIV disease, it is possible that certain of the physiological and structural abnormalities in the lungs of HIV-infected individuals may be attributed to some distortion in the integrity of these nonhematopoietic cells.

B. Relation Between Load of HIV and Disease Progression

General

The hallmark of disease pathogenesis in HIV infection is successive depletion of CD4 T cells, which correlates inextricably with development of opportunistic infections and death of the infected host. One of the important concepts to have emerged from studies of HIV infection of blood (and lymphoid) cells is that there is a direct relation between the decline of CD4 T cells and viral load (reviewed in Refs. 19 and 20). Early after infection, the level of virus in the plasma rises precipitously as the number of peripheral CD4 T cells declines. Plasma viremia, however, decreases as the number of CD4 T cells stabilizes. During this period of relative stabilization of CD4 T-cell numbers, the infected individual remains asymptomatic for several years, a situation known as clinical latency. Plasma viremia rises again, however, as opportunistic infections are acquired after 7–10 years, suggesting a relation between load of virus and development of the complications inflicted by HIV disease. Indeed, a large body of literature has now been amassed that suggests that disease progression is driven by increasing viral burden within peripheral blood CD4 T cells (19,20).

Nevertheless, in spite of the rise in viral load, one of the enigmas about HIV disease is that the relentless development of clinical complications seems out of proportion to the low frequency of infected T cells and low level of HIV DNA per cell, even in advanced stages of disease. Two related recent developments help explain this mystery: First, there is now clear evidence that active viral transcription is an ongoing, persistent process, even during the period of clinical latency, as determined by expression of viral mRNA by RT-PCR (26,28,58–60). Thus, in spite of low levels of viral DNA load and frequency of infected blood cells, virus is being produced at all stages of clinical disease. Second, the findings of Pantaleo et al. that aggressive viral transcription also occurs in the lymphoid organs, even during early, asymptomatic stages of HIV disease, convincingly demonstrate that there is probably never a stage of true microbiological latency in the HIV-infected host (28). The virus is being actively produced throughout the course of disease.

Pantaleo et al. further demonstrate that the architecture of lymph nodes changes dramatically during disease progression, showing involution of the germinal centers and follicular dendritic cells in late stages of HIV disease (28). Because these are precisely the anatomical areas in which high levels of viral particles are observed in earlier stages of disease, these authors pose the hypothesis that the late-stage increase in viral load observed in peripheral blood cells results when the lymphoid organs are no longer able to contain the virus (28). Thus, the paradox of low peripheral blood viral DNA load in spite of disease progression in most infected individuals may be partly explained by the findings that during early disease stages viral production is both active and is contained primarily within lymphoid organs where newly recruited lymphocytes from the blood may be destroyed after viral infection.

Both peripheral blood mononuclear cells and the lymphoid tissue from long-term survivors of HIV infection show strikingly less viral RNA than do cells from similar compartments from individuals whose disease is progressive (61,62). These data indicate that far less active viral production is occurring in long-term survivors. Whether host immune responses or differences in viral factors, or both, are responsible for controlling the active production of HIV in long-term survivors has not been fully determined, although evidence for host and viral factors exists (61,62). Complete elucidation of how viral activation is contained in these fortunate individuals likely will help in development of therapeutic interventions to control HIV production in others.

Relation Between Load of HIV in Lung Cells and Disease Progression

To begin to understand the relation between load of HIV in lung cells, clinical stage of disease, and cellular function, Sierra-Madero in my laboratory studied 14 HIV-infected subjects during an early (6 subjects, 435 $\pm$ 171 peripheral CD4 cells per microliter, mean $\pm$ SD) and a late stage of disease (8 subjects, 43 $\pm$ 43 peripheral CD4 cells per microliter; 30). Importantly, none of the subjects studied had concurrent pulmonary symptoms or disease that could be detected clinically, and this is as yet the only study of HIV load in lung cells of HIV-infected patients without concurrent opportunistic infection or other pulmonary complications. The load of HIV was determined in peripheral blood mononuclear cells (PBMC), which comprise both total lymphocytes and monocytes; blood nonadherent (NA) cells, which are enriched for lymphocytes; monocytes; unseparated bronchoalveolar cells (BAC); and AM. The MN and AM were treated twice with anti–CD2-labeled magnetic beads to assure depletion of contaminating T lymphocytes.

Viral titer in each of these cell populations was determined by end-point dilution viral cultures. Various dilutions of cells were added to phytohemagglutinin (PHA)-stimulated PBMC from a healthy HIV-negative donor. Supernatants of cocultures were collected weekly for 4 weeks and assayed for HIV p24 antigen by enzyme-linked immunosorbant assay (ELISA); Figure 2 shows the results. Among blood cells, HIV was comparable in PBMC and NA and significantly higher than in MN, indicating that lymphocytes were the predominant infected cell. The HIV titer in PBMC and NA also were significantly higher than in BAC or AM. There was no difference in viral titer between BAC and purified AM, suggesting that most HIV in BAC resides within the macrophage population. The most surprising finding in this study was that AM from all of the asymptomatic subjects were culture-negative, indicating that AM from these subjects could not be a reservoir of HIV. In contrast, AMs from six of the eight subjects with AIDS were culture positive.

To assess total HIV load in our study, we performed a semiquantitative PCR using ^{32}P-labeled 5′ primers. To ensure that the DNA content was

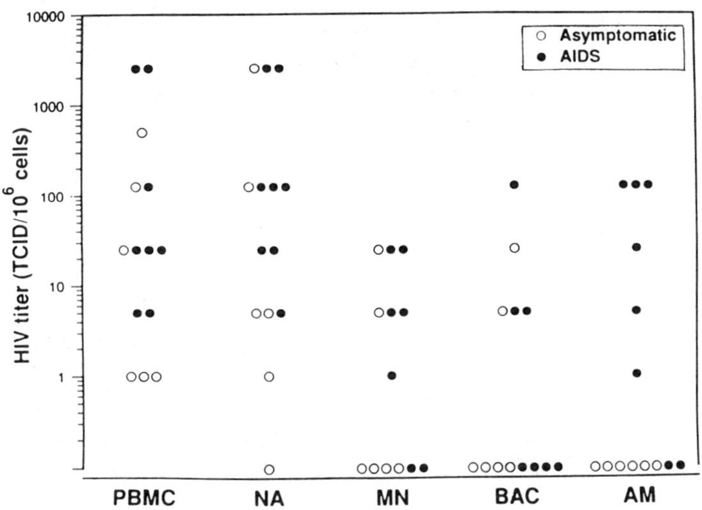

Figure 2 Virus titer in blood and alveolar mononuclear cells from subjects with early and late clinical stages of HIV infection. PBMC, peripheral blood mononuclear cells; NA, nonadherent cells; MN, monocytes; BAC, bronchoalveolar cells; AM, alveolar macrophages; asymptomatic subjects, more than 200 CD4$^+$ per microliter; subjects with AIDS, fewer than 200 CD4$^+$ cells per microliter. (From Ref. 30.)

comparable among our samples, we first amplified each sample with a β-globin primer pair. An R/U5 primer pair (M667/AA55) and a *gag* primer pair (SK 38/39) were used to amplify HIV sequences. The R/U5 primer pair is particularly sensitive because it is at the start site of reverse transcription (at the primer-binding site) and thus amplifies all transcripts including those that are incompletely reverse transcribed (63). In each PCR reaction, HIV of known copy number (or DNA of a known microgram quantity for globin controls) was amplified concurrently for comparison with the samples. Figure 3 shows the results using R/U5 as copy numbers of HIV per microgram DNA. As for the viral titer data, the load of HIV DNA in PBMC and NA cells was greater than in MN, BAC, or AM. The load of HIV among BAC and AM did not differ. The level of HIV DNA was greater, however, in AM than MN from subjects with AIDS, but not than asymptomatic subjects. Results were comparable using the primer pair SK 38/39 (data not shown).

Thus, by both viral titer and HIV DNA copy number, blood lymphocytes harbored more HIV per cell than MN or AM cells. The AM from asymptomatic subjects demonstrated little or no evidence of HIV infection and the level increased by the stage at which AIDS had been defined;

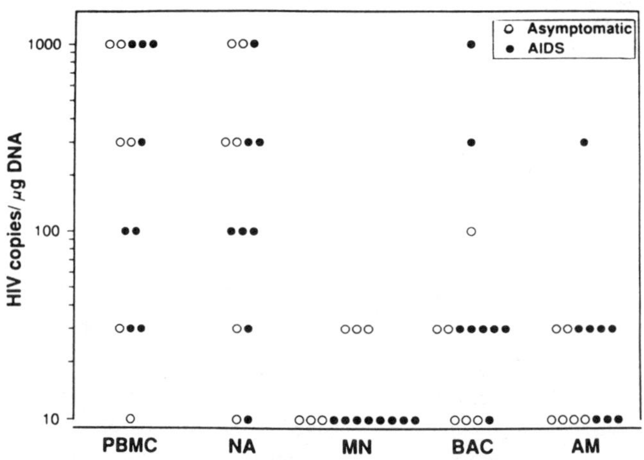

Figure 3 Load of HIV DNA in blood and alveolar mononuclear cells from subjects with early and late clinical stages of HIV infection, as shown by semiquantitative PCR using β-globin primers to normalize for cellular DNA and R/U5 HIV primers. Values less than 10 were undetectable. PBMC, peripheral blood mononuclear cells; NA, nonadherent cells; MN, monocytes; BAC, bronchoalveolar cells; AM, alveolar macrophages. (From Ref. 30.)

Therefore, AM do not appear to be major reservoirs of HIV, at least in the early stages of disease, although they become infected during later stages.

Tumor necrosis factor (TNF) production was increased in AM from both the asymptomatic and AIDS groups of subjects as determined by ELISA and by bioassay (30). Thus, there was no relation between the level of virus in these cells and the production of this important cytokine. Several other studies also show increased cytokine production by AM from HIV-infected subjects (reviewed in Ref. 30). Twigg and colleagues found increased accessory cell function at an early (AIDS-related complex; ARC) as well as late stage of disease (AIDS; 64). Buhl et al. reported an increase in expression of markers of activation on alveolar macrophages from asymptomatic HIV-infected individuals (65). Thus, many functions and properties of AM are upregulated in HIV disease and are increased at a time when the virus cannot be detected in the cells, suggesting either that very low levels of viral infection (undetectable) may activate the cells, or that other factors, such as HIV products, may be activating the cells early in the course of HIV disease.

C. Mechanisms of CD4 Lymphocyte Depletion

General

The relation between depletion of CD4 T cells, viral load, and disease progression is unquestionable (66; reviewed in 19). The mechanisms for the inexorable destruction of these immunocytes, however, are not entirely clear. Several hypotheses have been postulated and are summarized in Table 2 (19,51). The direct cytopathic ways that HIV might destroy CD4 T lymphocytes include formation of holes in the cell membrane during viral budding; insertion of HIV envelope proteins into the cell membrane, altering its integrity; and accumulation of unintegrated HIV DNA in the cell cyto-

Table 2 Possible Mechanisms of Cytotoxicity by HIV

Direct
Formation of holes in cell membrane during viral budding
Insertion of HIV envelope proteins into the cell membrane
Accumulation of unintegrated HIV DNA in the cell cytoplasm
Indirect
Syncytia formation
Production of toxic substances
Autoimmune phenomena
Destruction by immune responses (ADCC, CTL)
Superantigen effects
Apoptosis

plasm. The very high viral loads in lymphoid organs, even in early disease, also may explain depletion of peripheral CD4 T cells, for these cells migrate to these organs in an effort to exert an immune response against viral antigens.

Several indirect mechanisms of death of CD4 T cells have also been suggested. Syncytia formation between infected and uninfected CD4 T cells may contribute to cell death of uninfected cells. Infected cells could induce substances that are toxic to uninfected cells. Autoimmune phenomena may occur by which, for example, antibodies directed against viral epitopes cross-react with the CD4 molecule. Free viral antigens, such as gp120, may bind to uninfected CD4 T cells, rendering these uninfected cells susceptible to antibody-dependent cellular cytotoxicity. Another indirect mechanism to explain CD4 T-cell depletion is that certain viral antigens may act as superantigens, stimulating massive proliferation, followed by depletion of T cells carrying specific variable β-chains on the T-cell receptor (67,68). More recently, several studies have demonstrated evidence that apoptosis may contribute to CD4 T-cell death (19). Apoptosis is a process of programmed cell death, rather than death caused by gross lysis or necrosis of the cell. CD4 T cells from HIV-infected subjects, in fact, undergo increased apoptosis in vitro both when unstimulated or stimulated with superantigens or mitogens (19).

If any or all of the foregoing possible mechanisms of CD4 depletion are directed at precursor stem cells, then a major mechanism for progressive loss of CD4 T cells could be at the level of impaired production, rather than direct destruction of these cells. Recent studies, however, almost entirely exclude problems in T-cell production as a mechanism for their loss. By using potent inhibitors of viral replication as a tool to calculate the kinetics of viral turnover, Wei et al. (69) and Ho et al. (70) demonstrated that extraordinarily high levels of viral production and destruction occur daily. These investigators estimated that 2 billion CD4 T cells are turned over daily in HIV-infected individuals, even during asymptomatic stages of disease when peripheral CD4 T-cells numbers are stable. Thus, it is highly unlikely that production of CD4 T cells is impaired during the prolonged asymptomatic period in the HIV-infected host because production keeps up with destruction for many years. Apparently, this high level of cellular production, in the end, is not able to maintain levels adequate for immune homeostasis.

CD8 cytotoxic T cells (CTL) are increased early in HIV disease and are directed against cells expressing a variety of HIV antigens, including envelope, core, and regulatory proteins (51). This action of CTL may be an important immune mechanism against HIV but also, as a consequence, may contribute to depletion of CD4 cells. Walker et al. demonstrated that

CD8 T cells contribute to control of HIV infection by suppressing virus replication (71). CTL activity, however, fails to provide adequate protection during HIV disease, and cytotoxic activity decreases with disease progression.

Lung-Related Mechanisms

The mechanisms of depletion of CD4 lymphocytes in the lung are unknown, but the mechanisms may be quite effective because, even in early stages of HIV disease, most alveolar lymphocytes are CD8 T cells. Plata et al. (72) and Autran et al. (47) demonstrated unequivocally that alveolar CD8 T cells are cytotoxic against HIV-infected alveolar macrophages and that cytotoxic activity is directed against HIV envelope antigens. The CTL activity of alveolar lymphocytes in HIV disease may also decrease with disease progression (73). $CD8^+CD57^+$ alveolar lymphocytes increase during disease progression, mirroring the decrease in CTL activity (72). Sadat-Sowti demonstrated that $CD8^+CD57^+$ alveolar lymphocytes from HIV-infected individuals produce an inhibitor of cytotoxic function of not only $CD8^+CD44^+$ T cells, but also of natural killer (NK) cells and lymphokine-activated killer (LAK) cells (74). An increase in such an inhibitor during disease progression conceivably could contribute to the rise in viral load in the lung, with progression to AIDS. Studies are necessary to determine how CD4 T cells or macrophages are depleted in the lung during HIV disease and the relations between viral load and CTL functions.

D. Viral Determinants of Pathogenesis

General

Another major concept that has emerged from studies of HIV infection of blood cells is that variations in the virus may influence pathogenesis of disease as well as response to therapy (reviewed in Ref. 51). The heterogeneity of HIV strains is at several levels, including serological, biological, and genetic (Table 3). Serological variations in HIV are demonstrated as differences in susceptibility of HIV strains to serum neutralization and to enhancing antibodies.

There are many biological differences in HIV strains. The findings that some strains of HIV are capable of infecting certain cell types more than others is called cellular tropism. In general, there are HIV strains that preferentially infect T cells (T-cell tropic strains) and HIV strains that infect both T cells and macrophages. Most HIV strains that dually infect T cells and macrophages show great differences in efficiency of infection, such that some productively infect macrophages to a much greater extent

Table 3 Heterogeneity of HIV Strains

Serological	
	Differences in neutralization by antibodies
	Differences in facilitation of entry by enhancing antibodies
Biological	
	Cell tropism
	Level of virus replication
	Level of latency
	Cytopathicity
Genetic structure	
	V3 domain of gp120 envelope protein (*env* gene)
	Reverse transcriptase (*pol* gene)

(macrophage tropic) and others infect T cells better. Differences in cellular tropism are partly determined at the level of entry of virus into the cell.

The HIV heterogeneity can also be reflected in differences in the ability of various strains to replicate in various cell types. Such differences in replication may reflect the influence of the intracellular milieu, as well as exogenous influences, such as cytokines, that may act preferentially on certain HIV strains. Certain strains of HIV enter a state of latency more than do others. The extent of cytopathology produced by a variety of HIV strains can also differ, as manifested by their capacity to form syncytia in in vitro infection assays. During early stages of HIV disease, viral isolates from the peripheral blood of infected individuals may grow more slowly, do not induce syncytia, and are tropic for monocyte lineage cells (75). Such strains also may be found in tissue macrophages. In contrast, progression of HIV infection is associated with the emergence of syncytium-inducing strains that are more T-cell tropic (51,75).

It is now recognized that such differences in biological activities of HIV strains is reflected by the genetic structure of these strains. For example, tropism of HIV for T cells and macrophages partly correlates with structural differences in HIV gp120 envelope protein, most clearly with the presence of certain residues in a 35-amino acid region within the highly variable principal neutralizing V3 domain of gp120 (76–78). Importantly, the V3 loop of gp120 also is a target of both neutralizing antibodies and cytotoxic T cells (79–81). It is believed that mutations in the *env* gene encoding this region results in evasion of host immune defenses by HIV and, thereby, further propagation of the virus. A high rate of mutation of the *pol* gene that codes for reverse transcriptase also confers heterogeneity to the HIV genome and is the principal reason for development of resistance to antiretroviral drugs such as zidovudine (azidothymidine; AZT).

Viral Determinants in the Lung

The non–syncytium-forming or relatively noncytopathic, macrophage tropic strains that predominate in the blood of many HIV-infected individuals in early stages of disease can also be found in the lung (82) as well as other tissues, including the brain and salivary glands (51). Schuitemaker et al. further found that such relatively noncytopathic strains are found in the lung, even once T-cell tropic, syncytium-forming strains are established in the blood at later stages of disease (83).

Potash et al. examined whether viral fusion with the membrane was a determinant in the infectability and replication of a macrophage tropic (ADA) or lymphocyte tropic (NIT) strain of HIV in human alveolar macrophages (84). The two strains fused equally well with alveolar macrophage membranes. Soluble CD4 locked infection of alveolar macrophages by either strain. Infection by the ADA strain was productive in alveolar macrophages from each of 14 healthy subjects, whereas productive infection was noted in only 8 of 14 subjects whose cells were infected with NIT; the failure of virus to replicate correlated with failure to accumulate HIV DNA after several days in culture. Thus, the difference in the capacity of macrophage and lymphocyte tropic strains to replicat in alveolar macrophages was not attributable to membrane fusion.

It is possible that the macrophage tropic strains found in the lung reflect those present concurrently in blood monocytes. Alternatively, HIV strains in the lung may evolve independently from those in blood cells, perhaps as influenced by the local milieu. To test these considerations, Itescu et al. determined the structure of the V3 domain of gp120 (a major determinant of macrophage tropism) in mononuclear cells from the blood and BAL fluid of the same HIV-infected individuals (85). HIV strains among bronchoalveolar cells differed from those of blood mononuclear cells in that the V3 domain nucleotide sequences were more homogeneous in the COOH-terminal region and contained a highly conserved, negatively charged amino acid motif. The authors speculated that this V3 loop COOH-terminal structure could be important in the capacity of HIV to infect alveolar macrophages.

Itescu et al. further performed phylogenetic analyses of the V3 domain nucleotide sequences in monocytes from the blood and alveolar macrophages from the lung (85). Results suggested that the strains in alveolar macrophages independently evolved from a presumed ancestral strain that might have originated with strains in blood monocytes. This important study provides further credence to the likelihood that the pulmonary complications of HIV disease are, at least partly, dictated by the microenvironment of the lung. Clearly, much more work needs to be done to fully understand HIV heterogeneity in the lung and the consequences of such strain differences on local pathogenesis.

E. Cellular Activation and HIV Replication

General

Replication of retroviruses including HIV in cells requires cellular activation (86–89). The exogenous stimuli capable of activating cells, and thereby, HIV production, include antigens, mitogens, and other viruses including HTLV-1, herpes simplex virus, and cytomegalovirus. Endogenous stimuli that can activate cells and thus HIV include growth and differentiation factors such as interleukin (IL)-2, granulocyte–macrophage colony-stimulating factor (GM)-CSF, macrophage (M)-GSF and IL-3, and cytokines, such as TNF-α and IL-6 (19,20). Transforming growth factor (TGF)-β, interferon-α (IFN-α) and IL-13, are cytokines that can inhibit HIV replication in vitro (19,20,51,75). There is increased expression of several cytokines in particular TNF-α during HIV disease, as detected in blood, lymph nodes, and other tissue compartments. These cytokines, in turn, may then increase HIV replication through autocrine or paracrine mechanisms.

Cellular activation affects HIV replication at several stages in the life cycle of the virus. It appears that cellular activation does not increase entry of the virus, although data are conflicting (63). Activation of T cells, however, induces completion of reverse transcription of RNA into DNA (62) and increases the rate of reverse transcription (90). The rate of reverse transcription is slowed in macrophages partly by a decrease in nucleotide pools; such slowed kinetics may influence viral replication in these cells (91). Integration of viral DNA into the host genome is also increased substantially by activation of T cells (92). Cellular proliferation likely is a concomitant of activation of T cells and likely is necessary for HIV production. Whether cellular proliferation of macrophages, which are generally nonreplicating cells, is necessary for HIV to grow is controversial (93), but factors, such as GM-CSF, may promote viral replication in macrophages through effects on proliferation. Several studies indicate that during an immune reaction macrophages infected in vivo can transmit latent HIV in vitro to T cells if the T cell is activated (94–96).

A large amount of work has focused on the mechanisms by which cytokines enhance HIV replication (reviewed in Refs. 19,20,51). Although probably many stages of viral growth may be altered by cytokines, the two best studied are at the level of transcriptional activation of DNA into RNA and posttranscriptional activation. TNF-α promotes HIV replication through activation of cellular-binding proteins, such as NF-κB which is bound to inhibitors in quiescent cells. Release of NF-κB from its inhibitor by TNF-α allows this cellular protein to translocate to the nucleus and bind to specific regions in the promoter (LTR) of HIV. On binding of NF-κB, transcription of HIV is initiated and new virions are formed. Other cytokines or differentiation factors such as IL-6 and GM-CSF act to promote HIV expression through posttranscriptional mechanisms. TGF-β, which is a cytokine that inhibits T-cell activation and proliferation, has variable effects on HIV replication, depending on the experimental conditions, but its suppressive effect may be both at the transcriptional and posttranscriptional levels.

Most of the studies of effects of exogenous or endogenous stimuli on HIV replication have been performing using T- or macrophage cell lines or primary cells infected with HIV in vitro. The extent to which these cellular activators promote HIV replication in vivo remains to be determined. Nevertheless, given the absolute necessity of cellular activation for HIV growth, it seems of extreme medical importance to fully understand the mechanisms of activation of cells and consequent HIV replication in vitro and in vivo so that improved therapeutic strategies can be implemented to control the growth of HIV.

Cellular Activation and HIV Replication in Lung Cells

Blood Monocytes Versus Alveolar Macrophages

In other lentiviral infections tissue macrophages are much more susceptible to support of viral replication than are blood monocytes, from which tissue macrophages are derived. We investigated whether the process of differentiation or of activation of macrophages increases the susceptibility of macrophages to productive infection with HIV (97). Blood monocytes from healthy subjects were cultured for 5–7 days to allow differentiation. Freshly isolated monocytes and alveolar macrophages from the same subject then were obtained. These alveolar macrophages, freshly isolated monocytes, and cultured monocytes were infected concurrently with a macrophage tropic strain ($HIV\text{-}1_{JR\text{-}FL}$). Figure 4 shows the kinetics of production of HIV as measured by p24 ELISA in culture supernatants of cells collected over 24 hr every 4 days. Monocytes failed to support infection with this strain of HIV; both CM and AM did support infection. Similar results were obtained in 12 experiments; HIV production was highest in cultured monocytes (9,216 $\pm$ 3,118 pg/mL), lowest in freshly isolated monocytes (9 $\pm$ 6) and intermediate, but significant in alveolar macrophages (4,145 $\pm$ 1,456).

Thus, the process of differentiation or activation, or both, increases the susceptibility to productive infection by mononuclear phagocytes.

To assess the basis for the increased susceptibility of cultured monocytes and alveolar macrophages for support of HIV growth, a semiquantitative DNA PCR assay was used to determine entry of HIV into the cells and the extent of reverse transcription of viral RNA into DNA. Cells were infected with HIV-$1_{JR\text{-}FL}$ or heat-inactivated virus, lysed at various times after infection, and PCR performed on cell lysates. DNA synthesis was barely detectable at 6 hr after infection, but increased and peaked at 24–48 hr after infection. Figure 5 shows the results at 24 hr after infection. Globin DNA levels were comparable among the cell types infected with live or heat-inactivated virus, indicating that host cell DNA did not differ (see Fig. 5a).

To assess entry and initiation of reverse transcription, a set of HIV primers (M667/AA55 in the R/U5 region of the LTR) was used (see Fig. 5b). This primer pair amplifies the first region of the HIV genome synthesized during reverse transcription (because the pair binds to sequences immediately 5′ to the primer-binding site where reverse transcription is initiated) and detects all viral DNA, including incomplete reverse transcripts (63). Cells infected with heat-inactivated virus showed no HIV DNA by

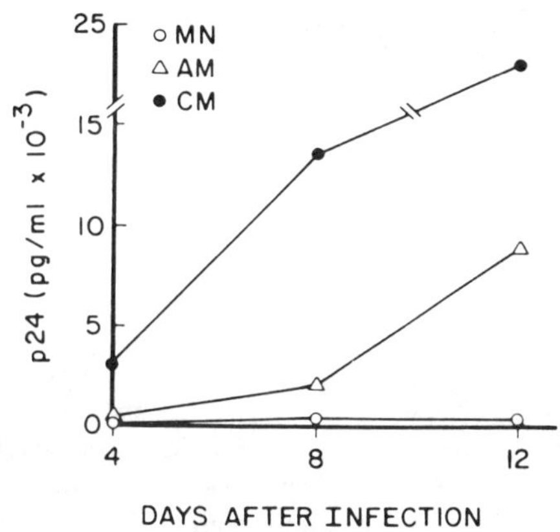

Figure 4 Kinetics of HIV production from mononuclear phagocytes: MN (monocytes), AM (alveolar macrophages), and CM (cultured monocytes) were infected with HIV-$1_{JR\text{-}FL}$ or heat-inactivated virus and cultured in 24-well plates. Supernatants were collected every 4 days after infection, with changing of the medium 24 hr before harvest. The p24 *gag* protein levels in culture supernatants were determined by ELISA. The p24 levels in supernatants of cells exposed to heat-inativated virus were always undetectable (not shown). Representative of 12 experiments. (From Ref. 97.)

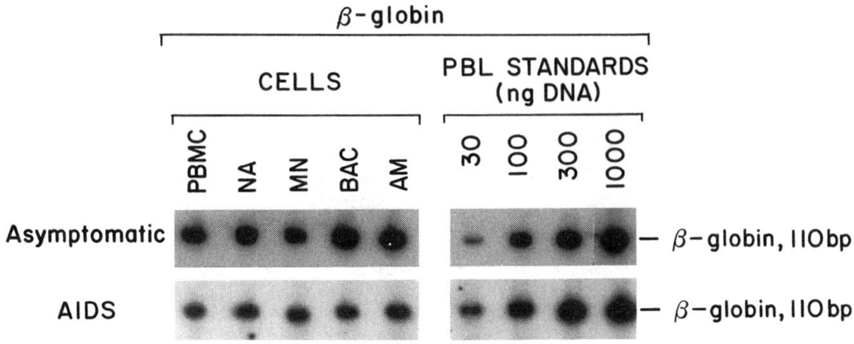

(a)

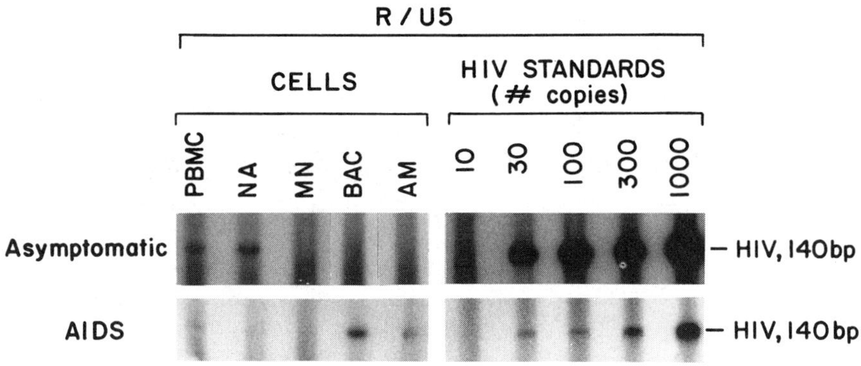

(b)

Figure 5 Quantification of cellular and HIV DNA, by PCR analysis, in mononuclear phagocytes infected in vitro. (a) Quantification of cellular DNA in HIV-infected mononuclear phagocytes. MN (monocytes), AM (alveolar macrophages), and CM (cultured monocytes) were infected with HIV-$1_{JR\text{-}FL}$ or HI (heat-inactivated) virus, washed, and transferred to 24-well plates at 2.5×10^5 cells per well. After 24 hr at 37°C, cells were lysed and PCR performed using β-globin–specific oligonucleotide primers. Known amounts of peripheral blood lymphocyte (PBL) DNA were amplified concurrently to quantify cellular DNA levels in experimental samples, and these are indicated. Amplified products were loaded onto gels and detected by autoradiography. (b) Quantification of initiation of reverse transcripts in infected mononuclear phagocytes. Amplification was performed using R/U5 primer pairs. HIV standards were amplified in parallel. (From Ref. 97.)

PCR, indicating that no contaminating proviral DNA was in the HIV stock used for the infection. Monocytes, alveolar macrophages, and cultured monocytes showed evidence of entry of HIV and initiation of reverse transcription, but levels were significantly higher in cultured monocytes and alveolar macrophages than in freshly isolated monocytes. A primer pair that amplifies intermediate-length reverse transcripts in the *tat/rev* region showed a pattern similar to that obtained with the R/U5 primers (data not shown). A primer pair (M667/M661) that flanks the primer binding site in the LTR/*gag* region, at which reverse transcription begins and ends, was used to detect evidence of completion of reverse transcription, because this primer pair detects only full-length double-stranded DNA (62). With this LTR/*gag* primer pair, we demonstrated that 10–30% of reverse transcripts that were initiated were completed and that there was no difference among cultured monocytes, alveolar macrophages, and freshly isolated monocytes in their ability to complete reverse transcription.

Thus, the uptake or initiation of reverse transcription was higher in cultured monocytes and alveolar macrophages than in freshly isolated monocytes, indicating that the increase in HIV production in these cells is partly because of these early events after infection. Freshly isolated monocytes did allow entry of HIV and extent of the process of reverse transcription was the same as for the more differentiated or activated mononuclear phagocytes. Together these results indicate that the increased production of HIV by CM and AM can be attributed to both increased uptake and some step or steps after reverse transcription. Current studies are focused on the role of integration and transcriptional activation in the replication of HIV in well-differentiated macrophages. The implication for the lung is that resident macrophages may be predisposed to support HIV replication because the cellular machinery is primed for better viral growth, perhaps owing to environmental exposures, to occult infection, or to the cytokine milieu. In fact, alveolar macrophages from patients with AIDS (but not patients with early stages of HIV) preferentially harbor more HIV than do blood monocytes (30).

Activation of HIV in Alveolar Macrophages by Smoking

Smoking causes large increases in the number of alveolar macrophages, and these cells are morphologicically and metabolically activated (98,99). Therefore, we hypothesized that alveolar macrophages from smokers might support HIV replication better in vitro than those from nonsmokers. Abbud in my laboratory thus examined the relative capacity of alveolar macrophages from healthy smokers and nonsmokers to support the growth of HIV-$1_{JR\text{-}FL}$ in culture (100). HIV peak p24 levels in culture supernatants of infected alveolar macrophages from 13 smokers was significantly higher than that of 13 nonsmokers: alveolar macrophages, nonsmokers 7037 ± 2550 pg/mL; alveolar macrophages, smokers 31,394 ± 8295, mean ± SE, $p < 0.002$. Representatives of six paired experiments are shown in Figure 6. These differences in susceptibility to HIV production could not be explained on the basis of viral entry, extent of reverse transcription, or release of monokines, including TNF-α, IL-1β, IL-6, and GM-CSF (100). HIV production by blood monocytes from smokers and nonsmokers infected in vitro was negligible. Thus, cigarette smoking selectively increases the susceptibility of alveolar macrophages to productive infection with HIV.

Clarke et al. reported an increase in burden of HIV in bronchoalveolar cells from HIV-infected smokers compared with nonsmokers (101). Several studies suggest either that smoking is a marker of high-risk behavior or that a biological effect of smoking may increase the risk of infection with HIV (102–104). Whether smoking increases progression of HIV-infected individuals to AIDS is controversial, with some studies showing no effect and others showing an effect of smoking on disease progression

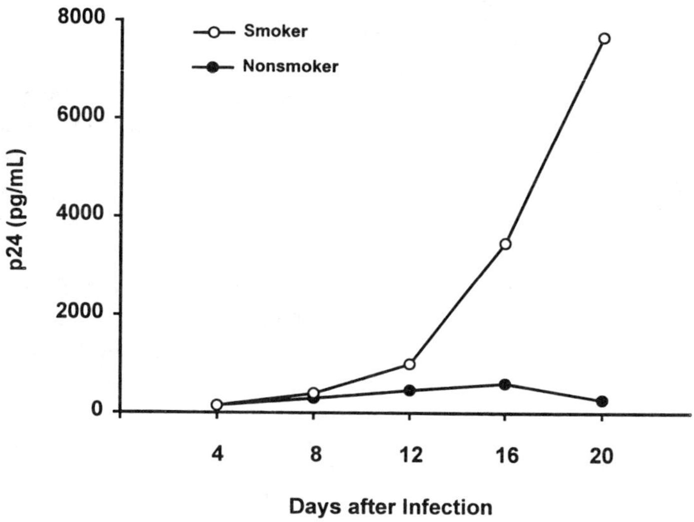

Figure 6 Kinetics of HIV production by alveolar macrophages from smokers and nonsmokers: Alveolar macrophages from six pairs of healthy smoking and nonsmoking volunteers were infected with HIV-$1_{JR\text{-}FL}$ and cultured in 24-well plates. Supernatants were collected over 24 hr every 4 days after infection for up to 20 days, and p24 *gag* protein was determined by ELISA. (Note: p24 levels from alveolar macrophages of nonsmoker 3 reached 100 pg/mL at day 12, but the scale fails to demonstrate this point.) (From Ref. 100.)

(101,102,105–109). There have, however, been non prospective epidemiological studies of the effect of smoking on progression of AIDS among well-defined smokers and nonsmokers at similar CD4 levels at entry into the study. Our in vitro study of markedly enhanced susceptibility to HIV production in alveolar macrophages from smokers provides the biological impetus for further epidemiological and virological longitudinal studies to resolve the issue of the influence of smoking on the pathogenesis of HIV disease, in general, and in the lung specifically.

Activation of HIV by Other Infections

Bacterial pneumonia and opportunistic infections of the lung remain among the most common complications of HIV disease. These infectious complications, in turn, may increase the rate of replication of HIV through mechanisms such as induction of cytokines. Both in vitro and in vivo studies of infectious agents that commonly involve the lung, including *Pneumocystis carinii* (PC) and mycobacteria, support this hypothesis.

Pneumocystis carinii pneumonia (PCP) is the most common opportunistic infection in HIV disease. The HIV load is higher in the lungs of individuals with PCP than from patients with non-PCP lung infections (38). Alveolar lymphocytes from HIV-infected patients with PCP are more commonly culture-positive for HIV, and viral production is higher than in alveolar lymphocytes from patients without lung infection or from their autologous blood lymphocytes (110). Thus, PC may increase the total level of HIV in the lungs. These results, however, need to be confirmed. Also, TNF-α production is increased in alveolar macrophages of HIV-infected patients, and production of this cytokine correlates with presence of lung opportunistic infections in general and with expression of HIV by these cells (44).

Monocytes from patients with tuberculosis express markers of activation, such as surface IL-2 receptor, and release increased amounts of TFN-α, IL-1, and IL-6 in response to lipopolysaccharide (111,112). These cytokines could function in an autocrine fashion to amplify HIV replication. Monocytes from patients with active pulmonary tuberculosis support productive infection with $HIV\text{-}1_{JR\text{-}FL}$ to a much greater extent than monocytes from healthy subjects, suggesting that concurrent infection increases the capacity of HIV to grow in mononuclear phagocytes (112). The kinetics of replication of HIV are enhanced in the U937 macrophage cell line coinfected with a strain of *M. avium* complex and HIV (113). Alveolar macrophages from healthy subjects coinfected with HIV and *M. avium* in vitro show enhanced production of HIV after several days in culture, suggesting that mycobacterial growth may act as an important cofactor for HIV replication in the lung (114). Whether dual infection with *M. tuberculosis* and HIV impinges on survival was studied by Whalen et al. in a retrospective, case-control study at four US Veterans Administration hospitals (115). Survival was shortened in dually infected patients when compared with CD4-matched HIV-infected controls. Thus, both in vitro and in vivo evidence supports the possibility that chronic mycobacterial infection may increase the rate of progression of disease through effects on viral replication.

IV. Summary and Future Directions

Much has been learned about the cellular targets of HIV infection in the lung, and some generalizations can be drawn. Bronchoalveolar cells from many, but not all, patients with AIDS harbor HIV, and alveolar macrophages appear to be the major cell type infected in alveolar spaces. The level of HIV in alveolar macrophages from AIDS patients is greater than in blood monocytes, but less than in blood lymphocytes. It appears that strains of HIV in alveolar macrophages evolved independently from strains in blood monocytes, suggesting local microenvironmental factors may be involved in infection of lung cells. Data now indicate that the virus is not actively replicating in alveolar macrophages, suggesting that local mechanisms to control the growth of HIV in the lung may be highly efficient. Surprisingly, HIV is not present in alveolar macrophages from asymptomatic patients at a relatively early stage of disease (peripheral CD4 cell levels of approximately 400/μl), further suggesting efficient mechanisms of killing or containment of HIV in the lung. Expression of cytokines, such as TNF-α is increased in alveolar macrophages from HIV-infected individuals at both an early and late stage of disease and does not correlate with absolute levels of HIV in the cells. Thus, indirect effects of HIV, such as that possibly induced by protein products of HIV, may alter the function of immune cells in an autocrine fashion or may cause injury to local structural cells.

Alveolar lymphocytes from AIDS patients also may be infected with HIV, but studies using highly purified alveolar lymphocytes have not been performed. CD8 alveolar lymphocytes dominate over CD4 cells even during early stages of disease. CD8 alveolar lymphocytes are cytotoxic to HIV-infected alveolar macrophages and may serve as a major mechanism of depletion of HIV in the lung.

Infection of lung fibroblasts may occur, but direct demonstration of infection of cells of the alveolocapillary membrane has not been reported. Evidence of damage to alveolar structural cells exists, however, suggesting at least indirect consequences of HIV infection on lung cells. Whether direct or indirect effects of HIV on alveolar epithelial or endothelial cells or of lung fibroblasts contribute to the development of lung disease remains to be determined.

In any compartment, cells must be activated for HIV replication to occur. The increased susceptibility to support of HIV replication in vitro by alveolar macrophages may be a consequence of activation of cells in vivo by chronic exposure to inhaled substances. Cigarette smoking causes a striking increase in growth of HIV in alveolar macrophages infected in vitro. Evidence supports the concept that local infections, such as by *P. carinii* and *M. tuberculosis*, also may enhance the replication of HIV in lung cells. The balance, however, between mechanisms that result in growth inhibition of HIV in lung cells and those that enhance viral replication are far from understood. Future directions to address the pathogenesis of pulmonary disease in HIV infection could best be addressed by the following approaches: longitudinal studies of pathogenesis of HIV in the lung to include relations among viral load, activation of viral infection, and cellular function; improved in vitro and ex vivo models of microbicidal activity of cells against opportunistic infections during HIV disease; and animal models of pathogenesis of HIV in the lung.

Acknowledgments

This work was supported by U.S. Public Health Service grants HL-53247, MO1RR0080, AI25879, and AI36219.

References

1. Greene WC. The molecular biology of human immunodeficiency virus type 1 infection. N Engl J Med 1991; 324:308–317.
2. Feinberg MB, Greene WC. Molecular insights into human immunodeficiency virus type-1 pathogenesis. Curr Opin Immunol 1992; 4:466–474.
3. Duh EJ, Maury WJ, Folks TM, Fauci AS, Rabson AB. Tumor necrosis factor α activates human immunodeficiency virus type 1 through induction of nuclear factor binding to the NF-κB sites in the long terminal repeat. Proc Natl Acad Sci USA 1989; 86:5974–5978.
4. Kestler HW, Ringler DJ, Mori K, Panicali DL, Sehgal PK, Daniel MD, Desrosiers RC. Importance of the *nef* gene for maintenance of high virus loads and for development of AIDS. Cell 1991; 65:651–662.
5. Daniel MD, Kirchoff F, Czajak SC, Sehgal PK., Desrosiers RC. Protective effects of a live attenuated SIV vaccine with a deletion in the *nef* gene. Science 1992; 258:1938–1941.
6. Malim MH, Cullen BR. Rev and the fate of pre-mRNA in the nucleus: implica-

tions for the regulation of RNA processing in eukaryotes. Mol Cell Biol 1993; 13:6180–6189.

7. Klatzmann D, Barre-Sinoussi F, Nugeyre MT, Dauguet C, Vilmer E, Griscelli C, Brun-Vezinet F, Rouzious C, Gluckman JC, Chermann JC, Montagnier L. Selective tropism of lymphadenopathy associated virus (LAV) for helper–inducer T lymphocytes. Science 1984; 225:59–62.
8. Popovic M, Read-Connole E, Gallo RC. T4 positive human neoplastic cell lines susceptible to and permissive for HTLV-III. Lancet 1984; 2:1472–1473.
9. Levy JA, Shimabukuro J, McHugh T, Casavant C, Stites D, Oshiro L. AIDS-associated retroviruses (ARV) can productively infect other cells besides human T helper cells. Virology 1984; 47:441–448.
10. Gartner S, Markovits P, Markovitz DM, Kaplan MH, Gallo RC, Popovic M. The role of mononuclear phagocytes in HTLV-III/LAV infection. Science 1986; 233:215–219.
11. Ho DD, Rota TR, Hirsch MS. Infection of monocyte/macrophages by human T lymphocytes virus type III. J Clin Invest 1986; 77:1712–1715.
12. Valentin A, Albert J, Fenyo, Åsio. HIV-1 infection of normal human macrophage cultures: implication for silent infection. Virology 1990; 177:790–794.
13. Nicholson JKA, Cross GD, Callaway CS, McDougal JS. In vitro infection of human monocytes with human T lymphotropic virus type III/lymphadenopathy-associated virus (HTLV-III/LAV). J Immunol 1986; 137:323–329.
14. Pauza CD. HIV persistence in monocytes leads to pathogenesis and AIDS. Cell Immunol 1988; 112:414–424.
15. Meltzer MS, Skillman DR, Gomatos PJ, Kalter DC, Gendelman HE. Role of mononuclear phagocytes in the pathogenesis of human immunodeficiency virus infection. Annu Rev Immunol 1990; 8:169–194.
16. McElrath MJ, Pruett JE, Cohn ZA. Mononuclear phagocytes of blood and bone marrow: comparative roles as viral reservoirs in human immunodeficiency virus type 1 infections. Proc Natl Acad Sci USA 1989; 86:675–679.
17. Schnittman SM, Psallidopoulos MC, Lane HC, Thompson L, Baseler M, Massari F, Fox CH, Salzman NP, Fauci AS. The reservoir for HIV-1 in human peripheral blood is a T cell that maintains expression of CD4. Science 1989; 41:305–308.
18. Spear GT, Ou C-Y, Kessler HA, Moore JL, Schochetman G, Landay AL. Analysis of lymphocytes, monocytes and neutrophils from human immunodeficiency virus (HIV)-infected persons for HIV DNA. J Infect Dis 1990; 162:1239–1244.
19. Schnittman SM, Fauci AS. Human immunodeficiency virus and acquired immunodeficiency syndrome: an update. Adv Intern Med 1994; 39:305–355.
20. Fauci AS. Immunopathogenesis of HIV infection. J Acquir Immune Defic Syndr 1993; 6:655–662.
21. Witmer MD, Steinman RM. The anatomy of peripheral lymphoid organs with emphasis on accessory cells: light-microscopic immunocytochemical studies of mouse spleen, lymph nodes, and Peyer's patch. Am J Anat 1984; 170:465–481.
22. Cameron PU, Lowe MG, Crowe SM, O'Doherty U, Pope M, Gezelter S,

Steinman RM. Susceptibility of dendritic cells to HIV-1 infection in vitro. J Leukoc Biol 1994; 56:257–265.
23. Cameron PU, Freudenthal PS, Barker JM, Gezelter S, Inaba K, Steinman RM. Dendritic cells exposed to human immunodeficiency virus-1 transmit a vigorous cytopathic infection to $CD4^+$ cells. Science 1992; 257:383–386.
24. Cameron PU, Pope M, Gezelter S, Barker JM, Steinman RM. Infection and apoptotic cell death of $CD4^+$ T cells during an immune response to HIV-1 pulsed dendritic cells. AIDS Res Hum Retroviruses 1994; 10:61–71.
25. von Stemm AMR, Ramsauer J, Tenner-Rácz K, Schmidt HF, Gigli I, Rácz P. Langerhans cells and interdigitating cells in HIV-1 infection. In: Kamperdijk EWA, Nieuwenhuis P, Hoefsmit ECM, eds. Dendritic Cells in Fundamental and Clinical Immunology. New York; Plenum, 1993:539–544.
26. Embretson J, Zupancic M, Ribas JL, Burke A, Rácz P, Tenner-Rácz K., Haase AT. Massive covert infection of helper T lymphocytes and macrophages by HIV during the incubation period of AIDS. Nature 1993; 362:359–362.
27. Schmitz J, van Lunzen J, Tenner-Rácz K, Grossschupff, Rácz P, Schmitz H, Dietrich M, Hufert FT. Follicular dendritic cells retain HIV-1 particles on their plasma membrane, but are not productively infected in asymptomatic patients with follicular hyperplasia. J Immunol 1994; 153:1352–1359.
28. Pantaleo G, Graziosi C, Demarest JF, Butini L, Montroni M, Fox CH, Orenstein JM, Kotler DP, Fauci AS. HIV infection is active and progressive in lymphoid tissue during the clinically latent stage of disease. Nature 1993; 362:355–358.
29. Fox CH, Tenner-Rácz K, Rácz P, Firpo A, Pizzo PA, Fauci AS. Lymphoid germinal centers are reservoirs of human immunodeficiency virus type 1 RNA. J Infect Dis 1991; 164:1051–1057.
30. Sierra-Madero JG, Toossi Z, Hom DL, Finegan CK, Hoenig E, Rich EA. Relationship between load of virus in alveolar macrophages from human immunodeficiency virus type-1 infected persons, production of cytokines, and clinical status. J Infect Dis 1994; 169:18–27.
31. Chayt KJ, Harper ME, Marselle LM, Lewin EB, Rose RM, Oleske JM, Epstine LG, Wong-Staal F, Gallo RC. Detection of HTLV-III RNA in lungs of patients with AIDS and pulmonary involvement. JAMA 1986; 256:2356–2359.
32. Plata F, Garcia-Pons F, Ryter A, Lebargy F, Goodenow M, Quan Dat MH, Autran B, Mayaud C. HIV-1 infection of lung alveolar fibroblasts and macrophages in humans. AIDS Res Hum Retroviruses 1990; 6:979–985.
33. Rose RM, Krivine A, Pinkston P, Gillis JM, Huang A, Hammer SM. Frequent identification of HIV-1 DNA in bronchoalveolar lavage cells obtained from individuals with the acquired immunodeficiency syndrome. Am Rev Respir Dis 1991; 143:850–854.
34. Lebargy F, Branellec A, Deforges L, Bignon J, Bernaudin J-F. HIV-1 in human alveolar macrophages from infected patients is latent in vivo but replicates after in vitro stimulation. Am J Repir Cell Mol Biol 1994; 10:72–78.
35. Dean NC, Golden JA, Evans LA, Warnock ML, Addison TE, Hopewell PC, Levy JA. Human immunodeficiency virus recovery from bronchoalveolar lavage fluid in patients with AIDS. Chest 1988; 93:1176–1179.

36. Resnick L, Pitchenik AE, Fisher E, Croney R. Detection of HTLV-III/LAV-specific IgG and antigen in bronchoalveolar lavage fluid from two patients with lymphocytic interstitial pneumonitis associated with AIDS-related complex. Am J Med 1987; 82:553–556.
37. Linnemann CC, Baughman RP, Frame PT, Floyd R. Recovery of human immunodeficiency virus and detection of p24 antigen in bronchoalveolar lavage fluid from adult patients with AIDS. Chest 1989; 96:64–67.
38. Clarke JR, Williamson JD, Mitchell DM. Comparative study of the isolation of human immunodeficiency virus from the lung and peripheral blood of AIDS patients. J Med Virol 1993; 39:196–199.
39. Landay AL, Schade SZ, Takefman DM, Kuhns MC, McNamara AL, Rosen RL, Kessler HA, Spear GT. Detection of HIV-1 provirus in bronchoalveolar lavage cells by polymerase chain reaction. J Acquir Immune Defic Syndr 1993; 6:171–175.
40. Clarke JR, Gates AJ, Coker RJ, Douglass JA, Williamson JD, Mitchell DM. HIV-1 proviral DNA copy number in peripheral blood leukocytes and bronchoalveolar lavage cells of AIDS patients. Clin Exp Immunol 1994; 96:182–186.
41. Harbison MA, Gillis P, Pinkston P, Byrn RA, Rose RM, Hammer SM. Effects of recombinant soluble CD4 (rCD4) on HIV-1 infection of monocyte/macrophages. J Infect Dis 1990; 161:1–6.
42. Gendelman HE, Narayan O, Kennedy-Stoskopf S, Kennedy PGE, Ghotbi Z, Clements JE, Stanley J, Pezeshpour G. Tropism of sheep lentiviruses for monocytes: susceptibility to infection and virus gene expression increase during maturation of monocytes to macrophages. J Virol 1986; 58:67–74.
43. Salahuddin SZ, Rose RM, Groopman JE, Markham PD, Gallo RC. Human T lymphotropic virus type III infection of human alveolar macrophages. Blood 1986; 68:281–284.
44. Israel-Biet D, Cadranel J, Beldjord K, Andrieu J-M, Jeffrey A, Even P. Tumor necrosis factor production in HIV seropositive subjects. Relationship with lung opportunistic infections and HIV expression in alveolar macrophages. J Immunol 1991; 147:490–494.
45. Jeffrey AA, Israel-Biet D, Andrieu J-M, Even P, Venet A. HIV isolation from pulmonary cells derived from bronchoalveolar lavage. Clin Exp Immunol 1991; 85:488–492.
46. Clarke JR, Krishnan V, Bennett J, Mitchell D, Jeffries DJ. Detection of HIV-1 in human lung macrophages using the polymerase chain reaction. AIDS 1990; 4:1133–1136.
47. Autran B, Sadat-Sowti B., Hadida F, Parrot A, Guillon J-M, Plata F, Mayaud C, Debré P. HIV-specific cytotoxic T lymphocytes against alveolar macrophages: specificities and downregulation. Res Virol 1991; 142:113–118.
48a. Semenzato G, Agostini C, Ometto L, Zambello R, Trentin L, Chieco-Bianchi L, de De Rossi A. $CD8^+$ T lymphocytes in the lung of acquired immunodeficiency syndrome patients harbor human immunodeficiency virus type 1. Blood 1995; 85:2308–2314.

48b. White DA, Matthay RA. Noninfectious pulmonary complications of infection with the human immunodeficiency virus. Am Rev Respir Dis 1989; 140:1763–1787.
49. Diaz PT, Clanton TL, Pacht ER. Emphysema-like pulmonary disease associated with human immunodeficiency virus infection. Ann Intern Med 116:124–128, 1992.
50. Meignan M, Guillon J-M, Denis M, Joly P, Rosso J, Carette M-F, Baud L, Parquin F, Plata F, Debre P, Akoun G, Autran B, Mayaud C. Increased lung epithelial permeability in HIV-infected patients with isolated cytotoxic T-lymphocytic alveolitis. Am Rev Respir Dis 1990; 141:1241–1248.
51. Levy JA. Pathogenesis of human immunodeficiency virus infection. Microbiol Rev 1993; 57:183–289.
52. Gilles PN, Lathey JL, Spector SA. Replication of macrophage-tropic and T–cell-tropic strains of human immunodeficiency virus type 1 is augmented by macrophage–endothelial cell contact. J Virol 1995; 69:2133–2139.
53. Dhawan S, Weeks BS, Soderland C, Schnaper HW, Toro LA, Asthana SP, Hewlett IK, Stetler-Stevenson WG, Yamada SS, Yamada KM, Meltzer MS. HIV-1 infection alters monocyte interactions with human microvascular endothelial cells. J Immunol 1995; 154:442–432.
54. Bourinbaiar AS, Phillips DM. Transmission of human immunodeficiency virus from monocytes to epithelia. J Acquir Immune Defic Syndr 1991; 4:56–63.
55. Ikeuchi K, Kim S, Byrn RA, Goldring SR, Groopman JE. Infection of nonlymphoid cells by human immunodeficiency virus type 1 or type 2. J Virol 1990; 64:4226–4231.
56. Mellert W, Kleinschmidt A, Schmidt J, Festl H, Emler S, Roth WK, Erfle V. Infection of human fibroblasts and osteoblast-like cells with HIV-1. AIDS 1990; 4:527–535.
57. Dolei A, Serra C, Arca MV, Toniolo A. Acute HIV-1 infection of $CD4^+$ human lung fibroblasts. AIDS 1992; 6:232–233.
58. Pantaleo G, Graziosi C, Fauci AS. The immunopathogenesis of human immunodeficiency virus infection. N Engl J Med 1993; 328:327–335.
59. Schnittman SM, Greenhouse JJ, Lane HC, Pierce PF, Fauci AS. Frequent detection of HIV-1 specific mRNAs in infected individuals suggests ongoing active viral expression in all stages of disease. AIDS Res Hum Retroviruses 1991; 7:361–367.
60. Piatek MJ Jr, Saag MS, Yang LC, Clark SJ, Kappes JC, Luk K-C, Hahn BH, Shaw GM, Lifson JD. High levels of HIV-1 in plasma during all stages of infection determined by competitive PCR. Science 1993; 259:1749–1754.
61. Cao Y, Qun L, Zhang L, Safrit J, Ho DD. Virologic and immunologic characterization of long-term survivors of human immunodeficiency virus type 1 infection. N Engl J Med 1995; 332:201–208.
62. Pantaleo G, Menzo S, Vaccarezza M, Graziosi C, Cohen OJ, Demarest JF, Montefiori D, Orenstein JM, Fox C, Schrager LK, Margolic JB, Buchbinder S, Giorgi JV, Fauci AS. Studies in subjects with long-term nonprogressive human immunodeficiency virus infection. N Engl J Med 1995; 332:209–216.

63. Zack JA, Arrigo SJ, Weitsman SR, Go AS, Haislip A, Chen ISY. HIV-1 entry into quiescent primary lymphocytes: molecular analysis reveals a labile, latent viral structure. Cell 1990; 61:213–222.
64. Twigg HL, Lipscomb ML, Yoffe B, Barbaro DJ, Weissler JC. Enhanced accessory cell function by alveolar macrophages from patients infected with the human immunodeficiency virus: potential role for depletion of $CD4^+$ cells in the lung. Am J Respir Cell Mol Biol 1989; 7:391–400.
65. Buhl R, Jaffe HA, Holyroyd KJ, Borok Z, Roum JH, Mastrangeli A, Wells FB, Kirby M, Saltini C, Crystal RG. Activation of alveolar macrophages in asymptomatic HIV-infected individuals. J Immunol 1993; 150:1019–1028.
66. Ho DD, Moudgil T, Alam M. Quantitation of human immunodeficiency virus type 1 in the blood of infected persons. N Engl J Med 1989; 321:1621–1625.
67. Dalgleish AG, Wilson S, Gompels M, Ludlam C, Gazzard B, Coates AM, Habeshaw J. T-cell receptor variable gene products and early HIV-1 infection. Lancet 1992; 339:824–828.
68. Imberti L, Sottini A, Bettinardi A, Puoti M, Primi D. Selective depletion in HIV infection of T cells that bear specific T cell receptor V beta sequences. Science 1991; 254:860–862.
69. Wei X, Ghosh SK, Taylor ME, Johnson VA, Emini EA, Deutsch P, Lifson JD, Bonhoeffer S, Nowak MA, Hahn BH, Saag MS, Shaw GM. Viral dynamics in human immunodeficiency virus type 1 infection. Nature 1995; 373:117–122.
70. Ho DD, Neumann AU, Perelson AS, Chen W, Leonard JM, Markowitz M. Rapid turnover of plasma virions and CD4 lymphocytes in HIV-1 infection. Nature 1995; 373:123–126.
71. Walker CM, Moody DJ, Stites DP, Levy JA. $CD8^+$ lymphocytes can control HIV infection in vitro by suppressing virus replication. Science 1986; 234:1563–1566.
72. Plata F, Autran B, Martins LP, Wain-Hobson S, Raphaël M, Mayaud C, Denis M, Guilon J-M, Debré P. AIDS virus-specific cytotoxic T lymphocytes in lung disorders. Nature 1987; 328:348–351.
73. Hoffenbach A, Langlade-Demoyen P, Dadaglio G, Vilmer E, Michel F, Mayaud C, Autran B, Plata F. Unusually high frequencies of HIV-specific cytotoxic lymphocytes in humans. J Immunol 1984; 142:452–462.
74. Sada-Sowti B, Parrot A, Quint L, Mayaud C, Debré, Autran B. Alveolar $CD8^+$-$CD57^+$ lymphocytes in human immunodeficiency virus infection produce an inhibitor of cytotoxic functions. Am J Respir Crit Care Med 1994; 149:972–980.
75. Meltzer MS, Skillman DR, Gomatos PJ, Klater DC, Gendelman HE. Role of mononuclear phagocytes in the pathogenesis of human immunodeficiency virus infection. Annu Rev Immunol 1990; 8:169–194.
76. O'Brien WA, Koyanagi Y, Namazie A, Zhao JQ, Diagne A, Idler K, Zack JA, Chen ISY. Nature 1990; 348:69–73.
77. Hwang SS, Boyle TJ, Lyerly HK, Cullen BR. Science 1991; 253:71–73.
78. Fouchier RA, Groenink M, Koostra NA, Tersmette M, Huisman HG, Miedema F, Schuitemaker H. J Virol 1992; 66:3183–3187.
79. Rusche JR, Javaherian K, McDanal C, Petro J, Lynn DL, Grimaila R, Langlois

A, Gallo RC, Arthur LO, Fischinger PJ, Bolognesi DP, Putney D, Matthews TJ. Antibodies that inhibit fusion of human immunodeficiency virus-infected cells bind a 24-amino acid sequence to the viral envelope, gp120. Proc Natl Acad Sci USA 1988; 85:3198–3202.

80. Looney DJ, Fisher AG, Putney SD, Rusche JR, Redfield RR, Burke DS, Gallo RC, Wong-Staal F. Type-restricted neutralization of molecular clones of human immunodeficiency virus. Science 1988; 241:357–359.
81. Takahashi H, Cohen J, Hosmalin A, Cease KB, Houghten R, Cornette JL, DeLisi C, Moss B, Germain RN, Berzofsky JA. Proc Natl Acad Sci USA 1988; 85:3105–3109.
82. Agostini C, Trentin L, Zambello R, Semenzato G. HIV-1 and the lung. Infectivity, pathogenic mechanisms, and cellular immune responses taking place in the lower respiratory tract. Am Rev Respir Dis 1993; 147:1038–1049.
83. Schuitemaker H, Koot M, Koostra NA, Dercksen MW, DeGoede REY, van Steenwijk RP, Lange JMA, Schattenkerk JKME, Miedema F, Tersmette M. Biological phenotype of human immunodeficiency virus type 1 clones at different stages of infection: progression of disease is associated with a shift from monocytotropic to T-cell-tropic virus populations. J Virol 1992; 66:1354–1360.
84. Potash MJ, Ziera M, Huang Z-B, Pearce TE, Eden E, Gendelman HE, Volsky DJ. Virus-cell membrane fusion does not predict efficient infection of alveolar macrophages by human immunodeficiency virus type (HIV-1). Virology 1992; 188:864–868.
85. Itescu S, Simonelli PF, Winchester RJ, Ginsberg HS. Human immunodeficiency virus type 1 strains in the lungs of infected individuals evolve independently from those in peripheral blood and are highly conserved in the C-terminal region of the envelope V3 loop. Proc Natl Acad Sci USA 1994; 91:11378–11382.
86. Temin HM. Studies on carcinogenesis by avian sarcoma viruses. V. Requirement for new DNA synthesis and for cell division. J Cell Physiol 1967; 69:53–64.
87. Folks T, Kelly J, Benn S, Kinter A, Justement J, Gold J, Redfield R, Sell KW, Fauci AS. Susceptibility of normal human lymphocytes to infection with HTLV-III/LAV. J Immunol 1986; 136:4049–4053.
88. Zagury D, Bernard J, Leonard R, Cheynier R, Feldman M, Sarin PS, Gallo RC. Long term cultures of HTLV-III infected T cells: a model of cytopathology of T-cell depletion in AIDS. Science 1986; 231:850–853.
89. Zack JA, Cann AJ, Lugo JP, Chen ISY. HIV-1 production from infected peripheral blood T cells after HTLV-1 induced mitogenic stimulation. Science 1988; 240:1026–1029.
90. Zack JA, Haislip AM, Krogstad P, Chen ISY. Incompletely reversed-transcribed human immunodeficiency virus type 1 genomes in quiescent cells can function as intermediates in the retroviral life cycle. J Virol 1992; 66:1717–1725.
91. O'Brien WA, Namazi A, Kalhor H, Mao S-H, Zack JA, Chen ISY. Kinetics of human immunodeficiency virus type 1 reverse transcription in blood mononuclear phagocytes are slowed by limitations of nucleotide precursors. J Virol 1994; 68:1258–1263.

92. Bukrinsky MI, Stanwick TL. Dempsey MP, Stevenson M. Quiescent T lymphocytes as an inducible virus reservoir in HIV-1 infection. Science 1991; 254:423-427.
93. Schuitemaker H, Kootstra NA, Koppelman MHGM, Bruisten SM, Huisman HG, Tersmette M, Miedema F. Proliferation-dependent HIV-1 infection of monocytes occurs during differentiation into macrophages. J Clin Invest 1992; 84:1154-1160.
94. Schrier RD, McCutchan JA, Wiley CA. Mechanisms of immune activation of human immunodeficiency virus in monocytes/macrophages. J Virol 1993; 67:5713-5720.
95. Mann DL, Gartner S, LeSane F, Buchow H, Popovic M. HIV-1 transmission and function of virus-infected monocytes/macrophages. J Immunol 1990; 144:2152-2158.
96. Mikovits JA, Lohrey NC, Schulof R, Courtless J, Ruscetti FW. Activation of infectious virus from latent human immunodeficiency virus infection of monocytes in vivo. J Clin Invest 1992; 90:1487-1491.
97. Rich EA, Chen ISY, Zack JA, Leonard ML, O'Brien WA. Increased susceptibility of differentiated mononuclear phagocytes to productive infection with human immunodeficiency virus-1 (HIV-1). J Clin Invest 1992; 89:176-183.
98. Martin RR. Altered morphology and increased acid hydrolase content of pulmonary macrophages from cigarette smokers. Am Rev Respir Dis 1973; 107:596-601.
99. Hoidal JR, Niewoehner DE. Lung phagocyte recruitment and metabolic alterations induced by cigarette smoke in humans and in hamsters. Am Rev Respir Dis 1982; 126:548-552.
100. Abbud RA, Finegan CK, Guay LA, Rich EA. Enhanced production of human immunodeficiency virus-1 (HIV-1) by in vitro infected alveolar macrophages from otherwise healthy cigarette smokers. J Infect Dis 1995; 172:859-863.
101. Clarke JR, Taylor IK, Fleming J, Nukuna A, Williamson JD, Mitchell DM. The epidemiology of HIV-1 infection of the lung in AIDS patients. AIDS 1993; 7:555-560.
102. Burns DN, Kramer A, Yellin F, Fuchs D, Wachter H, DiGioia RA, Sanchez WC, Grossman RJ, Gordin FM, Biggar RJ, Goedert JJ. Cigarette smoking: a modifier of human immunodeficiency virus type 1 infection. J Acquir Immune Defic Syndr 1991; 4:76-83.
103. Halsey NA, Coberly JS, Holt E, Coreil J, Kissinger P, Moulton LH, Brutus JR, Boulos R. Sexual behavior, smoking and HIV-1 infection in Haitian woman. JAMA 1992; 267:2062-2066.
104. Boulos R, Halsey NA, Holt E, the City Soleil/JHU AIDS Project Team. HIV-1 in Haitian woman 1982-1988. J Acquir Immune Defic Syndr 1990; 3:721-728.
105. Coates RA, Farewall VT, Raboud J, Read SE, MacFadden DK. Calzavara LM, Johnson JK, Sheperd FA, Fanning MM. Cofactors of progression to acquired immunodeficiency syndrome in a cohort of male sexual contacts of men with human immunodeficiency virus disease. Am J Epidemiol 1990; 132:717-722.
106. Goedert JJ, Biggar RJ, Melbye M, Mann DL, Wilson S, Gail MH, Grossman

RJ, DiGioia RA, Sanchez WC, Weiss SH, Blattner WA. Effect of T4 count and cofactors on the incidence of AIDS in homosexual men infected with human immunodeficiency virus. JAMA 1987; 257:331–334.

107. Craib KJP, Schecter MT, Montaner JSG, Le TN, Sestak P, Willoughby B, Voigt R, Haley L, O'Shaughnessy MV. The effect of cigarette smoking on lymphocyte subsets and progression to AIDS in a cohort of homosexual men. Clin Invest Med 1992; 15:301–308.
108. Newell GR, Mansell PWA, Wilson MB, Lynch HK, Spitz MR, Hersh EM. Risk factor analysis among men referred for possible acquired immune deficiency syndrome. Prev Med 1985; 14:81–89.
109. Nieman RB, Fleming J, Coker RJ, Harris JRW, Mitchell DM. The effect of cigarette smoking on the development of AIDS in HIV-1 seropositive individuals. AIDS 1993; 7:705–710.
110. Israel-Biet D, Cadranel J, Even P. Human immunodeficiency virus production by alveolar lymphocytes is increased during *Pneumocystis carinii* pneumonia. Am Rev Respir Dis 1993; 148:1308–1312.
111. Wallis RS, Ellner JJ, Shiratsuchi H. Macrophages, mycobacteria and HIV: the role of cytokines in determining mycobacterial virulence and regulating viral replication. Res Microbiol 1992; 143:398–405.
112. Toossi Z, Sierra-Madero JG, Blinkhorn RA, Mettler MA, Rich EA. Enhanced susceptibility of blood monocytes from patients with pulmonary tuberculosis to productive infection with human immunodeficiency virus type 1. J Exp Med 1993; 177:1511–1516.
113. Ghassemi M, Andersen BR, Reddy VM, Gangadharan PRJ, Spear GT, Novak RM. Human immunodeficiency virus and *Mycobacterium avium* complex coinfection of monocytoid cells results in reciprocal enhancement of multiplication. J Infect Dis 1995; 171:68–73.
114. Denis M, Ghadirian E. Interaction between *Mycobacterium avium* and human immunodeficiency virus type 1 (HIV-1) in bronchoalveolar macrophages of normal and HIV-1 infected subjects. Am J Respir Cell Mol Biol 1994; 11:487–495.
115. Whalen C, Horsburgh CR, Hom D, Lahart C, Simberkoff M, Ellner JJ. Accelerated course of human immunodeficiency virus infection after tuberculosis. Am J Respir Crit Care Med 1995; 151:129–135.

6

HIV and Lung Lymphocyte Function

CARLO AGOSTINI and GIANPIETRO SEMENZATO

Padua University School of Medicine
Padua, Italy

Introduction

Human immunodeficiency virus (HIV) is widely recognized to be equipped with the ability to infect a variety of lung cells, giving rise to a striking cell-mediated immune response in the pulmonary microenvironment (1–5). Infection of lung cells is an early event during HIV infection, as suggested by the fact that pulmonary cells from asymptomatic patients may contain proviral DNA, although at lower levels than during late stages of the disease (6–8). Following virion entry of the lung, the main pathological finding is the development of a massive leukocyte infiltration of the lower respiratory tract. Different factors facilitating the influx, activation, and proliferation of immunocompetent cells contribute to the pathogenesis of acquired immunodeficiency syndrome (AIDS)-associated inflammatory pulmonary disease. In particular, growing evidence supports the notion that alveolar macrophages represent the major source of several inflammatory cytokines and chemotactic factors that mediate infiltration of cytotoxic T lymphocytes (CTL) into lung parenchyma (3). These cells, accounting for the major effector arm of the lung immune system against HIV, show the capability of recognizing epitopes of structural proteins of HIV and contribute to the control of viral spreading in the surrounding microenvironment.

This chapter focuses on the pattern of immunological activities of pulmonary lymphocytes in the pulmonary immune mechanisms against HIV, reviewing the events leading to the recruitment, homing, expansion, and functional properties of lymphoid cells in the lung. Recent evidence will also be covered that indicates that not only $CD4^+$ T lymphocytes and macrophages, but also pulmonary $CD8^+$ cells represent a target or a reservoir for HIV in vivo. In the final section of the chapter we will provide the reader with a glimpse of the translation into the clinical setting of biological research, emphasizing the pathogenetic role envisaged for lung $CD8^+$ cells and their byproducts in the pathogenesis of AIDS-associated pulmonary complications.

It seems appropriate to conclude this brief introduction by mentioning that the technique of bronchoalveolar lavage (BAL) deserves full credit for having improved our knowledge on the effects of HIV infection on the lung microenvironment. By providing access to cell populations within the lower respiratory tract, BAL has allowed researchers to highlight the multidirectional communication networks between the retrovirus and cellular and soluble components of the pulmonary immune system.

II. Lymphocytic Alveolitis in HIV-Infected Patients

Human lymphocytes are functionally compartmentalized in the lung into secondary and tertiary lymphoid tissues (9). In particular, virtually all of the organized lymphoid tissue of the lung is represented by follicles that are located throughout the bronchial tree, as far down as the small bronchioles. These structures can be considered specialized sites for secondary lymphoid differentiation and are constituted by B-cell germinal centers surrounded by T cells, macrophages, and dendritic cells. In lung follicles naive B and T cells collect, differentiate into memory and effector lymphocytes, and continuously traffic until they respond to their cognate antigen.

The parenchyma of the lung represents a paradigmatic tertiary lymphoid tissue that normally contains only a few lymphoid elements. In fact, in the normal nonsmoking adult, more than 90% of the cells within the alveolar spaces and interstitium are macrophages, whereas lymphocytes account for 5–10% of the entire BAL cell population. As in other tertiary lymphoid organs, pulmonary lymphocytes are CD45RO "memory" cells, sparsely distributed along the submucosa and lamina propria, between the epithelial cells and within the interstitium.

An optimal host response against pathogenic stimuli depends on the rapid homing to sites of pulmonary inflammation by memory lymphocytes that have been previously primed in secondary lymphoid tissues. When an unwanted antigen enters the pulmonary tract, specialized antigen-presenting cells are engaged, and a complex cascade of intercellular communications occurs between accessory cells and effector T lymphocytes. Following antigen recognition, the clonal expansion of intra-alveolar T cells and the migration of memory T lymphocytes from secondary lymphoid tissues result in the accumulation and differentiation of antigen-specific T lymphocytes with effector specializations.

The AIDS-associated interstitial lung disease represents the prototype of a pulmonary disorder that is associated with a noticeable infiltration of antigen-specific T cells. In fact, following the spread of HIV into pulmonary parenchyma the cell-to-cell contact between accessory cells (i.e., alveolar macrophages) and memory T lymphocytes, recruited from secondary lymphoid tissue, leads to an adaptive increase in the number of antigen-specific and nonspecific T cells, with highly specialized effector functions (Fig. 1). In terms of frequency of this phenomenon, epidemiological studies have estimated that approximately 25–50% of patients with HIV infection show a high intensity alveolitis that is initiated and sustained by T cells (7,8). Interestingly, the alveolitis may be documented not only in the earlier stages of HIV infection, but also in patients with full-blown AIDS with severe T-cell depletion, suggesting that the immune function in the lung may be regulated differently from that in peripheral blood.

A. Phenotypic Characteristics of the Lymphoid Infiltrate

In the last few years several investigators have characterized lymphocytes recovered from the BAL of patients with AIDS by using a variety of monoclonal antibodies (MAbs). Phenotypic data have provided a great body of information directly related to the differentiation and functional activities of the pulmonary lymphoid system during HIV infection. For the reader's convenience, in Table 1 we have listed MAbs (both clustered and nonclustered) that will be discussed in this chapter, with related reactivities and specificities.

In normal individuals, lung T cells, which account for most lymphocytes resident in the lower respiratory tract, bear the T-cell receptor (TCR)-associated CD3 antigen and the receptor molecule for sheep red blood cells (CD2). $CD4^+$ helper-related and $CD8^+$ cytotoxic–suppressor-related cells are present in proportions superimposable on those observed in the peripheral blood (CD4/CD8 ratio ≈2; 9). In the BAL of patients with HIV infection $CD8^+$ lymphocytes dramatically increase both in percentage and in abso-

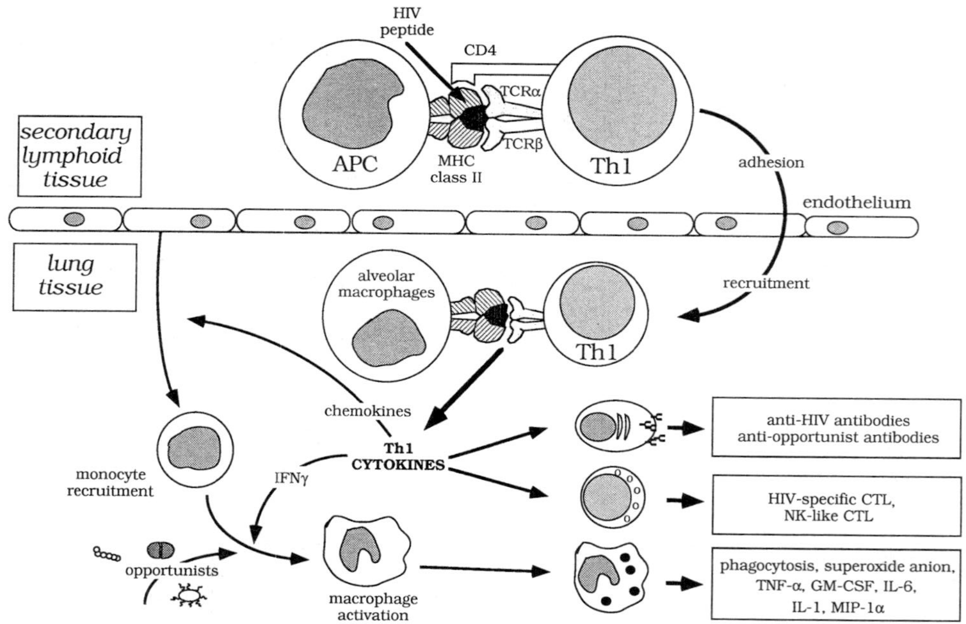

Figure 1 Putative role of the antigen-presenting cells and pulmonary CD4$^+$ T$_H$1 cells in the induction of the local immune response against HIV-1 during the early phases of the HIV disease. Following recognition of virions trapped in the follicular dendritic cell network in the lymph node, the migration of memory T lymphocytes from secondary lymphoid tissues results in the local release of T$_H$1 cytokines (including IL-2), which favor the accumulation and differentiation of HIV-specific T lymphocytes with effector specializations in the lung parenchyma. APC, antigen-presenting cells; CTL, cytotoxic T lymphocyte; GM-CSF, granulocyte–macrophage colony-stimulating factor; IFNγ, interferon-γ; IL, interleukin; MHC, major histocompatibility complex; MIP, macrophage inflammatory protein; NK, natural killer; TCR, T-cell receptor.

lute number, whereas the opposite behavior can be observed for the CD4 cell population (Fig. 2). Consistent with data obtained on cells retrieved from the BAL, immunohistological studies have clearly shown the presence of a generalized $CD8^+$ cell infiltration of the lung parenchyma. Helper-related pulmonary $CD4^+$ lymphocytes are virtually absent in biopsy specimens, even if remarkable differences are detectable in the absolute number of lung CD4 cells among HIV-infected patients at different disease stages (10,11). Other markers related to the activation and differentiation state of T cells are taken into account in the section devoted to the immunological role of T cells in the pulmonary microenvironment.

For B lymphocytes, the percentage of cells with surface immunoglobulins is equal in HIV-infected patients and in controls (less than 5% in the BAL). B cells do not display quantitative defects in the expression of B-related markers (CD19, CD20, CD23), but do produce increased amounts of immunoglobulins. As a consequence, the surfactant composition is altered, and high concentrations of immunoglobulins, including antibodies specific to HIV, and immune complexes are commonly present in lung epithelial lining fluid of these patients (12). Furthermore, immunoglobulin deposits are associated with the presence of rare plasma cells in involved tissues.

B. Mechanisms Leading to HIV Infection of Pulmonary Cells

Studies in lymphoid organs has favored the understanding and characterization of the pathogenetic events influencing and promoting HIV infection in the different stages of HIV disease. After primary infection, the retrovirus is disseminated throughout the body and compartmentalized in secondary lymphoid tissues, where a reservoir of viruses is established. Extracellular virions are trapped in the follicular dendritic cell network in the lymph node germinal centers, which then serve as a source of infection for lymphoid cells migrating through the secondary lymphoid tissue during the course of infection, even during the early asymptomatic period (13). As disease progresses, the architecture of secondary lymphoid tissue is destroyed (13). With the onset of AIDS, the dissolution of the follicular dendritic cell network in the lymph node leads to the inability to trap extracellular virions, and HIV redistributes massively outside the secondary lymphoid tissue to tertiary lymphoid tissue, including brain, lung, colon, and liver (14,15).

Several techniques have been used to search for the presence of HIV in the lung parenchyma, including virus culture of total and fractioned BAL cell subpopulations, in situ hybridization, p24 HIV protein detection in BAL cells and fluids, and evaluation of proviral load by the DNA–PCR tech-

Table 1 Clustered and Nonclustered Monoclonal Antibodies with Related Reactivity and Antigen Specificity That Have Been Discussed in This Chapter

Monoclonal antibody	Reactivity	Comments
Clustered monoclonal antibodies		
CD2	T cells, some NK cells	Receptor molecule for sheep red cells, involved in cell adherence after binding to LFA-3
CD3	T cells	Associated with the TCR
CD4	T-helper–inducer cells Some macrophages	Class II MHC receptor, receptor for HIV-1
CD8	T-suppressor–cytotoxic cells	Class I MHC receptor
CD11a	Leukocytes	α-Chain of the leukocyte function associated-1 antigen (LFA-1); binds ICAM-1 (CD54) and ICAM-2
CD16	NK cells, granulocytes, macrophages	Low affinity Fc receptor for IgG (FcγRIII)
CD18	Leukocytes	Integrin-β_2, mediates cell–cell and cell–matrix adhesion
CD19	All B cells	Transmembrane polypeptide
CD20	B cells after pro–B-cell stage	Putative involvement in ion transport
CD23	Strongly expressed on IL-4–activated B cells; weakly expressed on mature B cells	Low affinity receptor for IgE
CD25	Actiavated T cells, NK cells, some macrophages	p55 of IL-2R
CD45RA (220-kDa isoform)	T-cell subset; B cells, macrophages	T cells expressing this antigen are naive or virgin T cells
CD45RO (180-kDa isoform)	T-cell subset, B cells, macrophages	T cells expressing this antigen are memory or primed T cells

CD49d	T- and B-cell subset	Fibronectin and CD106 receptor
CD54	T cells, macrophages, endothelium cells, dendritic cells	Intercellular adhesion molecule 1 (ICAM-1), is the ligand for LFA-1, receptor for rhinovirus
CD56	NK cells	Isoform of neural adhesion molecule
CD57	Granular lymphocytes, some T and B cells	Unknown function
CD62E	Activated endothelial cells; activated platelets	Mediates leukocyte adhesion to endothelium in inflammation
CD95	Most cell types	FAS, APO-1 transduces apoptotic signal
CD102	Activated T cells	Intercellular adhesion molecule 2 (ICAM-2) is the ligand for CD11a/CD18 on endothelial cells
CD103	Activated T cells	Analogous to the integrin family
CD106	Activated endothelial cells	Vascular cell adhesion molecule, (VCAM), involved in adhesion of leukocytes on endothelia
CD120a	Most cell types	Type 1 receptor for TNF
CD120b	Most cell types	Type 2 receptor for TNF
CD122	NK cells, some T and B cells	Intermediate-affinity receptor for IL-2
Nonclustered monoclonal antibodies		
WT31	All α/β TCR cells	Associated with the TCR
TCRδ1, TCR-γδ-1	All γ/δ TCR cells	Associated with the TCR
A13, δTCS1	$V\delta1^+$ γ/δ TCR cells	Associated with the TCR
BB3	$V\delta2^+$ γ/δ TCR cells	Associated with the TCR
HLA-DR	T cells, B cells, macrophages, and other APC	Class II MHC antigen
Ki67	All proliferating cells	Antigen expressed during G_1,S,G_2, and M cell cycle phases
bcl-2	Most cell types	Involved in the control of activation-induced cell death

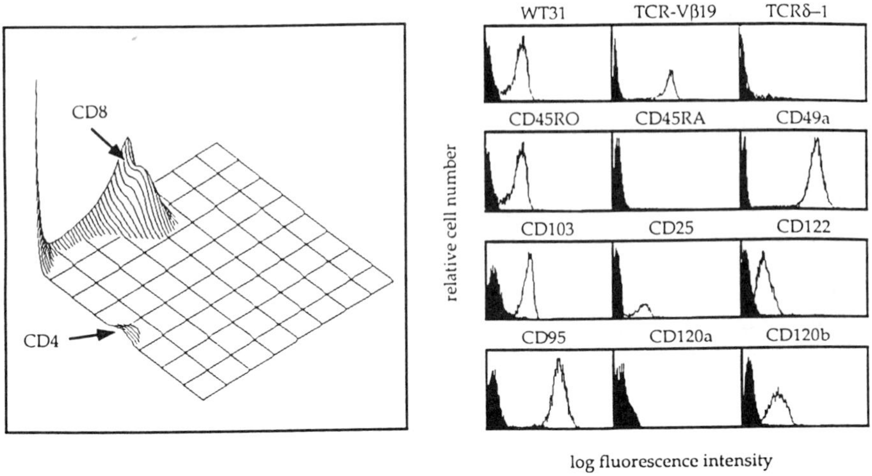

Figure 2 Flow cytometry profile of BAL T cells recovered from a patient with early HIV-1 infection and lymphocytic alveolitis (44% of BAL cells were lymphocytes, as determined by morphological evaluation of the cytospin). Pulmonary T lymphocytes were stained with phycoerythrin-conjugated anti-CD8 MAb and fluorescein-conjugated anti-CD4 MAb. $CD8^+$ cells (88% of BAL T lymphocytes) were gated, and the proportion of WT31, TCR-Vβ19, TCR-δ1, CD45RO, CD45RA, CD49a, CD103, CD25, CD122, CD95, CD120a, and CD120b-positive cells was determined by three-color fluorescence, following incubation with a biotinylated anti-IgG_1 or anti-IgG_2 antimouse MAb and streptoavidin-RED613. As shown in the figure, most BAL CD8 cells express the α/β TCR (recognized by the WT31 MAb), whereas γ/δ cells are scattered among BAL CD8 cells (less than 1% in this case). A bias in the usage of TCR–Vβ region was demonstrated, for 18% of α/β T cells are $V\beta19^+$ in this case. Furthermore, CD8 cells were CD45RO-activated "memory" T cells because they expressed activation markers (CD49a and CD103 determinants), cytokine receptors (including CD120b, CD122, and, in slight percentage, CD25), and the Fas antigen (CD95). (Phenotypic data from Refs. 3, 34, 39, 40, 43, and 46.)

nique (3,14,15). By means of these different approaches, it has been demonstrated that pulmonary tissues may represent reservoirs of HIV in vivo. In fact, HIV sequences and proteins have been detected in secondary lymphoid follicles of the lung. As discussed in Chapter 5, the integration of the HIV genome has been shown in different pulmonary cell populations, including alveolar macrophages, pulmonary T cells, and fibroblasts.

The mechanisms leading to the retroviral infection of the pulmonary microenvironment have, to some extent, been elucidated. Peripheral blood $CD4^+$-infected cells, predominantly monocyte–macrophages that harbor the provirus in a latent form, may enter the lung where they differentiate into resident cells, thereby facilitating the persistence of the retroviral infection

(2). Because secondary lymphoid follicles of the lung serve as reservoirs for HIV (10), the establishment of HIV infection of the pulmonary parenchyma may also be considered the consequence of a migratory process involving infected T cells originating from pulmonary lymphoid tissues. The recent demonstration that cell-free virus is carried by the microcirculation suggests that a third pathway may favor the invasiveness of HIV into the lung (16). In fact, it is possible that HIV may cross the alveolocapillary membrane as a free extracellular virion, entering the lung parenchyma, and infecting resident cells.

Clearly, the progressive fall of lung CD4 cells seen following HIV infection of pulmonary parenchyma at least partly reflects the marked depletion of $CD4^+$ lymphocytes that occurs in vivo in patients with AIDS. Several mechanisms have been proposed to explain the pulmonary depletion of $CD4^+$ cells, including the accumulation of unintegrated viral DNA. Within the lung a tissue homeostasis of the number of T cells occurs when the physiological cell death is balanced by the replacement of dead cells through cellular recruitment from the secondary follicles (9). Thus, microenvironmental mechanisms, including cell-to-cell contact and high local concentration of HIV in the follicular dendritic cell network of germinal centers, may contribute to enhancing the rate of infection of $CD4^+$ cells that are trafficking in the pulmonary lymph node. Because cytoplasmic retroviral DNA has been demonstrated in pulmonary cells (17), it is possible that the quantitative defect of $CD4^+$ lung T cells may at least partly be the result of the well-known direct cytopathic effect of the accumulation of cytoplasmic retroviral DNA.

As specified in detail later, a general state of activation of HIV-specific cell-mediated immune response (i.e., HIV-specific cytotoxicity) takes place in the lung of HIV-infected individuals (3). Accordingly, that the HIV-specific CTL response is responsible for the lysis of HIV-expressing cells may represent a major mechanism for the progressive clearance of pulmonary $CD4^+$ infected cells. Furthermore, there are data indicating that a dysregulation of the apoptosis control system takes place in the lung of HIV-infected patients (see later discussion). These observations led to the speculation that the process of activation-induced cell death might influence the gradual loss of lung $CD4^+$ cells. Finally, syncitia formation between HIV-infected alveolar macrophages and uninfected T cells (18) has been claimed as another possible cause for the depletion of $CD4^+$ T cells in the pulmonary microenvironment.

C. Lung $CD8^+$ Lymphocytes Represent a Reservoir for HIV Infection

Accumulating evidence indicates that HIV can also enter cells lacking the CD4 receptor, suggesting that, in theory, every human cell could be infected by this retrovirus. The fact that HIV can enter cells lacking the CD4 molecule (such as some neural cells, liver cells, or epithelia) makes the representation of the pathogenetic mechanisms of HIV infectivity more complex than previously thought (3). Despite the broad spectrum of HIV targets, the mechanisms by which the virus interacts with and affects the CD4-negative cells, as well as the pattern of infection (latent vs. productive) in these cells, have been poorly characterized.

Recently, we evaluated the proviral load by using the DNA–PCR technique on T-cell subsets retrieved by BAL (19). In addition to the hypothesis that HIV infection plays a central role in the decline of lung $CD4^+$ T cells, our data suggest an unexpected in vivo infectivity of HIV toward the pulmonary $CD8^+$ cell compartment. In fact, although most of the BAL proviral DNA is contained in the underrepresented $CD4^+$ cell subset, PCR analysis directly performed on the $CD8^+$ cell subset demonstrated that this population carries detectable amounts of HIV DNA. This finding was unexpected because BAL T cells accounting for the alveolitis in the lungs of AIDS patients express the $CD8^+$ phenotype. The presence of proviral DNA in $CD8^+$ cells was previously reported in in vitro models only, and attempts to infect highly purified populations of $CD8^+$ cells directly have as yet been unsuccessful (20,21).

This finding prompts several considerations for the pattern of infectivity of HIV and the pathways of viral spread to these cells. Among the mechanisms that make pulmonary $CD8^+$ cells susceptible to HIV infection in vivo, an obvious explanation can be deduced by recent in vitro studies showing that HIV transmission occurs through cell-to-cell contact between persistently infected $CD4^+$ cells and $CD8^+$ lymphocytes (21). In fact, recent studies demonstrate that the respiratory mucosa of patients with AIDS is equipped with a high number of CTL that recognize and lyse HIV-infected $CD4^+$ target cells (22). Because HIV can spread to $CD8^+$ CTL during the process of killing in vitro (21), it is conceivable that the repeated contact occurring in the lung microenvironment between activated HIV-specific CTL and relevant targets could ultimately lead to the infection of $CD8^+$ cells.

An additional, and not necessarily alternative, hypothesis that we provided rests on the fact that pulmonary HIV-specific CTL derive from precursors transiently coexpressing CD4 and CD8 in HIV-infected secondary lymphoid tissues (19). When we evaluated CD4 gene expression in highly purified $CD8^+$ cells obtained from the BAL of AIDS patients with CD8 high-intensity alveolitis, detectable amounts of RNA for the CD4 molecule were found, despite the lack of membrane CD4 reactivity. This finding supports the concept that lung CTL might at least in part originate from T precursors that transiently coexpress both CD4 and CD8 determinants in secondary follicles.

III. Role of Pulmonary CD8$^+$ Cells in the Pulmonary Microenvironment

A. Pulmonary CD8$^+$ Cells Are Involved in Virus–Host Conflict

The HIV and related proteins are capable of initiating a cellular-mediated immune response within the lung, ultimately leading to the local accumulation and differentiation of responding T cells (i.e., the AIDS-associated lymphocytic alveolitis). In fact, acting as antigen-presenting cells and secreting a variety of cytokines, such as interleukin-1 (IL-1), IL-6, tumor necrosis factor-α (TNF- α), granulocyte–macrophage colony-stimulating factor (GM-CSF), and macrophage inflammatory protein-1α (MIP-1α) (23–30), alveolar macrophages induce the expansion of intra-alveolar lymphoid precursors and the recruitment of memory lymphocytes from the secondary lymphoid tissue to the lung (see Fig. 2). Dual- and three-color flow-cytometry analysis performed on lung CD8$^+$ subsets have shown that the accumulation of T cells is mainly due to two functionally distinct populations of cytotoxic cells: (1) CD3$^+$/CD8$^+$/S6F1^{bright} CTL that express the D44 determinants and have anti-HIV activity (31); and (2) CD3$^+$/CD8$^+$/S6F1^{bright} T cells bearing the natural killer (NK)-related CD56 and CD57 markers, with NK and suppressor activity, respectively (31,33).

The hypothesis that CD8 lymphocytes are recruited in response to the presence of HIV proteins and HIV-infected cells within the lung parenchyma is substantiated by several functional studies. Plata et al. for the first time pointed out that CD3$^+$/CD8$^+$/D44$^+$ CTL may lyse ^{51}Cr-labeled HIV-infected autologous alveolar macrophages (AMs) (22). The T-cell–mediated lysis of AMs is major histocompatibility complex (MHC)-restricted because anti-HLA-A, B, C and MAbs are able to completely inhibit the cytolytic activity (31). Furthermore, the P815 target cell line experimentally transfected with HLA-A2 and the HIV-related gene *env*, can be selectively lysed by BAL CD8$^+$ CTL isolated from HLA-A2 cross-matched HIV-seropositive patients (22). Taken together, these data lead to the assumption that a major component within the lymphocytic alveolitis is represented by MHC-restricted CTL that are able to recognize and attack HIV structural proteins on the surface of infected cells.

The respiratory mucosa of patients with HIV infection is also equipped with a discrete number of cells expressing the CD56 NK-associated markers and showing NK-like activity (34). Non–MHC-restricted cells represent the first line of the pulmonary host defense against tumor and microbial infections, these cells are appointed to destroy foreign material in a nonspecific manner. In patients with AIDS the $CD56^+/CD8^+$ cellular component of the alveolitis does not seem to take part in host defence mechanisms against HIV, but rather, along with alveolar macrophages, contributes to the the resistance against pulmonary opportunistic infections (34). The importance of NK- and macrophage-mediated killing in controlling the infectivity of many of these microorganisms may vary from pathogen to pathogen and during the different phases of HIV disease (34). In particular, a relation between the modifications of MHC-restricted and NK-like CTL activity and the development of opportunistic pulmonary complications has been suggested (3). The $CD8^+/D44^+$ CTL activity prevails at an early stage of HIV infection, whereas opportunistic infections are generally controlled by the NK-like cells, which are more expanded in the advanced phases of the disease (3).

B. Cell Adhesion Molecules Initiate the Migration of $CD8^+$ Cytotoxic T Lymphocytes to Sites of Pulmonary Inflammation

As in other interstitial lung diseases, lung T lymphocytes scattered throughout the pulmonary parenchyma of patients with HIV infection have undergone prior activation. In fact, $CD8^+$ cells recirculating within the lung tissue of HIV-infected subjects express the CD45RO memory phenotype and high levels of adhesion receptors, selectins, and leukocyte integrins, including CD18, CD49d, CD69, and CD103 (3; see Fig. 2).

Recent data strengthened the emerging significance of the expression of adhesion molecules by endothelial cells in lung immunity. The expression of intercellular adhesion molecules (ICAMs; CD54 and CD102) and vascular cell adhesion molecule (VCAM-1; CD106) molecules on pulmonary endothelium is induced by inflammatory mediators that are locally released by lung immunocompetent cells following HIV infection (9; Fig. 3). Under certain conditions cytokines (such as IL-1 and TNF-α) and bacterial products (including lipopolysaccharide) upregulate the expression of mRNA for adhesion molecules on endothelial cells. Through the release of cytokines antigen-activated T cells, alveolar and interstitial macrophages, and other mucosal and intra-alveolar accessory cells (dendritic and endothelial cells) expand the pool of memory cells within the inflamed areas. Keeping in mind that adhesion molecules help the interaction of lymphocytes with the cellular and extracellular matrix components (35), it is likely that the heightened expression of CAMs in pulmonary vessels allows HIV-specific effector cells to extravasate efficiently from secondary lymphoid tissues to the inflamed pulmonary parenchyma. Conceivably, the local release of cytokines contributes to the magnitude of the cytotoxic response.

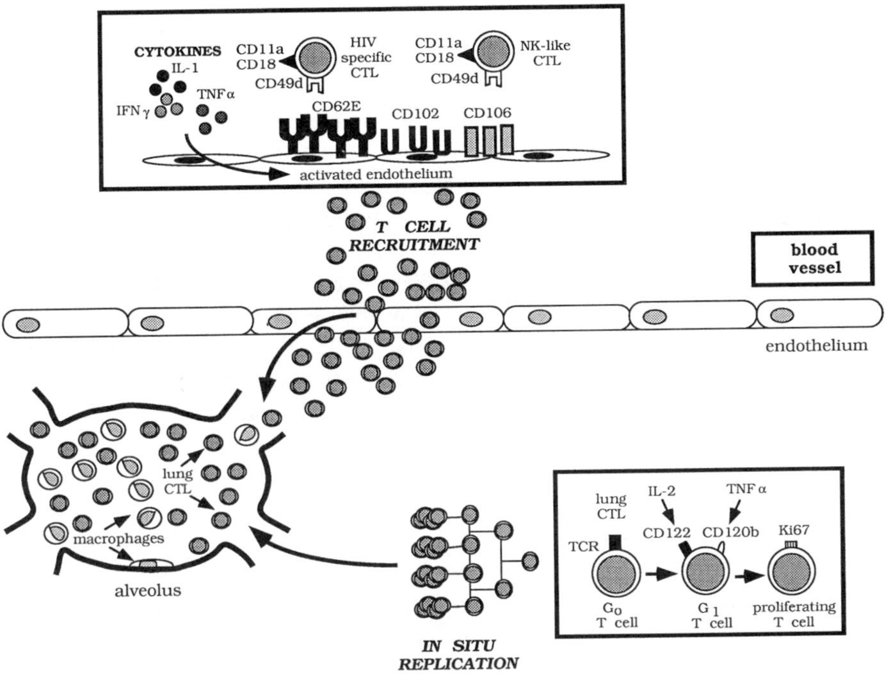

Figure 3 Mechanisms possibly involved in the development of T-cell alveolitis in patients with HIV infection. T-cell redistribution and in situ IL-2 and TNF-α-dependent proliferation of pulmonary T cells. T-cell recruitment is the result of the binding of CD11a and VD49d molecules expressed on the cell surface of primed lymphocytes to ligands expressed by the cytokine-activated endothelium (including CD62E, CD102, and CD106). The consequent binding of memory T cells to inflamed endothelium determines the tendency of primed lymphocytes to localize at sites of inflammation. Cytokine-mediated in situ replication of CTL involve the induction of IL-2 synthesis in pulmonary T_H1 cells as an early competence step likely triggered by HIV itself or related proteins. In parallel, alveolar macrophages release high amounts of TNF-α in response to HIV or opportunistic infections. Because of their repeated exposure to HIV-infected cells, CTL express maximal levels of the membrane receptors for IL-2 (CD122) and the p75 TNF-R (CD120b). The binding of IL-2 and TNF-α to their receptors initiates the progression of the cell cycles leading to the replication of the T cell.

C. Cytokine-Mediated T-Cell Proliferation Is Involved in the Pathogenesis of Alveolitis

In HIV disease, a high number of BAL T cells express the cell–cycle-related Ki67 antigen, supporting the possibility that an in situ lymphocyte proliferation occurs (3). Moreover, recent findings suggest that the interactions between cytokine receptors and their ligands might define regulatory networks that contribute to the lymphocyte proliferation in the pulmonary microenvironment. In particular, three cytokines (i.e., IL-2, TNF-α, and MIP-1α) have been involved in the development of CD8 alveolitis (see Fig. 3).

Direct evidence that IL-2 contributes to the growth of the T cells in alveolitis has been recently provided by studies showing that HIV-associated interstitial pneumonia is characterized by a compartmentalized IL-2 production within the lung and by discrete BAL levels of IL-2 (36,37). Furthermore, lung T cells of patients with HIV infection bear CD45RO and *bcl*-2 antigens, suggesting the persistence of IL-2 or stimulating antigens in the surrounding environment (3). In fact, recent reports emphasize the crucial role of *bcl*-2 in blocking apoptosis and selecting mature T cells for survival after IL-2–mediated activation (38). A high expression of this gene, which was first identified at the site of translocations common to follicular lymphoma, protects lymphoid cells from programmed cell death when IL-2 is withdrawn. By contrast, a reduced *bcl*-2 expression after immune stimulation of CD45RO T cells renders these cells prone to apoptosis and suicide, providing a physiological mechanism for the clearence of primed cells. As discussed in the previous sections, HIV-associated alveolitis is characterized by an accumulation of T cells, mostly bearing CD8 phenotype. Whether a dysregulation of the *bcl*-2 and Fas–fas-L apoptosis control systems may lead to an abnormal persistence of the CD8 immune response into the pulmonary microenvironment, favoring the development of the immune-mediated damage of the lung tissue (see later), still remains to be elucidated.

Other findings are consistent with the hypothesis that IL-2 might act as a growth factor for T lymphocytes infiltrating lung tissues of patients with AIDS. The BAL $CD8^+$ cells from patients with AIDS and T-cell alveolitis express the p75 and, to some extent, the p55 chains of the IL-2 receptor (CD122 and CD25, respectively; 39,40; see Fig. 2). Furthermore, more than 90% of BAL CD8 cells efficiently bind IL-2 (39). When one considers that the binding of IL-2 to its receptors initiates the progression of the cell cycle leading to the replication of the T cell, these data emphasize the potential role of the IL-2–IL-2R system in the mechanisms leading to the activation and amplification of the pulmonary inflammatory process during HIV infection. It is also possible that IL-2 binding might be important in the regulation of the potential capabilities of cytotoxic T cells. Clearly, the in situ release of IL-2 reaches its highest levels during the early phases of the infection, when the number of lung CD4 cells is near the normal range. It remains to be established whether HIV upregulates IL-2 release per se in the pulmonary environment by infecting activated pulmonary T cells (41).

The evidence that TNF-α is able to provide costimulatory proliferative signals for T cells and that high amounts of TNF-α are released by alveolar macrophages during HIV infection (24–26) raises a second intriguing possibility (i.e., that this proinflammatory cytokine may amplify the IL-2-mediated local proliferation of T cells). To test this hypothesis in a recent study we evaluated the expression of TNF receptors (TNF-R) by T cells and the effect of TNF-α on the local IL-2–mediated proliferative activity (40; see Fig. 3). The upregulation of the expression of some members of the TNF-R superfamily; specifically, CD120b (i.e., the type 2 receptor for TNF-α) was observed to be highly expressed by T cells retrieved by the BAL of patients with AIDS. Furthermore, lung CTL could be induced to proliferate by the costimulation with IL-2 and TNF-α.

When viewing these data as a whole it is tempting to draw the conclusion that, as in other interstitial lung disorders, the compartmentalization of IL-2 and TNF-α secretion may represent a crucial step in the expansion of the pulmonary HIV-specific CTL pool in the lung. Alternatively, CD120b could participate in the regulation of the lytic activity of pulmonary CTL. It is also possible that other cytokines may deliver a direct proliferative signal for lung CTL. In particular, Twigg et al. (23) provided detailed data showing that alveolar macrophages from HIV-infected subjects enhance the proliferative activity of allogeneic T cells through the release of IL-1 and IL-6 and other unknown factors.

Another member of the TNF-R superfamily expressed by pulmonary CTL is Fas antigen (CD95). This molecule is expressed at high levels by chronically stimulated T cells and is believed to play an important role in limiting the expansion of antigen-reactive T cells (42). Under appropriate conditions, Fas protein mediates T-cell apoptosis after ligation with a specific ligand (Fas-L), thereby preventing excessive accumulation of antigen-activated lymphocytes (42). Interestingly, Fas is overexpressed by pulmonary $CD8^+$ CTL (43; see Fig. 2). The high expression of this molecule is consistent with the pathophysiology of the high-intensity T-cell alveolitis during HIV disease and supports a role for the Fas/Fas-L control system in limiting the development of T-cell alveolitis.

D. Genomic and Expressed T-Cell Antigen Receptor Repertoire in Lung T Cells

A brief description of the molecular structure of TCR–CD3 complex genes and products is needed to introduce the issue of the genomic and expressed TCR repertoire in HIV infection. The specific recognition of antigens involves specific receptors on the surface of immunocompetent cells. Whereas in B cells the receptor that recognizes antigen in soluble form is represented by a surface immunoglobulin, the membrane-bound TCR represents the T-cell structure devoted to the recognition of foreign peptides of an antigen processed in the context of a MHC molecule by an antigen-presenting cell (APC). There are four distinct antigen-binding chains (α, β, γ, and δ) expressed as mutually exclusive heterodimers (i.e., the α/β and γ/δ receptors; 44); in humans, most mature T cells use the α/β TCR. These two complexes of transmembrane heterodimers are associated with at least six CD3 peptides, which are believed to trigger the cell when the TCR binds the antigen (44).

Similar to immunoglobulins on B cells, the antigen specificity and diversity of the TCR arise through the rearrangement of the large repertoire of variable (V), diversity (D), joining (J), and constant (C) gene regions of the TCR segments during T-cell ontogenity. More than 10^{16} possible V(D)J junctional combinations may exist for the α/β and γ/δ heterodimers. Use of MAbs to the α, β, γ, and δ chains of the TCR that have specificity for defined V regions, together with DNA molecular analysis of the α/β or the γ/δ TCR genes allow one to verify whether the cell population we are dealing with is composed of cells consistently possessing an identical TCR rearrangement (monoclonal expansion), by cells belonging to a limited number of clones (oligoclonal expansion), or by a multitude of cells that are different from each other (polyclonal expansion). Both these techniques have been applied to the study of the TCR repertoire in the lungs of patients with interstitial lung diseases.

With the aim of studying the model that governs the accumulation of T cells at the lung level, the expression and the configuration of CD3–TCR complex shown by pulmonary and peripheral blood T cells in patients with AIDS and high-intensity T-cell alveolits was recently investigated. By using the WT31 MAb that recognizes the α/β TCR, it has been demonstrated that most BAL T cells from healthy individuals coexpress the α/β TCR (3). By contrast, only a few normal lung cells (about 5%) stain with the TCRδl MAb that recognizes a common epitope of the δ-chain, apparently expressed by all γ/δ TCR cells (45). Most pulmonary $CD3^+$ cells accumulating in the lung of HIV-infected patients express the α/β TCR (3), as do normal T cells. However, in a subset of patients with AIDS a small, but definite, proportion of peripheral blood lymphocytes (ranging from 5 up to 40% of BAL T cells) stains with MAbs that recognize T-cells bearing γ/δ TCR (46–48). The γ/δ^+ TCR cell pool can be subdivided in two nonoverlapping cell populations, termed Vδ1 and Vδ2, based on the absence or presence of an interchain disulfide bond (45). The disulfide-linked form of γ/δ TCR is identified by the BB3 (Vδ2) MAb, whereas A13/TCS-δ1 MAbs define the non–disulfide-linked type of γ/δ TCR. Although in normal individuals BB3$^+$ Vδ2$^+$-related T cells account for two-thirds of the total γ/δ pool, in patients with AIDS and pulmonary complications, most circulating γ/δ TCR lymphocytes are TCS-δ1$^+$ (Vδ1$^+$) (46–48); this leads to a decrease in the peripheral blood Vδ2/Vδ1 ratio.

We have offered a putative explanation for the mechanisms leading to the alteration of the Vδ2/Vδ1 ratio in the peripheral blood of patients with AIDS. A selective expansion of γ/δ TCR lymphocytes takes place in the lungs of a subgroup of patients with AIDS and *Pneumocysits carinii* pneumonia (46,49–51). Specifically, we observed that BB3$^+$ Vδ2$^+$-related cells account for the most lung γ/δ TCR cells that can be recovered from the BAL of patients with HIV infection and PCP. The increase in the Vδ2$^+$ cells is observed in the microenvironment where the immune response against *P. carinii* takes place, strongly suggesting the hypothesis that target antigens (including *P. carinii* antigens) or environmental stimuli may favor the selective migration of Vδ2$^+$/BB3$^+$ cells from the peripheral blood to the lung (51). In this scenario, the depletion of BB3$^+$ cells in the peripheral blood (and the consequent increase in the relative percentage of A13$^+$/Vδ1$^+$ cells) is likely to represent an epiphenomenon, related to the redistribution of Vδ2$^+$ cells to the sites of PCP-associated inflammation (51).

To verify whether lung CD8 cells respond to one or more antigenic stimuli, the molecular structure of the TCR gene in patients with AIDS has been investigated. The large diversity of the α- and β-chains and, hence, the diversity of T cells toward vast numbers of antigens is based on the rearrangement of the large repertoire of V, D, J, and C segments (44). The study of the molecular organization of the TCR also makes it possible to determine whether proliferating cells show a preferential usage of definite gene regions in response to a specific antigenic stimulation, thereby indicating an ordered immune response in which the TCR has been stimulated. By using specific MAbs against different V regions of the TCR and the PCR analysis, we showed a marked quantitative skewing in the usage of Vβ chain regions of the TCR in the lungs of patients with HIV infection, with an overexpression of T cells bearing some Vβ region segments (52,53). Several data in humans suggest that T cells expressing certain V genes are preferentially stimulated by specific "superantigens," including those derived from *Staphylococcus aureus* and *Mycobacterium tuberculosis* (54). The discovery that retrovirus-derived "superantigens" are involved in the pathology of murine retrovirus infection (55) suggests the hypothesis that HIV-encoded superantigens, by activating or deleting relevant T-cell subsets, may contribute to the pathogenesis of T-cell alveolitis. Given the known similarities between HIV proteins and several known enterotoxins (56), it might also be hypothesized that bacterial products released during opportunistic and nonopportunistic pulmonary infections might drive T-cell selection by inducing either expansion or reduction of HIV-specific T cells bearing particular Vβ gene products. Proliferative studies, in presence of bacterial endotoxins, that show areas of sequence homology with HIV are needed to verify this hypothesis.

E. The Progressive Impairment of Cytotoxic T-Lymphocyte Activity Correlates with the Development of Opportunistic Infections

Despite the presence of cytotoxic T cells in BAL fluid, which theoretically should confer a resistant state against HIV, these highly specialized effectors fail to protect the patients against a progression toward AIDS. Indeed, an ongoing impairment of CTL efficiency can be demonstrated, with development of clinical AIDS (57). In addition, pulmonary NK-like CTL activity declines in advanced stages of HIV disease (34). It has thus been hypothesized that pathogens cause disseminated opportunistic infections in persons with waning immune function of pulmonary NK cells (3).

Various factors have been implicated in the downregulation of HIV-specific and NK-like CTL populations with time (Fig. 4). Likely, HIV infectiveness of CD8 cells may contribute to the fall in lytic activity (19). Other factors that could be involved with the loss of cytotoxic response along with progression toward AIDS include (1) the decrease or the functional impairment of $CD4^+$ cells; (2) the progressive inability to produce in situ biological response modifiers that are essential for the effectiveness of cytotoxic T cells (including IL-2 and TNF-α); (3) the inappropriate secretion of inhibitory cytokines (TGF-β, IL-10; 58); (4) the emergence of HIV variants; and (5) the in vivo production of soluble inhibitors of cytolytic function. Moreover, because there is a short region of sequence homology between Fas and gp120 HIV protein (59), it is also possible that anti-gp 120 antibodies might cross-react with Fas to transmit an apoptosis-inducing signal, thereby contributing to the progressive loss of the cytotoxic activity by lung $CD8^+$ cells, which overexpress CD95.

Concerning the in vivo production of soluble inhibitors of cytolytic function, a recent study has suggested the active role of suppressor T cells in the release of factors that downmodulate the cytotoxic immune responses against HIV. In a longitudinal analysis Sadat-Sowti et al. (60) demonstrated that $CD57^+/CD8^+$ suppressor T cells are expanded in the lung of patients with advanced HIV infection and that the accumulation of these cells mirrors the progressive decrease of pulmonary CTL efficiency. Interestingly, $CD57^+/CD8^+$ cells release a glycosylated non–antigen-specific soluble

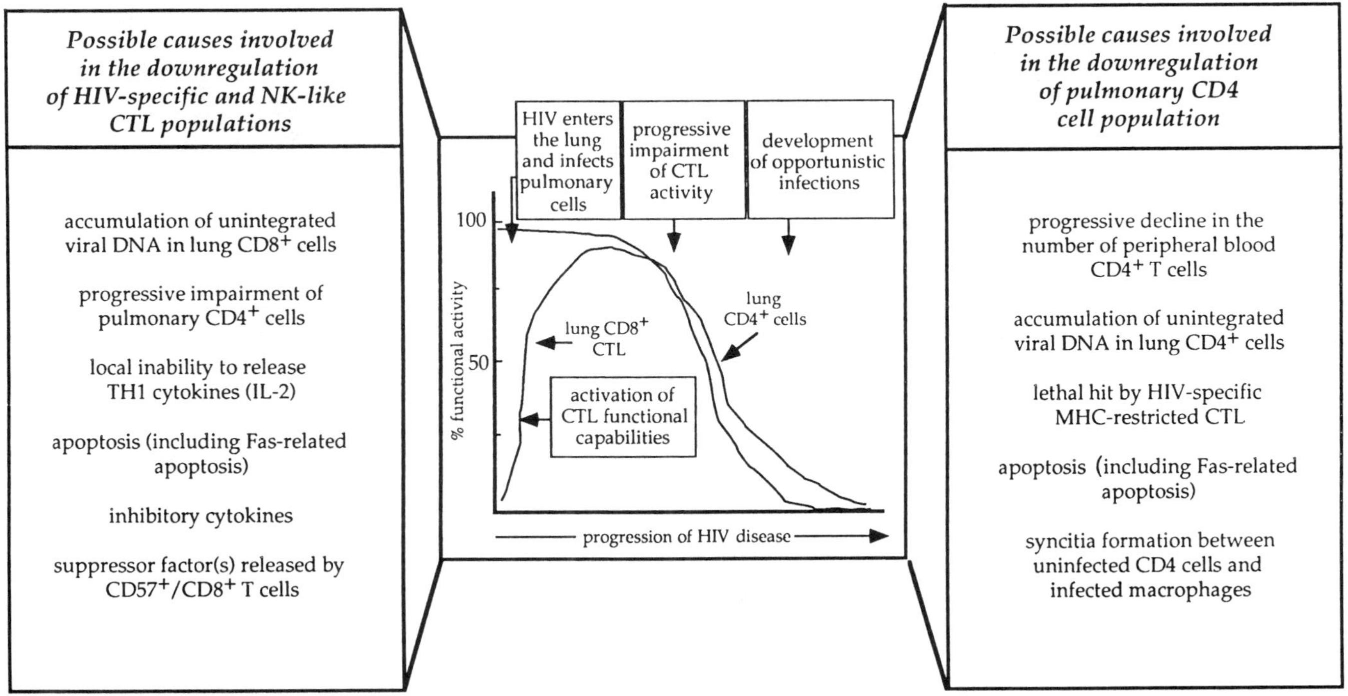

Figure 4 Mechanisms possibly involved in the impairment of cytotoxic machinery and in the progressive depletion of $CD4^+$ cells in the lung of HIV-infected patients. HIV-1 enters the lung and causes the gradual depletion of the $CD4^+$ cells and, as a consequence, the inability to produce in situ biological response modifiers that are essential for the effectiveness of cytotoxic cells. The in situ impairment of the helper population leads to the progressive reduction of the function of HIV-1-specific CTL, facilitating the spreading of the virus into the lung microenvironment. Inasmuch as cells with NK-like activity represent one of the first lines of natural resistance against infections, the lack of killing capacity of pulmonary NK cells leads to an enhanced susceptibility to serious opportunistic infections. The percentages on the abscissa are related to the absolute number of $CD4^+$ cells and the cytotoxic functions in a healthy HIV-1 seropositive individual. The relations between the time course of the absolute number of $CD4^+$ cells and the activity of cytotoxic cells are largely hypothetical. (From Refs. 10 and 34.)

inhibitor of cytotoxic function that has the capability of downregulating NK-, LAK-, and MHC-restricted CTL activities and is distinct from cytokines that have been described to induce negative effects on lymphocyte function (60).

Therefore, it is possible that this still-uncharacterized protein could block a common step of the cytolytic process in cytotoxic T cells, independently of the target cell-specific recognition. Noteworthy is that the cell-to-cell contact between pulmonary CTL and targets is not affected by HIV infection (34). Furthermore, the secretion of this soluble inhibitor of cytolytic function occurs irrespective of HIV infection and is not linked to the presence of HIV proteins (60). Efforts should be expanded to definitively characterize the inhibitor factor(s) produced by pulmonary $CD57^+$/$CD8^+$ cells during HIV infection.

IV. Relation Between $CD8^+$ Cell Alveolitis and the Development of Respiratory Failure

Abnormalities of pulmonary function tests are present not only in HIV-seropositive patients with diffuse disease of the lung parenchyma, but also in symptomless individuals without abnormalities on chest radiographs (61). In particular, common alterations throughout the course of HIV infection are a low carbon monoxide diffusing capacity (DL_{CO}), caused by an impairment of the exchanging ability of the alveolar capillary membrane and an abnormal oxygenation that is present in virtually all PCP patients after exercise. Additionally, patients infected with HIV, but without identifiable lung infections or neoplasms have a reduction in mean DL_{CO} values and accelerated DTPA clearance. Interestingly, abnormal DL_{CO} in the absence of lung disease represents a marker of HIV-induced immunosuppression and, therefore, is a predictor of a more rapid progression to AIDS (62).

The finding that HIV-seropositive individuals with no evidence of lung disease may have a high-intensity alveolitis associated with a reduction in DL_{CO} supports the suggestion that local inflammation plays a role in the progressive decline of pulmonary function tests. Phillips et al. recently showed that HIV may spread to epithelia (63), which may behave as target cells for HIV-specific effector T cells. This line of reasoning implies that the respiratory epithelium may represent a potential target for CTL that, during immune-mediated response against HIV, are recruited from blood to the interstitium and then to the epithelial surface. As a matter of fact, a strong correlation exists between the degree of $CD8^+$ alveolitis and the value of epithelia permeability, as determined by the pulmonary clearance of inhaled ^{99m}Tc-diethylenetriamine pentaacetate (DPTA-Cl; 64). Abnormalities of PaO_2 are also independently associated with the increase in the absolute number of alveolar CD8 cells (64).

The foregoing data raise the central issue of whether the study of BAL cells and products provides additional information relevant to survival among HIV-infected persons. The prognostic usefulness of morphological and immunological evaluations of BAL cell populations in determining the mortality risk in HIV infection has been taken into consideration by several groups (10,11,65,66). The risk of death is greatly increased in HIV-seropositive individuals with opportunistic infections and BAL neutrophilia, whereas in patients without histological, cultural, or cytological confirmation of pulmonary opportunistic infections, the most important variable with predictive value appears to be the number of pulmonary $CD8^+$ lymphocytes. Although the foregoing studies indicate the predictive value of BAL cell analysis, they were based on a restrospective evaluation of data obtained from selected groups of patients belonging to the IV CDC group who developed a fatal opportunistic infection after a variable period subsequent to the BAL analysis. However, the small number of patients made it impossible to obtain highly statistically significant values. Even more importantly, information on changes of the individual BAL parameters over time are still lacking. Longitudinal studies of BAL findings in a large number of HIV-infected patients followed from an asymptomatic stage until the diagnosis of AIDS are thus mandatory to clearly define the natural course of the respiratory illness in persons with HIV infection.

V. Concluding Remarks

Several pieces of evidence highlight the intriguing virus–host networks that take place in the lung of HIV-infected patients. A variety of studies now indicate that both lung $CD4^+$ and $CD8^+$ T cells represent a major reservoir for HIV infection. More knowledge is surely mandatory in the area of the complex relation between local T-cell–mediated immunity and AIDS-associated pulmonary diseases. Through virological and immunological studies we hope to gain new models of treatment for the disease state characterized by the functional impairment of the lung host defenses. In particular, investigations directly correlating HIV burden in BAL T cells, CTL activity, and clinical outcome appear to be warranted to accurately delineate the natural history of HIV infection in the lung. Another issue that needs to be solved in the near future is related to the possibility of modulating the pulmonary immune response against HIV. The recent availability of immunoregulatory drugs that alter the local production of biological response modifiers or effector functions of pulmonary lymphocyte subsets might help in attaining this goal. A more complete understanding of the synergies between cytokines and the local HIV load will also help in planning therapeutic interventions with combinations of cytokines.

Currently, there is also intensive investigation underway to uncover ways to develop a scoring system that will allow a risk stratification among HIV-infected patients with pulmonary complications. Multicentric cooperative studies were recently designed to examine the possibility of using BAL cell findings and other markers, such as viral burden or cytokine levels in the BAL fluid in determining mortality and morbidity risk (57). The BAL data should be correlated with demographic, clinical, and immunological variables of HIV infection. This approach will facilitate early recognition of cases that are at the greatest risk of death, and thus, most likely to benefit from early intervention with therapeutic agents that can prevent pulmonary complications, including pentamidine or other prophylactic agents. Given the high morbidity and mortality that is associated with the development of pulmonary complications in an asymptomatic HIV-seropositive patient, it will also be important to assess the validity and the possibility of extending the use of these prognostic determinants to individuals with early HIV disease. Such approaches should provide predictive information in a timely manner for those HIV-infected patients who are at risk for developing disabling illness without other unnecessary discomfort for those patients who show a low or no risk for respiratory complications.

Acknowledgments

The authors wish to thank their colleagues who contributed to the original studies discussed in this paper (Refs. 5, 9, 10, 19, 25, 27–29, 32, 34, 39, 40, 43, 46, and 51–53). We also wish to thank Mr. Martin Donach for his help in the preparation of the manuscript. Supported by a grant from Ministero della Sanità, Istituto Superiore di Sanità (MS/ISS), Progetto AIDS 1995 (Rome, Italy).

References

1. Semenzato G, Agostini C. [Editorial]. Human retroviruses and lung involvement. Am Rev Respir Dis 1989; 139:1317–1322.
2. Rankin JA, Collman R, Daniele RP. Acquired immunodeficiency syndrome and the lung. Chest 1988; 94:155–164.
3. Agostini C, Trentin L, Zambello R, Semenzato G. [State of the Art]. HIV-1 and lung. Infectivity, pathogenic mechanisms and cellular immune response taking place in the lower respiratory tract. Am Rev Respir Dis 1993; 147:1038–1041.

4. Davis L, Beck JM, Shellito J. Update: HIV infection and pulmonary host defenses. Semin Respir Infect 1993; 8:75–85.
5. Mayaud CM, Cadranel J. HIV in the lung: guilt or not guilt. Thorax 1993; 48:1191–1195.
6. Landay AL, Schade SZ, Takefman DM, Kuhns MC, McNamara AL, Rosen RL, Kessler HA, Spear GT. Detection of HIV-1 provirus in bronchoalveolar lavage cells by polymerase chain reaction. J Acquir Immune Defic Syndr 1993; 6:1721–1726.
7. Clarke JR, Taylor IK, Fleming J, Nukuna A, Williamson JD, Mitchell DM. The epidemiology of HIV-1 infection of the lung in AIDS patients. AIDS 1993; 7:555–560.
8. Sierra Madero JG, Toossi Z, Hom DL, Finegan CK, Hoenig E, Rich EA. Relationship between load of virus in alveolar macrophages from human immunodeficiency virus type 1-infected persons, production of cytokines, and clinical status. J Infect Dis 1994; 169:18–27.
9. Agostini C, Chilosi M, Trentin L, Zambello R, Semenzato G. Pulmonary immune cells in health and disease. Lymphocytes. Eur Respir J 1993; 6:1378–1401.
10. Agostini C, Zambello R, Trentin L, Poletti V, Spiga L, Gritti F, Cipriani A, Salmaso L, Cadrobbi P, Semenzato G. Prognostic significance of the evaluation of bronchoalveolar lavage populations in patients with HIV-1 infection and pulmonary involvement. Chest 1991; 100:1601–1606.
11. Guillon JM Autran B, Denis M, Fouret P, Plata F, Mayaud CM, Akoun GM. Human immunodeficiency virus-related lymphocytic alveolitis. Chest 1988; 94:1264–1270.
12. Young KR, Rankin JA, Naegel GP, Paul ES, Reynolds HY. Bronchoalveolar lavage cells and proteins in patients with the acquired immunodeficiency syndrome: an immunological analysis. Ann Intern mMed 1985; 103:522–533.
13. Pantaleo G, Graziosi C, Demarest JF, Cohen OJ, Vaccarezza M, Gantt K, Muro-Cacho C, Fauci AS. Role of lymphoid organs in the pathogenesis of human immunodeficiency virus (HIV) infection. Immunol Rev 1994; 140:105–130.
14. Donaldson YK, Bell JE, Ironside JW, Brettle RP, Robertson JR, Busuttil A, Simmonds P. Redistribution of HIV outside the lymphoid system with onset of AIDS. Lancet 1994; 343:383–385.
15. Sei S, Kleiner DE, Kopp JB, Chandra R, Klotman PE, Yarchoan R, Pizzo PA, Mitsuya H. Quantitative analysis of viral burden in tissues from adults and children with symptomatic human immunodeficiency virus type 1 infection assessed by polymerase chain reaction. J Infect Dis 1994; 170:325–333.
16. Piatak M, Saag MS, Yang LC, Clark SJ, Kappes JC, Luk KC, Hahn BH, Shaw GM, Lifson JD. High levels of HIV-1 in plasma during all stages of infection determined by competitive PCR. Science 1993; 259:1749–1754.
17. Rose RM, Krivine A, Pinkston P, Gillis JM, Huang A, Hammer SM. Frequent identification of HIV-1 DNA in bronchoalveolar lavage cells obtained from individuals with the acquired immunodeficiency syndrome. Am Rev Respir Dis 1991; 143:850–854.
18. Twigg HL, Lipscomb MF, Yoffe B, Barbaro DJ, Weissler JC. Enhanced acces-

sory cell function by alveolar macrophages from patients infected with human immunodeficiency virus and its potential role for depletion of CD4+ cells in the lung. Am J Respir Cell Mol Biol 1989; 1:391–400.
19. Semenzato G, Agostini C, Ometto L, Zambello R, Trentin L, Chiecho-Bianchi L, De Rossi A. CD8+ T lymphocytes in the lung of AIDS patients harbor human immunodeficiency virus type 1. Blood 1995; 85:2308–2314.
20. De Maria A, Pantaleo G, Schnittman SM, Grenhouse JJ, Baseler M, Orenstein JM, Fauci AS. Infection of CD8+ T lymphocytes with HIV. Requirement for interaction with infected CD4+ cells and induction of infectious virus from chronically infected CD8+ cells. J Immunol 1991; 146:2220–2229.
21. De Maria A, Colombini S, Schnittman SM, Moretta L. CD8+ cytolytic T lymphocytes become infected in vitro in the process of killing HIV-1-infected targets cells. Eur J Immunol 1994; 24:531–537.
22. Plata F, Autran B, Martins LP, Wain-Hobson S, Raphael M, Mayaud C, Denis M, Guillon JM, Debre P. AIDS-virus specific cytotoxic T lymphocytes in lung disorders. Nature 1987; 328:348–351.
23. Twigg HL, Iwamoto GK, Soliman DM. Role of cytokines in alveolar macrophage accessory function in HIV-infected individuals. J Immunol 1992; 149:1462–1469.
24. Israel-Biet D, Cadranel J, Beldjord K, Andrieu M, Jeffrey A, Even P. Tumor necrosis factor production in HIV-seropositive subjects. Relationship with lung opportunistic infections and HIV expression in alveolar macrophages. J Immunol 1991; 147:490–494.
25. Agostini C, Zambello R, Trentin L, Garbisa S, Francia di Celle P, Bulian P, Onisto M, Poletti V, Spiga L, Raise E, Foà R, Semenzato G. Alveolar macrophages from patients with AIDS and AIDS-related complex constitutively synthesize and release tumor necrosis factor alpha. Am Rev Respir Dis 1991; 143:195–201.
26. Millar AB, Miller RF, Noeleen MF, Meager A, Semple SJG, Rook GAW. Production of tumor necrosis factor-α by blood and lung mononuclear phagocytes from patients with human immunodeficiency virus-related lung disease. Am J Respir Cell Mol Biol 1991; 5:144–148.
27. Trentin L, Garbisa S, Zambello R, Agostini C, Caenazzo C, Di Francesco C, Cipriani A, Francavilla E, Semenzato G. Spontaneous production of IL-6 by alveolar macrophages of HIV-1 seropositive patients. J Infect Dis 1992; 166:731–737.
28. Agostini C, Trentin L, Zambello R, Bulian P, Garbisa S, Cipriani A, Cadrobbi P, Semenzato G. Alveolar macrophages from patients with HIV-1 infection express accessory molecules, activation markers, and release increased amounts of biological response modifiers. Chest 1993; 102 (suppl):108–112.
29. Agostini C, Trentin L, Zambello R, Bulian P, Caenazzo C, Cipriani A, Cadrobbi P, Garbisa S, Semenzato G. Release of GM-CSF by alveolar macrophages in the lung of HIV-1 infected patients. A mechanism accounting for macrophage and neutrophil accumulation. J Immunol 1992; 149:3379–3385.
30. Denis M. Ghadirian E. Alveolar macrophages from subjects infected with HIV-1 express macrophage inflammatory protein-1α (MIP-1α): contribution to CD8+ alveolitis. Clin Exp Immunol 1994; 96:187–192.

31. Autran B, Plata F, Guillon JM, Joly P, Mayaud C, Debrè P. HIV-specific cytotoxic T lymphocytes directed against alveolar macrophages in HIV-1 infected patients. Res Virol 1990; 141:131–136.
32. Agostini C, Poletti V, Zambello R, Trentin L, Siviero F, Spiga L, Gritti F, Semenzato G. Phenotypical and functional analysis of bronchoalveolar lavage lymphocytes in patients with HIV infection. Am Rev Respir Dis 1988; 138:1609–1615.
33. Joly P, Guillon JM, Mayaud C, Plata C, Theodorou I, Denis M, Debré P, Autran B. Cell-mediated suppression of HIV-specific cytotoxic T lymphocytes. J Immunol 1988; 143:2193–2202.
34. Agostini C, Zambello R, Trentin L, Feruglio C, Masciarelli M, Siviero F, Poletti V, Spiga L, Gritti F, Semenzato G. Cytotoxic events taking place in the lung of patients with HIV-1 infection. Evidence for an intrinsic defect of the MHC-unrestricted killing partially restored by incubation with rIL-2. Am Rev Respir Dis 1990; 142:516–522.
35. Furfaro S, Berman JS. The relation between cell migration and activation in inflammation: beyond adherence. Am J Respir Cell Mol Biol 1992; 7:248–250.
36. Spain BA, Soliman DM, Twigg HL III. Enhanced interleukin-2 production by lymphocytes from HIV-infected patients with lymphocytic alveolitis is compartmentalized within the lung. 1994 International Conference of the American Lung Association and the American Thoracic Society, Boston, MA, Am J Respir Crit Care Med 1994; 149:A264.
37. Biglino A, Forno B, Pollono AM, Ghio P, Albera C. Alveolar immune mediators in HIV-related pneumonia. Different role of IL-2 and IL-1 in inducing lung damage. Chest 1993; 103:439–443.
38. Akbar AN, Salmon M, Savill J, Janossy G. The role of *bcl*-2 in T cell memory a "balancing act" between cell death and survival. Immunol Today 1993; 14:256–260.
39. Zambello R, Trentin L, Benetti R, Cipriani A, Crivellaro C, Cadrobbi P, Agostini C, Semenzato G. Expression of a functional p75 interleukin-2 receptor on lung lymphocytes from patients with HIV-1 infection. J Clin Immunol 1992; 12:371–377.
40. Agostini C, Zambello R, Trentin L, Cerutti A, Enthammer C, Facco M, Milani A, Sancetta R, Garbisa S, Semenzato G. Expression of TNF receptors by T cells and membrane TNFα by alveolar macrophages suggests a role for TNFα in the regulation of the local immune responses in the lung of HIV-1–infected patients. J Immunol 1995; 155:2928–2938.
41. Westendorp MO, Li-Weber M, Frank RW, Krammer PH. Human immunodeficiency virus type 1 *tat* upregulates interleukin-2 secretion in activated T cells. J Virol 1994; 68:4177–4185.
42. Alderson MR, Tough TW, Davis-Smith T, Braddy S, Falk B, Schooley KA, Goodwin RG, Smith CA, Ramsdell F, Lynch DH. Fas ligand mediates activation induced cell death in human T lymphocytes. J Exp Med 1995; 181:71–82.
43. Agostini C, Zambello R, Sancetta R, Cerutti A, Milani A, Tassinari C, Cipriani A, Trentin L, Semenzato G. Expression of TNF-receptor superfamily members

by lung T lymphocytes. A putative role in the maintenance of the T cell alveolitis in patients with interstitial lung disease. (submitted).
44. Moss PAH, Rosenberg WMC, Bell JI. The human T cell receptor in health and disease. Annu Rev Immunol 1992; 10:71–96.
45. Moretta L, Ciccone E, Ferrini S, Pelicci PG, Mingari MC, Zeromski J, Bottino C, Grossi C, Moretta A. Molecular and cellular analysis of human T lymphocytes expressing γδ T-cell receptor. Immunol Rev 1991; 120:117–135.
46. Agostini C, Zambello R, Trentin L, Cerutti A, Bulian P, Crivellaro C, Cipriani A, Semenzato G. γ/δ T cell receptor subsets in the lung of patients with HIV-1 infection. Cell Immunol 1994; 153:194–205.
47. Autran B, Triebel F, Katlama C, Rozenbaum W, Hercend T, Debre P. T-cell receptor gamma/delta lymphocyte subsets during HIV infection. Clin Exp Immunol 1989; 75:206–210.
48. De Maria A, Ferrazin A, Ferrini S, Ciccone E, Terragna A, Moretta L. Selective increase of a subset of T cell receptor γδ T lymphocytes in the peripheral blood of patients with human immunodeficiency virus type 1 infection. J Infect Dis 1992; 164:917–919.
49. Kagi MK, Fierz W, Grob PJ, Russi EW. High proportion of gamma–delta T cell receptor positive T cells in bronchoalveolar lavage and peripheral blood of HIV-infected patients with *Pneumocystis carinii* pneumonias. Respiration 1993; 60:170–177.
50. Perrella O, Perrella A, Soscia E, Marinelli A, Minnini V, Guerriero S, Briante R, Finelli L. What is the role of T-lymphocytes with gamma/delta receptors in *Pneumocystis carinii* pneumonia in AIDS patients? AIDS 1994; 8:395–396.
51. Agostini C, Zambello R, Trentin L, Semenzato G. T-lymphocytes with γ/δ T cell receptors in patients with AIDS and *Pneumocystis carinii* pneumonia. AIDS 1995; 9:203–204.
52. Semenzato G, Zambello R, Trentin L, Sancetta R, Enthammer C, Facco M, Tassinari C, Agostini C. Immune mechanisms in the lung during human immunodeficiency virus infection. Reg Immunol 1995; (in press).
53. Trentin L, Zambello R, Cerutti A, Enthammer C, Sancetta R, Facco M, Cipriani A, Agostini C, Semenzato G. Discrete usage of T-cell receptor Vβ gene regions in the lung of patients with interstitial lung diseases. Lymphocyte Activation, Keystone Symposia on Molecular and Cellular Biology. Keystone, CO. J Cell Biochem 1994; 18D:348.
54. Gascoigne NRJ. Interaction of the T cell receptor with bacterial superantigens. Semin Immunol 1993; 5:13–19.
55. Hugin AW, Vacchio MS, Morse HC. A virus-encoded "superantigen" in a retrovirus-induced immunodeficiency syndrome in mice. Science 1991; 252:424–427.
56. Bisset LR, Fierz W. Areas of sequence homology between several staphylococcal exotoxin "superantigens" and the HIV-1 *pol* protein. AIDS Res Hum Retroviruses 1992; 8:1543–1545.
57. Hoffenbach A, Langlade-Demoyen P, Dadaglio G, Vilmer E, Michel F, Mayaud

C, Autran B, Plata F. Unusually high frequencies of HIV-specific cytotoxic T lymphocytes in humans. J Immunol 1989; 142:452–462.
58. Akridge RE, Oyafuso LKM, Reed SG. IL-10 is induced during HIV-1 infection and is capable of decreasing viral replication in human macrophages. J Immunol 1994; 153:5782–5789.
59. Szawlowski PWS, Hanke T, Randall RE. Sequence homology between HIV-1 gp 120 and the apoptosis mediating Fas protein. AIDS 1993; 7:1018–1025.
60. Sadat-Sowti B, Parrot A, Quint L, Mayaud C, Debre P, Autran B. Alveolar $CD8^+/CD57^+$ lymphocytes in human immunodeficiency virus infection produce an inhibitor of cytotoxic function. Am J Respir Crit Care Med 1994; 149:972–980.
61. Agostini C, Semenzato G. Does bronchoalveolar lavage analysis provide a tool to monitor disease progression or predict survival in patients with HIV-1 infection? Thorax 1994; 49:848–851.
62. Nieman RB, Fleming J, Coker RJ, Harris JR, Mitchell DM. Reduced carbon monoxide transfer factor (TLCO) in human immunodeficiency virus type I (HIV-I) infection as a predictor for faster progression of AIDS. Thorax 1993; 48:481–485.
63. Phillips DM, Bourinbaiar AS. Mechanisms of HIV spread to epithelia. Virology 1992; 186:261–267.
64. Meignan M, Guilon JM, Denis M, Joly P, Rosso J, Carette MF. Increased lung epithelia permeability in HIV-infected patients with isolated cytotoxic T lymphocytic alveolitis. Am Rev Respir Dis 1990; 141:1241–1248.
65. Mason GR, Hashimoto CH, Dickman PS, Foutty LF, Cobb CJ. Prognostic implications of bronchoalveolar lavage neutrophilia in patients with *Pneumocystis carinii* pneumonia and AIDS. Am Rev Respir Dis 1989; 139:1336–1342.
66. Jensen BN, Lisse IM, Gerstoft J, Borgeskov S, Skinhoj P. Cellular profiles in bronchoalveolar lavage fluid of HIV-infected patients with pulmonary symptoms: relation to diagnosis and prognosis. AIDS 1991; 5:527–533.

7

HIV and Alveolar Macrophage Function

HOMER L. TWIGG III

Indiana University Medical Center
Indianapolis, Indiana

I. Introduction

Perhaps nowhere else in the body is the relation between HIV and host cells more critical than in the lung. Cells in the alveolar space must constantly differentiate potential pathogenic organisms and particles they are exposed to from the vast array of nonspecific antigens and pollutants inhaled with each breath. Evolution has led to the current state in which cells present in the alveolar milieu are generally poor initiators of immune and inflammatory responses. This protective adaptation allows the lung to continue to serve its primary function—namely, gas exchange—in the absence of chronic inflammation induced by inhaled foreign material.

The alveolar macrophage (AM), being the principal cell found in the alveolar space, plays a central role in regulating pulmonary inflammatory and immune responses. After appropriate stimulation, AM can carry out a wide variety of functions. However, in response to evolutionary pressures to minimize unnecessary inflammation in the lower respiratory tract, these cells have developed relatively poor inflammatory and immunological capabilities. For example, although they have exceptional phagocytic abilities, AMs have a poor capacity to mount subsequent inflammatory processes required for killing of intracellular organisms. The alveolar macrophage is also a relatively inactive immune cell, compared with other cells of monocyte–macrophage lineage. This does not imply that the AM cannot participate in immune and inflammatory responses. In certain conditions, usually resulting in cellular activation, the AM can demonstrate potent function in these areas.

Human immunodeficiency virus (HIV) infection has profound effects on alveolar macrophage function, thereby threatening the homeostatic balance between proinflammatory and suppressive responses. This chapter will focus on the effects of HIV infection on alveolar macrophage function and examine potential implications of these changes. It should be stated that most studies examining the effects of HIV on macrophage function have been performed in monocytes or monocyte-derived macrophages. Few studies have specifically examined alveolar macrophage function. From the foregoing discussion, it is apparent that the alveolar compartment represents an unique environment in which macrophages must function. Thus, extrapolation from studies performed on other cells of monocyte–macrophage lineage must be made with caution. This distinction will be emphasized throughout this chapter.

II. Mechanisms of HIV Effects on Alveolar Macrophages

HIV can affect alveolar macrophage function through many potential mechanisms (Table 1). As discussed in Chapter 5, AM can be infected by HIV

Table 1 Mechanisms by Which HIV May Affect Alveolar Macrophages

1. Direct effect of HIV infection
   - A. On macrophage accessory cell function
   - B. On macrophage cytokine secretion
2. HIV-induced alterations in the alveolar milieu
   - A. Decreased $CD4^+$ T cells
     - Potential decreased interferon-γ
   - B. Increased $CD8^+$ T cells
     - Potential increased interferon-γ
     - Cytotoxic to HIV-infected macrophages
   - C. Increased secretion of macrophage cytokines
   - D. Alterations in surfactant
3. Direct effect of HIV proteins
   - A. On cellular (especially T-cell) proliferation
   - B. On T-cell and macrophage cytokine secretion

(1–3). Numerous studies have documented a direct effect of HIV infection on AM cytokine secretion and expression of surface molecules important in immunological responses. However, this infection is usually in the latent form, with very little detectable viral mRNA or protein found unless AM are stimulated in vitro (3,4). In addition, the actual number of infected AM varies with the stage of infection, being low early and increasing as patients progress to the acquired immunodeficiency syndrome (AIDS) (5). Because AMs demonstrate functional alterations even early in infection, other HIV effects must be operational.

A second mechanism by which HIV may effect AM function is through alterations in the cellular and biochemical makeup of the alveolar environment. HIV infection is accompanied by a decrease in the percentage of $CD4^+$ lymphocytes and an increase in the percentage and absolute number of $CD8^+$ lymphocytes in bronchoalveolar lavage (BAL; 6–8). Because $CD4^+$ memory cells are preferentially infected early in HIV infection (9,10) and they are an important source of interferon gamma (IFN-γ) (11), early HIV infection could be characterized by a relative lack of this important macrophage-activating cytokine. On the other hand, studies show that the $CD8^+$ lymphocytes that accumulate in the alveolar space of HIV-infected individuals are HIV-specific cytotoxic T cells (12,13). Because HIV-specific cytotoxic T lymphocytes release IFN-γ when they encounter infected target cells (14), they may make up for the loss of IFN-γ–secreting $CD4^+$ T cells. However, this may be accompanied by killing of HIV-infected AM (13). Thus, there is a myriad of potential lymphocyte-mediated effects on AM function in HIV-infected patients. When one adds to this mixture the many AM-derived cytokines that are produced in increased amounts by HIV-infected AM (15), it is easy to see how the alveolar milieu in HIV infection is vastly different from the normal one.

A third mechanism by which HIV can alter AM function is through effects of viral proteins. The HIV proteins *nef*, gp120, p24, and *tat*, all have been reported to directly affect cellular function: *nef* inhibits NF-κB expression in human T cells (16). Similar inhibition of this important DNA-binding protein in macrophages could have significant effects on cellular activation and cytokine secretion. Soluble gp120 directly impairs accessory cell-dependent T-cell proliferation (17,18). This protein also inhibits AM activity against *Cryptococcus neoformans* (19). p24 impairs IFN-γ–induced activation of the monocyte cell line THP1 (20). Finally, the HIV *tat* protein affects a wide variety of cellular functions, from inhibition of T-cell proliferation (21), to induction of cytokine secretion in tissue macrophages and macrophage cell lines (22,23).

III. Morphological Changes

In addition to an increased number of lymphocytes, one-third of HIV-infected individuals have an elevated number of AM in bronchoalveolar lavage (24). Whether this is due to in situ proliferation of AM or to recruitment of monocytes into the alveolar space is unknown. Agostini and colleagues (25) have shown that AMs from HIV-infected patients spontaneously produce granulocyte–macrophage colony-stimulating factor (GM-CSF) and proliferate in the presence of this factor. On the other hand, monocytes are likely constantly being recruited to the lung in response to the numerous infections seen in these patients. Evidence suggests that HIV itself can promote differentiation of monocytes into more mature forms (26). It is likely both monocyte recruitment and in situ proliferation account for the increased number of AM in HIV infection.

Once in the lung, HIV-infected AM appear to have a normal life span. Viability of AM from normal volunteers and HIV-infected individuals without active pneumonia is similar (27). Ultrastructurally, AMs from these patients appear to have increased numbers of microvilli on the cell surface, consistent with a functionally active phagocyte (27). These cells have increased phagocytic vacuoles, some of which contain lymphocytic debris.

Although it is clear AMs can be infected with HIV, there is controversy over the amount of viral protein these cells harbor. Most investigators have readily detected proviral HIV DNA in AM (2–5). However, active transcription of the HIV provirus, as measured by viral mRNA levels, has been much more difficult to document (3,4). By using immunohistochemical techniques, one group of investigators has shown that 12–58% of AM from HIV-infected patients with lymphocytic alveolitis or lymphocytic interstitial pneumonitis express viral proteins (13). By similar techniques another group found very few freshly isolated AMs contained viral proteins (4). The clinical status of the patients was not described. However, when AMs were cultured for 6 days in the presence of tumor necrosis factor-α (TNF-α) and GM-CSF, 30–60% of cells expressed viral proteins, and 60–80% contained HIV-1 RNA, as assessed by in situ hybridization. These findings are consistent with the wealth of information documenting that cytokines and coinfections can upregulate HIV expression in latently infected cells (28–35). Viral burden in the lung increases with disease progression (5). Thus, it is likely that the ability to detect viral proteins in AM depends on the stage of disease and the presence or absence of coexisting conditions at the time of study. Whether viral proteins are confined to intracellular vacuoles, as has been demonstrated in other tissue macrophages (36), or are more evenly distributed in the cytoplasm or on the cell surface is not yet known.

Regardless of the degree of infection by HIV, it is now apparent that monocytes and AMs isolated from these individuals are activated. This can be demonstrated by the presence of surface molecules associated with cellular activation. Infection of monocytes and macrophages, including AM, is associated with increased expression of MHC class II molecules, especially HLA-DR (37–40). Likewise, expression of β2 integrins, particularly LFA-1 (CD11α/CD18), and one of its ligands, intercellular adhesion molecule (ICAM-1; CD54), are upregulated in HIV-infected AM and monocytic cell lines (39,41,42). Other markers of activation, such as GM_1 ganglioside (43) and the IgG Fc receptor type 1 (44) are also upregulated in monocytes from HIV-infected individuals. Whether similar findings occur in AMs is unknown.

Other surface markers that can be altered in HIV infection include the CD4 molecule. Several studies have shown that CD4 is down-modulated in monocytic cells infected with HIV in vitro (37,45). In contrast, CD4 appears to be upregulated in AM from HIV-infected individuals (39). Because down-modulation of CD4 is associated with binding of HIV gp120 (18), increased expression of CD4 on AM may reflect both cellular activation and a relative paucity of free virus in the alveolar milieu. Finally, alterations in the AM mannose receptor have been found that may contribute to an impaired ability to clear *Pneumocystis carinii* in the alveolar space (46).

Why are AMs from HIV-infected subjects activated? Buhl and colleagues have shown that freshly isolated AM from these individuals express IP-10 gene transcripts, a gene specifically induced by IFN-γ, whereas normal AM do not (40). This suggests the presence of IFN-γ in the lower respiratory tract of HIV-infected subjects. The concept that AMs in HIV-infected individuals are being activated by IFN-γ at first appears contradictory to standard dogma. Early studies suggested IFN-γ production was impaired in patients with AIDS (47–49), likely owing to loss of $CD4^+$ memory T lymphocytes responsible for the bulk production of this cytokine (11). However, early in HIV infection before the loss of memory cells, IFN-γ production by $CD4^+$ T cells is upregulated (50,51). As HIV infection progresses and $CD4^+$ T cells decline, cytotoxic T lymphocytes (CTL) become an important source of IFN-γ (14). HIV-specific CTL can be expected to accumulate in areas where there is increased expression of viral antigens. Although the number of infected peripheral blood mononuclear cells (PBMC) is low and exists mainly in a latent stage (52), tissues containing differentiated macrophages appear to contain substantially more infected cells (13,36). Increased expression of viral antigens in various organs can be expected to result in accumulation of HIV-specific CTL within that tissue; $CD8^+$ cells actively producing IFN-γ have been demonstrated in lymph nodes from HIV-infected patients (53). Because HIV-specific CTL are readily detectable in the lungs of infected subjects (13), they could provide a source of IFN-γ. Indeed, recent studies have suggested that $CD8^+$ lymphocytes isolated from BAL of asymptomatic HIV-infected patients with lymphocytic alveolitis are a rich source of IFN-γ (54). However, with time, even these cells decline in the lungs of HIV-infected patients and are replaced by suppressor $CD8^+$ T cells (55). Thus, a scenario can be hypothesized whereby IFN-γ is present in high concentrations in the lungs of HIV-infected individuals until late in the disease process (Fig. 1). Only very late in HIV infection does the amount of IFN-γ in the lungs fall to levels inadequate to activate AM, leading to the late infectious pulmonary complications of AIDS.

IV. Phagocytosis

Macrophage phagocytosis can be divided into four parts, each of which can be altered by HIV infection (Fig. 2). First, the macrophage must move toward the material to be phagocytosed (chemotaxis). Second, it must adhere to the object to be ingested. Third, the foreign material must be taken up by the macrophage into phagocytic vacuoles. Finally, the material must be broken down through a variety of cellular digestive mechanisms. Some of these functions have been examined directly in AM. Others have been

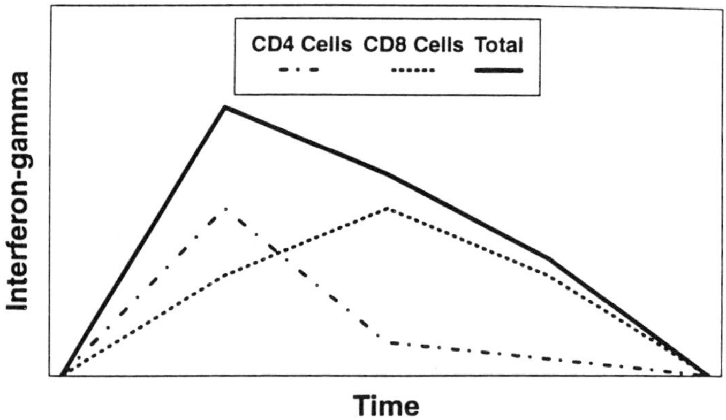

Figure 1 Potential source of IFN-γ in the lungs of HIV-infected subjects. Early in HIV infection $CD4^+$ memory T cells are an important source of this cytokine. As disease progresses CD4 counts fall and $CD8^+$ cytotoxic T lymphocytes accumulating in the lung become an important source of IFN-γ. As a result, IFN-γ concentrations have the potential to remain high in the lung of HIV-infected patients until late in the disease process.

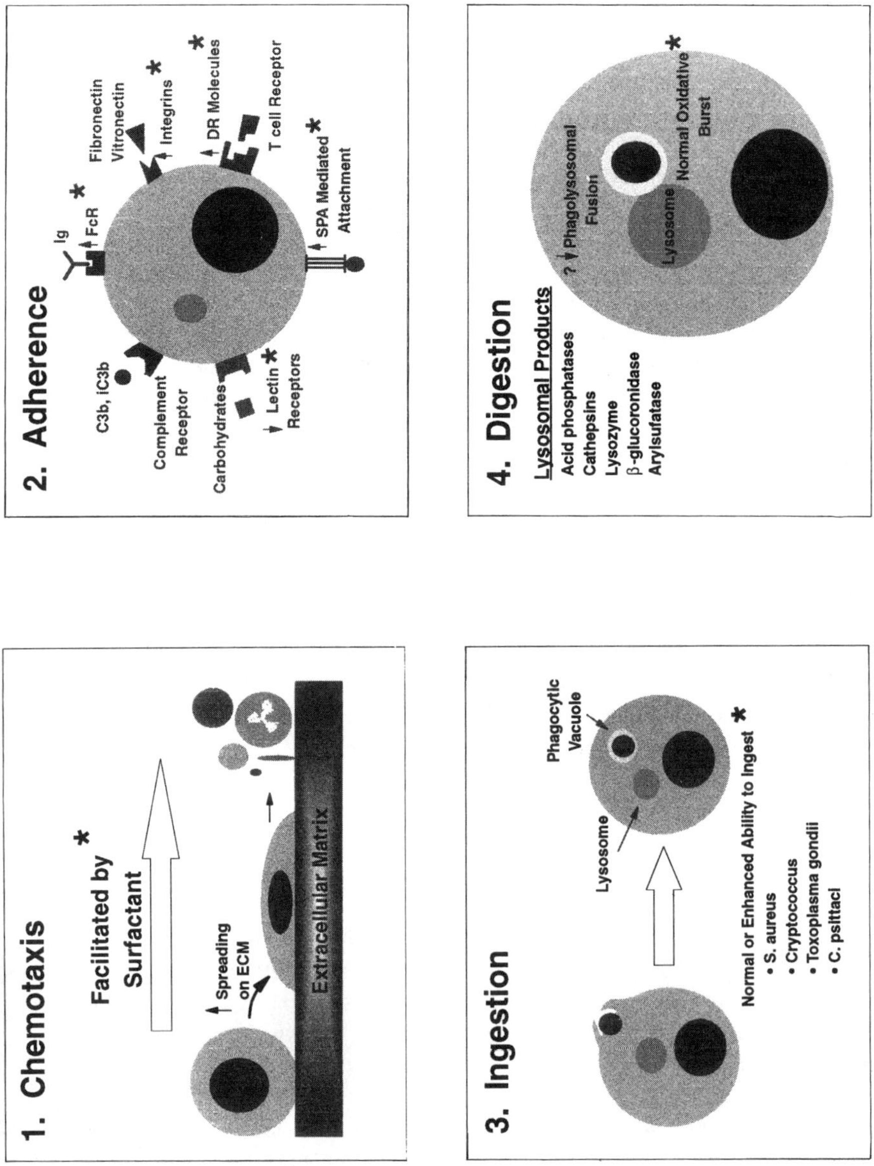

Figure 2 Four steps of alveolar macrophage phagocytosis that may be modified by HIV infection. Information from studies that were done on material (i.e., cells, bronchoalveolar lavage fluid) obtained from HIV-infected subjects is signified by an asterisk (*).

studied mainly in monocytes, and extrapolation to AM must be done with caution.

One of the earliest studies performed with monocytes in HIV-infected patients demonstrated impaired chemotaxis in response to FMLP, C5a, and the protozoan *Giardia lamblia* when compared with normal monocytes (56). This defect was most profound in patients with AIDS. Other investigators have shown that HIV infection affects the manner in which monocytes interact with extracellular matrix (57). HIV-infected monocytes bound to extracellular matrix more avidly than uninfected cells. Furthermore, infected cells tended to spread out more readily. Alveolar macrophages are less mobile than monocytes, but still possess the capability to migrate. Whether the foregoing observations apply to AM or other tissue macrophages is unknown. However, any analysis of AM chemotaxis in HIV infection will have to separate viral effects on AM from potential effects on surfactant, which facilitates AMs migration (58). This latter point is critical because surfactant protein A, the component responsible for enhancing AM chemotaxis (58), is increased in HIV-infected individuals with (59), and without (60), pneumonia.

Once an AM has migrated into the vicinity of the material to phagocytosed, binding must occur between the particle and cell surface. Many of the molecules described previously that are potentially upregulated on AM in HIV infection (DR, β_2-integrins, Fc receptors) can promote adherence to other cells or foreign material. In contrast, alterations in other molecules can impair AMs' binding to antigens (46). Thus, whether AMs from HIV-infected patients bind targets efficiently will depend on the pathway used by the AM to bind the material to be ingested. Many ingestable particles are taken up through Fc and complement receptor-mediated processes. Interestingly, surfactant protein A enhances both Fc and complement receptor-mediated phagocytosis (61). Because surfactant protein A is increased in HIV infection, one might speculate that AMs from these individuals efficiently bind and phagocytose material taken up by these pathways. In support of this hypothesis, Downing and colleagues (60) have shown that *M. tuberculosis* binds more avidly to AM in the presence of BAL fluid from HIV-infected patients compared with normal BAL (Fig. 3). Furthermore, removal of surfactant protein A from BAL by immunoprecipitation reduced AM–*M. tuberculosis* binding to normal levels. Surfactant protein A also binds avidly to *P. carinii* (62) and thus may be important in AM uptake of this organism. However, uptake of *P. carinii* is also mediated by the macrophage mannose receptor (63), a molecule that is altered in HIV infection (46). It must be emphasized that most studies examining AM binding to *P. carinii* have been performed on animal macrophages, normal human AM, or normal AM exposed to HIV BAL. Very few studies

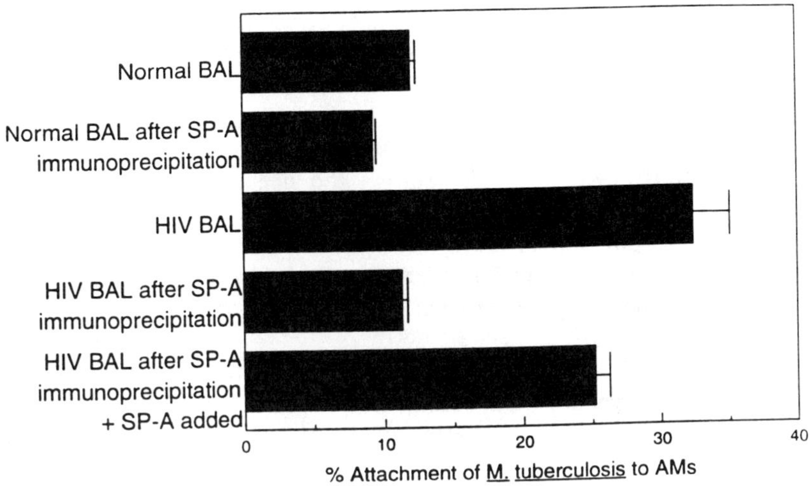

Figure 3 Evidence that surfactant protein A (SP-A) in bronchoalveolar lavage (BAL) from HIV-infected individuals promotes *M. tuberculosis* attachment to alveolar macrophages. Normal and HIV BAL were added to murine AM 30 min before the addition of ^{51}Cr-labeled *M. tuberculosis* and the percentage attachment was determined. Attachment was significantly higher using BAL from HIV-infected individuals compared with normal BAL ($p < 0.001$). Removal of SP-A from the BAL of both groups by immunoprecipitation resulted in a significant decrease in *M. tuberculosis* attachment. Addition of highly purified human SP-A restored the enhanced attachment observed in the HIV-infected group.

have examined AM from HIV-infected patients directly. Thus, the question of how well HIV AMs bind this organism remains unresolved.

Once the AM has bound the material to be phagocytosed, it must be ingested. Although it may seem logical that binding leads to internalization of bound material, this is not always true. For example, gp120 inhibits ingestion of *Cryptococcus neoformans* by normal AM, without altering initial binding of the organism (19). This study emphasizes the need to separate these two important steps when analyzing phagocytosis.

With the foregoing caveat in mind, numerous studies have examined the ability of monocytes and macrophages from HIV-infected patients to phagocytose various organisms. In general studies have shown normal or decreased monocyte phagocytic function, but normal to enhanced AM function, again demonstrating the danger in extrapolating monocyte studies to tissue macrophages. Monocytes from symptomatic HIV-infected patients have an impaired ability to phagocytose *Staphylococcus aureus* (64) and antibody-coated sheep red blood cells (65). Normal monocytes infected in vitro with HIV^{Bal} retain the ability to phagocytose *C. neoformans* (66). In contrast, AM from HIV-infected patients without pneumonia demonstrate an enhanced ability to phagocytose *S. aureus* (27). Several other studies have shown that AM phagocytic function is normal in HIV infection (66,67). Only one study has suggested that AMs' phagocytic function is impaired in HIV infection (19). This may reflect the organism studied (C. neoformans), the cell studied (normal AM), or the conditions examined (exposure to gp120, rather than intact virus). Although the reasons for differential effects of HIV infection on monocyte and AMs' phagocytic function remain unclear, one likely explanation involves the cytokine milieu in which each cell must operate.

The last step in efficient phagocytosis is digestion of the material taken up into phagocytic vacuoles, resulting in degradation of inert material and killing of viable organisms. Ingested material is destroyed by lysosomal enzymes, reactive oxygen species, and reactive nitrogen species. Numerous investigators have examined the effect of HIV on monocyte and macrophage oxidative metabolism. Studies on oxidative burst responses in monocytes are conflicting. Several studies demonstrate an impaired ability of monocytes and monocyte-derived macrophages from HIV-infected individuals to produce reactive oxygen species spontaneously or in response to appropriate stimuli (68,69). Other investigators have found this function is intact in HIV-infected subjects (66,67,70,71). Studies in AM are fewer but consistent. In general, AM oxidative burst potential in HIV-infected patients appears to be normal, especially in the presence of appropriate macrophage-activating cytokines (40,67,72).

Studies on lysosomal function in HIV infection are lacking. One group of investigators found that monocyte phagolysosomal fusion was impaired late in HIV infection (73). Recombinant gp120 induced similar defects in normal monocytes. Whether similar effects are seen in tissue macrophages is unknown. Studies looking at lysosomal enzymes in HIV infection are also scarce. Clearly, much work needs to be done in this area.

Provided all four steps involved in phagocytosis are intact, the end result should be killing of ingested organisms. Despite the wide discrepancies between some of the studies described in the foregoing, the end results (killing of organisms) are remarkably uniform. In general, monocytes or monocyte-derived macrophages from HIV-infected patients kill ingested organisms poorly (64,65,70). In contrast, killing of ingested bacteria, parasites, and fungi is largely preserved in AM (27,67,72). In the one study in which monocytes and macrophages were directly compared, HIV-infected monocytes had reduced anticryptococcal activity, whereas similarly infected AM retained this function (66). Several mechanisms could explain this dichotomy between monocytes and AM. Hypothesis center around differences between the vascular compartment and alveolar space relative to infectious viral burden, presence of coinfections, and cytokine concentrations. As described earlier, the end result is AM activation (40). Murray has shown that IFN-γ activates HIV-infected AMs to function efficiently as phagocytes (67,72). Thus, it is likely that AM from HIV-infected patients retain their phagocytic capabilities owing to chronic activation, either by IFN-γ, HIV itself, or coinfection present in the lower respiratory tract.

V. Secretory Products

Macrophages are a rich source of a wide variety of secretory products (74). These products can be loosely grouped into five categories (Table 2): reactive oxygen and nitrogen species, enzymes and proteases, antiproteases and free radical scavengers, metabolites or arachidonic acid, and cytokines. The ability of AM from HIV-infected subjects to secrete reactive oxygen species was described earlier. Very little is known about HIV AM function relative to the next three categories. Only a few studies have been performed in monocytes and, even these, present conflicting data. For example, whereas one group found that monocytes from HIV-infected subjects had impaired prostaglandin (PG)E_2 production induced by mitogens (70), another group demonstrated that normal monocytes infected with HIV in vitro produced increased amounts of this prostaglandin (75). In contrast

Table 2 Alveolar Macrophage Secretory Products[a]

1. Reactive free radicals
    - **Reactive oxygen species**
    - Reactive nitrogen species
2. Enzymes and proteases
3. Antiproteases and free radical scavengers
4. Arachidonic acid metabolites
    - Cyclooxygenase products
    - **Lipoxygenase products**
5. Cytokines
    - **IL-1**
    - **IL-6**
    - **IL-8**
    - **GM-CSF**
    - **TNF-α**

[a]Items in bold are produced in normal or increased amounts in the lungs of HIV-infected subjects.

with monocytes, in which cyclooxygenase products are the major consequence of arachidonic acid metabolism, AMs preferentially produce lipoxygenase products (76). Interestingly, leukotriene B_4 concentrations have been elevated in BAL from HIV-infected patients with nonspecific interstitial pneumonitis (77). Phospholipase A_2 concentrations were also elevated in these patients, as well as in asymptomatic HIV-positive individuals, suggesting a generalized increase in arachidonic acid metabolism. The cells responsible for these findings were not defined. Thus, it is possible that HIV infection is associated with a generalized increase in arachidonic acid metabolism in monocytes and tissue macrophages. More research is needed in this area.

A. Cytokines

In contrast with other macrophage secretory products, perhaps no aspect of AM biology in HIV infection has been studied as intensely as cytokine production. Virtually every AM-derived cytokine yet studied has been secreted in increased amounts in HIV-infected patients, including IL-1 (5,78), IL-6 (5,78,79), IL-8 (77), GM-CSF (25), and tumor necrosis factor-α; 5,80–83). Importantly, enhanced secretion of these cytokines can occur in the absence of any recognized inflammatory or infectious process, as well as in response to low concentrations of nonspecific stimuli (i.e., lipopolysaccharides or phorbol esters). This implies that AMs from HIV-infected individuals not only spontaneously synthesize and secrete these factors, but also possess the ability to respond in an augmented fashion to stimuli that would otherwise have no, or only minimal, effects on nonactivated cells.

There are several possible explanations for the increased AM cytokine secretion observed in HIV-positive individuals (Fig. 4). It is possible that enhanced cytokine secretion reflects AM exposure to pathogens in the lungs of these individuals. Clearly, enhanced AM cytokine secretion occurs in HIV-infected subjects with pulmonary disease (25,79,81,83); however, enhanced cytokine secretion is seen even in asymptomatic HIV-infected individuals (5,78,80), suggesting this alteration is a direct consequence of HIV infection.

A second explanation for the enhanced cytokine secretion demonstrated by AMs from HIV-infected individuals could be direct stimulation by the virus itself. Merrill et al. demonstrated that HIV could induce secretion of IL-1 and TNF from monocytes (84). Secretion of these cytokines was induced immediately after exposure of monocytes to heat-inactivated HIV, indicating that this effect occurred in the absence of productive viral infection. Isolated HIV envelope glycoproteins gp120 and gp160 can induce IL-6 secretion from CD4 T cells (85). In both these studies cytokine

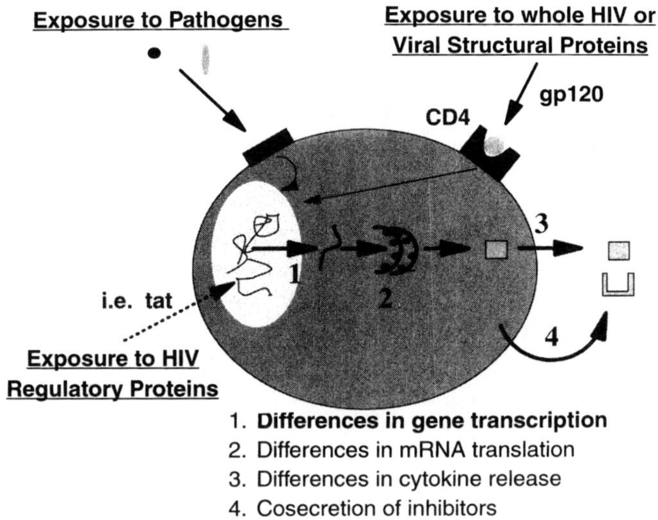

Figure 4 Potential mechanisms for enhanced cytokine secretion by AM from HIV-infected individuals. The AMs may be stimulated to produce cytokines through their normal pathway by usual or opportunistic pathogens, HIV itself, or viral structural proteins. Alternatively, HIV regulatory proteins can directly initiate cytokine gene transcription. Note that increased cytokine secretion can result from enhanced gene transcription, enhanced mRNA translation and posttranslational processing, enhanced secretion of the finished product, or alteration in the secretion of cytokine inhibitors. Increased cytokine gene transcription appears to be the major mechanism whereby HIV upregulates AM cytokine production.

secretion was blocked by soluble CD4, indicating that actual contact between cell surface CD4 and HIV envelope proteins was necessary for stimulation. Studies correlating AM cytokine secretion with pulmonary viral load are conflicting: AM TNF secretion was greater in cells shown to express HIV, as documented by coculture techniques with T-cell blasts (80); in contrast, there was no correlation between viral load, as determined by PCR techniques, and production of TNF-α, IL-1β, or IL-6 (5).

A third explanation for the enhanced cytokine secretion observed in HIV AMs involves the interaction of viral regulatory proteins with the host cells' genome. Cytomegalovirus immediate–early gene products can induce IL-1 transcription in the monocytic cell line THP-1 (86); HIV-1 *trans*-activating proteins, such as *tat*, might likewise induce cytokine gene transcription in HIV-infected cells (87). In support of this hypothesis, THP-1 cells transfected with the HIV-1 *tat* gene demonstrated enhanced unstimulated as well as LPS-induced IL-6 secretion (23) associated with accumulation of IL-6 mRNA transcripts. In fact, most studies documenting enhanced cytokine secretion by HIV-infected macrophages also demonstrate concomitant increases in cytokine mRNA (5,25,79,81,87). Thus, increased mRNA induced by HIV regulatory proteins may explain increased cytokine secretion by HIV-infected cells. Whether the accumulation of mRNA is due to increased gene transcription or enhanced RNA stability is unknown.

Finally, increased cytokine secretion by HIV-infected AM could reflect enhanced translational and posttranslational machinery in these cells. The secretory process could be facilitated. However, one study showed no difference in intracellular IL-1β and IL-6 between normal and HIV-infected AM, suggesting translation and secretion was not affected (78).

Whatever the mechanism, increased macrophage cytokine secretion has been implicated as playing a central role in the pathogenesis of HIV-related diseases (88–91). TNF-α, in particular, has been signaled out for its ability to be upregulated by HIV, induce other macrophage cytokines, and causes many of the processes associated with HIV infection, such as the wasting syndrome, AIDS encephalopathy, and Kaposi's sarcoma. Not only does HIV induce macrophage cytokines, but also these cytokines, in turn, may upregulate viral expression in other monocytes or macrophages (28–33) or nearby T cells (92,93), thereby propagating the virus in an autocrine or paracrine manner. This process can be modulated at several points. For example, other infections can either directly upregulate HIV expression (35,80,94) or themselves induce cytokines capable of upregulating viral expression (95). Furthermore, the foregoing discussion does not consider potential effects HIV may have on cytokine receptors. In fact, the HIV *tat* gene can modify the TNF receptor in a human B-cell line (96). In another study, HIV infection induced release of the soluble IL-6 receptor from a promonocytic cell line (97). Because IL-6 complexed to the soluble IL-6 receptor can bind to gp130 (an IL-6 signal-transducing membrane glycoprotein found on many cells) and behaves as a cytokine agonist (98), secretion of this receptor could serve as another mechanism to upregulate the effects of cytokines in HIV infection.

From the foregoing discussion, it is apparent that BAL fluid from HIV-seropositive patients can be a veritable "cytokine soup," containing increased concentrations of any number of different cytokines. To this hodgepodge one must factor in the effect of cytokines on other lung cells, especially T-cell and AM proliferation. The increased concentration of cytokines and resultant increase in cellular components renders the alveolar space an ideal medium for immune and inflammatory reactions in response to specific and nonspecific antigenic challenges. More importantly, increases in cytokine and cell concentrations can occur spontaneously, thereby causing symptoms in the absence of recognized pulmonary disease. It is important to recognize that augmented cytokine secretion and the increased number of immune cells in the alveolar space does not necessarily translate into enhanced immunological function. Clearly, HIV infection is characterized by impaired immune responses to various infectious agents. It is likely that cytokines with negative regulatory functions, or even cytokine inhibitors, are similarly upregulated in the alveolar space. For example, monocytes secreted an IL-1 inhibitor that masked detection of bioactive IL-1 in bioassays (99). Also, adherent cells from HIV-infected subjects secreted a 29-kDa protein that inhibits T-cell proliferation by decreasing expression of the IL-2 receptor and IL-2 secretion (100).

In summary, the cellular constituents of the lower respiratory tract in HIV-infected individuals are likely to depend on the prevailing cytokine profile in the alveolar milieu which, in turn, is affected by many variables, including the presence or absence of specific infectious agents, the degree of AM infection by HIV, and the degree of continued immune stimulation by potential environmental antigens. The presence of increased cytokine levels and cell numbers in the alveolar space can be expected to have multiple clinical consequences, depending on which of these components are up- or downregulated.

VI. Immune Function

Besides phagocytosis, the major immune function of AMs involves their role as accessory cells in the generation of cellular and humoral immune responses. An accessory cell (AC) is a cell that induces lymphoproliferation in the presence of antigens, mitogens, and alloantigens, leading to subsequent production of effector T cells capable of enhancing antibody production or performing cytotoxic functions. Although several cell types possess AC capabilities, cells of the monocyte–macrophage lineage are classically thought of as the major AC in the body. In this section AM function in B-cell and T-cell responses will be examined.

A. AM–B-Cell Interactions

Despite the presence of a polyclonal hypergammaglobulinemia in individuals infected with HIV, these patients are predisposed to pulmonary infections with encapsulated bacterial pathogens (101). These infections typically reflect an inability to generate opsonizing antibodies, specifically of the IgG isotype, that are directed against the infecting pathogens. In vitro, local immunoglobulin production by B lymphocytes depends on stimulation by T-cell cytokines secreted as a result of interactions with antigen-primed accessory cells (102). In the normal lung, this results in the local production of concentrations of IgG higher than those of IgA. In that the primary opsonizing antibody activity resides in the IgG isotype, it is possible that the increased susceptibility to pulmonary infections caused by encapsulated organisms in HIV-infected patients might be secondary to decreased local IgG concentrations in the lung.

Alveolar macrophages induce IgG production from PBMC in response to alloantigens, a process that requires IL-4 and IFN-γ (103), whereas IgA production is augmented by IL-5 and TGF-β; 104). TGF-β, which is derived from mononuclear phagocytes, has reciprocal activity that results in the inhibition of IgG production. Normally, IgG in the alveolar space is at a higher concentration than IgA which, in turn, is much higher than IgM. If, in HIV-infected individuals, the concentration of opsonizing antibodies is decreased in the alveolar space, this might be reflected in a decrease in the concentration of IgG relative to IgA. In fact, some of the earliest studies on lung immunoglobulin levels in HIV infection demonstrated increased IgA production in individuals with pneumonitis (105). Studies from our laboratory have also shown that despite the ability of AM from HIV-infected patients to secrete cytokines that enhance B-cell proliferation and differentiation (i.e., IL-6), BAL from HIV-infected subjects contains increased IgA and decreased IgG concentrations (105a). In that local concentrations of immunoglobulin are the result of AM interactions between T and B lymphocytes, the ability of AM from HIV-infected patients to stimulate alloantigen-induced immunoglobulin production in normal PBMC was determined. Although normal AM stimulated much greater IgG than IgA production in response to alloantigens (103), AM from HIV-infected patients stimulated IgA production, without stimulating any IgG or IgM production (Fig. 5). Preliminary studies suggest this may be due to AM overproduction of TGF-β, which is a potent inhibitor of IgG production, while augmenting IgA production (104).

B. AM–T-Cell Interactions

Alveolar macrophages are poor stimulators of T-cell proliferation, compared with blood monocytes; this was speculated to be beneficial, for the lung is constantly exposed to airborne mitogenic and antigenic stimuli (106–108). However, AM from HIV-infected individuals are significantly better AC compared with normal AM in stimulating a mitogen response (109). Initial studies included only HIV-infected patients who were undergoing diagnostic bronchoscopy to evaluate pulmonary symptoms. Because these patients may have had an active pulmonary inflammatory process, it was important to determine whether the enhanced stimulation of mitogenic responses oc-

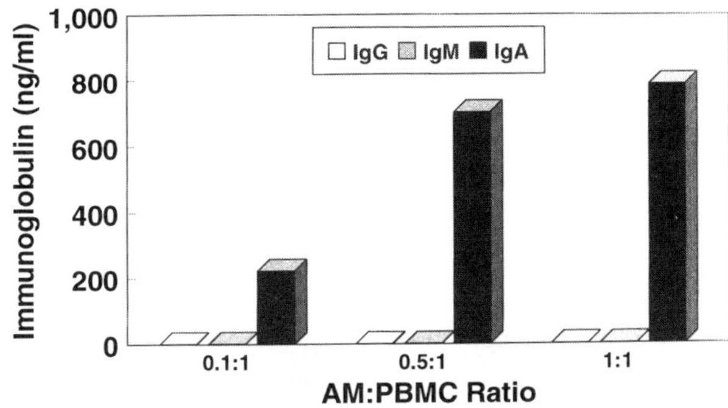

Figure 5 Ability of AM from HIV-infected patients to stimulate alloantigen-induced immunoglobulin production in normal PBMC. Fifty thousand PBMC were cultured with varying ratios of AM as shown. After 6 days, supernatants were harvested and immunoglobulin levels measured by ELISA. Although it was previously shown that normal AM stimulate much greater IgG than IgA production in response to alloantigens (103), AM from HIV-infected patients stimulated IgA production without stimulating any IgG or IgM production

curred in clinically well, asymptomatic HIV-infected individuals and, thus, reflected a direct effect of the virus. Interestingly, in studies of HIV-infected patients the major group of patients with enhanced AM AC function are asymptomatic (Fig. 6), indicating that nonspecific pulmonary inflammation is unlikely to explain the enhanced AC function (109). Unlike normal AMs, AMs from HIV-infected subjects were as capable as autologous blood monocytes at stimulating mitogen responses. That AMs from HIV-infected subjects show enhanced AC capabilities should not be surprising, for these cells are activated (40). Individuals with other disease states characterized by cellular activation in the lower respiratory tract (e.g., sarcoidosis) also have AMs with enhanced AC function (110).

Three potential mechanisms exist to explain the enhanced AM AC function in HIV-infected patients: (1) enhanced AM–T-cell adherence in HIV-infected patients; (2) increased secretion of T-cell stimulatory factors by HIV AM, and (3) decreased inhibitory properties of HIV AM. Optimal AC function requires secretion of macrophage cytokines important in T-cell proliferation and efficient AC–T-cell contact (111,112). For the latter requirement, AM AC function in normal volunteers correlates with their ability to bind T cells (106). Given the increased expression of HLA-DR and adhesion molecules on the surface of HIV-infected AM (37–42), one would speculate that these cells possess an enhanced ability to bind T cells. However, mitogen-induced T-cell–AM adherence is identical in normal volun-

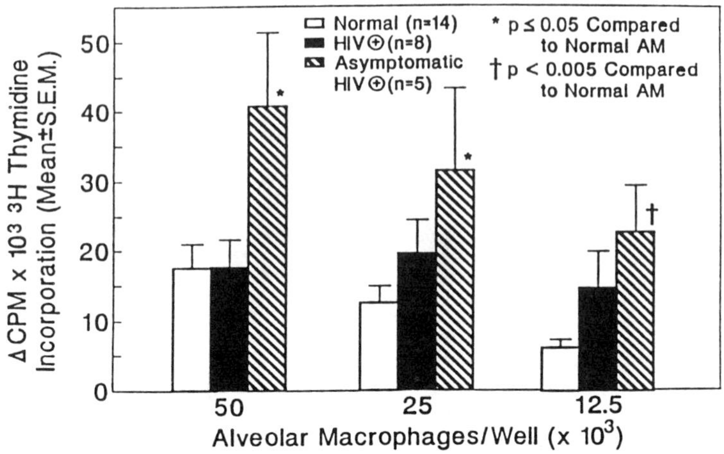

Figure 6 Alveolar macrophage accessory cell function in normal volunteers (white bars), symptomatic HIV-infected patients undergoing diagnostic bronchoscopy, and asymptomatic HIV-infected subjects with no pulmonary symptoms. AM in the concentrations shown were cultured with 10^5 normal T cells in the presence of concanavalin A (con-A) for 3 days, and lymphoproliferation was quantitated by tritiated thymidine incorporation. Enhanced AM accessory cell function in HIV-infected subjects is most pronounced in asymptomatic individuals. These findings make it less likely that concurrent pulmonary infection explains the enhanced AM AC function in these patients.

teers and HIV-positive patients (113). These findings do not imply that increased expression of surface adhesion molecules is not facilitating HIV AM AC function. Many receptor–counterreceptor interactions between AC and T lymphocytes serve dual purposes: first, to hold T cells in close proximity to AC so that secreted AC factors can have an optimal effect, and second, to act as a direct costimulatory signal for T-cell activation (114–119). Thus, increased expression of HLA-DR molecules and β_2-integrins could still contribute significantly to the enhanced AC function of HIV AM.

In further studies, unlike in normal AM, an inverse relation is seen between AM–T-cell binding and AC function in HIV-positive patients, suggesting that close AM–T-cell contact may be detrimental in this setting (Fig. 7; 113). Although these studies suggest that factors, other than adherence, are more important in determining maximal AC function of HIV AM, AM–T-cell contact is still essential for optimal AC function in HIV-infected patients. This was demonstrated by showing that adhesion molecule antibodies capable of abrogating AM–T-cell adherence also effectively blocked AC function when added at the beginning of culture. When these antibodies were added 4 hr after the initiation of culture, accessory cell

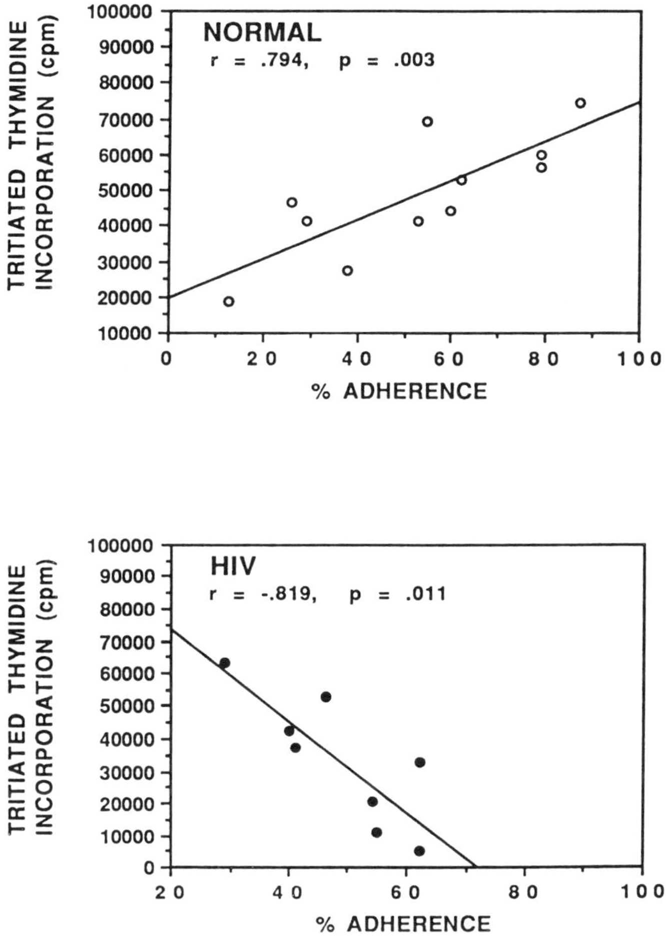

Figure 7 Correlation between AM AC function and AM–T-cell adherence in normal volunteers and HIV-positive patients. T-cell adherence to normal AM or HIV AM in the presence of con-A was determined at 4 hr of culture and correlated with the ability of 25,000 AMs to induce proliferation in 10^5 normal T cells in response to the same mitogens. There was a direct correlation between normal AM AC function in con-A assays and their ability to bind T cells. In contrast, HIV AM AC function in con-A assays was inversely correlated with their ability to bind T cells.

function in normal volunteers was still completely inhibited; however, significantly less inhibition of accessory cell function was noted in HIV-positive individuals. When antibodies were added after 24 hr of culture there was a modest inhibitory effect in both groups. These data indicate that augmented AM–T-cell adherence, although still critical for optimal AC function, does not explain the enhanced AC function of HIV-infected AM.

The second and third possibilities explaining enhanced AC function by HIV AM involve soluble factors, either as inhibitory factors, secreted by normal AM, or as stimulatory factors, secreted by AM from HIV-positive individuals. Alveolar macrophage supernatants from normal volunteers and HIV-positive patients, when added to mitogen assays using normal AM as AC, enhance the lymphoproliferation induced by normal AM (78). The HIV-positive supernatants are significantly better enhancers of normal mitogen responses than normal supernatants. In contrast, both normal and HIV supernatants have negligible effects when added to mitogen assays using AM from HIV patients as AC, suggesting HIV AM are already secreting optimal amounts of T-cell stimulatory factors: IL-1 and IL-6 are likely candidates for these factors, for they enhance AC function (120). Alveolar macrophages from HIV-infected patients secrete greater amounts of IL-1 and IL-6 than do normal AM, both spontaneously and in response to LPS or mitogenic stimuli (5,78,79).

These data demonstrate that secretion of important soluble factors involved in T-cell proliferation is enhanced in AM from HIV-positive patients. Working in concert, augmented IL-6 and IL-1 production and secretion may partly explain the enhanced AC function demonstrated by AMs from HIV-positive individuals. This conclusion is further supported by data demonstrating that passage of AM supernatants over protein G immunoaffinity columns coupled with anti-IL-1 and anti-IL-6 antibodies, effectively removes the ability of both normal and HIV AM supernatants to enhance mitogen assays (78).

Finally, it is possible that HIV AMs are "less inhibitory" than normal AMs. Normal AMs inhibit increases in intracellular calcium in stimulated T cells (121). Inhibition appears to be mediated by a membrane-bound signal on the AMs. Subsequent work has shown that this signal is membrane-bound surfactant components (122). Because surfactant is altered in HIV infection (59,60), it is possible that surfactant is "less suppressive" in HIV-infected patients. Interestingly, AMs isolated from patients with idiopathic pulmonary fibrosis, another immune-mediated disease, characterized by activation of AMs, were less suppressive than normal AMs (122); GM-CSF abrogates the natural inhibitory properties of normal AMs (123). This might have important effects on AMs from HIV-infected patients in whom secretion of this cytokine is upregulated (25). Other factors, such as prostaglandins and nitric oxide, can inhibit AC function (124,125). It is possible that AM production of these mediators is altered in HIV infection. Finally, it is possible that secretion of inhibitory cytokines such as

IL-10, which inhibits AC function (126), is downregulated in HIV infection.

From studies of AM–T-cell adhesion and AM cytokine secretion, a model for AM AC function in normal volunteers and HIV-positive patients can be proposed (Fig. 8). In normal volunteers it is important to maintain alveolar macrophage T-cell adherence so that T cells may be held in close proximity to the cytokine-secreting macrophage. Because normal AMs secrete relatively small amounts of important T-cell cytokines, such as IL-1 and IL-6, T cells that are not in close proximity to AMs will not prolifer-

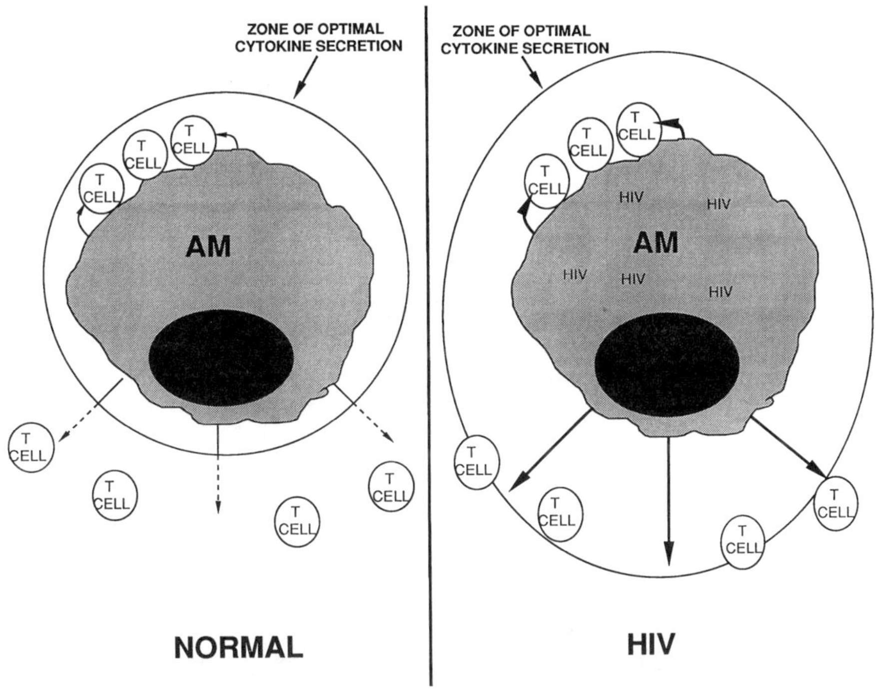

Figure 8 Proposed model of AM accessory cell function in normal volunteers and HIV-positive patients. Initial AM–T-cell contact is required in both groups to initiate cellular immune responses. However, owing to enhanced secretion of T-cell stimulatory cytokines (i.e., IL-1 and IL-6) by HIV AM, a zone of optimal cytokine secretion extends further from the HIV AM microenvironment than from normal AM. Thus, more T cells that have been activated and subsequently disengaged from AC can be optimally stimulated by AM cytokines in HIV-positive patients. Note that AM–T-cell contact is potentially detrimental in HIV-positive individuals if passage of HIV is facilitated from the infected AM to uninfected T cells.

ate, even if they have been previously activated. A corollary to this would be that the more T cells that remain in contact with AMs the more T cells will proliferate. In contrast, HIV AMs secrete greater amounts of IL-1 and IL-6; therefore, cells that have been activated, but are no longer in contact with AMs, are still able to proliferate in the presence of these T-cell stimulatory cytokines. The greater the cytokine secretion the greater this sphere of influence extends. In contrast with normal volunteers, AM–T-cell adherence may actually be detrimental in HIV-positive patients owing to viral passage from infected macrophages to noninfected T cells.

VII. Implications

What are the theoretical implications of enhanced AC function of AM in the lungs of HIV-infected patients? There are five potential sequelae whereby enhanced AM AC function in HIV-infected patients may ultimately lead to $CD4^+$ T-cell depletion in the lung (Fig. 9). The first is formation of syncytia between infected AM and T cells (109). This process would be facilitated by the increased expression of β_2-integrins on HIV-infected AM (127,128). Second, AM may infect $CD4^+$ T cells directly when these cells come in contact with infected AM (129–131). Third, increased T-cell proliferation as a result of enhanced secretion of AM cytokines makes T cells more susceptible to infection by free virus (132). Fourth, as described previously, these same cytokines upregulate HIV replication in latently infected $CD4^+$ T cells and other macrophages. Lastly, enhanced AM–$CD4^+$ T-cell interactions may ultimately lead to increased production of $CD8^+$ CTL active against viral antigens that can then kill AM and virally infected or uninfected $CD4^+$ T cells. The alveolar environment may be especially suitable for generating a CTL response for reasons already described; namely, enhanced AM activation and the potential for greater exposure to HIV than occurs in the vascular compartment.

All the responses described in the foregoing would be expected to result in depletion of $CD4^+$ T cells in the lung (133,134). Recent emphasis has focused on lymphoid organs as the predominant site at which HIV's propagation and destruction of $CD4^+$ T cells occur. If enhanced AM AC function reflects processes going on in other tissue macrophages, including those in lymphoid organs, then systemic $CD4^+$ T-cell depletion would be facilitated as well through these mechanisms. Indirect support for this hypothesis comes from the observation that an inverse relation exists between AM AC function and peripheral blood $CD4^+$ T-cell counts or CD4/CD8 ratio in HIV-infected patients (Fig. 10; 109).

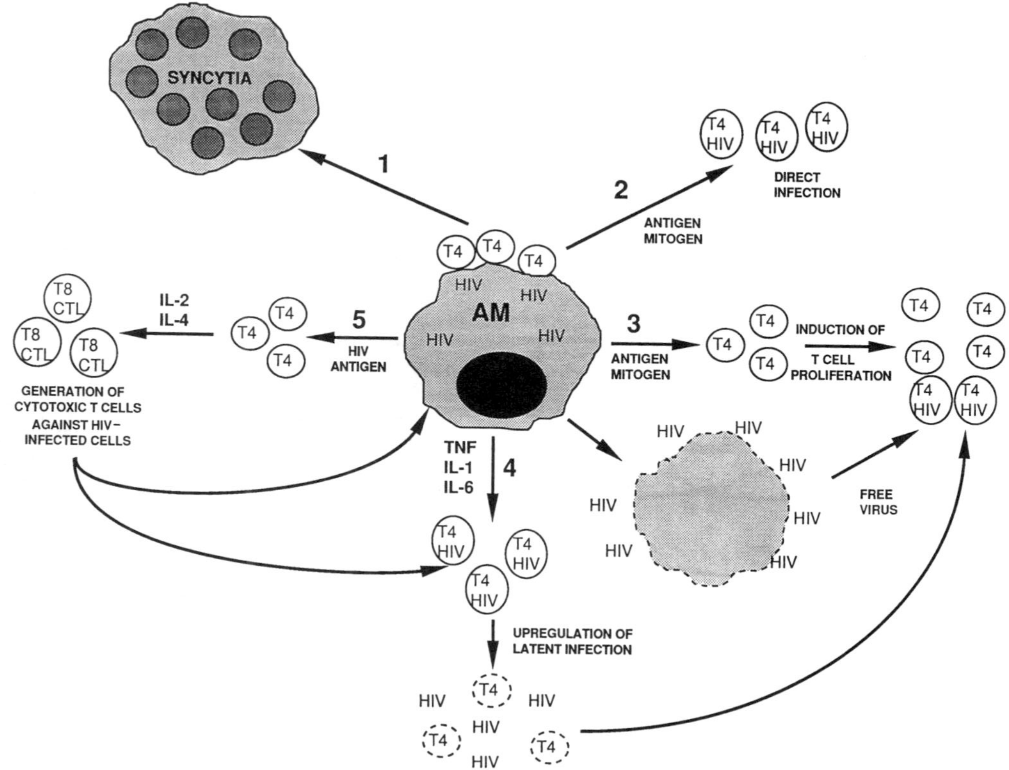

Figure 9 Five potential mechanisms by which enhanced AM accessory cell function may lead to $CD4^+$ T-cell depletion in the lung: (1) formation of syncytia, (2) infection of uninfected T cells through AM–T-cell contact, (3) induction of proliferation in uninfected T cells, thus rendering them more susceptible to infection by free virus, (4) upregulation of viral replication in latently infected T cells, and (5) enhanced ability to facilitate formation of HIV-specific cytotoxic T cells.

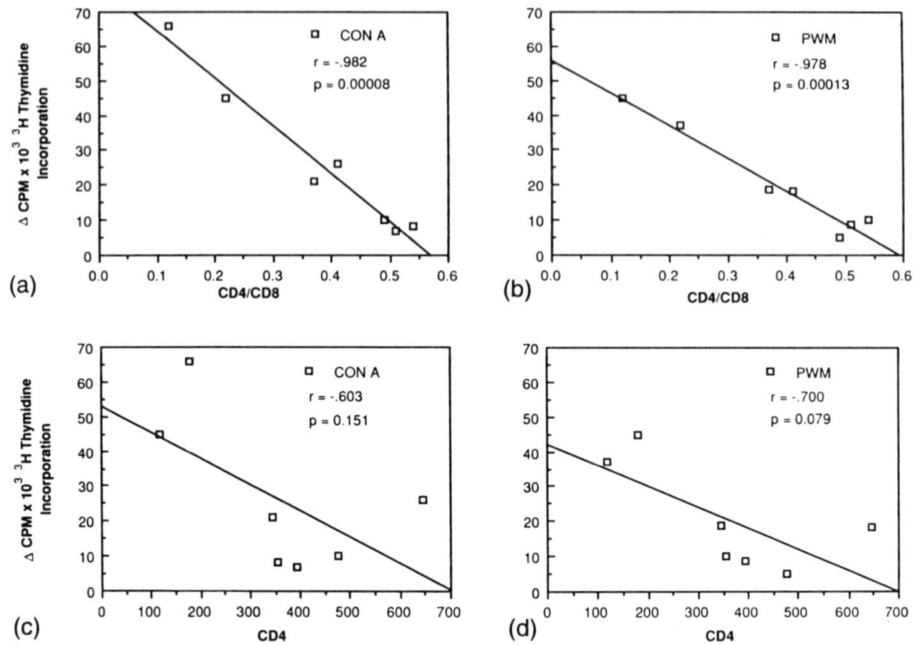

Figure 10 Relation between the ability of AM from HIV-positive patients to stimulate a mitogen response and their CD4/CD8 ratios (a, b) and absolute CD4 counts (c, d). Highly significant negative correlations exist between the CD4/CD8 ratio and the ability of AM to stimulate a (a) con-A and (b) pokeweed mitogen response. There was weaker but suggestive negative correlations between the absolute CD4 counts and AM accessory cell function in (c) con-A and (d) pokeweed mitogen assays.

Besides contributing to the depletion of $CD4^+$ T cells, HIV-infected AM may play a central role in the development of the lymphocytic alveolitis that is so prevalent in these individuals (7,8). One could hypothesize that lymphocytic alveolitis is mediated by chronically infected and activated AM that have augmented abilities to secrete T-cell stimulatory cytokines, such as IL-1 and IL-6 spontaneously and in response to nonspecific stimuli (Fig. 11), resulting in enhanced AC function. Responding activated CTL then secrete IL-2 (135) which may perpetuate T-cell proliferation in the absence of further AC involvement. Furthermore, IFN-γ secretion by CTL may feed back and further activate AM. Enhanced GM-CSF further enhances AM AC function (123). What perpetuates this response is the apparent inability of HIV-specific CTL to clear infected cells, especially AM, from the alveolar space. In support of this immune hypothesis concerning the develop-

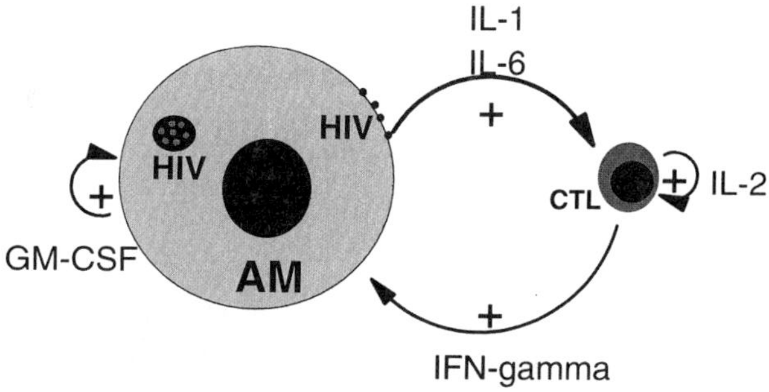

Figure 11 Potential mechanism for the development of lymphocytic alveolitis in HIV infection. Lymphocytic alveolitis could be mediated by chronically infected and activated AM that have augmented abilities to secrete T-cell stimulatory cytokines, such as IL-1 and IL-6 spontaneously and in response to nonspecific stimuli, resulting in enhanced AC function. Responding activated CTL then secrete IL-2, which may perpetuate T-cell proliferation in the absence of further AC involvement. Furthermore, IFN-γ secretion by CTL may feedback and further activate AM. Increased GM-CSF secretion further enhances AM accessory cell function. What perpetuates this response is the apparent inability of HIV-specific CTL to clear infected cells, especially AM, from the alveolar space.

ment of lymphocytic alveolitis is the recent finding that the incidence of lymphocytic alveolitis is reduced in HIV-infected subjects who smoke (Fig. 12; 136). Smoking has immunosuppressive effects on AM function, both in decreasing AC function (137) and impairing cytokine secretion (138–140). In concordance with this data, AM from HIV-infected patients have a reduced ability to stimulating mitogen-induced lymphoproliferation and secrete IL-1 and IL-6 when compared with AM from nonsmoking patients (136). It is tempting to speculate that cigarette smoking impairs the generation of cellular immune responses in the lungs of HIV-infected individuals and subsequent development of lymphocytic alveolitis.

VIII. Concluding Remarks

Most HIV-infected individuals will have pulmonary complications during the course of their illness. The pathogenesis of many of these complications involves an exuberant immune or inflammatory response, either to

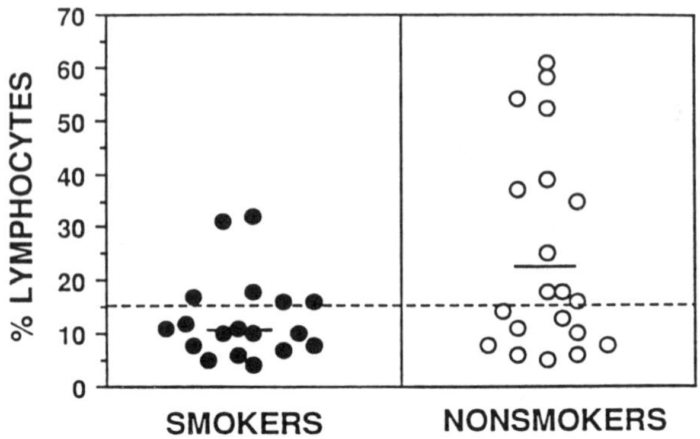

Figure 12 Percentage of lymphocytes in BAL of smoking (dark circles) and nonsmoking (white circles) HIV-positive individuals. BAL from smoking HIV-infected individuals contained a lower percentage of lymphocytes than BAL from nonsmokers (smokers 12.9 ± 1.9%, nonsmokers 24.7 ± 4.3%, $p < 0.05$). The incidence of lymphocytic alveolitis, defined as percentage lymphocytes in BAL ≥ 15% (dotted line), was significantly lower in HIV-positive smokers (6/18 or 33%) compared with nonsmokers (11/20 or 55%).

infecting organisms, nonspecific stimuli, or HIV itself. Activated AMs play a central role in mediating these responses. Macrophages, by virtue of their resistance to the cytopathic effect of HIV, are a natural reservoir for the virus. Thus, the lower respiratory tract in HIV-infected individuals contains a mixture of activated AM, T cells, stimulatory cytokines, infectious organisms, nonspecific inhaled antigens, and HIV itself (cell-associated or latent). Given this rich medium for immune and inflammatory responses, it is not surprising that pulmonary complications are so common in HIV infection, even in the absence of recognized infections. A better understanding of how HIV affects the AM, a cell central in the pathogenesis of immune and inflammatory responses in the lung, will allow the development of novel therapeutic strategies directed at the pulmonary complications of HIV infection.

References

1. Salahuddin SZ, Rose RM, Groopman JE, Markham PD, Gallo RC. Human T lymphotropic virus type III infection of human alveolar macrophages. Blood 1986; 68:281–284.
2. Clarke JR, Krishnan V, Bennett J, Mitchell D, Jeffries DJ. Detection of HIV-1 in human lung macrophages using the polymerase chain reaction. AIDS 1990; 4:1133–1136.

3. Rose RM, Krivine A, Pinkston P, Gillis JM, Huang A, Hammer SM. Frequent identification of HIV-1 DNA in bronchoalveolar lavage cells obtained from individuals with the acquired immunodeficiency syndrome. Am Rev Respir Dis 1991; 143:850–854.
4. Lebargy F, Branellec A, Deforges L, Bignon J, Bernaudin JF. HIV-1 in human alveolar macrophages from infected patients is latent in vivo but replicates after in vitro stimulation. Am J Respir Cell Mol Biol 1994; 10:72–78.
5. Sierra-Madero JG, Toossi Z, Hom DL, Finegan CK, Hoenig E, Rich EA. Relationship between load of virus in alveolar macrophages from human immunodeficiency virus type 1-infected persons, production of cytokines, and clincal status. J Infect Dis 1994; 169:18–27.
6. Wallace JM, Barbers RG, Oishi JS, Prince H. Cellular and T-lymphocyte subpopulation profiles in bronchoalveolar lavage fluid from patients with acquired immunodeficiency syndrome and pneumonitis. Am Rev Respir Dis 1984; 130:786–790.
7. Guillon JM, Autran B, Denis M, Fouret P, Plata F, Mayaud CM, Akoun GM. Human immunodeficiency virus-related lymphocytic alveolitis. Chest 1988; 94:1264–1270.
8. Agostini C, Poletti V, Zambello R, Trentin L, Siviero F, Spiga L, Gritti F, Semenzato G. Phenotypical and functional analysis of bronchoalveolar lavage lymphocytes in patients with HIV infection. Am Rev Respir Dis 1988; 138:1609–1615.
9. Schnittman SM, Lane HC, Greenhouse J, Justement JS, Baseler M, Fauci AS. Preferential infection of $CD4^+$ memory T cells by human immunodeficiency virus type 1: evidence for a role in the selective T-cell functional defects observed in infected individuals. Proc Natl Acad Sci USA 1990; 87:6058–6062.
10. van Noesel CJM, Gruters RA, Terpstra FG, Schellekens PTA, van Lier RAW, Miedema F. Functional and phenotypic evidence for a selective loss of memory T cells in asymptomatic human immunodeficiency virus-infected men. J Clin Invest 1990; 86:293–299.
11. Sanders ME, Makgoba MW, Sharrow SO, Stephany D, Springer TA, Young HA, Shaw S. Human memory T lymphocytes express increased levels of three cell adhesion molecules (LFA-3, CD2, and LFA-1) and three other molecules (UCHL1, CDw29, and Pgp-1) and have enhanced IFN-γ production. J Immunol 1988; 140:1401–1407.
12. Agostini C, Zambello R, Trentin L, Feruglio C, Masciarelli M, Siviero F, Poletti V, Spiga L, Gritti F, Semenzato G. Cytotoxic events taking place in the lung of patients with HIV-1 infection. Am Rev Respir Dis 1990; 142:516–522.
13. Plata F, Autran B, Martins LP, Wain-Hobson S, Raphael M, Mayaud C, Denis M, Guillon JM, Debre P. AIDS virus-specific cytotoxic T lymphocytes in lung disorders. Nature 1987; 328:348–351.
14. Jassoy C, Harrer T, Rosenthal T, Navia BA, Worth J, Johnson RP, Walker BD. Human immunodeficiency virus type 1-specific cytotoxic T lymphocytes release gamma interferon, tumor necrosis factor alpha (TNF-α) and TNF-β when they encounter their target antigens. J Virol 1993; 67:2844–2852.

15. Twigg HL. Bronchoalveolar lavage fluid in HIV-infected patients: "cytokine soup." Chest 1993; 104:659–661.
16. Niederman TMJ, Garcia JV, Hastings WR, Luria S, Ratner L. Human immunodeficiency virus type 1 *nef* protein inhibits NF-κB induction in human T cells. J Virol 1992; 66:6213–6219.
17. Chirmule N, Kalyanaraman VS, Oyaizu N, Slade HB, Pahwa H. Inhibition of functional properties of tetanus antigen-specific T-cell clones by envelope glycoprotein gp120 of human immunodeficiency virus. Blood 1990; 75:152–159.
18. Cefai D, Ferrer M, Serpente N, Idziorek T, Dautry-Varsat A, Debre P, Bismuth G. Internalization of HIV glycoprotein gp120 is associated with down-modulation of membrane CD4 and $p56^{ick}$ together with impairment of T cell activation. J Immunol 1992; 149:285–294.
19. Wagner RP, Levitz SM, Tabuni A, Kornfeld H. HIV-1 envelope protein (gp120) inhibits the activity of human bronchoalveolar macrophages against *Cryptococcus neoformans*. Am Rev Respir Dis 1992; 146:1434–1438.
20. Nong Y, Kandil O, Tobin EH, Rose RM, Remold HG. The HIV core protein p24 inhibits interferon-γ-induced increase of HLA-DR and cytochrome *b* heavy chanin mRNA levels in the human monocyte-like cell line THP1. Cell Immunol 1991; 132:10–16.
21. Viscidi RP, Mayur K, Lederman HM, Frankel AD. Inhibition of antigen-induced lymphocyte proliferation by *tat* protein from HIV-1. Science 1989; 246:1606–1608.
22. Zauli G, Davis BR, Re MC, Visani G, Furlini G, La Placa M. *tat* protein stimulates production of transforming growth factor-β1 by marrow macrophages: a potential mechanism for human immunodeficiency virus-1-induced hematopoietic suppression. Blood 1992; 80:3036–3043.
23. Iwamoto GK, Konicek SA, Twigg HL. Modulation of accessory cell function and interleukin-6 production by the HIV-1 *tat* gene. Am J Respir Cell Mol Biol 1994; 10:580–585.
24. Agostini C, Zambello R, Trentin L, Poletti V, Spiga L, Gritti F, Cipriani A, Salmaso L, Cadrobbi P, Senenzato G. Prognostic significance of the evaluation of bronchoalveolar lavage cell populations in patients with HIV-1 infection and pulmonary involvement. Chest 1991; 100:1601–1606.
25. Agostini C, Trentin L, Zambello R, Bulian P, Caenazzo C, Cipriani A, Cadrobbi P, Garbisa S, Semenzato G. Release of granulocyte–macrophage colony-stimulating factor by alveolar macrophages in the lung of HIV-1-infected patients. J Immunol 1992; 149:3379–3385.
26. Roulston A, D'Addario M, Boulerice F, Caplan S, Wainberg MA, Hiscott J. Induction of monocytic differentiation and NF-κB activities by human immunodeficiency virus 1 infection of myelomonoblastic cells. J Exp Med 1992; 175:751–763.
27. Musher DM, Watson DA, Nickeson D, Gyorkey F, Lahart C, Rossen RD. The effect of HIV infection on phagocytosis and killing of *Staphylococcus aureaus* by human pulmonary alveolar macrophages. Am J Med Sci 1990; 299:158–163.
28. Biswas P, Poli G, Kinter AL, Justement JS, Stanley SK, Maury WJ, Bressler P,

Orenstein JM, Fauci AS. Interferon γ induces the expression of human immunodeficiency virus in persistently infected promonocytic cells (U1) and redirects the production of virions to intracytoplasmic vacuoles in phorbol myristate acetate-differentiated U1 cells. J Exp Med 1992; 176:739–750.
29. Kazazi F, Mathijs JM, Chang J, Malafiej P, Lopez A, Dowton D, Sorrell TC, Vadas MA, Cunningham AL. Recombinant interleukin 4 stimulates human immunodeficiency virus production by infected monocytes and macrophages. J Gen Virol 1992; 73:941–949.
30. Poli G, Bressler P, Kinter A, Duh E, Timmer WC, Rabson A, Justement JS, Stanley S, Fauci AS. Interleukin 6 induces human immunodeficiency virus expression in infected monocytic cells alone and in synergy with tumor necrosis factor α by transcriptional and post-transcriptional mechanisms. J Exp Med 1990; 172:151–158.
31. Poli G, Kinter A, Justement JS, Kehrl JH, Bressler P, Stanley S, Fauci AS. Tumor necrosis factor α functions in an autocrine manner in the induction of human immunodeficiency virus expression. Proc Natl Acad Sci USA 1990; 87:782–785.
32. Mellors JW, Griffith BP, Ortiz MA, Landry ML, Ryan JL. Tumor necrosis factor-α/cachectin enhances human immunodeficiency virus type 1 replication in primary macrophages. J Infect Dis 1991; 163:78–82.
33. Kalter DC, Nakamura M, Turpin JA, Baca LM, Hoover DL, Dieffenbach C, Ralph P, Gendelman HE, Meltzer MS. Enhanced HIV replication in macrophage colony-stimulating factor-treated monocytes. J Immunol 1991; 146:298–306.
34. Israel-Biet D, Cadranel J, Even P. Human immunodeficiency virus production by alveolar lymphocytes is increased during *Pneumocystis carinii* pneumonia. Am Rev Respir Dis 1993; 148:1308–1312.
35. Golden MP, Kim S, Hammer SM, Ladd EA, Schaffer PA, DeLuca N, Albrecht MA. Activation of human immunodeficiency virus by herpes simples virus. J Infect Dis 1992; 166:494–499.
36. Meltzer MS, Skillman DR, Gomatos PJ, Kalter DC, Gendelman HE. Role of mononuclear phagocytes in the pathogenisis of human immunodeficiency virus infection. Ann Rev Immunol 1990; 8:169–194,
37. Mann DL, Gartner S, LeSane F, Blattner WA, Popovic M. Cell surface antigens and function of monocytes and a monocyte-like cell line before and afer infection with HIV. Clin Immunol Immunopathol 1990; 54:174–183.
38. Koethe SM, Carrigan DR, Turner PA. Increased density of HLA-DR antigen on monocytes of patients infected with the human immunodeficiency virus. J Med Virol 1989; 29:82–87.
39. Agostini C, Trentin L, Zambello R, Bulian P, Garbisa S, Cipriani A, Cadrobbi P, Semenzato G. Alveolar macrophages in HIV-1 infection express accessory molecules, activation markers, and release increased biological response modifiers. Chest 1993; 103(suppl2):108S–111S.
40. Buhl R, Jaffe HA, Holroyd KJ, Borok Z, Roum JH, Mastrangeli A, Wells FB,

Kirby M, Saltini C, Crystal RG. Activation of alveolar macrophages in asymptomatic HIV-infected individuals. J Immunol 1993; 150:1019–1028.
41. Petit AJC, Terpstra FG, Miedema F. Human immunodeficiency virus infection downregulates HLA class II expression and induces differentiation in promonocytic U937 cells. J Clin Invest 1987; 79:1883–1889.
42. Rossen RD, Smith CW, Laughter AH, Noonan CA, Anderson DC, McShan WM, Hurvitz MY, Orson FM. HIV-1 stimulated expression of CD11/CD18 integrins and ICAM-1: a possible mechanism for extravascular dissemination of HIV-1 infected cells. Trans Assoc Am Physicians 1989; 102:117–130.
43. Auci DL, Chice SM, Durkin HG, Murali MR. Constitutive production of PAI-II and increased surface expression of GM_1 ganglioside by peripheral blood monocytes from patients with AIDS: evidence of monocyte activation in vivo. J Leukoc Biol 1992; 52:282–286.
44. Capsoni F, Minonzio F, Ongari AM, Colombo G, Rizzardi GP, Bonara P, D'Arminio-Monforte A, Zanussi C. Increased expression of IgG Fc receptor type I on neutrophils and monocytes from HIV-infected subjects. Clin Exp Immunol 1992; 90:175–180.
45. Geleziunas R, Bour S, Boulerice F, Hiscott J, Wainberg MA. Diminution of CD4 surface protein but not CD4 messenger RNA levels in monocytic cells infected by HIV-1. AIDS 1991; 5:29–33.
46. Koziel H, Kruskal BA, Ezekowitz RAB, Rose RM. HIV impairs alveolar macrophage mannose receptor function against *Pneumocystis carinii*. Chest 1993; 103(suppl 2):111S–112S.
47. Murray HW, Rubin BY, Masur H, Roberts RB. Impaired production of lymphokines and immune (gamma) interferon in the acquired immunodeficiency syndrome. N Engl J Med 1984; 310:883–889.
48. Murray HW, Hillman JK, Rubin BY, Kelly CK, Jacobs JL, Tyler LW, Donelly DM, Carriero SM, Godbold JH, Roberts RB. Patients at risk for AIDS-related opportunistic infections: clinical manifestations and impaired gamma interferon production. N Engl J Med 1985; 313:1504–1510.
49. Maggi E, Macchia D, Parronchi P, Mazzetti M, Ravina A, Milo D, Romagnani S. Reduced production of interleukin 2 and interferon-gamma and enhanced helper activity for IgG synthesis by cloned $CD4^+$ T cells from patients with AIDS. Eur J Immunol 1987; 17:1685–1690.
50. Rinaldo C, Piazza P, Wang Y, Armstrong J, Gupta P, Ho M, Petteway S, Reed D, Lyter D, Kingsley L. HIV-1-specific production of IFN-γ and modulation by recombinant IL-2 during early HIV-1 infection. J Immunol 1988; 140:3389–3393.
51. Fan J, Bass HZ, Fahey JL. Elevated IFN-γ and decreased IL-2 gene expression are associated with HIV infection. J Immunol 1993; 151:5031–5040.
52. McElrath MJ., Steinman RM, Cohn ZA. Latent HIV-1 infection in enriched populations of blood monocytes and T cells from seropositive patients. J Clin Invest 1991; 87:27–30.
53. Emilie D, Peuchmaur M, Maillot MC, Crevon MC, Brousse N, Delfraissy JF, Dormont J, Galanaud P. Production of interleukins in human immunodeficiency virus-1-replicating lymph nodes. J Clin Invest 1990; 86:148–159.

54. Spain BA, Soliman DM, Konicek SA, Iwamoto GK, Twigg HL. Interferon-gamma production is upregulated in lung lymphocytes from asymptomatic HIV-infected individuals with lymphocytic alveolitis (abstract). Clin Res 1994; 42:425A.
55. Joly P, Guillon GM, Mayaud C, Plata F, Theodorou I, Denis M, Debre P, Autran B. Cell-mediated suppression of HIV-specific cytotoxic T lymphocytes. J Immunol 1989; 143:2193–2201.
56. Smith PD, Ohura K, Masur H, Lane HC, Fauci AS, Wahl SM. Monocyte function in the acquired immune deficiency syndrome: defective chemotaxis. J Clin Invest 1984; 74:2121–2128.
57. Dhawan S, Vargo M, Meltzer MS. Interactions between HIV-infected monocytes and the extracellular matrix: increased capacity of HIV-infected monocytes to adhere to and spread on extracellular matrix associated with changes in extent of virus replication and cytopathic effects in infected cells. J Leukoc Biol 1992; 52:62–69.
58. Wright JR, Youmas DC. Pulmonary surfactant protein A stimulates chemotaxis of alveolar macrophages. Am J Physiol 1993; 264:L338–L344.
59. Phelps DS, Rose RM. Increased recovery of surfactant protein A in AIDS-related pneumonia. Am Rev Respir Dis 1991; 143:1072–1075.
60. Downing JF, Pasula R, Wright JR, Twigg HL III, Martin II WJ. Surfactant protein A promotes attachment of *Mycobacterium tuberculosis* to alveolar macrophages during infection with human immunodeficiency virus. Proc Natl Acad Sci USA 1995; 92:4848–4852.
61. Tenner AJ, Robinson SL, Borchelt J, Wright JR. Human pulmonary surfactant protein (SP-A), a protein structurally homologous to C19, can enhance FcR- and CR1-mediated phagocytosis. J Biol Chem 1989; 264:13923–13928.
62. Zimmerman PE, Voelker DR, McCormack FX, Paulsrud JR, Martin WJ II. 120-kd surface glycoprotein of *Pneumocystis carinii* is a ligand for surfactant protein A. J Clin Invest 1992; 89:143–149.
63. Ezekowitz RAB, Williams DJ, Koziel H, Armstrong MYK, Warner A, Richards FF, Rose RM. Uptake of *Pneumocystis carinii* mediated by the macrophage mannose receptor. Nature 1991; 351:155–158.
64. Szkaradkiewicz A. Phagocytosis and microbicidal capacity of human monocytes in the course of HIV infection. Immunol Let 1992; 33:145–150.
65. Capsoni F, Minonzio F, Ongari AM, Rizzardi GP, Lazzarin A, Zanussi C. Monocyte-derived macrophage function in HIV-infected subjects: in vitro modulation by rIFN-γ and rGM-CSF. Clin Immunol Immunopathol 1992; 62:176–182.
66. Cameron ML, Granger DL, Matthews TJ, Weinberg JB. Human immunodeficiency virus (HIV)-infected human blood monocytes and peritoneal macrophages have reduced anticryptococcal activity whereas HIV-infected alveolar macrophages retain normal activity. J Infect Dis 1994; 170:60–67.
67. Murray HW. Macrophage activation in the acquired immunodeficiency syndrome. In: Steinman RM, North RJ, eds. Mechanisms of Host Resistance to Infectious Agents, Tumors and Allografts. New York: Rockefeller University Press, 1986:321–332.

68. Muller F, Rollag H, Froland SS. Reduced oxidative burst responses in monocytes and monocyte-derived macrophages from HIV-infected subjects. Clin Exp Immunol 1990; 82:10–15.
69. Spear GT, Kessler HA, Rothberg L, Phair J, Landay AL. Decreased oxidative burst activity of monocytes from asymptomatic HIV-infected individuals. Clin Immunol Immunopathol 1990; 54:184–191.
70. Roux-Lombard P, Aladjem D, Balavoine JF, Chofflon M, Despont JP, Hirschel B, Jeannet M, Kapanci Y, Lang R, Toccanier MF, Voinier B, Wilhelm A, Dayer JM, Cruchaud A. Altered functions of peripheral blood monocytes in homosexual males and intravenous drug users with persistent generalized lymphadenopathy. Eur J Clin Invest 1986; 16:262–270.
71. Dukes CS, Matthes TJ, Weinberg JB. Human immunodeficiency virus type 1 infection of human monocytes and macrophages does not alter their ability to generate an oxidative burst. J Infect Dis 1993; 168:459–462.
72. Murray HW, Gellene RA, Libby DM, Rothermel CD, Rubin BY. Activation of tissue macrophages from AIDS patients: in vitro response of AIDS alveolar macrophages to lymphokines and interferon-γ. J Immunol 1985; 135:2374–2377.
73. Pittis MG, Sternik G, Sen L, Diez RA, Planes N, Pirola D, Estevez ME. Impaired phagolysomal fusion of peripheral blood monocytes from HIV-infected subjects. Scand J Immunol 1993; 38:423–427.
74. Nathan CF. Secretory products of macrophages. J Clin Invest 1987; 79:319–326.
75. Foley P, Kazazi F, Biti R, Sorrell TC, Cunningham AL. HIV infection of monocytes inhibits the T-lymphocyte proliferative response to recall antigens, via production of eicosanoids. Immunology 1992; 75:391–397.
76. Balter MS, Toews GB, Peters-Golden M. Different patterns of arachidonate metabolism in autologous human blood monocytes and alveolar macrophages. J Immunol 1989; 142:602–608.
77. Lipschik GY, Doerfler ME, Kovacs JA, Travis WD, Andrawis VA, Lawrence MG, Dichter JR, Ognibene FP, Shelhamer JH. Leukotriene B_4 and interleukin-8 in human immunodeficiency virus-related pulmonary disease. Chest 1993; 104:763–769.
78. Twigg HL, Iwamoto GK, Soliman DM. Role of cytokines in alveolar macrophage accessory cell function in HIV-infected individuals. J Immunol 1992; 149:1462–1469.
79. Trentin L, Garbisa S, Zambello R, Agostini C, Caenazzo C, Di Francesco C, Cipriani A, Francavilla E, Semenzato G. Spontaneous production of IL-6 by alveolar macrophages of HIV-1 seropositive patients. J Infect Dis 1992; 166:731–737.
80. Israel-Biet D, Cadranel J, Beldjord K, Andrieu JM, Jeffrey A, Even P. Tumor necrosis factor production in HIV-seropositive subjects; relationship with lung opportunistic infections and HIV expression in alveolar macrophages. J Immunol 1991; 147:490–494.
81. Agostini C, Zambello R, Trentin L, Garbisa S, Francia Di Celle P, Bulian P, Onisto M, Poletti V, Spiga L, Raise E, Foa R, Semenzato G. Alveolar macroph-

ages from patients with AIDS and AIDS-related complex constitutively synthesize and release tumor necrosis factor alpha. Am Rev Respir Dis 1991; 144:195–201.
82. Cox RA, Anders GT, Cappelli PJ, Johnson JE, Blanton HM, Seaworth BJ, Treasure RL. Production of tumor necrosis factor-alpha and interleukin-1 by alveolar macrophages from HIV-1-infected persons. AIDS Res Hum Retroviruses 1990; 6:431–441.
83. Millar AB, Miller RF, Foley NM, Meager A, Semple SJG, Rook GAW. Production of tumor necrosis factor-α by blood and lung mononuclear phagocytes from patients with human immunodeficiency virus-related lung disease. Am J Respir Cell Mol Biol 1991; 5:144–148.
84. Merrill JE, Koyanagi Y, Chen ISY. Interleukin-1 and tumor necrosis factor α can be induced from mononuclear phagocytes by human immunodeficiency virus type 1 binding to the CD4 receptor. J Virol 1989; 63:4404–4408.
85. Oyaizu N, Chirmule N, Ohnishi Y, Kalyanaraman VS, Pahwa S. Human immunodeficiency virus type 1 envelope glycoproteins gp120 and gp160 induce interleukin-6 production in $CD4^+$ T-cell clones. J Virol 1991; 65:6277–6282.
86. Iwamoto GK, Monick MM, Clark BD, Auron PE, Stinski MF, Hunninghake GW. Modulation of interleukin 1 beta gene expression by the immediate early genes of human cytomegalovirus. J Clin Invest 1990; 85:1853–1857.
87. Yamato K, El-Hajjaoui Z, Simon K, Koeffler HP. Modulation of interleukin-1β RNA in monocytic cells infected with human immunodeficiency virus-1. J Clin Invest 1990; 86:1109–1114.
88. Matsuyama T, Kobayashi N, Yamamoto N. Cytokines and HIV infection: is AIDS a tumor necrosis factor disease? AIDS 1991; 5:1405–1417.
89. Merrill JE. Cytokines and retroviruses. Clin Immunol Immunopathol 1992; 64:23–27.
90. Rosenberg ZF, Fauci AS. Immunopathogenic mechanisms of HIV infection: cytokine induction of HIV expression. Immunol Today 1990; 11:176–180.
91. Butera ST. Cytokine involvement in viral permissiveness and the progression of HIV disease. J Cell Biochem 1993; 53:336–342.
92. Israel N, Hazan U, Alcami J, Munier A., Arenzana-Seisdedos F, Bachelerie F, Israel A, Virelizier JL. Tumor necrosis factor stimulates transcription of HIV-1 in human T lymphocytes, independently and synergistically with mitogens. J Immunol 1989; 143:3956–3960.
93. Clouse KA, Powell D, Washington I, Poli G, Strebel K, Farrar W, Barstad P, Kovacs J, Fauci AS, Folks TM. Monokine regulation of human immunodeficiency virus-1 expression in a chronically infected human T cell clone. J Immunol 1989; 142:431–438.
94. Brinchmann JE, Gaudernack G, Thorsby E, Vartdal F. Staphylococcal exotoxin superantigens induce human immunodeficiency virus type 1 expression in naturally infected $CD4^+$ T cells. J Virol 1992; 66:5924–5928.
95. Clouse KA, Robbins PB, Fernie B, Ostrove JM, Fauci AS. Viral antigen stimulation of the production of human monokines capable of regulating HIV1 expression. J Immunol 1989; 143:470–475.

96. Pocsik E, Higuchi M, Aggarwal BB. Down-modulation of cell surface expression of p80 form of the tumor necrosis factor receptor by human immunodeficiency virus-1 *tat* gene. Lymphokine Cytokine Res 1992; 11:317–325.
97. Honda M, Yamamoto S, Cheng M, Yasukawa K, Suzuki H, Saito T, Osugi Y, Tokunaga T, Kishimoto T. Human soluble IL-6 receptor: its detection and enhanced release by HIV infection. J Immunol 1992; 148:2175–2180.
98. Taga T, Hibi M, Hirata Y, Yamasaki K, Uasukawa K, Matsuda T, Hirano T, Kishimoto T. Interleukin-6 triggers the association of its receptor with a possible signal transducer, gp130. Cell 1989; 58:573–581.
99. Berman MA, Sandborg CI, Calabia BS, Andrews BS, Friou GJ. Interleukin 1 inhibitor masks high interleukin 1 production in acquired immunodeficiency syndrome. Clin Immunol Immunopathol 1987; 42:133–140.
100. Ammar A, Sahraoui Y, Tsapis A, Bertoli AM, Jasmin C, Georgoulias V. Human immunodeficiency virus-infected adherent cell-derived inhibitory factor (p29) inhibits normal T cell proliferation through decreased expression of high affinity interleukin-2 receptors and production of interleukin-2. J Clin Invest 1992; 90:8–14.
101. Janoff EN, Breiman RF, Daley CL, Hopewell PC. Pneumococcal disease during HIV infection: epidemiologic, clinical, and immunologic perspectives. Ann Intern Med 1992; 117:314–324.
102. Jelinek DF, Lipsky PE. Ther roles of T cell factors in activation, cell cycle progression, and differentiation of human B cells. J Immunol 1985; 134:1690–1696.
103. Wilkes DS, Weissler JC. Alloantigen-induced immunoglobulin production in human lung: differential effects of accessory cell populations in IgG synthesis. Am J Respir Cell Mol Biol 1994; 10:339–346.
104. Sonoda E, Matsumoto R, Hitoshi Y, Ishii T, Sugimoto M, Araki S, Tominaga A, Yamaguchi N, Takatsu K. Transforming growth factor B induces IgA production and acts additively with interleukin 5 for IgA production. Exp Med 1989; 170:1415–1420.
105. Rankin JA, Walzer PD, Dwyer JM, Schrader CE, Enriquez RE, Merrill WW. Immunologic alterations in bronchoalveolar lavage fluid in the acquired immunodeficiency syndrome (AIDS). Am Rev Respir Dis 1983; 128:189–194.
105a. Twigg HL, Spain BA, Soliman DM, Bowen LK, Heidler KM, Wilkes DS. Impaired IgG production in the lungs of HIV-infected individuals. Cell Immunol 1996; 170:127–133.
106. Lyons CR, Ball EJ, Toews GB, Weissler JC, Stastny P, Lipscomb MF. Inability of human alveolar macrophages to stimulate resting T cells correlates with decreased antigen-specific T cell-macrophage binding. J Immunol 1986; 137:1173–1180.
107. Lipscomb MF, Lyons CR, Nunez G, Ball EJ, Stastny P, Vial W, Lem V, Weissler J, Miller LM, Toews GB. Human alveolar macrophages: HLA-DR-positive macrophages that are poor stimulators of a primary mixed leukocyte reaction. J Immunol 1986; 136:497–504.
108. Toews GB, Vial WC, Dunn MM, Guzzetta P, Nunez G, Stastny P, Lipscomb

MF. The accessory cell function of human alveolar macrophages in specific T cell proliferation. J Immunol 1984; 132:181–186.

109. Twigg HL, Lipscomb MF, Yoffe B, Barbaro DJ, Weissler JC. Enhanced accessory cell function by alveolar macrophages from patients infected with the human immunodeficiency virus: potential role for depletion of $CD4^+$ cells in the lung. Am J Respir Cell Mol Biol 1989; 1:391–400.
110. Lem VM, Lipscomb MF, Weissler JC, Nunez G, Ball EJ, Stastny P, Toews GB. Bronchoalveolar cells from sarcoid patients demonstrate enhanced antigen presentation. J Immunol 1985; 135:1766–1771.
111. Chatila TA, Schwartz DH, Miller R, Geha RS. Requirement for mitogen, T cell-accessory cell contact, and interleukin 1 in the induction of resting T-cell proliferation. Clin Immunol Immunopathol 1987; 44:235–247.
112. Kawakami K, Yamamoto Y, Kakimoto K, Onoue K. Requirement for delivery of signals by physical interaction and soluble factors from accessory cells in the induction of receptor-mediated T cell proliferation. J Immunol 1989; 142:1818–1825.
113. Twigg HL, Soliman DM. Role of alveolar macrophage–T cell contact in accessory cell function in HIV-infected individuals. Am J Respir Cell Mol Biol 1994; 11:138–146.
114. Hynes RO. Integrins: a family of cell surface receptors. Cell 1987; 48:549–554.
115. Arnaout MA. Structure and function of the leukocyte adhesion molecules CD11/CD18. Blood 1990; 75:1037–1050.
116. Dougherty GJ, Hogg N. The role of monocyte lymphocyte function-associated antigen 1 (LFA-1) in accessory cell function. Eur J Immunol 1987; 17:943–947.
117. Haverstick DM, Gray LS. Lymphocyte adhesion mediated by lymphocyte function-associated antigen-1. I. Long term augmentation by transient increases in intracellular cAMP. J Immunol 1992; 149:389–396.
118. Damle NK, Klussman K, Linsley P, Aruffo A. Differential costimulatory effects of adhesion molecules B7, ICAM-1, LFA-3, and VCAM-1 on resting and antigen-primed $CD4^+$ T lymphocytes. J Immunol 1992; 148:1985–1992.
119. Van Seventer GA, Shimizu Y, Horgan KJ, Shaw S. The LFA-1 ligand ICAM-1 provides an important costimulatory signal for T cell receptor-mediated activation of resting T cells. J Immunol 1990; 144:4579–4586.
120. Ruppert J, Peters JH. IL-6 and IL-1 enhance the accessory activity of human blood monocytes during differentiation to macrophages. J Immunol 1991; 146:144–149.
121. Yarbrough WC, Wilkes DS, Weissler JC. Human alveolar macrophages inhibit receptor-mediated increases in intracellular–calcium concentration in lymphocytes. Am J Respir Cell Mol Biol 1991; 5:411–415.
122. Weissler JC, Mendelson C, Moya F, Yarbrough WC. Effect of interstitial lung disease macrophages on T-cell signal transduction. Am J Respir Crit Care Med 1994; 149:191–196.
123. Bilyk N, Holt PG. Inhibition of the immunosuppressive activity of resident pulmonary alveolar macrophages by granulocyte/macrophage colony-stimulating factor. J Exp Med 1993; 177:1773–1777.

124. Metzger Z, Hoffeld JT, Oppenheim JJ. Macrophage-mediated suppression. I. evidence for participation of both hydrogen peroxide and prostaglandins in suppression of murine lymphocyte proliferation. J Immunol 1980; 124:983–988.
125. Denhma S, Rowland IJ. Inhibition of the reactive proliferation of lymphocytes by activated macrophages: the role of nitric oxide. Clin Exp Immunol 1992; 87:157–162.
126. Ding L, Shevach EM. IL-10 inhibits mitogen-induced T cell proliferation by selectively inhibiting macrophage costimulatory function. J Immunol 1992; 148:3133–3139.
127. Valentin A, Lundin K, Patarroyo M, Asjo B. The leukocyte adhesion glycoprotein CD18 participates in HIV-1-induced syncytia formation in monocytoid and T cells. J Immunol 1990; 144:934–937.
128. Pantaleo G, Butini L, Graziosi C, Poli G, Schnittman SM, Greenhouse JJ, Gallin JI, Fauci AS. Human immunodeficiency virus (HIV) infection in $CD4^+$ T lymphocytes genetically deficient in LFA-1: LFA-1 is required for HIV-mediated cell fusion but not for viral transmission. J Exp Med 1991; 173:511–514.
129. Mann DL, Gartner S, LeSane F, Buchow H, Popovic M. HIV-1 transmission and function of virus-infected monocytes/macrophages. J Immunol 1990; 144:2152–2158.
130. Lewis DE, Yoffe B, Bosworth CG, Holling FB, Rich RR. Human immunodeficiency virus-induced pathology favored by cellular transmission and activation. FASEB J 1988; 2:251–255.
131. Lyerly HK, Ohen OJ, Weinhold KJ. Transmission of HIV by antigen presenting cells during T-cell activation: prevention by 3′-azido-3′-deoxythymidine. AIDS Res Hum Retroviruses 1987; 3:87–94.
132. Folks T, Kelly J, Benn S, Kinter A, Justement J, Gold J, Redfield R, Sell KW, Fauci AS. Susceptibility of normal human lymphocytes to infection with HTLV-III/LAV. J Immunol 1986; 136:4049–4053.
133. Pantaleo G, Graziosi C, Fauci AS. The immunopathogenesis of human immunodeficiency virus infection. N Engl J Med 1993; 328:327–335.
134. Fox CH, Cottler-Fox M. The pathobiology of HIV infection. Immunol Today 1992; 13:353–356.
135. Spain BA, Soliman DM, Sidner RA, Twigg HL.Enhanced proliferation and IL-2 secretion by lung subjects. Am J Physiol 1995; 269 (Lung Cell Mol Physiol 13): L498–L506.
136. Twigg HL, Soliman DM, Spain BA. Impaired alveolar macrophage accessory cell function and reduced incidence of lymphocytic alveolitis in HIV-infected patients who smoke. AIDS 1994; 8:611–618.
137. Laughter AH, Martin RR, Twomey JJ. Lymphoproliferative responses to antigens mediated by human pulmonary alveolar macrophages. J Lab Clin Med 1977; 89:1326–1332.
138. Brown GP, Iwamoto GK, Monick MM, Hunninghake GW. Cigarette smoking decreases interleukin 1 release by human alveolar macrophages. Am J Physiol 1989; 256:C260–C264.

139. Soliman DM, Twigg HL. Cigarette smoking decreases bioactive interleukin-6 secretion by alveolar macrophages. Am J Physiol 1992; 263:L471–L478.
140. McCrea KA, Ensor JE, Nall K, Bleecker ER, Hasday JD. Altered cytokine regulation in the lungs of cigarette smokers. Am J Respir Crit Care Med 1994; 150:696–703.

Part Three

DIAGNOSIS OF PULMONARY DISORDERS

8

Bronchoscopic and Other Invasive Sampling Techniques in the Diagnosis of Pulmonary Complications of HIV Infection

STEVE H. SALZMAN

Albert Einstein College of Medicine
and Beth Israel Medical Center
New York, New York

I. Introduction

Bronchoscopy has played the central role in defining the spectrum of pulmonary disorders that occur in patients with human immunodeficiency virus (HIV) infection. More than 15 years into the epidemic, there is now controversy over the continuing role of bronchoscopy in the evaluation of pulmonary illnesses in this patient group. Given the knowledge and experience we have gained, some recommend initial empiric therapy for *Pneumocystis carinii* pneumonia (PCP) or bacterial pneumonia, the two most common pulmonary complications, reserving bronchoscopy only for those who have not responded to the empiric therapy and have negative studies of induced sputum. A second controversy relates to the necessity of including transbronchial lung biopsies (TBBs), in addition to bronchoalveolar lavage (BAL), at the time of bronchoscopy.

At our institution, it is our practice that hospitalized patients with the acquired immunodeficiency syndrome (AIDS) with diffuse ground-glass opacities on chest radiographs are treated for PCP, followed by studies that will confirm a specific diagnosis. Our bias is that bronchoscopy should include TBB, in addition to BAL, to optimize the diagnostic yield, particularly for diagnoses other than PCP. The data relating to these controversies will form the basis of this chapter.

II. Overall Yield of Bronchoscopy

Since the beginning of the AIDS epidemic, bronchoscopy has had a central role in the diagnosis of pulmonary diseases. Studies published through 1985 suggest that the diagnostic yield of bronchoscopy ranges from 65 to 96% (1–4). These early studies were important because the high rate of open lung biopsy (OLB) procedures, follow-up bronchoscopy, and autopsy allow an accurate assessment of the false-negative rate of bronchoscopy. However, analysis of these data with our current knowledge raises doubts about the certainty of their conclusions. We now know that culture of *Mycobacterium avium–intracellulare* (MAI) or cytomegalovirus (CMV) from a pulmonary source, or even the presence of CMV intracellular inclusion bodies, are not sufficient to diagnose pulmonary infection (5,6). Currently, parenchymal Kaposi's sarcoma (KS) is inferred by the presence of bronchial KS, identified by inspection alone (7–10). Another problem was failure to distinguish between the yield for a rapid diagnosis by stains and histological features, from the later diagnosis by culture growth (2). This is a particularly important distinction for slow-growing organisms, such as mycobacteria and most fungi (11–14). Failure to make this distinction may overstate the sensitivity of bronchoscopy for the clinically important *rapid* diagnosis based on stained samples. Lastly, as we learned more about pulmonary complications of AIDS, recurrent bacterial pneumonia and tuberculosis were included as AIDS-defining illnesses in HIV-infected patients (15); these infections were largely omitted in early reports of bronchoscopy in AIDS.

Despite these limitations, clinical experience and the literature confirm that bronchoscopy is very useful for establishing the diagnosis of treatable complications of HIV infection. Excluding bacterial pneumonia, which is generally diagnosed presumptively from clinical findings and response to antimicrobial therapy, the overall yield of bronchoscopy appears to exceed 85% (16).

III. Bronchoalveolar Lavage and Transbronchial Biopsy

A. Technique

Bronchoalveolar lavage plays a central role in the diagnosis of pulmonary infectious complications in HIV-infected patients. In patients with diffuse disease, BAL has usually been performed by wedging the bronchoscope in a subsegmental bronchus of the right middle lobe or lingula, because their position in the supine patient allows good return of lavage fluid. Sterile normal saline solution is instilled in 20- to 60-mL aliquots, up to a volume of 100–200 mL, and suction is applied for sample collection (7,17). A sample of 40–50% of the instilled volume, with a minimum of 50 mL, is considered acceptable. Recent studies show that bilobar BAL sampling of an upper lobe and a second site, either the area of greatest radiographic abnormality, or the middle lobe or lingula in diffuse disease, enhances the yield for *P. carinii* (PC), particularly in patients receiving aerosol pentamidine antipneumocystis prophylaxis (18–24); Tables 1 and 2). Others have not found the sensitivity of BAL to be reduced by pentamidine prophylaxis (25,26). Although the general trend has been toward larger volume bilobar BAL, a small recent study suggested that a single 60-mL aliquot, with a returned volume of 15–25 mL was adequate to diagnose PCP when an immunofluorescent stain was used (27). We have adopted the larger-volume, bilobar approach in our practice. The pooled specimen should be submitted for cytological studies, stained for PC, and stained and cultured for mycobacteria and fungi. At most centers, studies for viruses and *Legionella* spp. are not performed routinely (7). In patients with focal disease, the area of radiopacity is sampled in a similar fashion. BAL can be performed safely, even in patients with thrombocytopenia and coagulopathy, in whom we prefer the transoral approach with a biteplate.

The TBBs are obtained from the involved area in focal disease, and from the lateral basal segment of the right lower lobe in diffuse disease, unless another area has a denser radiographic appearance. The optimal number of biopsies is unknown. One study suggests that the optimal number of TBBs to diagnose PCP varied from two in severe disease to four with a normal chest radiograph; however, this analysis excluded biopsies not containing alveoli (28). Because the adequacy of specimens is not known in advance, and the optimal number of biopsies is not known for

Table 1 Bronchoalveolar Lavage Technique

Focal disease: wedge in subsegmental bronchus in area of greatest involvement

Diffuse disease: sample two lobes (upper lobe and middle lobe/lingula), wedge in subsegmental bronchus, choose nondependent segments (e.g., anterior or apical segment of upper lobe); bilobar sampling most important for patients receiving inhaled pentamidine prophylaxis

Normal saline, 100–200 mL in 20- to 60-mL aliquots, in each lobe sampled; sample should be 40–50% of instilled volume and minimum of 50 mL

Processing: cytology, *Pneumocystis* stains and mycobacterial and fungal stains and cultures

Table 2 Modifications to Bronchoalveolar Lavage (BAL) Procedures to Improve Sensitivity for *Pneumocystis carinii:* The Effect of Aerosolized Pentamidine, Site, and Number of Lobes Lavaged, and Immunofluorescence Staining

	Site of BAL[a]					
	Right middle lobe or lingula		Upper lobe		Bilobar	
Ref.	AP+[b]	AP–[c]	AP+[b]	AP–[c]	AP+[b]	AP–[c]
18	62	100				
26	71–75	76–78				
19		86				93
22	86		100			
21	85	91	100	96		
23	80	95			98[d]	100[d]
24	65		95			

[a]Percentage of specimens positive.
[b]AP+, patients receiving aerosolized pentamidine antipneumocystis prophylaxis.
[b]AP–, patients not receiving aerosolized pentamidine antipneumocystis prophylaxis.
[d]Immunofluorescence staining.

other complications of HIV, we generally obtain at least five to six biopsy specimens. In addition to histological studies, the biopsy sample should be routinely cultured for mycobacteria and fungi (Table 3).

B. Diagnostic Yield

Both BAL and TBB are useful in the diagnosis of pulmonary disorders in patients with HIV infection. Broaddus et al. found an overall sensitivity for pulmonary infections of 86% for BAL, compared with 87% for TBB (2). Together, their yield was 96%. However, this study was limited by diagnostic criteria that make it applicable to PCP alone, for which the sensitivity of BAL and TBB were 89% and 93%, respectively. All cases of PCP were diagnosed when both BAL and TBB were performed, which is consistent with the 94–100% sensitivity for *P. carinii* of these combined procedures reported by others (1,3,4). BAL alone is 79–100% sensitive in the diagnosis of PCP, the most common condition diagnosed by bronchoscopy (1–4,16,18–24,29–32). Recent studies with upper lobe or bilobar BAL indicate sensitivities for PC of 93–100% for BAL alone (19,21–24; see Table 1). TBB will generally not be needed to confirm a diagnosis of PCP.

Pneumocystis carinii pneumonia is the most frequent diagnosis from bronchoscopy; consequently, some studies and reviews suggest that BAL without TBB is adequate at the time of bronchoscopy (33–39). However, studies showing the high yield of BAL alone typically had few patients with other diagnoses, or rarely performed TBB (40).

The additive yield of TBB appears to be most important in conditions other than PCP. Francis et al. found that TBB and BAL were equally sensitive for PCP (85 and 79%, respectively), although biopsy was more useful than cytology in the diagnosis of other infections and KS (31). In a study designed to determine the relative yield of BAL and TBB in the diagnosis of HIV-associated tuberculosis, Salzman et al. reviewed 31 patients who had both procedures performed (11). A TBB acid-fast smear or histology

Table 3 Transbronchial Biopsy Technique

Optimal number of biopsy specimens unknown; however we recommend a minimum of five to six.
Sample the area of focal disease, or right lower lobe, lateral basal segment in diffuse disease (safe and convenient).
Processing: histology, *Pneumocystis* stains, and mycobacterial and fungal stains and cultures.

was positive in 39%, compared with 10% of BAL smears. Furthermore, TBB was the exclusive source of a positive culture in 16% of patients. Similarly, Salzman et al. reported that TBB established an immediate diagnosis of histoplasmosis in 9 of 13 (69%) patients with HIV infection, whereas BAL stains were positive in only 2 of 14 (14%; 13). Our analysis of 205 bronchoscopic procedures in 182 patients with HIV infection revealed that 26% of diagnoses were established exclusively by TBB (16). The additive role of TBB was most important in noninfectious diagnoses, for which it was the exclusive source of diagnostic material in 54%. It was the source of the only diagnostic result in 40% of infections other than PC, and had its least helpful role for PCP, for which it provided the only positive test in 8% of cases.

Batungwanayo et al. reported (41) that TBB and BAL have overall diagnostic yields of 82 and 26%, respectively. This reflects the spectrum of pulmonary complications of HIV in Africa, where PCP is rare, and nonspecific interstitial pneumonitis (NIP), tuberculosis, and cryptococcal pneumonia were the three most common diagnoses. Cazzadori and colleagues, studying immunocompromised patients with HIV infection, renal transplants, and leukemia, found that the addition of TBB was important for overall yield, especially for the diagnosis of mycoses, tuberculosis, and malignant infiltration of the lung (42). The yield of bronchoscopy, TBB, and BAL in 84 bronchoscopic procedures in HIV-infected patients was 80, 77, and 48%, respectively ($p < 0.01$ for TBB versus BAL).

Taken together, these data show that, despite the high sensitivity of BAL for PC, the overall diagnostic yield is highest when both TBB and BAL are performed. Some perform BAL alone on an initial bronchoscopy because TBB procedures increase the risk of complications, especially pneumothorax, and prolongs procedure time (34,38,43,44). We routinely obtain both samples unless a hemorrhagic diathesis is present or the patient is supported by mechanical ventilation. With fluoroscopic guidance, our rate of pneumothorax is near 1% when performing TBB.

A sequential approach of using BAL on the initial bronchoscopic procedure, followed by TBB and BAL, if necessary, is supported by the study of Cadranel and associates (43). BAL alone was performed on 194 HIV-infected patients, followed by empiric β-lactam or macrolide therapy for 10 days if nondiagnostic. Only 29 (15%) patients failed to respond, and underwent a site-directed BAL and TBB at a site determined by chest computed tomography (CT). Of note, 22 of 29 (76%) requiring repeat bronchoscopy had received antipneumocystis prophylaxis. The repeat bronchoscopy was diagnostic in 90% of cases. BAL and TBB were complementary, each positive in 62% of patients.

IV. Other Procedures

Brush Biopsy

The value of brush biopsy of pulmonary infiltrates has been evaluated in detail only for PCP. The sensitivity is low (40–55%) compared with BAL and TBB, and there is no additive yield (4,20,30). This procedure has been abandoned at most centers in the evaluation of pulmonary disorders complicating HIV infection (5,7).

B. Transbronchoscopic Needle Aspiration Biopsy

Mediastinal lymphadenopathy is often seen in HIV-infected patients with mycobacterial and fungal infections, lymphoma, and KS. Except for KS, all of these conditions might be identified from the cytological or small-core specimens that are obtained with transbronchoscopic needle aspiration biopsy (TBNA). Infections with *M. tuberculosis*, MAI, and *Cryptococcus* causing mediastinal lymphadenopathy have been confirmed with this technique (45–48). By using a 19-gauge histology/aspiration needle in 41 HIV-infected patients with mediastinal or hilar adenopathy, Harkin and colleagues obtained diagnostic material in 23 of 44 (52%) procedures (48). TBNA was the exclusive means of diagnosis in 13 of 41 (32%) patients. The procedure was most useful in mycobacterial infection, which was the final diagnosis in 23 of 44 (52%) procedures. TBNA was diagnostic in 20 of 23 (87%) mycobacterial infections, including a rapid diagnosis by visualization of acid-fast bacilli, or granuloma in 17/23 (74%).

C. Endobronchial Biopsy

The most common condition causing endobronchial abnormalities in HIV-infected patients is KS (49). Bronchial KS is usually diagnosed by its characteristic appearance in patients who also have cutaneous disease. Other conditions, including tuberculosis, atypical mycobacterioses, cryptococcosis, aspergillosis, and bronchogenic carcinoma, may cause endobronchial abnormalities (50–56). Biopsy should be performed on any endobronchial abnormalities that are not typical of KS, especially in patients without obvious cutaneous involvement. Sufficient material should be obtained for both histological evaluation and culture for mycobacteria and fungi, for infectious endobronchial diseases may mimic bronchogenic carcinoma (51,53; see Table 4 on p. 212).

D. Percutaneous Needle Biopsy

An early study showed that needle biopsy of HIV-infected patients with diffuse lung disease has a high yield, but carries a relatively high risk of pneumothorax (57), so bronchoscopy has been the preferred procedure in this setting. Percutaneous needle aspiration is most helpful in the evaluation of focal mass lesions and lymphadenopathy (54,58). In a recent study of 45 HIV-infected patients, lung aspiration with a 25-gauge needle, without premedication or fluoroscopy, established a diagnosis (mostly PCP, tuberculosis, and bacterial pneumonia) in 62% of procedures (59). Only one of the eight pneumothoraces required chest tube drainage. This technique may be superior to bronchoscopy for the diagnosis of bacterial infections.

E. Repeat Bronchoscopy

Repeat bronchoscopy has its highest yield in patients with a new pulmonary presentation after recovery from the initial illness. Repeat bronchoscopy within 30 days has a lower yield, but is occasionally useful, especially when the first bronchoscopy was nondiagnostic. The yield of repeat bronchoscopy was 38% after an initial nondiagnostic bronchoscopy, compared with 15% when a patient was deteriorating despite treatment for a confirmed infection (60). In contrast with the relatively low yield of early repeat procedures, 80% of patients who had a second bronchoscopy after 1 month because of new pulmonary symptoms had a diagnosis established.

The low likelihood of establishing a new, treatable diagnosis by repeat bronchoscopy in patients who do not respond to therapy is supported by Stover et al. (1). Eight patients with PCP on their initial bronchoscopy underwent 11 additional bronchoscopic procedures because of a lack of response to therapy. In only 1 was a new pathogen, CMV, found. The usefulness of repeat bronchoscopy is uncertain because these studies were limited by use of bronchial wash, rather than BAL (60) and small study size (1). Despite its probable low yield, some pulmonologists would repeat bronchoscopy before obtaining an open lung biopsy (OLB) because of its lower morbidity.

F. Open Lung Biopsy

An OLB is most helpful when an initial bronchoscopy is nondiagnostic or is not performed because of bleeding disorders or respiratory failure (61). As in repeat bronchoscopy, OLB has a lower yield in patients who deteriorate despite treatment for an established diagnosis. KS was the most frequent finding of OLB after nondiagnostic bronchoscopy (61–63). Other disorders that may require OLB for diagnosis include CMV pneumonitis, lymphoma, lymphocytic interstitial pneumonitis (LIP), and NIP.

The indications for OLB are diminishing because of the high yield of BAL and TBB for treatable opportunistic infections (64), the safety of

BAL even in those with coagulopathy, and our current acceptance of a diagnosis of pulmonary KS based on bronchoscopic inspection alone (8). Most would reserve OLB for the following situations: (1) progressive pulmonary disease with negative BAL and TBB, (2) progressive pulmonary disease with a negative BAL and uncorrectable coagulopathy, and (3) mechanical ventilation with negative BAL or TBB. Although the yield of OLB is low in patients who deteriorate despite an established diagnosis, new diagnoses may occasionally be discovered.

V. Bronchoscopy in Infectious Diseases

A. Bacterial Pneumonia

The role of quantitative BAL and protected-catheter brushing in the diagnosis of bacterial pneumonia in non-HIV–infected patients is controversial, and is currently not recommended as a routine practice (65). In a prospective study of fever and pulmonary infiltrates in HIV-infected patients, 30% of patients were considered to have bacterial pneumonia based on clinical criteria (66). With quantitative cultures of telescoping plugged catheter specimens, and a diagnostic cutoff of 10^3 colony-forming units (CFU)/ml, this method of diagnosis was 53% sensitive and 76% specific. From clinical criteria, Magnenat et al. found that 45% of pulmonary episodes in HIV-infected patients were due to bacterial pneumonia. They found that quantitative BAL culture, using a cutoff of 10^5/mL, had a sensitivity of 83% in patients who did not receive antibiotics before bronchoscopy and 23% in those who did, and the specificity was 80.5% (67). Further studies are needed to clarify the role of bronchoscopic methods for the diagnosis of bacterial pneumonia.

Until these issues are resolved, empiric treatment for bacterial pneumonia is warranted for patients who have focal infiltrates and a compatible clinical illness. If the patient does not improve, and if acid-fast bacilli (AFB) smears of sputum are negative, bronchoscopy that includes BAL and TBB should be performed. Some would perform sputum induction for *P. carinii* and AFB before bronchoscopy. If bronchoscopic specimens are nondiagnostic, but the patient improves with a continued or modified antibacterial regimen, then a clinical diagnosis of bacterial pneumonia is inferred.

B. *Pneumocystis carinii* Pneumonia

The diagnosis of PCP depends on identification of the organism from specimens derived from the lung. The least invasive diagnostic modality is the induction of sputum with 3% saline delivered by ultrasonic nebulization.

In some centers, *P. carinii* can be identified by modified Giemsa, methenamine silver, or immunofluorescent staining in up to 80% of cases (68–70), although many centers have a much lower yield. Spontaneously produced sputum should not be stained for *P. carinii* because of a very low yield. If sputum induction is not diagnostic, the next step to establish a diagnosis should be bronchoscopy. Even though BAL cell differentials are of no diagnostic value in AIDS, BAL neutrophilia indicates a worse prognosis in PCP (71,72).

The high sensitivity of BAL for *P. carinii* led to investigations of the role of lavage that is not performed with the bronchoscope (73–77). The major advantages are convenience and lower expense, especially if performed by nonphysician personnel. In patients who have endotracheal tubes, PCP was diagnosed in 19 of 20 cases simply by instilling 60 mL of saline in 10-mL aliquots and collecting the specimen 30 sec after each aliquot into a sputum trap using standard suction catheters (75).

C. Mycobacterial Infections

In a study that included non-HIV–infected patients, bronchial wash and BAL were complementary (78). The reported sensitivity of BAL AFB smear, 68%, overstates the yield of BAL because 34% of patients had positive smears from spontaneous sputum and underwent bronchoscopy for research purposes. TBB was not performed in this study.

In a study that included BAL and TBB in all patients (11), when smears were negative, or when patients failed to produce sputum, 48% of patients with HIV and tuberculosis had a rapid presumptive diagnosis by stains or identification of granulomata from bronchoscopy specimens that included BAL, TBB, and postprocedure sputum analysis. TBB was more sensitive than BAL for this purpose (39 and 10%, respectively). Half of the immediate diagnoses were derived exclusively from TBB specimens. By contrast, only 10% of smears were positive from bronchoscopy that yielded MAI (11). Because tuberculosis is more commonly smear-positive, communicable, and more easily treated than MAI, treatment for tuberculosis should be initiated when microscopy reveals AFB or granulomata.

In the same study, sputum obtained both before and after bronchoscopy had a higher yield on culture (78 and 79%, respectively) than BAL or TBB, although sputum could not always be obtained. Taken together, BAL, TBB, and sputum produced after bronchoscopy provided important information in 65% of cases by providing an immediate diagnosis or as the exclusive source of a positive culture. Testing the sensitivities to antituberculous agents is especially important in areas with a high prevalence of resistant organisms.

This and a similar study (12) show that bronchoscopy is important to establish an early diagnosis of tuberculosis in sputum smear-negative patients and enhances the yield on culture, especially in patients who do not produce sputum. BAL, TBB, and sputum after bronchoscopy should be obtained. Inclusion of TBB is warranted because of the incremental diagnostic yield over BAL and sputum alone.

The isolation of MAI from respiratory specimens is not considered diagnostic of invasive pulmonary or disseminated disease (5). Bronchoscopy should include TBB, endobronchial biopsy, or TBNA so that histological evidence of tissue invasion may be found.

TBNA with an histology needle should be included in patients with mediastinal or hilar adenopathy, for this has been diagnostic in 87% of patients when the lymphadenopathy was due to mycobacterial infection (48).

Both tuberculosis and MAI may infect the bronchi in HIV-infected patients, mimicking bronchogenic carcinoma in clinical presentation, chest radiographic features, and bronchoscopic findings (51–53). Although most patients are febrile, some present with wheeze or hemoptysis alone. Radiographs typically demonstrate thoracic lymphadenopathy, with focal infiltrates, atelectasis, or pleural effusions present in some. Endobronchial masses often obstruct the airway and have ranged from exophytic, lobulated lesions with white, pink, or necrotic surfaces, to sessile polypoid lesions.

Calpe and associates found bronchial abnormalities in 6 (24%) of 25 bronchoscopic procedures diagnostic of TB, emphasizing some subtle findings that may be overlooked (55). The bronchoscopic findings were (1) diffusely reddened mucosa in 5, localized in 1; (2) exophytic mass with superficial necrotic tissue in 3; (3) localized, raised whitish plaques in 4; (4) small miliary lesions in the bronchial mucosa in 2; and (5) extrinsic compression of the trachea and main bronchi in 3. Radiographic patterns differed in the groups with and without endobronchial tuberculosis (TB). Mediastinal adenopathy without parenchymal disease was typical of endobronchial involvement. The opposite radiographic pattern was seen in those with normal bronchoscopic examinations. When adenopathy is present, the bronchoscopist should be alert for subtle mucosal disease, and include endobronchial biopsy and TBNA when appropriate.

Acid-fast smears of sputum and bronchoscopic specimens may be negative in many patients with pulmonary tuberculosis, despite an appropriate diagnostic evaluation. Empiric therapy should be considered while awaiting culture results in patients with roentgenographic abnormalities that are consistent with tuberculosis who do not have another plausible disorder identified. Alternatively, OLB or mediastinoscopy can be performed.

Current techniques to identify tuberculosis are either insensitive (AFB stain) or delayed (culture). Highly sensitive techniques, such as those employing the polymerase chain reaction (PCR), may be useful to identify smear-negative, culture-positive cases (79). However, specificity and positive predictive value has been variable. Previously treated, inactive tuberculosis and tuberculous infection without disease (tuberculin-positive only) may result in a positive PCR test (the test is "too sensitive"). This is likely to limit the usefulness of PCR in the diagnosis of active tuberculosis.

D. Cytomegalovirus Pneumonia

Although CMV can often be isolated from the lung, in the past it rarely caused significant pneumonitis in patients with HIV infection (80). Cultures of BAL fluid of patients with AIDS who have pneumonia caused by various pathogens are positive for CMV in up to 50% of cases, viral inclusion bodies may be seen within lavage cells, and cytopathic changes may be found in pulmonary parenchymal specimens. When treatment is directed at coexisting pathogens, such as *P. carinii*, without agents active against CMV, the presence of CMV has not appeared to alter the prognosis (6,80–82).

Given these data, a diagnosis of CMV pneumonia in patients with AIDS has depended on demonstration of characteristic intranuclear or cytoplasmic inclusion bodies within lung cells, including alveolar macrophages, and preferably when no other pulmonary pathogen is identified (5,80). Consequently, bronchoscopy should include TBB, but OLB is sometimes required (1,4,5,60–63).

Recent data suggest that the role of CMV as a pathogen has been augmented by the use of adjunctive corticosteroids for PCP and, in this group, isolation of CMV may be significant. In a group of 159 consecutive AIDS patients with PCP, patients treated with corticosteroids had a 2.1 mortality ratio ($p = 0.08$) when BAL was culture-positive for CMV, when compared with the groups not treated with corticosteroids or not culture-positive for CMV, or both (83). Multivariate analysis indicated that corticosteroid use and isolation of CMV did not independently predict mortality, although their combination was predictive of increased mortality risk. The difference in mortality was not explained by differences in CD4 cell counts or severity of PCP based on Po_2 values. Another group has reported that 10 of 65 (15%) inpatients treated for PCP died, all with CMV coinfection and treated with steroids (84). There were not deaths in the 20 patients without CMV present.

Other data suggest that the significance of CMV in BAL may have been underestimated (85). Although evidence for CMV did not predict 3-

week mortality, this study found that long-term survival (3 and 6 months) was predicted by the presence of CMV cytopathic changes together with a positive culture of BAL; 6-month mortality was predicted by positive culture alone. The effect was not explained by CD4 counts or *P. carinii* coinfection. The role of steroids was not evaluated.

These data suggest that any evidence of CMV pulmonary infection should be considered possibly significant in a deteriorating patient, although firm diagnosis continues to require cytopathological evidence and absence of coinfection.

E. Fungal Diseases

Although less common than bacterial infections and PCP, serious fungal infections also occur in the setting of severe immunocompromise, both as new infections and as reactivation of latent disease. The types of fungal infections that occur in patients with AIDS depend on the severity of immunodeficiency and whether the patient has lived in endemic areas.

Baughman and colleagues reported that BAL smear was positive in 14 of 41 (34%) patients, and culture-positive in 35 (85%) in a patient group that included 19 HIV-infected patients with a variety of pulmonary fungal infections (78). They also point out that sputum smears and cultures were rarely helpful for diagnosis in fungal infections, and that bronchial wash was complementry to BAL. This study may overstate the usefulness of BAL, for TBB was not performed.

Cryptococcosis

A review of fungal disease in HIV-infected patients reports that cryptococcal cultures and wet preparation of expectorated sputum are positive for *C. neoformans* in less than 25% of cases (14). They state that bronchoscopy with biopsy for both culture and histopathology is usually necessary for diagnosis, and that serum cryptococcal antigen is almost always positive in high titer in cryptococcal lung disease.

Two separate reports from a single institution evaluated the diagnostic yield of bronchoscopic procedures in HIV-related cryptococcal pulmonary disease in 21 patients (47,50). An early diagnosis by microscopy was obtained from sputum (9%), BAL (60–82%), bronchial wash (70%), TBB (67–75%), bronchial brush (66%), and in endobronchial and transbronchial needle biopsies. Serum cryptococcal antigen was positive in 14 (93%) of 15 patients tested. Whereas no sputum culture was positive, positive cultures were obtained from BAL (63–100%), bronchial wash (40%), TBB (25%), and endobronchial biopsies (67%). Endobronchial abnormalities included red and white thrush-like plaques, and mucosal granularity (50).

A report of 37 cases in Rwanda emphasized the usefulness of BAL, which was positive on culture in 27 of 33 (82%) procedures, compared with 10 of 21 (48%) TBBs (86). Stains of histophathological specimens from TBB were positive in 10/21 (48%), although BAL cytology results were not reported. This group reports that serum cryptococcal antigen was detected in only 8 of 26 (31%) patients, and these all had extrapulmonary disease.

Baughman and colleagues report that a high titer of cryptococcal antigen in serum is strongly suggestive, and an antigen titer of 1:8 or higher in bronchoalveolar lavage fluid is diagnostic of cryptococcal pneumonia (87). The cost-effectiveness of routine assay of BAL for this antigen is likely to be low because cryptococcal pneumonia is relatively uncommon.

Although none of these studies report on the additive role of TBB, BAL alone appears to be highly useful, particularly because this is a relatively rapidly growing fungus.

Histoplasmosis

Patients with HIV infection who come from endemic areas may develop disseminated disease when immunodeficiency permits reactivation of latent infection (13). The diagnosis is established by identification or culture of the organism from lung-derived specimens, bone marrow, lymph node, blood, liver, or skin. Serological tests are positive in about half the patients (88).

Although bone marrow is a common site of diagnostic specimens for histoplasmosis in AIDS (89,90), it appears that bronchoscopy has a higher overall yield. Bronchoscopy was positive by stains or culture in 87% of patients, compared with 71% of bone marrow evaluations (13). TBB was important for establishing a rapid diagnosis. A *Histoplasma* sp. was identified by stain of the TBB in 69% of patients, whereas BAL stains were positive in only 14%. However, culture of BAL was more sensitive than TBB culture (69 and 20%, respectively).

Radioimmunoassay for *H. capsulatum* polysaccharide antigen in the urine was positive in 59 of 61 (97%) patients with AIDS and disseminated histoplasmosis (91), and was useful in detecting relapse (92). When this diagnosis is suspected, and the test is available, this noninvasive test can establish the diagnosis.

Aspergillosis

Virtually all patients with this infection have pulmonary involvement, either as the sole site or as part of disseminated infection. Although most patients have the classic risk factors of severe neutropenia, glucocorticoid administration, hematological malignancy, and prior antibiotic use, it is becoming increasingly clear that severe immunosuppression itself may be the only risk factor (14,93,94). Almost all patients have CD4 counts of fewer than 50 (93) or fewer than 100 (94).

Two types of pulmonary disease have been identified: an invasive parenchymal infection, and less frequently, a predominantly bronchial disease (14,54,93–95). Bronchi are visibly abnormal in some patients. These patients may present with wheeze or prominent cough. Ulcerative or plaque-like tracheobronchitis was well characterized in four patients (95). Patients had mild to moderate diffuse tracheobronchitis, with erythematous, edematous mucosa. Multiple, white 2- to 3-mm plaques to nodules were seen, with exudate-covered ulceration in some patients. Biopsy of lesions revealed typical branching hyphae in all four patients, and tissue invasion in three. BAL cytology and culture were positive in two (50%) of four, and three (100%) of three, respectively. There is also a noninvasive form of "obstructing bronchial aspergillosis," with large mucoid casts full of *Aspergillus* organisms expectorated or found at bronchoscopy (54). These may result in segmental or lobal atelectasis, and progress to invasive pseudomembranous tracheobronchitis (54).

The vast majority of patients with aspergillosis have lung parenchymal involvement. Diagnosis requires the documentation of tissue invasion with biopsy, or recovery of the fungus from usually sterile sites. Recovery of *Aspergillus* sp. from respiratory secretion appears to be common in AIDS patients who do not have clinical evidence of infection with the fungus. A retrospective review of 972 AIDS patients seen over 10 years, identified 45 with *Aspergillus* spp. isolated from a respiratory site (31 sputum and 14 bronchoscopy specimens; 96). Invasive aspergillosis was felt to be present based on autospy in 4 (26 autopsies performed) and clinical course in 1. Colonization was suspected in the remaining 40 patients (89%). Bronchoscopy should include bronchial and TBB to confirm tissue invasion, although isolation of aspergillus from a patient with AIDS and a compatible clinical picture should be considered as probable invasive disease, particularly when risk factors for aspergillosis are present and no alternative diagnosis is established.

The relative sensitivity of BAL and TBB has not been systematically evaluated. Denning et al. reported that BAL and percutaneous aspirates were more useful than TBB (54), Lotholary emphasized the usefulness of BAL (93), but Singh et al. found TBB to be particularly useful (95). These authors observations reflect the frequency of isolation from that specimen, rather than the sensitivity of the procedure, because TBB was frequently not performed.

Denning et al. found percutaneous needle cytology and culture were diagnostic in four (100%) of four obtained; BAL cytology and culture, in two (40%) of five, and five (100%) of five, respectively; TBB stains were negative in the three obtained, and cultures of this specimen are not reported (54). Lotholary and colleagues emphasize the usefulness of BAL, from which an *Aspergillus* sp. was isolated in 28 (100%) of 28 patients (93). Results of BAL stains were not reported. However, 6 (86%) of the 7 patients who had histological specimens obtained antemortem had diagnostic findings. These included bronchial biopsy in 2, tracheal biopsy in 2, bronchial and TBB in 1, and OLB in 1. Klapholz et al. (98). found that specimen stains had a higher yield from BAL (7/8, 88%), compared with TBB (3/6, 50%). Although these studies suggest that BAL has a higher yield than TBB, the latter should be routinely included to distinguish invasive disease from colonization.

Techniques using PCR of BAL appears unlikely to be helpful, owing to poor positive predictive value, related to the inability to distinguish colonization from infection ("too sensitive"). There is also risk for environmental contamination of reagents from this ubiquitous fungus (99). Serology has been unhelpful except for the rare case of aspergilloma, in which serum precipitins (antiaspergillus IgG) are useful (93,94). Serum and BAL antigen detection has been positive in 25% (four of six tested), and 100% (three of three tested), respectively (93).

Coccidioidomycosis

In endemic areas, pulmonary coccidioidomycosis, with or without disseminated disease, is common in HIV-infected patients with CD4 lymphocyte counts of fewer than 250/mm^3 (14). Diagnosis requires culture or visualization in biological material or histopathological sections. The fungus is rarely identified by KOH wet mount or Papanicolaou stain of spontaneous sputum (14). Bronnimann et al. reported that spherules of *Coccidioides* were seen more often in bronchial wash and TBB specimens than in BAL or sputum samples (100). Culture of bronchoscopic specimens was positive more often than sputum cultures. Graham et al. showed that the addition of TBB to BAL improves the diagnostic yield (101).

A recent study has defined the relative usefulness of bronchoscopic specimens for this fungus (102). BAL or bronchial wash cytology was diagnostic in 18 of 42 (42%) AIDS patients and 11 of 35 (31%) non-AIDS patients ($p = 0.63$). The BAL or bronchial wash culture had a sensitivity of 100%. The median time to definitive identification was 25 days, although growth on the fungal medium and preliminary identification was available in a median of 3.5 days in the 10 patients for whom data were available.

TBB performed simultaneously in 7 AIDS patients yielded morphological identification of the fungus in all (100% sensitivity). The major role of TBB is in establishing an early diagnosis in the most acutely ill patients with miliary disease.

Fish et al. found that 83% of patients had positive serology; 74% by complement fixation, but tube precipitin was positive in only 39% (103). However, serology is not specific for active disease, so the main role is in monitoring the success of therapy (14).

Blastomycosis

Blastomycosis is uncommon in HIV-infected patients, occurring sporadically in those who have lived in endemic areas and have CD4 lymphocyte counts of fewer than 200 (104). Diagnosis requires growth in culture or visualization of the organism in biological material or histopathological sections (14). Culture growth is slow, so a rapid diagnosis requires visualization of the organism. Pappas et al. emphasized the important role of cytological or histological examination of sputum, BAL fluid, cerebrospinal fluid, and tissue biopsies in obtaining a rapid diagnosis in 93% of patients (104). Serology is not helpful. The role of bronchoscopy and relative sensitivity of BAL and TBB were not addressed.

VI. Neoplastic Diseases of the Lung

A. Kaposi's Sarcoma

Kaposi's sarcoma is the most common malignancy occurring in persons with HIV infection, and the skin is the major site of involvement. KS can involve the parenchyma, airways, pleura, and intrathoracic lymph nodes, leading to a diverse range of symptoms and radiographic findings (8,9,105–111). Patients with pulmonary KS had a median CD4 count of 19 in a recent large study (112). Patients with KS may undergo bronchoscopy because of symptoms suggesting airway involvement (wheezing, hoarseness, stridor, or hemoptysis) or, more commonly, because of chest radiographic abnormalities, with or without cough, dyspnea, and fever. The major usefulness of bronchoscopy in these settings is the visual identification of typical lesions in the airways. Bronchial lesions are irregular macular to slightly raised patches that are similar in appearance to skin KS, except that they are often bright red, rather than purple. Their distribution ranges from the larynx to the segmental bronchi, with an avidity for the bronchial division (113,114). The extent of involvement varies from scattered discrete nodular or macular foci to numerous confluent erthematous areas. These lesions may resemble suction trauma. Occasionally, they are bulky enough to cause obstruction in the upper airway or bronchial lumen.

The frequency of visible endobronchial abnormalities in patients with thoracic KS is reported to be 87–97% (10,108,109), although one study found visible abnormalities in only 35% (105). This variability is probably explained by the frequency with which more invasive procedures, such as OLB, mediastinoscopy, and autopsy were used to obtain a final diagnosis of KS. Patients with clinically significant parenchymal KS usually have typical endobronchial abnormalities, the extent of which correlates with the degree of radiographic abnormality (10,115). However, parenchymal disease may be present without bronchial involvement (9,115).

The histological diagnosis of thoracic KS may be difficult to establish. Most reports indicate a diagnostic yield less than 20% from biopsy of endobronchial lesions (10,105,109,110,113). The yield may be enhanced by the use of "alligator"-toothed forceps and choice of location for biopsies (111). Selecting lesions at carinas subdividing lobar or segmental orifices allows deeper forceps biopsy of submucosal lesions. Bronchial brushing and other cytological methods are not helpful because histological interpretation is required for diagnosis (109).

Some authors consider biopsy contraindicated because of a high risk of bleeding from this vascular tumor (108,109), but larger and more recent reports indicate a low rate of bleeding from either endobronchial or transbroncial biopsy (8,113,114). The finding of typical lesions on inspection of the airways in patients with previously diagnosed skin KS should be considered diagnostic, because the diagnostic yield of forceps biopsy is low, and may occasionally cause significant hemorrhage. However, a similar-appearing, although solitary, endobronchial lesion caused by a *Cryptococcus* sp. was reported (50). When an endobronchial abnormality typical of KS is solitary or not associated with skin or other previous site of KS, biopsy should be performed (Table 4).

Although most patients with endobronchial KS have cutaneous disease, patients occasionally have a pulmonary presentation of KS first (105,110,116,117). In Huang and colleagues' large study of 168 patients

Table 4 Endobronchial Disease in HIV Infection

Kaposi's sarcoma (KS) is most common, red macular to slightly raised patches, not solitary.
Visual diagnosis of KS is adequate when typical appearance and nonpulmonary KS is established.
Mycobacteria, fungi, and bronchogenic carcinoma all occur less often.
Perform biopsy when not clearly KS; biopsy is *not* contraindicated in KS.

with pulmonary KS, 15% had bronchial KS without mucocutaneous involvement (112). The patients without skin or oral mucosal involvement were more likely to have isolated tracheal KS, and a greater incidence of concurrent opportunistic infection (50% vs. 23%, $p < 0.01$). These features suggest that bronchial KS unassociated with skin KS is usually less extensive and often an incidental finding in a patient with opportunistic pneumonia. However, extensive bronchial KS can occur without skin involvement.

The yield of TBB for parenchymal disease caused by KS is reported to be less than 15% (9,10,106,109,113). Explanations include patchy involvement of the parenchyma resulting in sampling error, and insufficient size to assess architecture. On the other hand, false-positive diagnoses from small biopsies taken with the bronchoscope may occur, because crush artifact, hemorrhage, granulation tissue, and fibrosis may mimic the histological features of KS (106). We recently found a 40% yield of TBB, perhaps because of the accumulated experience of the pathologists (16).

Even in the presence of endobronchial KS, evaluation of the parenchyma with BAL and TBB is usually indicated because of high rates of simultaneous opportunistic infections (9,105–109). The confirmation of parenchymal KS is less important because its presence correlates well with the finding of endobronchial involvement (7,9,10). In 76 patients with pulmonary KS, but without simultaneous pulmonary infection, tumor extent at bronchoscopy (grade 1–3) correlated with severity of parenchymal disease on chest radiographs (stage 0–3; $p < 0.01$: 115). In this study, 12% had lesions confined to the trachea, epiglottis, or larynx without tumor at or below the tracheal carina (grade 1); 41% had lesions within the bronchi, limited to three or fewer lobes (of the six "lobes," including lingula; grade 2); 47% had diffuse, extensive, or confluent disease in four or more lobes (grade 3).

An OLB increases the diagnostic yield for KS, and KS has been reported to be the most common diagnosis in patients undergoing the procedure for a nondiagnostic bronchoscopy that included TBB (61,63). This partly reflects a period when the visual identification of bronchial KS was not known to predict parenchymal involvement. However, even OLB is not 100% sensitive for KS when compared with autopsy, presumably because of patchy parenchymal involvement. A presumptive diagnosis of pulmonary KS, without bronchoscopic confirmation, is sometimes made in the appropriate setting. Clinical clues that suggest pulmonary KS in a patient with respiratory symptoms and an abnormal chest radiograph include the presence of cutaneous involvement, absence of fever, absence of pulmonary uptake on gallium scan, and nodular densities (8,118).

B. Other Malignant Neoplasms

Non-Hodgkin's lymphoma occurs with increased frequency in patients with HIV infection and may involve the intrathoracic lymph nodes, pleura, and pulmonary parenchyma, the latter revealing multiple nodules or interstitial infiltrates on chest roentgenogram (119). Few data are available on diagnostic techniques for thoracic lymphoma in AIDS (8). TBB, thoracentesis, and pleural biopsy are sometimes diagnostic, but OLB or mediastinoscopy are often required. Solid tumors, including primary lung cancers, are now believed to occur with increased frequency in HIV-infected persons (120, 121). The role of bronchoscopy in this setting has not been reported.

VII. Idiopathic Pulmonary Disorders

Many HIV-infected patients have pulmonary disorders without defined infectious or neoplastic etiology. These include LIP, NIP, bronchiolitis obliterans-organizing pneumonia (BOOP), and primary pulmonary hypertension (122–126). LIP, NIP, and BOOP require histological diagnosis, confirmed with TBB or OLB (8,123,125). BAL has no role in the diagnosis of these disorders. The diagnosis of primary pulmonary hypertension is established by OLB or clinical criteria.

VIII. Infection Control

The HIV can be isolated from most body fluids of infected patients, including saliva, alveolar fluid, and lung tissue (127,128), so there is concern about proper infection control practices in the bronchoscopy suite. There are no reports of transmission of HIV infection by the bronchoscope to patients, or by aerosol to the bronchoscopist (128). Nevertheless, clinicians should use effective precautions to avoid transmission of other airborne pathogens, especially *M. tuberculosis*. Bronchoscopy should be performed in rooms that have adequate air exchanges, and all personnel should wear tight-fitting protective respirator masks (129). To avoid contact of infected secretions with skin and mucosa, clean gloves, protective eyewear, and a gown should be worn (130,131). The principle of universal precautions dictates that masks and other environmental controls should be used uniformly during all bronchoscopic procedures.

Because unrecognized HIV infection may be present in any patient, all bronchoscopes should be cleaned and disinfected using techniques adequate to eliminate HIV and other important pathogens. Glutaraldehyde is an effective disinfectant of HIV-contaminated endoscopes (128). Although it appears that proper cleaning with detergent alone is adequate to eliminate HIV from contaminated bronchoscopes (130), thorough disinfection should also be performed. With strict adherence to proper cleaning and disinfection protocols (128,130,131), separate instruments are not needed for HIV-infected patients. Manual cleaning of the surface, valves, and channels with detergent and water immediately after the procedure is necessary to avoid drying of secretions and formation of a biofilm, which can be hard to remove. Disinfection consists of soaking the bronchoscope and all internal channels in 2% glutaraldehyde for at least 20 min. After soaking, the channel should be rinsed with sterile water or 70% alcohol. In the era of infection with HIV and other transmissible pathogens, nonimmersible bronchoscopes should be phased out as soon as possible.

IX. Suggested Diagnostic Algorithm: Empiric Therapy or Early Bronchoscopy?

Some recommend initial empiric therapy for PCP in patients with diffuse infiltrates, because it is the most common disease causing this presentation (33,132–136). They reserve bronchoscopy for patients who do not respond to 5 days of empiric therapy. Delay in bronchoscopy, even after weeks of treatment, does not appreciably reduce the diagnostic yield for *P. carinii* (137).

However, when PCP occurs, coinfection with other organisms is common (40). In addition, the adjunctive use of steroids may cause nonspecific improvement in patients with other diagnoses, and contribute to the emergence of other opportunistic infections, such as aspergillosis and CMV, although the incidence of TB does not appear to be increased (54,83,84, 97,138,139). If PCP is the most likely diagnosis, therapy should be started while the diagnostic evaluation is in progress. We and others (5,7,35,134,140) prefer to establish a definitive diagnosis initially by noninvasive specimens (spontaneous and induced sputum), followed by bronchoscopy if sputum studies are nondiagnostic. This issue has been the subject of recent articles and editorials (35,136,140–143).

We are unaware of a prospective trial comparing empiric treatment with and without bronchoscopic confirmation. An important retrospective study from 56 hospitals in five cities suggests that empiric treatment for PCP without bronchoscopic confirmation is associated with increased mortality (odds ratio 1.64 compared with confirmed cases; 143). Mortality, in this study of 1021 patients with a final diagnosis of PCP, was 22% in those who did not undergo bronchoscopy, 14% in those with positive bronchoscopy, and 11% in those with negative bronchoscopy, but still treated for

PCP ($p < 0.05$). Multivariate analysis showed the major predictor of in-hospital mortality was severity of illness based primarily on $P(A\text{-}a)O_2$, and secondarily on lymphocyte count. The other predictors were no bronchoscopy (odds ratio 1.64) and black or Hispanic race–ethnicity (odds ratios, 1.77 and 1.71, respectively). Multivariate analysis showed that factors associated with lower bronchoscopy rates were Medicaid insurance (odds ratio 0.69), treatment at a county hospital (odds ratio 0.57), and prior PCP prophylaxis (odds ratio 0.60). This latter group would have an increased likelihood not to have PCP, so empiric therapy was ill-advised. Severity of illness was not a significant predictor of bronchoscopy use in multivariate analysis, indicating that reluctance to perform bronchoscopy on the most hypoxemic, unstable patients was not the reason that lack of bronchoscopic evaluation predicted mortality. The authors concluded that severity of illness was the major predictor of mortality in patients treated for PCP. The better outcome of those proved by bronchoscopy, even when adjusted for severity of illness, suggests that bronchoscopy contributed to this improved outcome. This may have been by excluding other treatable conditions.

Masur and Shelhamer have proposed that empiric therapy for PCP without confirmation is appropriate when the following criteria are met (136): mild disease ($Po_2 > 70$–80, or pulse oximetry above 95%); symptoms not severe or rapidly progressive; typical chest radiograph for PCP (if lobar consolidation, empiric treatment for bacterial organisms instead); no radiologic features atypical for PCP (pleural effusion, adenopathy, nodules); patient not receiving PCP prophylaxis, or a preventive regimen other than trimethoprim–sulfamethoxazole (because this would decrease the likelihood of PCP and probably infection with *S. pneumoniae* and *H. influenzae*); able to tolerate oral medications, compliant, and reliable; local epidemiology does not substantially increase the likelihood of tuberculosis, histoplasmosis, or coccidioidomycosis as in certain North American cities and areas of the developing world; patient not hospitalized, where the costs of hospitalization outweigh the savings of empiric therapy. We feel this is a sensible approach, but note that we consult on few patients who meet these criteria.

Because of different local epidemiology, a different approach to empiric therapy without bronchoscopic confirmation has been suggested in Tanzania (144). This study of 127 HIV-infected patients with acute respiratory disease used a staged approach of initial AFB sputum smear, empiric treatment for bacterial pneumonia, followed by bronchoscopy with BAL alone in those who did not respond. They found that bronchoscopy added little to management because very few patients had PCP, 75% had tuberculosis, and 14% had bacterial pneumonia. They advocate empiric

Table 5 Suggested Diagnostic Algorithm in HIV Infection: Focal Pulmonary Disease

Step 1	
	Blood cultures, pleural fluid studies if effusion present.
	Empiric therapy for bacterial pneumonia.
	Stain and culture sputum for mycobacteria.
Step 2	
	If not improving or no diagnosis: sputum induction for *Pneumocystis* and mycobacteria is an option before bronchoscopy.
Step 3	
	If not improving or no diagnosis: bronchoscopy with bronchoalveolar lavage and transbronchial biopsy.

tuberculosis therapy in those with negative AFB smears who fail to improve with antibacterial therapy.

Our local diagnostic approach considers the relatively high incidence of tuberculosis in New York City, although we feel this approach is appropriate to most North American and European countries. HIV-infected patients with acute febrile illnesses and focal consolidation on chest radiographs should be treated for bacterial pneumonia, and sputum should be stained and cultured for mycobacteria. If empiric treatment is unsuccessful, or if there is diffuse radiographic involvement, sputum induced with hypertonic saline aerosol should be examined for PC, AFB, and possibly fungi. If these studies yield no diagnosis, bronchoscopy should be performed (Tables 5 and 6).

Table 6 Suggested Diagnostic Algorithm in HIV Infection: Diffuse Pulmonary Disease

Step 1	
	Empiric therapy for *Pneumocystis*.
	Nodules, adenopathy, or pleural effusion make *Pneumocystis* less likely.
	Sputum induction for *Pneumocystis* and mycobacteria (spontaneous sputum, if produced, is best for acid-fast bacilli).
Step 2	
	If no diagnosis, bronchoscopy with bronchoalveolar lavage (BAL) and transbronchial biopsy (TBB)[a]

[a]Some practitioners perform bronchoscopy only if the patient fails to improve on empiric antipneumocystis therapy; some do BAL without TBB on an initial bronchoscopy.

Table 7 Reasons to Perform Transbronchial Biopsy (TBB) During Bronchoscopy of HIV-Infected Patients

Enhances yield for early diagnosis (stains for organism or histology) or culture, or both: *M. tuberculosis*, *Histoplasma*, *Coccidioides*, *Pneumocystis*.
Histology needed to establish significance of culture or BAL stain: cytomegalovirus, *M. avium-intracellulare*, *Aspergillus*.
Histology required for diagnosis: lymphocytic interstitial pneumonitis, nonspecific interstitial pneumonitis, lymphoma, Kaposi's sarcoma[a].
The patient may be too ill for TBB after a first bronchoscopy with negative bronchoalveolar lavage.

[a]A presumptive diagnosis of parenchymal involvement can be made by bronchial inspection.

X. Bronchoalveolar Lavage with or Without Transbronchial Biopsy?

In addition to BAL we routinely obtain TBB specimens to optimize the overall diagnostic yield, particularly for disorders other than PCP (Table 7). Because the incidence of PCP is declining with the use of anti-pneumocystis prophylaxis (145), and most with the disease are diagnosed by sputum induction, a lower proportion of patients who undergo bronchoscopy will have PCP than in previous years.

Some perform BAL alone on an initial bronchoscopy because of its relatively high yield, rapidity of performance, and lower risk for pneumothorax and other complications. In our experience, the pneumothorax rate when we do TBB is only 1%. We believe that the increased diagnostic yield afforded by TBB, particularly for conditions other than PCP, supports its routine use when performing bronchoscopy in patients with HIV infection. Those who perform BAL alone on the initial bronchoscopy should promptly repeat the procedure with TBB when patients fail to respond to treatment. In the future, newer diagnostic techniques, such as immunohistochemistry and PCR, should improve the sensitivity of both biopsy and BAL-sampling techniques (33,79).

References

1. Stover DE, White DA, Romano PA, Gellene RA. Diagnosis of pulmonary disease in acquired immune deficiency syndrome (AIDS). Am Rev Respir Dis 1984; 130:659–662.
2. Broaddus C, Dake MD, Stulbarg MS, et al. Bronchoalveolar lavage and transbronchial biopsy for the diagnosis of pulmonary infections in the acquired immunodeficiency syndrome. Ann Intern Med 1985; 102:747–752.
3. Rosen MJ, Tow TW, Teirstein AS, Chuang MT, Marchevsky A, Bottone EJ.

Diagnosis of pulmonary complications of the acquired immune deficiency syndrome. Thorax 1985; 40:571–575.
4. Murray JF, Felton CP, Garay SM, et al. Pulmonary complications of the acquired immunodeficiency syndrome. Report of National Heart, Lung and Blood Institute Workshop. N Engl J Med 1984; 310:1682–1688.
5. Murray JF, Mills J. Pulmonary infectious complications of human immunodeficiency virus infection. Am Rev Respir Dis 1990; 141:1356–1372, 1582–1598.
6. Jacobson MA, Mills J, Rush J, et al. Morbidity and mortality of patients with AIDS and first-episode *Pneumocystis carinii* pneumonia unaffected by concomitant pulmonary cytomegalovirus infection. Am Rev Respir Dis 1991; 144:6–9.
7. Murray JF, Garay SM, Hopewell PC, Mills J, Snider GL, Stover DE. Pulmonary complications of the acquired immunodeficiency syndrome: an update. Report of the Second National Heart, Lung and Blood Institute Workshop. Am Rev Respir Dis 1987; 135:504–509.
8. White DA, Matthay RA. Noninfectious pulmonary complications of infection with the human immunodeficiency virus. Am Rev Respir Dis 1989; 140:1763–1787.
9. Meduri GU, Stover DE, Lee M, Myskowski PL, Caravelli JF, Zaman MB. Pulmonary Kaposi's sarcoma in the acquired immune deficiency syndrome. Clinical, radiographic, and pathologic manifestations. Am J Med 1986; 81:11–18.
10. Pozniak AL, Latiff AS, Neill P, Houston S, Chen K, Robertson V. Pulmonary Kaposi's sarcoma in Africa. Thorax 1992; 47:730–733.
11. Salzman SH, Schindel ML, Aranda CP, Smith RL, Lewis ML. The role of bronchoscopy in the diagnosis of pulmonary tuberculosis in patients at risk of HIV infection. Chest 1992; 102:143–146.
12. Kennedy DJ, Lewis WP, Barnes PF. Yield of bronchoscopy for the diagnosis of tuberculosis in patients with human immunodeficiency virus infection. Chest 1992; 102:1040–1044.
13. Salzman SH, Smith RL, Aranda CP. Histoplasmosis in patients at risk for the acquired immunodeficiency syndrome in a nonendemic setting. Chest 1988; 93:916–921.
14. Sarosi GA, Ampel NA, Cohn DL, et al. Fungal infection in HIV-infected persons. Statement of the American Thoracic Society. Am J Respir Dis 1995; 152:816–822.
15. Centers for Disease Control and Prevention (CDC). 1993 revised classification system for HIV infection and expanded surveillance case definition for AIDS among adolescents and adults. MMWR 1992; 41(RR-17):1–19.
16. Salzman SH, Bernstein LE, Villamena PC, Schneider RF, Mayo PH, Rosen MJ. Bronchoscopic lung biopsy improves the diagnostic yield of bronchoscopy in patients with known or suspected HIV infection. J Bronchol 1996; 3:88–95.
17. Miller RF, Leigh TR, Collins JV, Mitchell DM. Tests giving an aetiological diagnosis in pulmonary disease in patients infected with the human immunodeficiency virus. Thorax 1990; 45:62–65.
18. Jules-Elysee KM, Stover DE, Zaman MB, Bernard EM, White DA. Aerosolized

pentamidine: effect on diagnosis and presentation of *Pneumocystis carinii* pneumonia. Ann Intern Med 1990; 112:750–757.
19. Meduri GU, Stover DE, Greeno RA, Nash T, Zaman MB. Bilateral bronchoalveolar lavage in the diagnosis of opportunistic pulmonary infections. Chest 1991; 100:1272–1276.
20. Metersky JL, Harrell JH II, Moser KM. Lack of utility of bronchial brush biopsy in patients infected with the human immunodeficiency virus. Chest 1992; 101:680–683.
21. Baughman RP, Dohn MN, Shipley R, Buchsbaum JA, Frame PT. Increased *Pneumocystis carinii* recovery from the upper lobes in *Pneumocystis* pneumonia. The effect of inhaled pentamidine prophylaxis. Chest 1993; 103:426–432.
22. Read CA, Cerrone F, Busseniers AE, Waldhorn RE, Lavelle JP, Pierce PF. Differential lobe lavage for diagnosis of acute *Pneumocystis carinii* pneumonia in patients receiving prophylactic aerosolized pentamidine therapy. Chest 1993; 103:1520–1523.
23. Levine SJ, Kennedy D, Shelhamer JH, et al. Diagnosis of *Pneumocystis carinii* pneumonia by multiple lobe, site-directed bronchoalveloar lavage with immunofluorescent monoclonal antibody staining in human immunodeficiency virus-infected patients receiving aerosolized pentamidine chemoprophylaxis. Am Rev Respir Dis 1992; 146:838–843.
24. Yung RC, Weinacker AB, Steiger DJ, et al. Upper and middle lobe bronchoalveolar lavage to diagnose *Pneumocystis carinii* pneumonia. Am Rev Respir Dis 1993; 148:1563–1566.
25. Teuscher AU, Opraveill M, Theiler R, et al. Predictive value of bronchoalveolar lavage in excluding a diagnosis of *Pneumocystis carinii* pneumonia during prophylaxis with aerosolized pentamidine. Clin Infect Dis 1993; 16:519–522.
26. Ng VL, Geaghan SM, Leoung G, et al. Lack of effect of prophylactic aerosolized pentamidine on the detection of *Pneumocystis carinii* in induced sputum or bronchoalveolar lavage specimens. Arch Pathol Lab Med 1993; 117:493–496.
27. Torrington KG, Finelli MR. Small volume bronchoalveolar lavage used in diagnosing *Pneumocystis carinii* pneumonia in HIV-infected patients. Chest 1995; 107:1013–1017.
28. Mones JM, Saldana MJ, Oldham SA. Diagnosis of *Pneumocystis carinii* pneumonia: roentgenographic–pathologic correlates based on fiberoptic bronchoscopy specimens from patients with the acquired immunodeficiency syndrome. Chest 1986; 89:522–526.
29. Golden JA, Hollander H, Stulbarg MS, Gamsu G. Bronchoalveolar lavage as the exclusive diagnostic modality for *Pneumocystis carinii* pneumonia. A prospective study among patients with acquired immunodeficiency syndrome. Chest 1986; 90:18–22.
30. Orenstein M, Webber CA, Cash M, Heurich AE. Value of bronchoalveolar lavage in the diagnosis of pulmonary infection in acquired immune deficiency syndrome. Thorax 1986; 41:345–349.
31. Francis ND, Goldin RD, Forster SM, et al. Diagnosis of lung disease in acquired immune deficiency syndrome: biopsy or cytology and implications for management. J Clin Pathol 1987; 40:1269–1273.

32. Weldon-Linne CM, Rhone DP, Bourassa R. Bronchoscopy specimens in adults with AIDS. Comparative yields of cytology, histology and culture for diagnosis of infectious agents. Chest 1990; 98:24–28.
33. Miller RF, Mitchell DM. AIDS and the lung: update 1995: 1. *Pneumocystis carinii* pneumonia. Thorax 1995; 50:191–200.
34. Meduri GU, Stein DS. Pulmonary manifestations of acquired immunodeficiency syndrome. Clin Infect Dis 1992; 14:98–113.
35. Kvale PK. How much bronchoscopic sampling is enough (for HIV-infected patients)? J Bronchol 1996; 3:83–84.
36. Bigby TD. Diagnosis of *Pneumocystis carinii* pneumonia. How invasive? Chest 1994; 105:650–651.
37. Griffiths MH, Kocjan G, Miller RF, Godfrey-Fausset P. Diagnosis of pulmonary disease in human immunodeficiency virus infection: role of transbronchial biopsy and bronchoalveolar lavage. Thorax 1989; 44:554–558.
38. Limper AH. Diagnosis of *Pneumocystis carinii* pneumonia: does use of only bronchoalveolar lavage suffice? Mayo Clin Proc 1996; 71:1121–1123.
39. Fraser JL, Lilly C, Israel E, Hulme P, Hanff PA. Diagnostic yield of bronchoalveolar lavage and bronchoscopic lung biopsy for detection of *Pneumocystis carinii*. Mayo Clin Proc 1996; 71:1025–1029.
40. Baughman RP, Dohn MN, Frame PT. The continuing utility of bronchoalveloar lavage to diagnose opportunistic infection in AIDS patients. Am J Med 1994; 97:515–522.
41. Batungwanayo J, Taelman H, Lucas S, et al. Pulmonary disease associated with the human immunodeficiency virus in Kigali, Rwanda: a fiberoptic bronchoscopy study of 111 cases of undetermined etiology. Am J Respir Crit Care Med 1994; 149:1591–1596.
42. Cazzadori A, Di Perii G, Todeschini G, Luzzati R, Boschiero L, Perona G, Concia E. Transbronchial biopsy in the diagnosis of pulmonary infiltrates in immunocompromised patients. Chest 1995; 107:101–106.
43. Cadranel J, Gillet-Juvin K, Antoine M, et al. Site-directed bronchoalveolar lavage and transbronchial biopsy in HIV-infected patients with pneumonia. Am J Respir Crit Care Med 1995; 152:1103–1106.
44. Huang L, Hecht FM, Stansell JD, Montanti R, Hadley WH, Hopewell PC. Suspected *Pneumocystis carinii* pneumonia with a negative sputum examination: is bronchoscopy useful? Am J Respir Crit Care Med 1995; 151:1866–1871.
45. Serda GJ, Rodriguez de Castro F, Sanchez-Alarcos JMF, Luna JC, Lopez FD, Navarro PC. Transcarinal needle aspiration in the diagnosis of mediastinal adenitis in a patient infected with the human immunodeficiency virus. Thorax 1990; 45:414–415.
46. Baron KM, Aranda CP. Diagnosis of mediastinal mycobacterial lymphadenopathy by transbronchial needle aspiration. Chest 1991; 100:1723–1724.
47. Malabonga VM, Basti J, Kamholz SL. Utility of bronchoscopic sampling techniques for cryptococcal disease in AIDS. Chest 1991; 99:370–372.
48. Harkin TJ, Ciotoli C, Addrizzo-Harris DJ, Naidich DP, Jagirdar J, Rom WN. Transbronchial needle aspiration in patients infected with HIV. Am J Respir Crit Care Med. In press.

49. Judson MA, Sahn SA. Endobronchial lesions in HIV-infected individuals. Chest 1994; 105:1314–1323.
50. Chechani V, Kamholz SL. Pulmonary manifestations of disseminated cryptococcosis in patients with AIDS. Chest 1990; 98:1060–1066.
51. Packer SJ, Cesario T, Williams JH Jr. *Mycobacterium avium* complex infection presenting as endobronchial lesions in immunosuppressed patients. Ann Intern Med 1988; 109:389–393.
52. Mehle ME, Adamo JP, Mehta AC, Wiedemann HP, Keys T, Longwoth DL. Endobronchial *Mycobacterium avium–intracellulare* infection in a patient with AIDS. Chest 1989; 96:119–200.
53. Wasser LS, Shaw GW, Talavera W. Endobronchial tuberculosis in the acquired immunodeficiency syndrome. Chest 1988; 94:1240–1244.
54. Denning DW, Follansbee SE, Scolaro M, Norris S, Edlestein H, Stevens DA. Pulmonary aspergillosis in the acquired immunodeficiency syndrome. N Engl J Med 1991; 324:654–662.
55. Calpe JL, Chiner E, Larramendi CH. Endobronchial tuberculosis in HIV-infected patients. AIDS 1995; 9:1159–1164.
56. Connoly MG Jr, Baughman RP, Dohn MN. *Mycobacterium kansasii* presenting as an endobronchial lesion. Am Rev Respir Dis 1993; 148:1405–1407.
57. Wallace JM, Batra P, Gong H Jr, Ovenfors C-O. Percutaneous needle lung aspiration for diagnosing pneumonitis in the patient with acquired immunodeficiency syndrome (AIDS). Am Rev Respir Dis 1985; 131:389–392.
58. Bottles K, McPhaul LW, Volberding P. Fine-needle aspiration in patients with acquired immunodeficiency syndrome (AIDS): experience in an outpatient clinic. Ann Intern Med 1988; 108:42–45.
59. Falguera M, Nogues A, Ruiz-Gonzalez A, Garcia M, Puig T, Rubio-Caballero M. Transthoracic needle aspiration in the study of pulmonary infections in patients with HIV. Chest 1994; 106:697–702.
60. Barrio JL, Harcup C, Baier JH, Pitchenik. Value of repeat fiberoptic bronchoscopies and significance of nondiagnostic bronchoscopic results in patients with the acquired immunodeficiency syndrome. Am Rev Respir Dis 1987; 135:422–425.
61. Fitzgerald W, Bevelaqua FA, Garay SM, Aranda CP. The role of open lung biopsy in patients with the acquired immunodeficiency syndrome. Chest 1987; 91:659–661.
62. McKenna RJ Jr, Campbell A, McMurtrey MJ, Mountain CF. Diagnosis for interstitial lung disease in patients with acquired immunodeficiency syndrome (AIDS): a prospective comparison of bronchial washing, alveolar lavage, transbronchial lung biopsy, and open-lung biopsy. Ann Thorac Surg 1986; 41:318–321.
63. Pass HI, Potter D, Shelhamer J, et al. Indications for and diagnostic efficacy of open-lung biopsy in the patient with acquired immunodeficiency syndrome (AIDS). Ann Thorac Surg 1986; 41:307–312.
64. Stulbarg MS, Golden JA. Open lung biopsy in the acquired immunodeficiency syndrome (AIDS). Chest 1987; 91:639–640.

65. Niederman MS, Bass JB Jr, Campbell GD, et al. Guidelines for the initial management of adults with community-acquired pneumonia: diagnosis, assessment of severity, and initial antimicrobial therapy. Am Rev Respir Dis 1993; 148:1418–1426.
66. Ferrer M, Torres A, Xaubet A, et al. Diagnostic value of telescoping plugged catheters in HIV-infected patients with pulmonary infiltrates. Chest 1992; 102:76–83.
67. Magnenat J-L, Nicod L, Aukenthaler R, Junod AF. Mode of presentation and diagnosis of bacterial pneumonia in human immunodeficiency virus-infected patients. Am Rev Respir Dis 1991; 144:917–922.
68. Bigby TD, Margolskee D, Curtis JL, et al. The usefulness of induced sputum in the diagnosis of *Pneumocystis carinii* pneumonia in patients with the acquired immunodeficiency syndrome. Am Rev Respir Dis 1986; 133:515–518.
69. Kovacs JA, Ng V, Masur H, et al. Diagnosis of *Pneumocystis carinii* pneumonia: improved detection in sputum with use of monoclonal antibodies. N Engl J Med 1988; 318:589–593.
70. Pitchenik AE, Ganjei P, Torres A, Evans DA, Rubin E, Baier H. Sputum examination for the diagnosis of *Pneumocystis carinii* pneumonia in the acquired immunodeficiency syndrome. Am Rev Respir Dis 1986; 133:226–229.
71. Mason GR, Hashimoto CH, Dickman PS, Foutty LF, Cobb CJ. Prognostic implications of bronchoalveolar lavage neutrophilia in patients with *Pneumocystis carinii* pneumonia and AIDS. Am Rev Respir Dis 1989; 139:1336–1342.
72. Smith RL, El-Sadr WM, Lewis ML. Correlation of bronchoalveolar lavage cell populations with clinical severity of *Pneumocystis carinii* pneumonia. Chest 1988; 92:60–64.
73. Caughey G, Wong H, Gamsu G, Golden J. Nonbronchoscopic bronchoalveolar lavage for the diagnosis of *Pneumocystis carinii* pneumonia in the acquired immunodeficiency syndrome. Chest 1985; 88:659–662.
74. Martin WR, Albertson TE, Siegel B. Tracheal catheters in patients with acquired immunodeficiency syndrome for the diagnosis of *Pneumocystis carinii* pneumonia. Chest 1990; 98:29–32.
75. Karpel JP, Prezant D, Appel D, Bezahler G. Endotracheal lavage for the diagnosis of *Pneumocystis carinii* pneumonia in intubated inpatients with acquired immune deficiency syndrome. Crit Care Med 1986; 14:741.
76. Larson RP, Ingalls-Severn KJ, Wright JR, Kiviat NC, Maunder RJ. Diagnosis of *Pneumocystis carinii* pneumonia by respiratory care practitioners: advantages of a nasotracheal suctioning method over sputum induction. Respir Care 1989; 34:249–253.
77. Bustamente EA, Levy H. Sputum induction compared with bronchoalveloar lavage by ballard catheter to diagnose *Pneumocystis carinii* pneumonia. Chest 1994; 105:816–822.
78. Baughman RP, Dohn MN, Loudon RG, Frame PT. Bronchoscopy with bronchoalveloar lavage in tuberculosis and fungal infections. Chest 1991; 99:92–97.
79. Schulger NW, Rom WN. The polymerase chain reaction in the diagnosis and

evaluation of pulmonary infection. Am J Respir Crit Care Med 1995; 152:11–16.
80. Drew WL. Cytomegalovirus infection in patients with AIDS. Clin Infect Dis 1992; 14:608–615.
81. Millar AB, Patou G, Miller RF, et al. Cytomegalovirus in the lungs of patients with AIDS. Respiratory pathogen or passenger? Am Rev Respir Dis 1990; 141:1474–1477.
82. Miles PR, Baughman RP, Linnemann CC Jr. Cytomagalovirus in the bronchoalveolar lavage fluid of patients with AIDS. Chest 1990; 97:1072–1076.
83. Jensen AB, Lundgren JD, Benfield T, Nielsen TL, Vestbo J. Does cytomegalovirus predict a poor prognosis in *Pneumocysitis carinii* pneumonia treated with corticosteroids? A note for caution. Chest 1995; 108:411–414.
84. Hyland M, Chan M, Hyland RH, Chan CK. Associating poor outcome with the presence of cytomegalovirus in bronchoalveolar lavage from HIV patients with *Pneumocystis carinii* pneumonia. Chest 1995; 107:595–597.
85. Hayner CE, Baughman RP, Linnemann CC Jr, Dohn MN. The relationship between cytomegalovirus retrieved by bronchoalveolar lavage and mortality in patients with HIV. Chest 1995; 107:735–740.
86. Batungwanayo J, Taelman H, Bogaerts J, et al. Pulmonary cryptococcosis associated with HIV-1 infection in Rwanda: a retrospective study of 37 cases. AIDS 1994; 8:1271–1276.
87. Baughman RP, Rhodes JC, Dohn MN, Henderson H, Frame PT. Detection of cryptococcal antigen in bronchoalveolar lavage fluid: a prospective study of diagnostic utility. Am Rev Respir Dis 1992; 145:1226–1229.
88. Wheat LJ, Connolly-Stringfield PA, Baker RL, et al. Disseminated histoplasmosis in the acquired immune deficiency syndrome: clinical findings, diagnosis and treatment, and review of the literature. Medicine 1990; 69:361–374.
89. Johnson PC, Khardori N, Najjar AF, Butt F, Mansell PWA, Sarosi GA. Progressive disseminated histoplasmosis in patients with acquired immunodeficiency syndrome. Am J Med 1988; 85:152–158.
90. Johnson PC, Hamill RJ, Sarosi GA. Clinical review: progressive disseminated histoplasmosis in the AIDS patient. Semin Respir Infect 1989; 4:139–146.
91. Wheat LJ, Connolly-Stringfield P, Kohler RB, Frame PT, Gupta MR. *Histoplasma capsulatum* polysaccharide antigen detection in diagnosis and management of disseminated histoplasmosis in patients with acquired immunodeficiency syndrome. Am J Med 1989; 87:396–400.
92. Wheat LJ, Connoly-Stringfield P, Blair R, Connoly K, Garringer T, Katz BP. Histoplasmosis relapse in patients with AIDS: detection using *Histoplasma capsulatum* variety *capsulatum* antigen levels. Ann Intern Med 1991; 115:936–941.
93. Lotholary O, Meyohas M, Dupont B, Cadranel J, Salmon-Ceron D, Peyramond D, Simonin D. Invasive aspergillosis in patients with acquired immunodeficiency syndrome: report of 33 cases. French Cooperative Study Group on Aspergillosis in AIDS. Am J Med 1993; 95:177–187.
94. Khoo SH, Denning DW. Invasive aspergillosis in patients with AIDS. Clin Infect Dis 1994; 19:S41–S48.

95. Kemper CA, Hostetler JS, Follansbee SE, et al. Ulcerative and plaque-like tracheobronchitis due to infection with *Aspergillus* in patients with AIDS. Clin Infect Dis 1993; 17:344–352.
96. Pursell KJ, Telzak EE, Armstrong D. *Aspergillus* species colonization and invasive disease in patients with AIDS. Clin Infect Dis 1992; 14:141–148.
97. Singh N, Yu VL, Rihs JD. Invasive aspergillosis in AIDS. South Med J 1991; 84:822–827.
98. Klapholz A, Solomon N, Perlman DC, Talavera W. Aspergillosis in the acquired immunodeficiency syndrome. Chest 1991; 100:1616–1618.
99. Bretagne S, Costa JM, Marmorat-Khuong A, et al. Detection of *Aspergillus* species DNA in bronchoalveolar lavage samples by competitive PCR. J Clin Microbiol 1995; 33:1164–1168.
100. Bronnimann DA, Adam RD, Galgiani JN, et al. Coccidioidomycosis in the acquired immunodeficiency syndrome. Ann Intern Med 1987; 106:372–379.
101. Graham AR, Sobonya RE, Bronnimann DA, Galgiani JN. Quantitative pathology of coccidioidomycosis in acquired immunodeficiency syndrome. Hum Pathol 1988; 19:800–806.
102. DiTomasso JP, Ampel NM, Sobonya RE, Bloom JW. Bronchoscopic diagnosis of pulmonary coccidioidomycosis. Comparison of cytology, culture, and transbronchial biopsy. Diagn Microbiol Infect Dis 1994; 18:83–87.
103. Fish DG, Ampel NM, Gagliani JN, et al. Coccidioidomycosis during human immunodeficiency virus infection. Medicine 1990; 69:384–391.
104. Pappas PG, Pottage JC, Powderly WG, et al. Blastomycosis in patients with the acquired immunodeficiency syndrome. Ann Intern Med 1992; 116:847–853.
105. Garay SM, Belenko M, Fazzini E, Schinella R. Pulmonary manifestations of Kaposi's sarcoma. Chest 1987; 91:39–43.
106. Ognibene FP, Steis RG, Macher AM, et al. Kaposi's sarcoma causing pulmonary infiltrates and respiratory failure in the acquired immunodeficiency syndrome. Ann Intern Med 1985; 102:471–475.
107. O'Brien RF, Cohn DL. Serosanguineous pleural effusions in AIDS-associated Kaposi's sarcoma. Chest 1989; 96:460–466.
108. Zibrak JD, Silvestri RC, Costello P, et al. Bronchoscopic and radiologic features of Kaposi's sarcoma involving the respiratory system. Chest 1986; 90:476–479.
109. Pitchenik AE, Fischl MA, Saldana MJ. Kaposi's sarcoma of the tracheobronchial tree. Chest 1985; 87:122–126.
110. Au JP, Krauthammer M, Lau KY, Rubin A. Kaposi's sarcoma presenting with endobronchial lesions. Heart Lung 1986; 15:411–413.
111. Greenberg JE, Fischl MA, Berger JR. Upper airway obstruction secondary to acquired immunodeficiency syndrome-related Kaposi's sarcoma. Chest 1985; 88:638–640.
112. Huang L, Schnapp LM, Gruden JF, Hopewell PC, Stansell JD. Presentation of AIDS-related pulmonary Kaposi's sarcoma diagnosed by bronchoscopy. Am J Respir Crit Care Med 1996; 153:1385–1390.
113. Vianna LA. Bronchoscopy in the diagnosis of pulmonary Kaposi's sarcoma in patients with AIDS. J Bronchol 1994; 1:9–14.
114. Hamm PG, Judson MA, Aranda CP. Diagnosis of pulmonary Kaposi's sarcoma

with fiberoptic bronchoscopy and endobronchial biopsy. Cancer 1987; 59:807–810.

115. Gruden JF, Hugan L, Webb WR, Gamsu G, Hopewell PC, Sides DM. AIDS-related Kaposi sarcoma of the lung: radiographic findings and staging system with bronchoscopic correlation. Radiology 1995; 195:545–552.
116. Bach MC, Bagwell SP, Fanning JP. Primary pulmonary Kaposi's sarcoma in the acquired immunodeficiency syndrome: a cause of persistent pyrexia. Am J Med 1988; 85:274–275.
117. Kornfeld H, Axelrod JL. Pulmonary presentation of Kaposi's sarcoma in a homosexual patient. Am Rev Respir Dis 1983; 127:248–249.
118. Kaplan LD, Hopewell PC, Jaffe H, et al. Kaposi's sarcoma involving the lung in patients with acquired immunodeficiency syndrome. J Acquir Immune Defic Syndr 1988; 1:23–30.
119. Polish LB, Cohn DL, Ryder JW, Myers AM, O'Brien RF. Pulmonary non-Hodgkin's lymphoma in AIDS. Chest 1989; 96:1321–1326.
120. Karp J, Profeta G, Marantz PR, Karpel JP. Lung cancer in patients with immunodeficiency syndrome. Chest 1993; 103:410–413.
121. Sridhar KS, Flores MR, Raub WA Jr, Saldana M. Lung cancer in patients with human immunodeficiency virus infection compared with historic control subjects. Chest 1992; 102:1704–1708.
122. Ognibene FP, Masur H, Rogers P, et al. Nonspecific interstitial pneumonitis without evidence of *Pneumocystis carinii* in asymptomatic patients infected with human immunodeficiency virus (HIV). Ann Intern Med 1988; 109:874–879.
123. Teirstein AS, Rosen MJ. Lymphocytic interstitial pneumonia. Clin Chest Med 1988; 9:467–471.
124. Allen JN, Wewers MD. HIV-associated bronchiolitis obliterans organizing pneumonia. Chest 1989; 96:197–198.
125. Joseph J, Harley RA, Frye MD. Bronchiolitis obliterans with organizing pneumonia in AIDS (letter). N Engl J Med 1995; 332:273.
126. Coplan NL, Shimony RY, Ioachim HL, et al. Primary pulmonary hypertension associated with human immunodeficiency viral infection. Am J Med 1990; 89:96–99.
127. Chayt KJ, Harper ME, Marselle LM, et al. Detection of HTLV-III RNA in lungs of patients with AIDS and pulmonary involvement. JAMA 1986; 256:2356–2359.
128. Spach DH, Silverstein FE, Stamm WE. Transmission of infection by gastrointestinal endoscopy and bronchoscopy. Ann Intern Med 1993; 118:117–128.
129. Centers for Disease Control and Prevention. Guidelines for preventing the transmission of tuberculosis in health-care settings, with special focus on HIV-related issues. MMWR 1990; 39(RR-17):1–7.
130. Hanson PJV, Collins JV. AIDS, aprons, and elbow grease: preventing the nosocomial spread of human immunodeficiency virus and associated organisms. Thorax 1989; 44:778–783.
131. Prakash UBS. Does the bronchoscope propagate infection? Chest 1993; 104:552–559.

132. Miller RF, Millar AB, Weller IVD, Semple SJG. Empirical treatment without bronchoscopy for *Pneumocystis carinii* pneumonia in the acquired immunodeficiency syndrome. Thorax 1989; 44:559–564.
133. Tu JV, Biem JH, Detsky AS. Bronchoscopy versus empirical therapy in HIV-infected patients with presumptive *Pneumocystis carinii* pneumonia. Am Rev Respir Dis 1993; 148:370–377.
134. Luce JM, Stover DE. Controversies in pulmonary medicine: presumed *Pneumocystis carinii* pneumonia should be treated empirically in patients with acquired immunodeficiency syndrome. Am Rev Respir Dis 1988; 138:1076–1077.
135. Miller RF, Mitchell DM. AIDS and the lung: update 1995: 1. *Pneumocystis carinii* pneumonia. Thorax 1995; 50:191–200.
136. Masur H, Shelhamer J. Empiric outpatient management of HIV-related pneumonia: economical or unwise? Ann Intern Med 1996; 124:451–453.
137. Shelhamer JH, Ognibene FP, Macher AM, et al. Persistence of *Pneumocystis carinii* in lung tissue of acquired immunodeficiency syndrome patients treated for pneumocystis pneumonia. Am Rev Respir Dis 1984; 130:1161–1165.
138. Jones BE, Taikwel EK, Mercado AL, Sian SU, Barnes PF. Tuberculosis in patients with HIV infection who receive corticosteroids for presumed *Pneumocystis carinii* pneumonia. Am J Respir Crit Care Med 1994; 149:1686–1688.
139. Martos A, Podzamczer D, Martinez-Lacasa J, Rufi G, Santin M, Gudiol F. Steroids do not enhance the risk of developing tuberculosis or other AIDS-related diseases in HIV-infected patients treated for *Pneumocystis carinii* pneumonia. AIDS 1995; 9:1037–1041.
140. Salzman SH, Rosen MJ. Bronchoscopy in patients with human immunodeficiency virus infection. J Bronchol 1994; 1:3–4.
141. Glassroth J. Empiric diagnosis of *Pneumocystis carinii* pneumonia: questions of accuracy and equity. Am J Respir Crit Care Med 1995; 152:1433–1434.
142. Horner RD, Bennett CL, Rodriguez D, et al. Relationship between procedures and health insurance for critically ill patients with *Pneumocystis carinii* pneumonia. Am J Respir Crit Care Med 1995; 152:1435–1442.
143. Bennett CL, Horner RD, Weinstein RA, et al. Empirically treated *Pneumocystis carinii* pneumonia in Los Angeles, Chicago and Miami: 1987–1990. J Infect Dis 1995; 172:312–315.
144. Daley EL, Muguis F, Chen LL, et al. Pulmonary complications of HIV infection in Dar es Salaam, Tanzania. Am J Respir Crit Care Med 1996; 154:105–110.
145. Hoover DR, Saah AJ, Bacellar H, et al. Clinical manifestations of AIDS in the era of pneumocystis prophylaxis. N Engl J Med 1993; 329:1922–1926.

9

Noninvasive Diagnostic Tests

ROSLYN F. SCHNEIDER

Albert Einstein College of Medicine and
Beth Israel Medical Center
New York, New York

I. Introduction

Noninvasive tests are used extensively in the diagnosis of human immunodeficiency virus (HIV)-related pulmonary diseases. In general, if a pattern of abnormality is specific for an illness, then invasive studies may be avoided. Pulmonary function tests, radiographic and nuclear radiographic studies are discussed in this chapter. Other invasive and noninvasive studies as they pertain to specific topics are discussed elsewhere.

II. Pulmonary Function Testing

Pulmonary function testing is often performed in the evaluation of pulmonary symptoms to identify and quantify pulmonary dysfunction. Resting arterial blood gases provide useful information on oxygenation and ventilation in chronic or acute disease. Exercise testing evaluates the metabolic, vascular, and ventilatory responses to an increased demand on these systems. The degree of limitation and patterns of response are assessed to identify dysfunction earlier. Accurate predicted values for comparable populations are essential for the interpretation of these tests.

A. Spirometry

Asymptomatic HIV-infected persons have normal forced vital capacity (FVC) and forced expiratory volume in 1 sec (FEV_1) measurements (1). In the Pulmonary Complications of HIV Infection Study, 1294 participants without an acquired immunodeficiency syndrome (AIDS)-defining diagnosis within 3 months of enrollment had measurements of FEV_1 and FVC that were almost 100% of predicted values for the group. HIV-infected injection drug users had lower measurements of FEV_1 and FVC than the other risk groups studied.

Pothoff et al. (2) also showed that asymptomatic persons with HIV infection had normal measurements of VC and FEV_1, but those with respiratory symptoms and pulmonary diagnoses had significantly lower measurements. Shaw et al. (3) studied a group of 169 HIV-seropositive persons: 33 without symptoms, 47 with persistent generalized adenopathy, 33 with AIDS-related complex (Centers for Disease Control; CDC group IV, subgroups A, B, C2, and E), 16 with cutaneous, nonpulmonary Kaposi's sarcoma, 6 with nonpulmonary Kaposi's sarcoma and another opportunistic infection affecting other organs, and 34 patients with pulmonary disorders related to AIDS. The FEV_1, peak expiratory flow rate, and maximal expiratory flow at 50% of the vital capacity were significantly reduced only in the group with *Pneumocystis carinii* pneumonia (PCP).

B. Diffusing Capacity

Several studies were performed to determine the expected diffusing capacity (D_Lco) measurements in persons with asymptomatic HIV infection, with active pulmonary disease, or with prior pulmonary disease (4). In the Pulmonary Complications of HIV Infection Study (1), persons with symptomatic HIV infection (thrush, weight loss, herpes zoster), but no AIDS-defining diagnosis had lower D_Lco measurements, compared with asymptomatic participants. HIV-infected injection drug users had lower D_Lco measurements than the other risk groups studied, but the difference was partially explained by other factors, including cigarette smoking and race. However, the D_Lco for the group with CD4 lymphocyte counts of fewer than 200/mm^3 was lower than in the other groups. In another investigation of the same cohort, the single-breath D_Lco was measured at 3- to 12-month intervals (5). A 20% reduction in corrected D_Lco did not predict the presence of PCP or other pulmonary infections in asymptomatic persons without new chest radiographic abnormalities.

Shaw et al. (3) also showed that the D_Lco was normal in subjects without symptoms, but with persistent generalized adenopathy. The mean values for D_Lco were significantly lower in those with AIDS-related complex (ARC), nonpulmonary Kaposi's sarcoma, and other nonpulmonary opportunistic infections. Low D_Lco measurements were observed during both the acute and recovery phase of PCP, as well as in those with pulmonary mycobacterial infection and pulmonary Kaposi's sarcoma.

In the investigation of Pothoff et al. (2), persons with HIV infection, respiratory symptoms, and a variety of pulmonary diagnoses had significantly lower D_Lco measurements compared with those without symptoms, even with prior pulmonary disease. In this study, the D_Lco measurements of asymptomatic persons with HIV infection, with or without prior pulmonary disease, were lower than those of the control group of persons not infected with HIV. Other studies also demonstrated that mean D_Lco measurements are reduced in HIV-infected persons with nonpulmonary manifestations of AIDS or absolute CD4 lymphocyte counts of fewer than 200/mm (3,6,7).

Patients with PCP usually have reductions in D_Lco. Coleman et al. (8) studied nine patients with PCP who were tested initially and at 105–258 days after diagnosis. Eight of nine patients had abnormalities of D_Lco, and there was significant improvement with long-term follow-up in four of the five who were available for study. Sankary et al. (9) evaluated 20 patients with low D_Lco and PCP, 20 with low D_Lco in whom PCP was excluded, and 20 nonsmoking healthy control subjects. They analyzed the data on membrane-diffusing capacity (D_M) and pulmonary capillary blood volume (V_C); there was a significantly larger reduction of D_M than V_C, accounting for the reduction of D_Lco in patients with PCP. After successful treatment for PCP, the mean D_M returned to normal, whereas the V_C was unchanged. This was in contrast with the subjects with other pulmonary disorders who had reduction of D_L owing to the more common proportional reduction of D_M and V_C.

In summary, persons with HIV infection and no identified pulmonary disease may have slightly reduced D_Lco measurements, especially when the CD4 lymphocyte count is low. The D_Lco is typically reduced in patients with pulmonary symptoms.

C. Exercise Testing

Pothoff et al. (2) compared the exercise capacity of HIV-seronegative subjects with HIV-infected persons. Persons with HIV infection and no lung disease had a decline of D_Lco with normal spirometric measurements, and reduced exercise capacity with an abnormal pattern of exercise gas exchange. There was no significant difference between this group and the group with prior PCP. The breathing and heart reserves were abnormally high in both groups, making occult cardiac or pulmonary circulatory disorders unlikely. In persons with acute pulmonary disease, the findings that were most abnormal were spirometry, D_Lco, and alveolar-to-arteriolar oxygen $(A–a)o_2$, gradients. Oxygen consumption and anaerobic threshold determinations were not as sensitive in detecting disease.

D. Arterial Blood Gas Measurement and Oxygen Saturation

Arterial blood gas measurements at rest and during exercise are useful in the determination of severity of physiological impairment, and may suggest a specific diagnosis of PCP. When these tests are normal PCP is unlikely, but other pulmonary diseases are not excluded.

Stover et al. (10) studied 90 patients with AIDS, or who were suspected of having HIV infection, who were being evaluated for pulmonary symptoms. Resting arterial blood gas values and blood gas values following 1.5 min of exercise on the Master's two-step staircase were measured. Thirteen of 37 patients without PCP and 15 of 53 patients with PCP had a normal $(A–a)o_2$ gradient at rest (less than 15 mmHg). A normal exercise test was defined as a decrease of the $(A–a)o_2$ gradient from rest to exercise of 5 mmHg or more. None of the 53 patients with PCP had a normal exercise study, whereas 16 of the 37 patients without PCP had a normal exercise study.

In patients with PCP and normal or near-normal chest radiographs, 15 of 16 patients with low resting Pao_2 values showed oxygen desaturation to less than 90% within 10 min of exercise on an exercycle at a constant speed and resistance (average 79%; range 53–90%) (11). In the 24 patients with PPC and normal resting Po_2 values, 80% had a reduction of oxygen saturation to less than 90%within ten minutes of exercise. Only 2 of the 19 patients with a pulmonary disorder that was proved not to be PCP had a significant reduction of oxygen saturation with exercise.

In another study, exercise oximetry was performed with other outpatient studies (4). A fall of oxygen saturation to 90% or less during 10 min of exercise on a bicycle with a standard resistance and speed was defined as an abnormal result. An abnormal test was present in 127 of 154 patients with PCP, whereas the test was abnormal in only 36 of 118 patients without PCP.

Exercise studies may involve sophisticated equipment that is not practical in the acute, office, or emergency department setting. In another series, the exercise study consistent of pedaling motions in the air at 40 cycles per minute (cpm) in the stretcher bed for 2 min while measuring pulse oximetry (12). A positive test, defined as a decrement of 3% in oxygen saturation, was noted in 17 of the 22 patients subsequently proved to have PCP, whereas the test was positive in only 2 of the 23 patients who did not have PCP, 20 of whom had bacterial pneumonia. Overall, the sensitivity and specificity of the test for the diagnosis of PCP was 77 and 91%, respectively.

III. Chest Radiography

Hospitalized patients who are diagnosed with pulmonary diseases usually have abnormal chest radiographs (13,14). Patterns of abnormalities are suggestive, but not specific, for particular diagnoses. These are listed in Table 1 (13–47). Computerized tomography (CT) may localize suspicious lesions, identify bronchiectasis, and reveal patterns of abnormalities suggestive of specific etiologies such as PCP (45–47). The radiographic findings of specific diseases are described in other chapters.

IV. Nuclear Scans

The role of nuclear scans in the diagnosis of illness in HIV-infected individuals has been examined since early in the HIV epidemic (48–53). Gallium-67 is a cyclotron-produced radionucleide that emits gamma rays detected by a scanner or camera following intravenous injection (54). Most of the gallium-67 is bound to protein through transferrin, ferritin, or lactoferrin. The mechanism of abnormal gallium-67 uptake is unknown. It cannot be due to only leukocyte accumulation because abnormal uptake occurs in granulocytopenic patients and in acellular cavities (55). More recent studies suggest increased vascular permeability as a mechanism (56).

Kramer et al. (48) reviewed 237 scans, performed on 180 HIV-seropositive persons with fever, suspected infection, or respiratory symptoms. The sensitivity of any gallium-67 scan abnormality for the diagnosis of PCP was 98%; however, the specificity was only 79%. When only intensely abnormal scans were studied, the specificity increased to 95%, but the sensitivity was reduced. The positive predictive value of an abnormal study for PCP was 62%, but increased to 77% if only intensely abnormal scans were studied. Gallium-67 scan abnormalities may be less reliable in those who are receiving aerosolized pentamidine for prophylaxis (49). Other pulmonary illnesses that are associated with abnormal scans include lymphoma, lymphocytic interstitial pneumonitis, nonspecific interstitial pneumonitis, *Mycobacterium avium* complex (MAC), tuberculosis, fungal dis-

Table 1 Radiographic Patterns of Abnormality in HIV Infection (13–47)

Pattern	Infection
Consolidation	Bacterial pathogens
	Pneumocystis carinii
	Mycobacterium tuberculosis
	M. avium complex
	M. kansasii
	M. fortuitum
	Nocardia asteroides
	Coccidioides immitis
	Histoplasma capsulatum
	Aspergillus fumigatus
	Lymphocytic interstitial pneumonitis
	Kaposi's sarcoma
Linear opacities	Bacterial pathogens
	P. carinii
	Cryptococcus neoformans
	H. capsulatum
	A. fumigatus
	M. avium complex
	M. kansasii
	M. xenopi
	M. gordonae
	Lymphocytic interstitial pneumonitis
	Nonspecific interstitial pneumonitis
	Lymphoma
	Cytomegalovirus
Nodular opacities	*M. tuberculosis*
	Coccidioides immitis
	Cryptococcus neoformans
	H. capsulatum
	Nocardia asteroides
	M. avium complex
	M. kansasii
	Lymphocytic interstitial pneumonitis
	Nonspecific interstitial pneumonitis
	Lymphoma
	Kaposi's sarcoma
Cavities	*P. carinii* (thin-walled)
	M. tuberculosis
	Bacterial abscess (*Staphylococcus*, mixed infections, *Rhodococcus equi*)
	Coccidioides immitis
	H. capsulatum

Table 1 Continued

Pattern	Infection
	A. fumigatus
	M. avium complex
	M. kansasii
Pneumothorax	*P. carinii*
	Cavitary lung diseases
Intrathoracic adenopathy	*M. tuberculosis*
	M. avium complex
	M. kansasii
	M. fortuitum
	Cryptococcus neoformans
	H. capsulatum
	P. carinii
	lymphoma
	Kaposi's sarcoma
Pleural effusion	*M. tuberculosis*
	Kaposi's sarcoma
	P. carinii
	Coccidioides immitis
	Cryptococcus neoformans
	Lymphoma
Atelectasis	*A. fumigatus*
	Kaposi's sarcoma
	M. avium complex
	M. kansasii
	Rhodococcus equi
Kerley B lines and peribronchial cuffing	Kaposi's sarcoma
Normal radiograph	*P. carinii*
	Kaposi's sarcoma
	M. tuberculosis
	M. avium complex
	A. fumigatus
	H. capsulatum
	Nonspecific interstitial pneumonitis

ease, and bacterial infections. These are often associated with less intense or focal abnormalities (48).

Autologous-labeled white blood cell scintigraphy with indium-111 was compared with gallium-67 scanning in 36 febrile patients with AIDS without localizing signs (57). Abnormalities, including sinusitis and bacterial pneumonia, were more likely to be identified by indium-111 scans alone, whereas PCP cases were more likely to be seen on gallium-67 scanning alone.

Indium-111 scintigraphy requires the labeling of autologous freshly drawn blood that is then injected intravenously, which exposes both staff and patients to the risk of HIV and other blood-borne infections. Indium-111–DTPA–IgG is a new radiopharmaceutical that does not require in vitro cell labeling and imaging may be performed 24–48 hr sooner than with gallium injection (58). Seventeen of 18 patients with PCP had diffusely increased uptake, and 10 of 11 patients without PCP had normal uptake. Focal uptake was present in 2 of 4 patients suspected of having bacterial infections.

Thallium-201 uptake is demonstrated in Kaposi's sarcoma lesions, whereas there is no uptake on gallium-67 scanning (59,60). The thallium-201 uptake is usually focal, whereas a pattern of diffusely increased uptake is usually seen with PCP (29).

Despite years of clinical investigation and experience, the exact role of nuclear scanning in the diagnosis of HIV-associated pulmonary disease remains unclear. A reasonable approach is to use nuclear scanning when there is extrapulmonary Kaposi's sarcoma and pulmonary abnormalities suggestive of pulmonary Kaposi's sarcoma. A gallium scan, if normal, makes infectious etiologies unlikely. If there is abnormal uptake, infectious and other etiologies should be sought. In patients with pulmonary symptoms and normal chest radiographs who may have other reasons for dyspnea, such as deconditioning and extrapulmonary illness, the finding of a normal nuclear scan reduces the likelihood of pulmonary parenchymal disease, with the exception of Kaposi's sarcoma. Another use for these scans is in the search for etiologies of unexplained fever. Nuclear scans may point to a focus of infection that was clinically unsuspected.

References

1. Rosen MJ, Jordan MC, Kvale PA, Rao AV, Miller A, Meiselman L, Hopewell PC, Glassroth J, Reichman LB, Wallace JM, Pulmonary Complications of HIV Infection Study Group. Pulmonary function tests in HIV-infected persons without AIDS. Am J Respir Crit Care Med 1995; 152:738–745.
2. Pothoff G, Wasserman K, Ostmann H. Impairment of exercise capacity in various groups of HIV-infected patients. Respiration 1994; 61:80–85.
3. Shaw RJ, Roussak C, Forster SM, Harris JRW, Pinching AJ, Mitchell DM. Lung function abnormalities in patients infected with the human immunodeficiency virus with and without overt pneumonitis. Thorax 1988; 43:436–440.
4. Smith DE, Forbes A, Davies S, et al. Diagnosis of *Pneumocystis carinii* pneumo-

nia in HIV antibody-positive patients by simple outpatient assessments. Thorax 1992; 47:1005–1009.

5. Kvale PA, Rosen MJ, Hopewell PC, et al. A decline in the pulmonary diffusing capacity does not indicate opportunistic lung disease in asymptomatic persons infected with the human immunodeficiency virus. Am Rev Respir Dis 1993; 148:390–395.
6. Ognibene FP, Masur H, Rogers P, et al. Non-specific interstitial pneumonitis without evidence of *Pneumocystis carinii* in asymptomatic patients infected with human immunodeficiency virus (HIV). Ann Intern Med 1988; 109:874–879.
7. Guillon JM, Autran B, Denis M, Fouret P, Plata F, Mayaud CM, Akoun GM. Human immunodeficiency virus-related lymphocytic alveolitis. Chest 1988; 94:1264–1270.
8. Coleman DL, Dodek PM, Golden JA, et al. Correlation between serial pulmonary function tests and fiberoptic bronchoscopy in patients with *Pneumocystis carinii* pneumonia and the acquired immunodeficiency syndrome. Am Rev Respir Dis 1984; 129:491–493.
9. Sankary RM, Turner J, Lipavsky AJA, et al. Alveolar–capillary block in patients with AIDS and *Pneumocystis carinii* pneumonia. Am Rev Respir Dis 1988; 137:443–449.
10. Stover DE, Greeno RA, Gagliardi AJ. The use of a simple exercise test for the diagnosis of *Pneumocystis carinii* pneumonia in patients with AIDS. Am Rev Respir Dis 1989; 139:1343–1346.
11. Smith DE, McLuckie A, Wyatt J, et al. Severe exercise hypoxaemia with normal or near normal x-rays: a feature of *Pneumocystis carinii* pneumonia. Lancet 1988; 2:1049–1051.
12. Sauleda J, Gea J, Aran X, et al. Simplified exercise test for the initial differential diagnosis of *Pneumocystis carinii* pneumonia in HIV antibody positive patients. Thorax 1994; 49:112–114.
13. Suster B, Akerman M, Orenstein M, et al. Pulmonary manifestations of AIDS: review of 106 episodes. Radiology 1986; 161:87–93.
14. Cohen BA, Pomerantz S, Rabinowitz JG, et al. Pulmonary complications of AIDS: radiographic features. AJR 1984; 143:115–122.
15. Naidich DP, Garay SM, Leitman BS, et al. Radiographic manifestations of pulmonary disease in the acquired immunodeficiency syndrome. Semin Roentgenol 1987; 22:14–30.
16. Golden JA, Sollitto RA. The radiology of pulmonary disease. Clin Chest Med 1988; 9:481–495.
17. Magnenat J-L, Nicod LP, Auckenthaler R, et al. Mode of presentation and diagnosis of bacterial pneumonia in human immunodeficiency virus-infected patients. Am Rev Respir Dis 1991; 144:917–922.
18. Uttamchandani RB, Daikos GL, Reyes RR, et al. Nocardiosis in 30 patients with advanced human immunodeficiency virus infection: clinical features and outcome. Clin Infect Dis 1994; 18:348-353.
19. Baron AD, Hollander H. *Pseudomonals aeruginosa* bronchopulmonary infection

in late human immunodeficiency virus infection. Am Rev Respir Dis 1993; 148:992–996.
20. Shapiro JM, Romney BM, Weiden MD, et al. *Rhodococcus equi* endobronchial mass with lung abscess in a patient with AIDS. Thorax 1992; 47:62–63.
21. Kwon KY, Colby TV. *Rhodococcus equi* pneumonia and pulmonary malakoplakia in acquired immune deficiency syndrome. Arch Pathol Lab Med 1994; 118:744–748.
22. DeLorenzo LJ, Huang CT, Maguire GP, et al. Roentgenographic patterns of *Pneumocystis carinii* pneumonia in 104 patients with AIDS. Chest 1987; 91:323–327.
23. Opravil M, Marincek B, Fuch WA, et al. Shortcomings of chest radiography in detecting *Pneumocystis carinii* pneumonia. J Acquir Immune Defic Syndr 1994; 7:39–45.
24. Pitchenik AE, Rubinson HA. The radiographic appearance of tuberculosis in patients with the acquired immune deficiency syndrome (AIDS) and pre-AIDS. Am Rev Respir Disease 1985; 131:393–396.
25. Barnes PF, Bloch AB, Davidson PT, et al. Tuberculosis in patients with HIV infection. N Engl J Med 1991; 324:1644–1650.
26. Chaisson RE, Schecter GF, Theuer CP, et al. Tuberculosis in patients with the acquired immune deficiency syndrome: clinical features, response to therapy, and survival. Am Rev Respir Dis 1987; 136:570–574.
27. Rigsby MO, Curtis AM. Pulmonary disease from nontuberculous mycobacteria in patients with human immunodeficiency virus. Chest 1994; 106:913–919.
28. Horsburgh CR Jr. *Mycobacterium avium* complex infection in the acquired immune deficiency syndrome. N Engl J Med 1991; 324:1332–1338.
29. Salzman SH, Smith RL, Aranda CP. Histoplasmosis in patients at risk for the acquired immune deficiency syndrome. Chest 1988; 93:916–921.
30. Cameron ML, Bartlett JA, Gallis HA, et al. Manifestations of pulmonary cytococcosis in patients with acquired immune deficiency syndrome. Rev Infect Dis 1991; 13:64–67.
31. Fish DG, Ampel NM, Galgiani JN, et al. Coccidioidomycosis during human immunodeficiency virus infection. Medicine 1990; 69:384–390.
32. Miller WT, Sais GJ, Frank I, et al. Pulmonary aspergillosis in patients with AIDS. Chest 1994; 105:37–44.
33. Drew LW. Cytomegalovirus infection in patients with AIDS. Clin Infect Dis 1992; 14:608–615.
34. Gruden JF, Huang L, Webb WR, Gamsu G, Hopewell PC, Sides DM. Radiology 1995; 195:545–552.
35. Davis SD, Henschke CI, Chamides BK, et al. Intrathoracic Kaposi's sarcoma in AIDS patients: radiographic–pathologic correlation. Radiology 1987; 163:495–500.
36. Brown RKJ, Huberman RP, Vanley G. Pulmonary features of Kaposi's sarcoma. AJR 1982; 139:659–660.
37. Meduri GU, Stover DE, Lee M, et al. Pulmonary Kaposi's sarcoma in the acquired immune deficiency syndrome—clinical, radiographic, and pathologic manifestations. Am J Med 1986; 81:11–18.

38. Garay SM, Belenko M, Fazzini E, Schinella R. Pulmonary manifestations of Kaposi's sarcoma. Chest 1987; 91:39–43.
39. Polish LB, Cohn DL, Ryder JW, et al. Pulmonary non-Hodgkin's lymphoma in AIDS. Chest 1989; 96:1321–1326.
40. Sandrasegaran K, Robinson PJ, Selby P. Staging of lymphoma in adults. Clin Radiol 1994; 49:149–161.
41. Levine AM. Acquired immune deficiency syndrome-related lymphoma. Blood 1992; 80:8–20.
42. Morris JC, Rosen MJ, Marchevsky A, et al. Lymphocytic interstitial pneumonia in patients at risk for the acquired immune deficiency syndrome. Chest 1987; 91:63–67.
43. Suffredini AF, Ognibene FP, Lack EE, et al. Nonspecific interstitial pneumonitis: a common cause of pulmonary disease in the acquired immunodeficiency syndrome. Ann Intern Med 1987; 107:7–13.
44. Griffiths MH, Miller RF, Semple SJG. Interstitial pneumonitis in patients infected with the human immunodeficiency virus. Thorax 1995; 50:1141–1146.
45. McGuinness G, Naidich DP, Garay S, et al. AIDS associated bronchiectasis: CT features. J Comput Assist Tomogr 1993; 17:260–266.
46. Bergin CL, Wirth RL, Castellino RA. *Pneumocystis carinii* pneumonia: CT and HRCT observations. J Comput Assist Tomogr 1990; 14;756–759.
47. Kuhlman JE, Kavuru M, Fishman EK, et al. *Pneumocystis carinii* pneumonia: spectrum of parenchymal CT findings. Radiology 1990; 175:711–714.
48. Kramer EL, Sanger JH, Garay SM, Grossman RJ, Tiu S, Banner H. Diagnostic implications of Ga-67 chest-scan patterns in human immunodeficiency virus-seropositive patients. Radiology 1989; 170:671–676.
49. Jules-Elysee KM, Stover DE, Zaman MB, Bernard BA, White DA. Aerosolized pentamidine: effect on diagnosis and presentation of *Pneumocystis carinii* pneumonia. Ann Intern Med 1990; 112:750–757.
50. Woolfenden JM, Carrasquillo JA, Carson SM, et al. Acquired immunodeficiency syndrome: gallium-67 citrate imaging. Radiology 1987; 162:383–387.
51. Kramer EL, Sanger JH, Garay SM, et al. Gallium-67 scan of the chest in patients with acquired immunodeficiency syndrome. J Nucl Med 1987; 28:1107–1114.
52. Coleman DL, Hattner RS, Luce JM, Podek PM, Golden JA, Murray JF. Correlation between gallium lung scans and fiberoptic bronchoscopy in patients with suspected *Pneumocystis carinii* pneumonia and the acquired immunodeficiency syndrome. Am Rev Respir Dis 1984; 130:1166–1169.
53. Abdel-Dayem HM, Di Fabrizio L, Kowalsky W, et al. Diffuse thallium lung uptake in *Pneumocystis carinii* pneumonia. Clin Nucl Med 1994; 19:287–291.
54. Bourquest P, Dclaval PH, Herry JY. Direct quantification of thoracic gallium-67 uptake in sarcoidosis. J Nucl Med 1986; 27:1550–1556.
55. Tsan MF. Studies on gallium accumulation in inflammatory lesions: III. J Nucl Med 1978; 19:492–495.
56. Tsan MF. Studies on gallium accumulation in inflammatory lesions. J Nucl Med 1985; 26:88–92.
57. Fineman DS, Palestro CJ, Kim CK, et al. Detection of abnormalities in febrile

AIDS patients with In-111-labeled leukocyte and Ga-67 scintigraphy. Radiology 1989; 170:677–680.
58. Khalkhali I, Mena I, Rauh DA, et al. 111-Indium-DTPA-IgG lung imaging in patients with pulmonary and HIV infection. Chest 1995; 107:1336–1341.
59. Lee UW, Rosen MP, Baum A, et al. AIDS related Kaposi's sarcoma: finding in thallium-201 scintigraphy. AJR 1988; 151:1233–1235.
60. Lee UW, Fuller JD, O'Brien MJ, et al. Preliminary Kaposi's sarcoma in patients with AIDS: scintigraphic diagnosis with sequential thallium and gallium scanning. Radiology 1991; 180:409–412.

10

Pulmonary Illness in HIV-Infected Adults
Screening and Case Finding

ROSLYN F. SCHNEIDER

Albert Einstein College of Medicine and
Beth Israel Medical Center
New York, New York

PAUL A. KVALE

Case Western Reserve University School
of Medicine and
Henry Ford Hospital
Cleveland, Ohio

I. Introduction

Most patients with human immunodeficiency virus (HIV) infection develop symptoms that bring them to medical attention. The physician integrates the symptoms with other diagnostic studies to make a diagnosis, and chooses a course of treatment based on the results of such studies, or makes empiric decisions based on probabilities.

There exists among physicians and laypersons alike, a belief that earlier recognition of a disease allows more timely therapy, with a reduction in morbidity and improved survival. As attractive as this notion seems, the theory that earlier diagnosis necessarily improves outcome may not be true: either effective treatment does not exist, or the diagnostic studies are not sufficiently precise to alter the course of the disease. This lack of precision may be due to inadequate sensitivity or specificity of the additional tests designed to detect the disease.

In this chapter, we will review the evidence for screening HIV-infected patients with simple and readily available diagnostic tests, including chest radiographs, pulmonary function tests, and induced sputum. These tests are very useful for the diagnosis of pulmonary diseases among symptomatic HIV-infected patients, but their usefulness in the diagnosis of occult pulmonary diseases in asymptomatic persons has only recently been studied. We will concentrate on *Pneumocystis carinii* pneumonia (PCP) because of its historical importance as the most common pulmonary opportunistic infection among HIV-infected persons, and tuberculosis because of its potential for disability and death of persons with HIV infection, and also because of its public health importance. We will also examine the role of screening chest radiographs in asymptomatic HIV infection, because chest radiographs have long been considered a mainstay in the diagnosis of nearly all types of pulmonary disorders.

II. Definitions

In 1951, the Commission on Chronic Illness defined *screening* as

> the presumptive identification of unrecognized disease or defect by the application of tests, examinations, or other procedures which can be applied rapidly. Screening tests sort out apparently well persons who probably have a disease from those who probably do not. A screening test is not intended to be diagnostic. Persons with positive or suspicious findings must be referred to their physicians for diagnosis and necessary treatment (1).

The primary objectives of screening tests are to detect preclinical disease, to reduce morbidity and mortality by earlier identification of disease, and to reduce the public health hazards of unrecognized disease. Potential disadvantages of screening include a longer duration of morbidity, false reassurance with false-negative results, potential risks of the tests, and the cost of the tests. Other problems related to screening include lead time bias when screening does not lead to more effective treatment, length bias, overdiagnosis, and selection bias (2).

The term *case finding* is defined as

> the active search for and pursuit of cases of chronic disease and disability in both asymptomatic and more advanced stages—in order to provide, for the patients concerned, available techniques of secondary prevention appropriate to the stage of disease, and thus stop further progression of the disease or disability to a more severe, complicated, or disabling stage (3).

These are different from *diagnosis*, which is "the application of a variety of questions, examinations, and other tests to patients who have actively sought health services in order to identify the exact cause for their chief complaints" (4). In the setting of HIV infection, all tests are either case-finding evaluations or diagnostic tests. Nevertheless, in usual clinical practice and as defined in the literature, many of these tests are referred to as screening tests.

Lead time bias occurs when a disease is diagnosed earlier in an asymptomatic person than if there were no evaluation, but the patient dies on the same date as he or she would have without screening. Survival from the time of diagnosis to the time of death is increased, but the outcome is identical. *Length bias* occurs when diseases that are detected by screening identifies persons with a better or more prolonged natural history than those diagnosed following symptoms. *Overdiagnosis* occurs when screening detects a disease that may never have been discovered during life, because subjects will die of other causes. *Selection bias* in screening is present when those who choose to be screened are at different risk than a general population in whom the screening test may be implemented (2).

The natural history of any disease greatly influences the value of screening. For screening to be useful, there should be a defined preclinical phase during which intervention might be of benefit (2). In HIV-infected persons, *P. carinii* pneumonia occurs commonly and may present with a prolonged subacute course. Tuberculosis is also more common among HIV-infected persons; this disease, more than any other complication of HIV infection, poses considerable public health risk if it is undetected and untreated. Other opportunistic infections that are more common in HIV-infected persons, such as fungal pneumonias, also might respond better to treatment if the infection could be detected at an early stage. The duration of these secondary infections in HIV-infected persons before the development of symptoms is unknown. Screening tests to identify these and other pulmonary illnesses during a preclinical phase would be desirable, if such screening allowed the institution of prompt treatment and led to an improved outcome.

Recommendations have been made by the American Thoracic Society to focus on primary prevention of lung diseases. Specific screening with spirometry or chest roentgenography for occult lung disease is not recommended for the general population owing to a lack of evidence that this is useful (5). The Centers for Disease Control and Prevention (CDC) previously recommended that a chest radiograph be performed in all HIV-infected persons who are anergic or who have a tuberculin skin test reaction of 5 mm or greater (6). More recently, the recommendation for chest radiographs in anergic persons was omitted (7). Bellin et al. proposed that populations with a high prevalence of HIV infection, such as injection drug users admitted to prisons, should have a screening chest radiograph on admission.

Among the 1314 prisoners who were studied, 17 of the 26 patients with radiographs most suggestive of tuberculosis would have been missed with tuberculin testing alone (8). It is not clear from these data how many were symptomatic, how many had confirmed tuberculosis, or had other non-tuberculous disorders.

III. History and Physical Examination

A careful history and physical examination are traditional methods of finding disease, but their role in asymptomatic HIV-infected persons has never been systematically studied, nor has the appropriate interval between visits been established. The history may identify risk factors for specific pulmonary disorders or symptoms that the person may have ignored. Specific questions should include the symptoms of fever, weight loss, fatigue, dyspnea at rest or with exertion, cough, sputum production, chest pain, and wheezing, which focus on the identification of pulmonary diseases. During a screening visit, education concerning HIV transmission and symptom recognition should be addressed. The spectrum of illnesses that complicate HIV infection varies with the individual's risk. For example, current substance abuse predisposes patients to needle-induced infections and vascular injury, while unemployment and homelessness interfere with access to appropriate medical services. Kaposi's sarcoma, on the other hand, is more frequent in homosexual men (9,10). Tuberculosis is more common in injection drug users, and methadone treatment centers provide a unique setting for its screening and chemoprophylaxis (11).

A focused physical examination may suggest the stage of HIV infection (wasting syndrome, oral thrush), identify a pulmonary illness, or identify an illness that may have pulmonary involvement during its course. Fever or weight loss may initiate a diagnostic workup for pulmonary disease, but these findings in most instances may be elicited by a careful history. Cutaneous or mucosal Kaposi's sarcoma is likely to be present in persons with pulmonary involvement (9). Lymphadenopathy that is rapidly progressive or unilateral may indicate tuberculosis, lymphoma with or without pulmonary involvement, or other infectious or neoplastic processes (12). Fundoscopic examination may suggest cytomegalovirus (CMV), toxoplasma, or *P. carinii* infection. Neurological examination may reveal focal findings of central nervous system (CNS) toxoplasmosis, lymphoma, tuberculosis, nocardia, fungal infection, or other neoplasm. Abdominal findings of hepatomegaly or splenomegaly suggest diseases including *Mycobacterium avium* complex (MAC) infection, tuberculosis, lymphoma, and histoplasmosis.

IV. Screening Tests

Screening tests for preclinical lung disease in HIV-infected individuals were examined in the Pulmonary Complications of HIV Infection Study (13–16). The cohort included 1171 HIV-infected subjects at six clinical centers in the United States recruited between November 1988 and February 1990. Of these, 841 (72%) were homosexual or bisexual, 274 (23%) were injection drug users, and 56 (5%) were female partners of HIV-infected men (16). Subjects were followed for a mean of approximately 4 ½ years. The usefulness of chest radiographs, induced sputum, and diffusing capacity screening were evaluated.

A. Chest Radiographs

The protocol for the Pulmonary Complications of HIV Infection Study included a requirement for surveillance-screening chest radiographs to be performed (in the absence of symptoms) at baseline, 3-, 6-, and 12-month intervals throughout the study on 1065 of the HIV-infected subjects enrolled (13). Symptoms were defined as new or worsening cough, sputum production, fever, night sweats, wheezing, chest pain, or dyspnea of less than 26-weeks' duration. Subjects were also defined as symptomatic for this analysis if a new pulmonary diagnosis was identified within the 3 months before the visit. The chest radiographs were than interpreted by trained investigators who were unaware of the clinical status of the patient. The interpretations of abnormalities were defined as pulmonary parenchymal abnormalities, pleural processes, adenopathy, and nodules or masses.

There were 5263 evaluable surveillance chest radiographs performed while subjects were asymptomatic: 123 (2%) radiographs were abnormal, and of these only 11 were associated with 13 new pulmonary diagnoses identified within 2 months of the abnormal film. The pulmonary disorders that were diagnosed included 4 cases of PCP, 3 of bacterial pneumonia, and 1 each of nontuberculous pulmonary mycobacterial infection, pulmonary tuberculosis, lung cancer, nonspecific interstitial pneumonitis, cytomegalovirus pneumonia, and pulmonary embolism. Among the 5140 normal chest radiographs, a new pulmonary diagnosis was identified in 44 during the following 2 months. The sensitivity of the screening chest radiograph (the probability of having an abnormal chest radiograph in subjects who have a new diagnosis identified in the 2-month period after the film) was 20%. The overall yield was low, regardless of transmission group, CD4 lymphocyte category, and whether or not they were anergic. When the sensitivity for the diagnosis of tuberculosis was specifically analyzed, the screening chest radiograph alone failed to identify a single case of tuberculosis. One subject had pulmonary tuberculosis and an abnormal surveillance-screening chest radiograph, but he also had a 16-mm tuberculin skin test reaction, which would have prompted a chest radiograph. Two other asymptomatic patients were identified with pulmonary tuberculosis who had normal surveillance-screening chest radiographs.

Although the sensitivity of the screening chest radiographs was low for the detection of asymptomatic pulmonary processes, the finding of a normal chest radiograph in an asymptomatic HIV-infected patient almost always meant that the subject did not have a complicating pulmonary disorder. Among the 5208 asymptomatic subjects with normal chest radiographs, 5096 did not develop a new pulmonary disorder within the next 2 months (97.8% specificity). However, there were many false-negative screening chest radiographs (0.9%), for 44 new pulmonary disorders were identified within the 2 months of a normal film (12 cases of PCP, 10 cases of bacterial pneumonia, 5 cases of pneumonia of uncertain etiology, 8 rib fractures, 4 episodes of pleural effusion, 2 cases of pulmonary tuberculosis, 2 cases of septic emboli owing to endocarditis, and 1 each of adult respiratory distress syndrome and asthma). Even more disturbing was the frequency of false-positive screening chest radiographs among the asymptomatic HIV-infected subjects. We identified 124 new abnormalities in 112 chest radiographs that were not followed by a new pulmonary diagnosis. These included diffuse or focal interstitial infiltrates in 53 chest radiographs, focal alveolar infiltrates in 20, solitary pulmonary nodules in 20, intrathoracic adenopathy in 10, pleural effusions in 7, combinations of focal interstitial or alveolar or nodular processes in 7, multiple nodules in 5, and focal cavitary lesions in 2 patients.

To summarize the place of a screening chest radiograph in asymptomatic ambulatory HIV-infected patients, the data from this study strongly suggest that it has very limited value. Most chest radiographs in asymptomatic persons will be normal. When the screening chest radiograph is abnormal, it is four times as likely to be a false-positive result as it is to identify a new pulmonary disease. False-negative results are just as common, for four times as many patients with negative-screening chest radiographs will develop a new symptomatic pulmonary disease within the subsequent 2 months as will be detected by the abnormal-screening chest radiograph.

B. Sputum Analysis

For patients who present with acute respiratory symptoms that include a productive cough, with and without HIV infection, a Gram stain of the sputum provides rapidly available information about the microbiology of the lower respiratory tract. However, its clinical usefulness has recently been questioned (17). If no sputum is produced spontaneously by a patient with a suspected lower respiratory infection, it is possible to induce an adequate sputum specimen, in more than 90% of patients, by having them inhale hypertonic saline. Induced sputum is helpful for the diagnosis of pulmonary tuberculosis in patients without spontaneously expectorated sputum when there are characteristic clinical or chest radiographic abnormalities. Since the mid-1980s, analysis of induced sputum has also been useful for the diagnosis of PCP in HIV-infected persons (18–20).

Sputum analysis was not an efficient means to screen HIV-infected asymptomatic subjects for clinically occult tuberculosis or PCP, however (13). In the Pulmonary Complications of HIV Infection Study, a baseline routine specimen was obtained from 1113 subjects. After a baseline study, 1518 routine, induced sputum samples were collected from 631 HIV-infected subjects at 3- and 12-month intervals. Two occult cases of tuberculosis were identified at baseline, and none at follow-up in asymptomatic subjects. Two more induced sputum specimens were positive for *M. tuberculosis* at follow-up, but 1 patient was clearly symptomatic and had an abnormal chest radiograph, and the other was a false-positive specimen. No cases of occult PCP were identified in any subject, but one specimen was false-positive for PCP. Five pathogenic nontuberculous mycobacteria were recognized during follow-up.

In addition to false-positive specimens for *M. tuberculosis* and PCP, routine analysis of induced sputum in asymptomatic HIV-infected patients is often contaminated by nonpathogenic nontuberculous mycobacteria. The false-positive rate from these organisms in the Pulmonary Complications of HIV Infection Study was 4% (107/2631 specimens).

Thus, collection and analysis of induced sputum in the asymptomatic HIV-infected population is not an effective strategy to identify either tuberculosis or PCP at an early stage. False-positive results are common and may lead to inappropriate treatment and marked anxiety, and the cost to identify such a small percentage of patients with tuberculosis can hardly be justified as an appropriate utilization of resources.

C. Diffusing Capacity Measurement

Serial pulmonary function tests and diffusing capacity ($D_{L}co$) measurements in asymptomatic HIV-infected persons were also evaluated in the Pulmonary Complications of HIV Infection Study (15). Because the diffusing capacity is often low in patients with PCP, it was thought that a 20% reduction in corrected diffusing capacity from a previous value might indicate the presence of PCP or other pulmonary infections, in the absence of new pulmonary symptoms or new abnormalities on chest radiographs. There were 64 subjects with a decline of 20% or more from a previous value within 2 years of entry. A sputum induction was performed in 44, and fiberoptic bronchoscopy in 14, including 6 with transbronchial biopsies. The subjects were followed for an additional 3–12 months. In no case was the decline in diffusing capacity caused by PCP or other documented pulmonary infections. Of the 63 subjects who had follow-up diffusing capacity measurements, improvement was noted in 45 (71%), stability in 7 (11%), and further decline in 11 (17%). Lymphocytic alveolitis, lymphocytic interstitial pneumonitis, or nonspecific interstitial pneumonitis may have been the cause of the fall in diffusing capacity in these subjects, as open-lung biopsy was not done in any, and transbronchial biopsy in only a few.

Because these noninfectious disorders usually require no treatment while patients are asymptomatic, identifying HIV-infected persons with these disorders by serial D_Lco measurements is not important. Abnormalities of D_Lco in the absence of symptoms should not lead to the suspicion of tuberculosis, PCP, or other pulmonary infections in HIV-infected persons.

D. CD4 Lymphocyte Determination

Monitoring of CD4 lymphocyte counts periodically determines the stage of illness and the need for prophylaxis for certain opportunistic infections (PCP, MAC). Opportunistic infections, including PCP, CMV pneumonia, and MAC, are unlikely to occur in persons with CD4 lymphocyte counts of more than $200/mm^3$ (21). the optimal schedule of measuring CD4 lymphocyte counts is unknown. The CDC recommends that measurement of CD4 lymphocyte counts be performed initially, every 6 months when the count is more than $600/mm^3$, and at least every 3 months when the count is between 200 and $600/mm^3$. Additional monitoring every 3 months may be needed when CD4 counts are fewer than $200/mm^3$ to assess response to antiviral therapy or to assess the need for additional prophylaxis or therapy (6).

E. Measurement of Viral Burden

Recent studies showed that measurement of HIV RNA in the blood is a better surrogate marker of progression of disease, and is a more rapid and reliable indicator of response to antiviral therapy (22). In a study of HIV-infected persons with hemophilia, the number of RNA copies of HIV-1 per milliliter of serum correlated strongly with the development of AIDS within 10 years: 72% in those with more than 100,000 copies, and no cases in those were fewer than 1000 copies. The exact role of this test in clinical practice is not established.

V. Summary

Review of available data demonstrates no morbidity or mortality benefit with any screening test. It seems prudent to evaluate asymptomatic patients periodically with a careful history and focused physical examination, and to perform only those tests that are likely to alter the plan of management, such as tuberculin skin testing (discussed in Chap. 13), CD4 lymphocyte measurement, and now possibly measurement of viral burden. Diagnostic studies to detect pulmonary disease should be performed only if there are new pulmonary symptoms.

References

1. Commission on Chronic Illness. Proceedings of the Conference on Preventive Aspects of Chronic Disease. March 12–14, 1951:14 (out of print).
2. Morrison A. Screening in chronic disease. Monogr Epidemiol Biostat 1992; 19:3–20.
3. Commission Chronic Illness. Chronic Illness in the United States—Prevention of Chronic Illness. Cambridge, MA: Harvard University Press, 1957:28–44.
4. Sackett DL, Holland WW. Controversy in the detection of disease. Lancet, 1975; 2:357–359.
5. Task Group on Screening for Adult Respiratory Disease. Screening for adult respiratory disease. Am Rev Respir Dis 1983; 128:768–774.
6. El-Sadr W, Oleske JM, Agins BD, et al. Evaluation and Management of Early HIV Infection. Clinical Practice Guideline No. 7. AHCPR Publication 94-0572. Rockville, MD: Agency for Health Care Policy and Research, Public Health Service, US Department of Health and Human Services, January 1994:40–41.
7. Kaplan JE, Masur H, Holmes KK, McNeil MM, Schonberger LB, Navin TR, Hanson DL, Gross PA, Jaffe HW, and the USPHS/IDSA Prevention of Opportunistic Infection Working Group. USPHS/IDSA guidelines for the prevention of opportunistic infections in persons infected with human immunodeficiency virus. Clin Infect Dis 1995; 21(suppl):S32–S43.
8. Bellin E, Fletcher D, Safyer S. Abnormal chest x-rays in intravenous drug users: implications for tuberculosis screening programs. Am J Public Health May 1993; 83:698–700.
9. Garay SM, Belenko M, Fazzini E, Schinella R. Pulmonary manifestations of Kaposi's sarcoma. Chest 1987; 91:39–43.
10. O'Connor PG, Selwyn PA, Schottenfeld RS. Medical care for injection-drug users with human immunodeficiency virus infection. N Engl J Med 1994; 331:450–459.
11. Reichman LB, Felton CP, Edsall JR. Drug dependence, a possible new risk factor for tuberculous disease. Arch Intern Med 1979; 139:337–339.
12. Bottles K, McPhaul LW, Volberding P. Fine-needle aspiration biopsy of patients

with the acquired immunodeficiency syndrome (AIDS): experience in an outpatient clinic. Ann Intern Med 1988; 108:42–45.
13. Schneider RS, Hansen NI, Kvale PA, Rosen MJ, the Pulmonary Complications of HIV Infection Study Group. Lack of utility of chest x-ray screening in asymptomatic HIV-infected adults. Arch Intern Med 1996; 156:191–195.
14. Kvale PA, Hansen NI, Markowitz N, et al. Routine induced sputum analysis is not cost-effective to screen HIV-infected persons for tuberculosis or *Pneumocystis carinii*. Clin Infect Dis 1994; 19:410–416.
15. Kvale PA, Rosen JM, Hopewell PC, et al. A decline in the pulmonary diffusing capacity does not indicate opportunistic lung disease in asymptomatic persons infected with the human immunodeficiency virus. Am Rev Respir Dis 1993; 148:390–395.
16. The Pulmonary Complications of HIV Infection Study Group. Design of a prospective study of the pulmonary complications of human immunodeficiency virus infection. J Clin Epidemiol 1993; 46:497–507.
17. Niederman MS, Bass JB, Campbell GD, Fein AM, Grossman RF, Mandell LA, Marrie TJ, Sarosi GA, Torres A, Yu VL. Guidelines for the initial management of adults with community-acquired pneumonia: diagnosis, assessment of severity, and initial antimicrobial therapy. Am Rev Respir Dis 1993; 148:1418–1426.
18. Pitchenik AE, Gangei P, Torres A, Evans A, Rubin E, Baier H. Sputum examination for the diagnosis of *Pneumocystis carinii* pneumonia in the acquired immunodeficiency syndrome. Am Rev Respir Dis 1986; 133:226–229.
19. Bigby TD, Margolskee D, Curtis JL, Michael PF, Sheppard D, Hadley WK, Hopewell PC. The usefulness of induced sputum in the diagnosis of *Pneumocystis carinii* pneumonia in the acquired immunodeficiency syndrome. Am Rev Respir Dis 1986; 133:515–518.
20. Zaman MK, Woofen OJ, Suprahmnay B, Ankobiah W, Finch JP, Kamholz SL. Rapid noninvasive diagnosis of *Pneumocystis carinii* from induced liquefied sputum. Ann Intern Med 1988; 109:7–10.
21. Masur H, Ognibene FP, Yarchoan R, et al. CD4 counts as predictors of opportunistic pneumonias in human immunodeficiency virus infection. Ann Intern Med 1989; 111:223–231.
22. O'Brien TR, Blattner WA, Waters D, Eyster E, Hilgartner MW, Cohen AR, Luban N, Hatzakis A, Aledort LM, Rosenberg PS, Miley WH, Kroner BL, Goedert JJ, for the Multicenter Hemophilia Cohort Study: Serum HIV-1 RNA levels and time to development of AIDS in the Multicenter Hemophilia Cohort Study. JAMA 1996; 276:105–110.

Part Four

PULMONARY INFECTIONS

11

Bacterial Pneumonia in the Setting of Human Immunodeficiency Virus Infection

ROBERT E. HIRSCHTICK

Northwestern University Medical School
Chicago, Illinois

JEFFREY GLASSROTH

MCP-Hahnemann Medical School
Philadelphia, Pennsylvania

I. Introduction

It was recognized early in the epidemic of acquired immunodeficiency syndrome (AIDS) that, in addition to infection by unusual, opportunistic organisms, individuals infected with the human immunodeficiency virus (HIV) were also susceptible to pneumonia caused by common bacterial pathogens (1–3). More recently, bacterial pneumonia has been noted to occur more frequently than *Pneumocystis carinii* pneumonia (PCP) in a large cohort of HIV-infected persons (4). The importance of bacterial pneumonia in this population is reflected in the 1993 revision of the Centers for Disease Control and Prevention (CDC) definition of AIDS (5), which includes recurrent bacterial pneumonia as an AIDS-defining condition in HIV-infected individuals. Appreciation of the frequent occurrence of bacterial pneumonia in this patient population is essential because, with prompt diagnosis, the outcome of HIV-associated bacterial pneumonia is reasonably good when treated appropriately (2,6).

II. Immunology

Although deficiency of cell-mediated immunity is its hallmark, HIV infection also induces significant dysfunction of humoral immunity (7–9), thereby predisposing infected individuals to bacterial infections, especially with encapsulated organisms such as *Streptococcus pneumoniae* and *Haemophilus influenzae* (8,10). Impaired B-cell activation and polyclonal hypergammaglobulinemia are common (7,8,9,11) as is impairment of local pulmonary defenses by alveolar macrophage dysfunction (12). Reduced neutrophil bactericidal activity against *Staphylococcus aureus* has been noted (13) and may occur with other bacteria as well. CD4 lymphocytes are important regulators of B-cell differentiation and indirectly play a role in antibody production and phagocytosis (11). Thus, one would predict that the incidence of bacterial pneumonia would be higher in individuals with lower CD4 lymphocyte counts. This has, in fact, been shown to be true (4,14). Finally, pharyngeal colonization by *S. pneumoniae*, the most common cause of bacterial pneumonia in HIV-infected individuals (1,3,4,6,14–18) is no more common in HIV-infected individuals than in HIV-negative controls. This finding suggests that the increased rate of *S. pneumoniae* infection in HIV infection is due to host immune factors, rather than to increased exposure to this pathogen (19).

III. Epidemiology

In 1984 it was noted that homosexual men with AIDS were frequently hospitalized for bacterial pneumonia (1). Later reports confirmed that bacterial pneumonia occurred more frequently in HIV-infected persons than in the general population (2,3). These reports estimated the annual incidence rate of pneumococcal pneumonia to be 17.9:1000–45.5:1000 HIV-infected individuals compared with 2.6:1000 individuals in the general population (2,3). Additional reports have noted an especially high risk of bacterial pneumonia in HIV-infected injection drug users (4,14,15,17), which is higher than in injection drug users without HIV infection (14). Moreover, among seropositive patients, the rate of bacterial pneumonia is higher in injection drug users than in homosexual men or in women who were infected heterosexually (3,4,18). However, all HIV transmission groups appear to be highly susceptible to bacterial pneumonia. A recent multicenter study that examined epidemiological risk factors for bacterial pneumonia in HIV-infected persons from different transmission categories is instructive (4). Bacterial pneumonia occurs more frequently in HIV-seropositive than in HIV-seronegative individuals, even when CD4 lymphocyte counts are more than 500/mm^3. The rate of bacterial pneumonia is higher in persons with lower CD4 lymphocyte counts and is highest in individuals with a CD4 lymphocyte count of fewer than 200/mm^3 (Table 1). Of note, cigarette smokers have an even greater risk of bacterial pneumonia than nonsmokers when CD4 lymphocytes counts are fewer than 200/mm^3. There appears to be no increased risk of pneumonia based on race, gender, or alcohol consumption (4). It has been suggested that individuals of unknown HIV-serostatus who experience recurrent bacterial pneumonia or pneumonia with concomitant bacteremia should be evaluated for possible HIV infection (16,19).

IV. Bacteriology

As in the general population, the most common cause of bacterial pneumonia in the setting of HIV-infection is *S. pneumoniae* (1,3,4,6,14–18). Witt et al. (3) found the incidence of pneumococcal pneumonia in HIV-infected patients to be 17.5 times higher than in the general patient population of Boston City Hospital. Other bacteria frequently cause pneumonia as well. Farley et al. (20) reported a 24-fold higher incidence of invasive *H. influenzae* infection in HIV-infected adults compared with all adults. *S. aureus* accounted for 15% of cases of bacterial pneumonia (in which a cause was identified) in the largest series to date (4). Gram-negative bacilli also cause bacterial pneumonia, with significant frequency, in HIV-infected individuals (4,6,14). HIV-associated gram-negative pneumonias follow a pattern similar to that seen in the population without HIV. That is, they occur most often as a nosocomial condition. Although apparently uncommon, *Rhodococcus equi* has been implicated as a cause of pneumonia in numerous case reports. Other causes of bacterial pneumonias have been reported, such as group B streptococcis, *Nocardia asteroides*, *Moroxella catarrhalis*, and *Legionella pneumophila*, but they appear to be relatively infrequent causes of disease in the HIV-infected population.

Table 1 Risk Factors for Bacterial Pneumonia in HIV-Infected Individuals

Injection drug use
CD4 lymphocyte count fewer than 200/mm^3
Cigarette smoking
Corticosteroids (*P. aeruginosa*)
Neutropenia (*P. aeruginosa*)

V. Clinical Presentation and Diagnosis

The clinical presentation of bacterial pneumonia is similar in HIV-seropositive and HIV-seronegative patients. A short duration of symptoms, usually a few days, as well as fever and a productive cough are generally noted (3). This latter symptom may help distinguish bacterial pneumonia from the dry cough usually associated with *P. carinii* pneumonia. Physical examination findings vary with the extent of focal lung consolidation and the degree of focal consolidation.

Chest radiographs most often demonstrate either segmental or lobar alveolar infiltrates. Focal consolidation is typically observed with *S. pneumoniae* pneumonia, whereas *H. influenzae* may show interstitial infiltration. Cavitation may be seen with a variety of pneumonias, including those caused by *P. carinii*, *S. aureus*, *P. aeruginosa*, and *R. equi*, as well as tuberculosis. However, as in the general population, it is generally not possible to determine the etiology of pneumonia solely from the chest radiograph in the setting of HIV-infection (21).

Leukocytosis, with a left shift, is commonly seen (22,23), although the absolute neutrophil count may not be as high as in HIV-seronegative patients. Serum lactate dehydrogenase (LDH) is normal in most patients with bacterial pneumonia, in contrast with *P. carinii* pneumonia. Sputum Gram stain and culture often provide clues to the etiology of bacterial pneumonia, provided the patient is able to produce a satisfactory specimen (with more than 25 neutrophils and fewer than 10 epithelial cells per low power field). However, sputum culture yields a potential pathogen less than 40% of the time in HIV-infected patients who present acutely with fever, productive cough, and a focal infiltrate (4,17). Many patients are unable to produce a satisfactory sputum, and many others have received antibiotic therapy before sputum collection, thereby reducing its yield. It has been suggested that bronchoalveolar lavage (BAL) might be diagnostically useful in this setting (17). BAL has an estimated sensitivity of 62% and specificity of 77% in the setting of HIV-associated bacterial pneumonia. However, when antibiotics are administered before the procedure, which is the usual sequence of events, the sensitivity of BAL drops to 23% (17).

Bacteremia as a complication of bacterial pneumonia occurs frequently in the HIV-infected population (1,2). Pneumococcal bacteremia occurs approximately eight times more often in hospitalized HIV-infected patients than in the general hospital population.

Patients with *P. carinii* pneumonia typically have a nonproductive cough, as well as a longer prodrome, diffuse interstitial infiltrates on chest radiograph, and an elevated serum LDH concentration. These features can be used to distinguish between bacterial pneumonia and pneumonia caused by *P. carinii*, although the two conditions may coexist simultaneously (23,24).

VI. Specific Pathogens

A. *Streptococcus pneumoniae*

Pneumonia caused by *S. pneumoniae* occurs at a younger age in HIV-infected patients than in the non-HIV population (31 years versus 59 years, respectively, in one study; 16). Pneumococcal pneumonia may be the initial manifestation of HIV infection, and its occurrence in young persons lacking other predisposing factors, especially if recurrent or bacteremic, should prompt an evaluation for HIV infection. The pneumococcal serotypes 3, 9, and 23 are the predominant causes of pneumonia in both the HIV and non-HIV populations (16). The clinical presentation of *S. pneumoniae* pneumonia in HIV-seropositive individuals differs somewhat from that seen in the seronegative population (16). The duration of symptoms at presentation may be several days for HIV-infected persons, rather than the few days classically described. Leukocyte counts tend to be lower in HIV-seropositive patients than in seronegatives. In one study, only 28.6% of HIV-infected patients with proved *S. pneumoniae* pneumonia had leukocyte counts of more than 10,000/mm^3 (16). Bacteremia has been noted in one-third to one-half of episodes of HIV-associated pneumococcal pneumonia (2,3,16), compared with one-fourth in the non-HIV population. Fever, productive cough with purulent sputum, and dyspnea are the norm and are seen with equal frequency in both groups (16,22). Dyspnea occurs in 50% of cases, whereas chest pain is infrequent (22). Lobar consolidation on chest radiograph is the rule (2,16), although interstitial infiltrates may be seen (17). Bilateral infiltrates occur commonly, whereas pleural effusions are only occasionally observed (16,22). Mechanical ventilation is required less often in HIV-associated pneumococcal pneumonia than in the non-HIV population, presumably because of the younger age and lower incidence of chronic heart and lung disease in the former group. A desire for limited ventilator support by some patients with advanced HIV infection may also be a factor. Manifestations that harken back to the preantibiotic era, such as empyema, mediastinitis, and brain abscess, have been described (25), but appear to be infrequent. An association between recurrent *S. pneumoniae* pneumonia and adult lymphoid interstitial pneumonitis (LIP) has been reported (26). Treatment of *S. pneumoniae* pneumonia with standard antibiotic therapy is generally successful (2,3,16). Pneumococcal resistance to penicillin has been reported in HIV-infected patients, but appears to reflect regional resistance, similar to the general population (16). There is no difference in mortality caused by sensitive compared with resistant strains when high-dose penicillin or third-generation cephalosporin therapy is used (27). Thus, these agents remain reasonable treatment options for pneumococcal pneumonia. Overall mortality in HIV-associated pneumococcal pneumonia is actually somewhat lower than in the non-HIV population (16), again, presumably because of the younger age and better cardiopulmonary function of the HIV group. However, in patients with bacteremia and advanced HIV infection, a mortality rate of 57% has been reported (22). This mortality rate for pneumococcal pneumonia with bacteremia is twice that noted in the non-HIV–infected population (28,29). Recurrence of pneumonia caused by *S. pneumoniae* is common (2,26) and occurs more often in HIV-seropositive than HIV-seronegative individuals. Redd et al. (30) reported a recurrence rate of 16% in HIV-infected persons, compared with 7% in persons without HIV infection.

B. *Staphylococcus aureus*

Staphylococcus aureus was identified as the cause of pneumonia in 15% of cases of bacterial pneumonia (in which a cause was identified) in one multicenter study (4) and in 6% of all HIV-infected patients presenting with respiratory symptoms at one large center (24). It occurs primarily as a community-acquired infection (24) and has been associated with injection drug use, neutropenia, and central venous catheters (31). *S. aureus* pneumonia tends to present with productive cough, dyspnea, and fever, developing suddenly over a few days time (24). Hemoptysis and pleuritic chest pain have also been noted. The radiographic manifestations are varied, with no particularly pathognomonic findings yet defined. Lobar consolidation is noted most commonly, occasionally with cavitation. Both sputum Gram stain and culture appear to be fairly sensitive in clinical studies, with estimated sensitivities of 80–100%. However, patients may be unable to produce sputum. Moreover, the not infrequent finding of previously undiagnosed *S. aureus* pneumonia at autopsy (32), suggests a lower sensitivity for sputum studies. The specificity of a respiratory culture positive for *S. aureus* is uncertain. Levine et al. (24) concluded that among HIV-infected patients presenting with respiratory symptoms, 62% of respiratory cultures yielding *S. aureus* were of indeterminate significance. Among patients judged to have *S. aureus* pneumonia, 38% were bacteremic. In one of these cases, an infection at an indwelling central catheter site led to secondary hematogenous spread to the lungs. Other pulmonic processes, such as pulmonary Kaposi's sarcoma, *P. carinii* pneumonia, and cytomegalovirus (CMV) pneumonia have been noted to frequently coexist with *S. aureus* pneumonia (24,31). It has been suggested that the disruption of bronchial mucosa induced by these processes may have predisposed these individuals to *S. aureus* pneumonia (33). Overall mortality in HIV-associated *S. aureus* pneumonia is high; death occurred in 38% of patients in the largest reported series (24). Often, the condition is unrecognized clinically and diagnosed only at autopsy (32,34). It is unclear whether pneumonia in these instances was a significant clinical condition, as opposed to a late-stage, pretermi-nal development (35). A high index of suspicion appears warranted for *S. aureus* pneumonia. Certainly, *S. aureus* isolated from the respiratory se-cretions of an HIV-infected individual deserves careful consideration as a potential pathogen before being dismissed as a contaminant.

C. *Haemophilus influenzae*

Serious infections caused by *H. influenzae* occur approximately 80 times more often in men with AIDS than in the general population (36). *H. influenzae* was the third most frequent pathogen isolated, after *S. pneumoniae* and *S. aureus*, from patients with HIV infection and bacterial pneumonia in a recent prospective series (4). *H. influenzae* pneumonia in HIV-infected individuals usually presents with productive cough and fe-ver (23). Dyspnea and chest pain commonly occur. Focal segmental or lobar infiltrates are the most common abnormality on chest radiography (Fig. 1), but diffuse interstitial infiltrates may be seen (2,23,37). Diffuse infiltration may indicate the presence of concomitant *P. carinii* pneumonia (23). Pleural effusions are unusual, occurring in less than 10% of cases (23). Associated bacteremia occurs in about 12% of cases (2,23).

Antibiotic therapy results in successful resolution of the pneumonia in almost all cases (23,37), although relapse may be more common with *H. influenzae* than with other organisms (2). Because *H. influenzae* pneu-monia is uncommon in otherwise healthy young adults, it has been sug-gested that its occurrence should prompt an evaluation for HIV infection.

D. *Pseudomonas aeruginosa*

Pseudomonas aeruginosa has been identified as the causative agent in ap-proximately 7% of episodes of HIV-associated bacterial pneumonia (4). Several recent reports (38–42) have described *P. aeruginosa* infections occurring in the setting of HIV infection and suggest that such infections may be increasing in frequency over the past few years. Afflicted individuals typically have advanced HIV infection, usually with CD4 lymphocyte counts of 30/mm^3 or fewer, and multiple prior AIDS-defining illnesses. Other re-ported risk factors for the development of *P. aeruginosa* infection include neutropenia, recent antibiotic therapy, and aerosolized pentamidine prophy-laxis against PCP (38,39). Corticosteroids, which are frequently used in

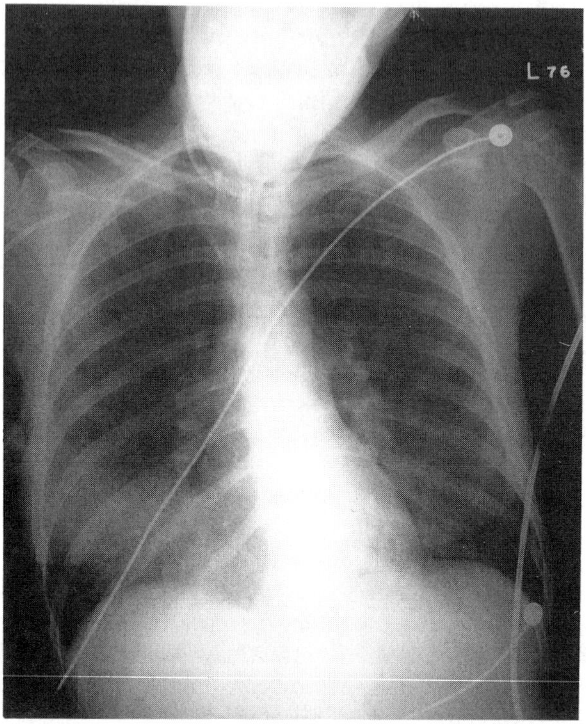

Figure 1 A 37-year-old woman with AIDS, a CD4 lymphocyte count of 4/mm^3, and a right middle lobe infiltrate caused by *H. influenzae* pneumonia. That patient required 5 days of ventilator support and survived the episode.

HIV-infected patients with PCP or immune thrombocytopenia, have also been associated with an increased risk (39,40). Traditionally associated with nosocomial acquisition in the general population, most (68–94%) of *P. aeruginosa* infections associated with HIV are community-acquired. However, as Fichtenbaum et al. point out (41), the frequent use of long-term central catheters and home intravenous antibiotic therapy in patients with advanced HIV infection blurs the distinction between community-acquired and nosocomial infection.

Patients with *P. aeruginosa* infection tend to present in one of two ways. Those with community-acquired infection have indolent symptoms, with a somewhat long duration (9–22 days). A smaller number of patients contract nosocomial infection and have a more fulminant presentation (42). As with other bacterial pneumonia, there appears to be no pathognomonic radiographic pattern, for single or multiple lobe involvement, diffuse infiltrates, and pleural effusions have been described (40). Cavitary infiltrates have been noted in 24–69% of chest radiographs (Fig. 2). Concomitant *P. aeruginosa* bacteremia is common, occurring in 19–56% of cases. About 20% of patients have empyema. Death of *P. aeruginosa* pneumonia occurs in 19–36% of cases. Patients with both pneumonia and bacteremia have a particularly high mortality rate (63%; 41). Early initiation of appropriate therapy (10–14 days of an antipseudomonal β-lactam antibiotic and an aminoglycoside intravenously, usually followed by another 2 weeks of oral or intravenous therapy) results in decreased mortality (13 vs. 57% in patients not receiving such therapy; 40). Antipseudomonal therapy is often not initiated in a timely fashion because of failure to consider this pathogen. Among survivors, the reported recurrence rates range from 23 to 86%

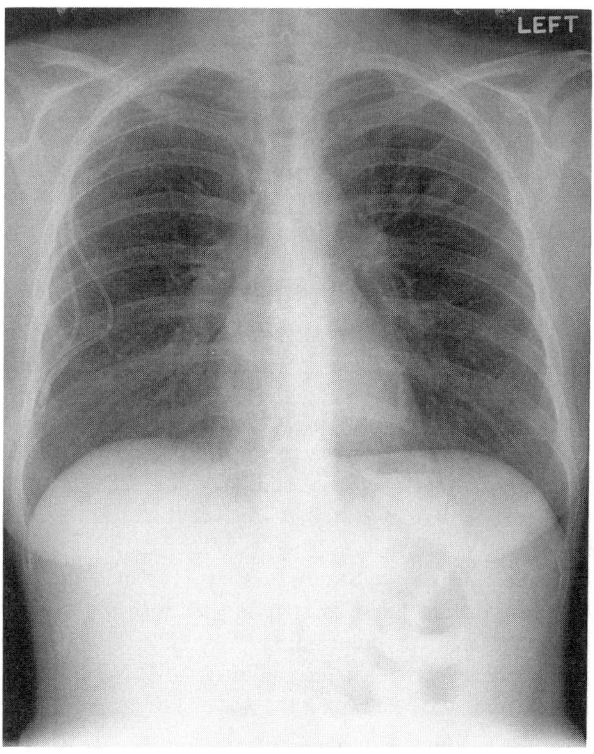

Figure 2 A 28-year-old woman with AIDS, a CD4 lymphocyte count of $12/mm^3$, and pneumonia caused by *P. aeruginosa*. Of note are the left upper lobe cavities with remarkably little surrounding infiltrate.

(39–42). The median duration of survival after diagnosis of infection with *P. aeruginosa* is approximately 80–130 days. This reflects not only the severity of the acute bacterial process, but also the advanced state of HIV disease in which *P. aeruginosa* infection typically occurs. Considering the relative frequency of community-acquired *P. aeruginosa* infection, strong consideration should be given to the institution of antipseudomonal therapy in HIV-infected patients with risk factors for this infection, such as advanced HIV infection, neutropenia, and steroid therapy, who present with pneumonia.

E. *Legionella pneumophila*

Pneumonia caused by *L. pneumophila* appears to be uncommon in HIV-infected individuals. Among 415 patients who underwent bronchoalveolar lavage for HIV-associated pulmonary disease at one institution, *L. pneumophila* was diagnosed in only 1 (43). The largest reported series consists of eight episodes in seven patients (44). These seven patients represented 1.7% of all patients with late-stage HIV disease in the study cohort. The range of CD4 lymphocyte count in these patients was 38–155/mm^3. Interestingly, four of the seven patients were receiving aerosolized pentamidine as prophylaxis against *P. carinii* pneumonia, three were receiving no prophylaxis, and no patient was receiving trimethoprim–sulfamethoxazole prophylaxis, even though trimethoprim-sulfamethoxazole was the most frequently used prophylactic agent in the study cohort. All patients presented with fever and cough. Chest radiography demonstrated focal infiltrates in six cases and diffuse infiltrates in two cases. The hospital drinking water was known to be contaminated with *L. pneumophila*, and five of the eight infections were hospital-acquired. Six cases occurred concomitantly with other pulmonary pathogens (*P. carinii* in four and *R. equi* in two). The diagnosis of *L. pneumophila* pneumonia was made by direct fluorescent antibody assay of BAL fluid in six of the eight cases and by indirect fluorescent antibody serology in two others. Antibiotic therapy (erythromycin in three cases, high-dose trimethoprim–sulfamethoxazole in three, ciprofloxacin in one, and doxycycline in one) resulted in a satisfactory response in all eight cases. The authors emphasized the need for routine testing for *L. pneumophila* in all HIV-infected persons with pneumonia in endemic locations (44). Other authors have reported a relapse of legionnaires' disease in an AIDS patient 4 months after completion of therapy (45) and a failure of quinolone therapy in HIV-associated legionnaires' disease (46).

F. *Rhodococcus equi*

Rhodococcus equi is an animal pathogen that causes pneumonia in horses and livestock. Human infection occurs in individuals with deficient cell-mediated immunity and exposure to animals or contaminated soil (47). Several reports have described *R. equi* pneumonia occurring in HIV-infected patients (47–55). The organism is an intracellular gram-positive pleomorphic rod. Because of its resemblance to a diphtheroid, it is often dismissed as a contaminant when cultured from blood or sputum (48). It weakly takes up acid-fast stain and may be confused with mycobacterial species. Pneumonia cause by *R. equi* usually presents as a focal pleural-based infiltrate in persons with reduced CD4 lymphocyte counts (mean 107/mm^3 in one report; 55). The chest radiograph may show a cavitary (49,51) or nodular infiltrate. The diagnostic yield of sputum culture appears to be low (52), and bronchoscopy is often required to establish the diagnosis. Resistance to β-lactam antibiotics is common. As many as 25–50% of HIV-infected patients with *R. equi* pneumonia die (53). Antibiotic monotherapy may lead to the development of microbial resistance (53). Double- or triple- antibiotic therapy administered over several weeks is required for successful resolution of the infection (50). Erythromycin, clarithromycin, rifampin, ciprofloxacin, vancomycin, tetracycline, trimethoprim–sulfamethoxazole, and aminoglycosides have the best reported activity against *R. equi*. Prolonged maintenance therapy has been advocated by several authors (53–55) to minimize the risk of relapse.

G. *Nocardia asteroides*

Nocardia asteroides is an aerobic actinomycete bacterium found in soil. Pneumonia that is due to *Nocardia asteroides* may present with any number of radiographic patterns in HIV-infected patients. Chest radiographs demonstrated solitary masses in 24% of cases, cavitation in 62%, and pleural effusions in 33%, in a series of 21 patients (56). *Nocardia asteroides* may be difficult to culture from sputum (57) and even from transbronchial biopsy (58). Transthoracic needle aspiration or open surgical biopsy may be required to confirm the diagnosis.

Sulfonamide therapy results in clinical improvement, but the incidence of sulfonamide intolerance is high in the setting of HIV infection, and alternative regimens are often required. Cefuroxime as monotherapy (59), minocycline and amikacin combination therapy (58), and minocyclin, netilmicin, and imipenem combination therapy (60) have been reported to be helpful in sulfa-intolerant patients.

VII. Outcome, Recurrence, and Prevention

A satisfactory response to appropriate antibiotic therapy can generally be anticipated. In cases of community-acquired pneumonia, reported cure rates are excellent: 88% in one series (2) and 100% in another (3). However, bacteremic patients with advanced HIV disease do not respond as well to antibiotic therapy and have a high mortality rate (22). The response to therapy is also poor and mortality high (62% in one series; 3) in cases of nosocomial bacterial pneumonia caused by gram-negative bacilli. The high mortality may be as much due to the original condition that led to hospitalization as to the pneumonia itself. Recurrence of community-acquired pneumonia appears to be common. Seven of 21 patients experienced a recurrence in one series (3), whereas 4 of 16 patients in another series had recurrent bacterial pneumonia, most often with *H. influenzae* (2).

The high incidence of pneumococcal disease in HIV-infected persons has prompted the Immunization Practices Advisory Committee of the CDC to recommend vaccination with 23-valent pneumococcal polysaccharide vaccine for all such individuals (61; Table 2). In individuals with relatively high numbers of CD4 lymphocytes, an appropriate antibody increase following vaccination has been demonstrated (62). However, in individuals with more advanced disease, a diminished antibody response has been noted (9,63,64). Thus, vaccination likely has a greater effect when administered earlier in the course of HIV infection. Moreover, antibody responses following vaccination are better in persons receiving zidovudine (AZT) therapy, suggesting that pneumococcal vaccination be delayed until 4 weeks after beginning this therapy (65). Despite the variability of antibody responses, vaccination against pneumococcal infection appears to be a reasonable preventative intervention in HIV-infected individuals. Rose et al. (66) have formulated the cost-effectiveness for pneumococcal vaccination in this population. These authors concluded that pneumococcal vaccination is an appropriate intervention, capable of reducing hospitalizations and death at all levels of CD4 lymphocyte count. They also estimated that pneumococcal vaccination has more effect in the HIV-infected population than in the general population older than 65 years (66). However, definitive data demonstrating the efficacy of pneumococcal vaccination in the HIV-infected population are lacking.

Table 2 Preventative Strategies for Bacterial Pneumonia in HIV-Infected Individuals

Beneficial
Trimethoprim–sulfamethoxazole prophylaxis against PCP
Possibly beneficial
Cessation of injection drug use
Cessation of smoking
Pneumococcal vaccination
Not beneficial
Alcohol cessation

There is observational evidence to support the use of antibiotic agents as prophylaxis against bacterial pneumonia. Hardy et al. (67) have demonstrated a lower incidence of bacterial infections, including pneumonia, in patients who received trimethoprim–sulfamethoxazole, as opposed to aerosolized pentamidine, for prophylaxis against *P. carinii* pneumonia. In addition, the time to first bacterial infection was also longer in the trimethoprim–sulfamethoxazole group. Data from a more recent study have shown a 32% lower rate of bacterial pneumonia in patients receiving trimethoprim–sulfamethoxazole prophylaxis (most commonly taken three times weekly) compared with other forms of prophylaxis (4).

Cigarette smoking has been associated with an increased risk of bacterial pneumonia in HIV-infected persons with CD4 lymphocyte counts of fewer than 200/mm^3 (4). Smoking cessation should be encouraged in this group.

VIII. Conclusions

Bacterial pneumonia occurs commonly in HIV-infected individuals and is particularly frequent in injection drug users and in persons with low CD4 lymphocytes levels. The causative organisms in this population are similar to the population at large: *S. pneumoniae*, *S. aureus*, *H. influenzae*, and gram-negative bacilli. Concomitant bacteremia is frequent in this population. Satisfactory treatment results are seen with standard antibiotic therapy in community-acquired pneumonia, but mortality is high in nosocomial pneumonia. Preventative strategies that can lower the risk of bacterial pneumonia include prophylaxis against *P. carinii* pneumonia with trimethoprim–sulfamethoxazole and possibly pneumococcal vaccination and smoking cessation.

References

1. Simberkoff MS, Sadr WE, Schiffman G, Rahal JJ. *Streptococcus pneumoniae* infections and bacteremia in patients with acquired immune deficiency syndrome with report of pneumococcal vaccine failure. Am Rev Respir Dis 1984; 130:1174–1176.
2. Polsky B, Gold JWM, Whimbey E, et al. Bacterial pneumonia in patients with the acquired immunodeficiency syndrome. Ann Intern Med 1986; 104:38–41.
3. Witt DJ, Craven DE, McCabe WR. Bacterial infections in adult patients with the acquired immune deficiency syndrome (AIDS) and AIDS-related complex. Am J Med 1987; 82:900-906.
4. Hirschtick RE, Glassroth J, Jordan MC, et al. Bacterial pneumonia in persons

infected with the human immunodeficiency virus. N Engl J Med 1995; 333:845–851.
5. Centers for Disease Control and Prevention (CDC). 1993 revised classification system for HIV infection and expanded surveillance definition for AIDS among adolescents and adults. MMWR 1992; 41(RR-17).
6. Cohn DL. Bacterial pneumonia in the HIV-infected patient. Infect Dis Clin North Am 1991; 5:485–507.
7. Janoff EN, Breiman RF, Daley CL, Hopewell PC. Pneumococcal disease during HIV infection; epidemiologic, clinical, and immunologic perspectives. Ann Intern Med 1992; 117:314–324.
8. Walsh TJ, Rubin M, Pizzo PA. Respiratory diseases in patients with malignant neoplasms. In: Shelhamer JH, Pizzo PA, Parrillo J, Masur H. Respiratory Disease in the Immunocompromised Host. Philadelphia: JB Lippincott, 1991:640–663.
9. Ammann AJ, Schiffman G, Abrams D, et al. B-cell deficiency in acquired immune deficiency syndrome. JAMA 1984; 251:1447–1449.
10. Walsh TJ, Pizzo PA. Treatment of respiratory infections in immunocompromised patients, pp 424–428. In: Shelhamer JH, moderator. Respiratory disease in the immunocompromised host. Ann Intern Med 1992; 117:415–431.
11. Toews GB. Predisposition to respiratory disease: immunologic and nonimmunologic factors, pp 415-418. In: Shelhamer JH, moderator. Respiratory disease in the immunocompromised patient. Ann Intern Med 1992; 117:415–431.
12. Rankin JA, Collman R, Daniele RP. Acquired immune deficiency syndrome and the lung. Chest 1988; 94:155–164.
13. Murphy PM, Lane HC, Fauci AS, Gallin JI. Impairment of neutrophil bactericidal capacity in patients wilth AIDS. J Infect Dis 1988; 158:627–630.
14. Selwyn PA, Feingold AR, Hartel D, et al. Increased risk of bacterial pneumonia in HIV-infected intravenous drug users without AIDS. AIDS 1988; 2:267–272.
15. Selwyn PA, Alcabes P, Hartel D, et al. Clinical manifestations and predictors of disease progression in drug users with human immunodeficieny virus infection. N Engl J Med 1992; 327:1697–1703.
16. Garcia-Leoni ME, Moreno S, Rodeno P, Cercenado E, Vicente T, Bouza E. Pneumococcal pneumonia in adult hospitalized patients infected with the human immunodeficiency virus. Arch Intern Med 1992; 152:1808–1812.
17. Magnenat J, Nicod LP, Auckenthaler R, Junod AF. Mode of presentation and diagnosis of bacterial pneumonia in human immunodeficiency virus-infected patients. Am Rev Respir Dis 1991; 144:917–922.
18. Wallace JM, Rao AV, Glassroth J, et al. Respiratory illness in persons with human immundeficiency virus infection. Am Rev Respir Dis 1993; 148:1523–1529.
19. Janoff EN, O'Brien J, Thompson P, et al. *Streptococcus pneumoniae* colonization, bacteremia, and immune response among persons with human immunodeficiency virus infection. J Infect Dis 1993; 167:49–56.
20. Farley MM, Stephens DS, Brachman PS, et al. Invasive *Haemophilus influenza*

disease in adults. A prospective, population-based surveillance. Ann Intern Med 1992; 116:808–812.
21. Marrie TJ. Community-acquired pneumonia. Clin Infect Dis 1994; 18:501–515.
22. Pesola GR, Charles A. Pneumococcal bacteremia with pneumonia; mortality in acquired immunodeficiency syndrome. Chest 1992; 101:150–155.
23. Schlamm HT, Yancovitz SR. *Haemophilus influenzae* pneumonia in young adults with AIDS, ARC, or risk of AIDS. Am J Med 1989: 86:11–14.
24. Levine SJ, White DA, Fels AO. The incidence and significance of *Staphylococcus aureus* in respiratory cultures from patients infected with the human immunodeficiency virus. Am Rev Respir Dis 1990; 141:89–93.
25. Rodriguez Barradas MC, Musher DM, Hamill RJ, et al. Unusual manifestations of pneumococcal infection in human immunodeficiency virus-infected individuals; the past revisited. Clin Infect Dis 1992; 14:192–199.
26. Harley W, Hoton JM, Corbin RP. Recurrent pneumococcal pneumonia in an HIV-positive patient with lymphoid interstitial pneumonitis. South Med J 1992; 85:1015–1016.
27. Pallares R, Linares J, Vadillo M, et al. Resistance to penicillin and cephalosporin and mortality from severe pneumococcal pneumonia in Barcelona, Spain. N Engl J Med 1995; 333:474–480.
28. Austrian R, Gold J. Pneumococcal bacteremia with especial reference to bacteremic pneumococcal pneumonia. Ann Intern Med 1964; 60:759–776.
29. Ruben FL, Norden CW, Korica Y. Pneumcoccal bacteremia at a medical/surgical hospital for adults between 1975 and 1980. Am J Med 1984;77: 1091–1094.
30. Redd SC, Rutherford GW, Sande M, et al. The role of human immunodeficiency virus infection in pneumococcal bacteremia in San Francisco residents. J Infect Dis 1990; 162:1012–1017.
31. Bedetti A, Bicocchi R, Pantaleoni M, Libanore M, Ghinelli F. Staphylococcal pneumonia in patients infected with HIV in northeastern Italy. Int Conf AIDS 1992; 8:abstr PuB 7029.
32. Marchevsky A, Rosen MJ, Chrystal G, Kleinerman J. Pulmonary complications of the acquired immunodeficiency syndrome: a clinicopathologic study of 70 cases. Hum Pathol 1985; 16:659–670.
33. Whimbey E, Gold JWM, Polsky B, et al. Bacteremia and fungemia in patients with the acquired immunodeficiency syndrome. Ann Intern Med 1986; 104:511–514.
34. Niedt GW, Schinella RA. Acquired immunodeficiency syndrome: clinicopathologic study of 56 autopsies. Arch Pathol Lab Med 1985; 109:727–734.
35. Dicpinigaitis PV, Levy DE, Gnass RD, Bernstein RG. Pneumonia due to *Staphylococcus aureus* in a patient with AIDS: review of incidence and report of an atypical roentgenographic presentation. South Med J 1995; 88:586–590.
36. Steinhart R, Reingold A, Taylor F, Anderson G, Wenger J. Invasive *Haemophilus influenzae* infections in men with HIV infection. JAMA 1992; 268:3350–3352.
37. Casadevall A, Dobroszycki J, Small C, Pirofski L. *Haemophilus influenzae* type b bacteremia in adults with AIDS and at risk for AIDS. Am J Med 1992; 92:587–590.

38. Schuster MG, Norris AH. Community-acquired *Pseudomonas aeruginosa* pneumonia in patients with HIV infection. AIDS 1994; 8:1437–1441.
39. Dropulic LK, Leslie JM, Eldred LJ, Zenilman J, Sears CL. Clinical manifestations and risk factors of *Pseudomonas aeruginosa* infection in patients with AIDS. J Infect Dis 1995; 171:930–937.
40. Shepp DH, Tang IT, Ramundo MB, Kaplan MH. Serious *Pseudomonas aeruginosa* infection in AIDS. J Acquir Immune Defic Syndr 1994; 7:823–831.
41. Fichtenbaum CJ, Woeltje KF, Powderly WG. Serious *Pseudomonas aeruginosa* infections in patients infected with human immunodeficiency virus: a case–control study. Clin Infect Dis 1994; 19:417–422.
42. Baron AD, Hollander, H. *Pseudomonas aeruginosa* bronchopulmonary infection in late human immunodeficiency virus disease. Am Rev Respir Dis 1993; 148:992–996.
43. Allam AA, Kamholz SL. *Legionella* pneumonia in AIDS. Chest 1989; 95:707–708.
44. Blatt SP, Dolan MJ, Hendrix CW, Melcher GP. Legionnaires' disease in human immunodeficiency virus-infected patients: eight cases and review. Clin Infect Dis 1994; 18:227–232.
45. Morley JN, Smith LC, Baltch AL, Smith RP. Recurrent infection due to *Legionella pneumophila* in a patient with AIDS. Clin Infect Dis 1994; 19:1130–1132.
46. Salord JM, Matsiota-Bernard P, Staikowsky F, et al. Unsuccessful treatment of *Legionella pneumophila* infection with a fluoroquinolone. Clin Infect Dis 1993; 17:518–519.
47. Emmons W, Reichwein B, Winslow DL. *Rhodococcus equi* infection in a patient with AIDS: literature review and report of an unusual case. Rev Infect Dis 1991; 13:91–96
48. Lasky JA, Pulkington N, Powers MA, Durack DT. *Rhodococcus equi* causing human pulmonary infection: review of 29 cases. South Med J 1991; 84:1217–1220.
49. Vestbo J, Lundgren JD, Gaub J, Roder B, Gutschik E. Severe *Rhodococcus equi* pneumonia: case report and literature review. Eur J Clin Microbiol Infect Dis 1991; 10:762–768.
50. Cury JD, Harrington PT, Hosein IK. Successful medical therapy of *Rhodococcus equi* pneumonia in a patient with HIV infection. Chest 1992; 102:1619–1621.
51. Magnani G, Elia GF, McNeil MM, et al. *Rhodococcus equi* cavitary pneumonia in HIV-infected patients; an unsuspected opportunistic pathogen. J Acquir Immune Defic Syndr 1992; 5:1059–1064.
52. Frame BC, Petkus AF. *Rhodococcus equi* pneumonia: case report and literature review. Ann Pharmacother 1993; 27:1340–1342.
53. Armbrecht C, Jablonowski H, Mauss S, et al. *Rhodococcus equi* pneumonia in an HIV infected patient. Int Conf AIDS 1993; 9:319 (abstr PO-BO6-1103).
54. Teding van Berkhout F, Boereboom F, Schneider MM, et al. Infection with *Rhodococcus equi* in an HIV-infected patient. Int Conf AIDS 1992; 8:139 (abstract PuB 7540).

55. Calzetti C, Elia G, Pizzaferri P, et al. *Rhodococcus equi* (R.E.) pneumonia in HIV infection: a 5 cases report. Int Conf AIDS 1992; 8:B115 (abstr PoB 3169).
56. Kramer MR, Uttamchandari RB. The radiographic appearance of pulmonary nocardiosis associated with AIDS. Chest 1990; 98:382–385.
57. Coker RJ, Bignardi G, Horner P, et al. *Nocardia* infection in AIDS: a clinical and microbiologic challenge. J Clin Pathol 1992; 45:821–822.
58. Rodriguez JL, Barrio JL, Pitchenik AE. Pulmonary nocardiosis in the acquired immunodeficiency syndrome. Diagnosis with bronchoalveolar lavage and treatment with non-sulphur containing drugs. Chest 1986; 90:912–914.
59. Telzak EE, Hii J, Polsky B, Kiehn TE, Armstrong D. *Nocardia* infection in the acquired immunodeficiency syndrome. Diagn Microbiol Infect Dis 1989; 12:517–519.
60. Cone L, Polkinghorn G, Woodard D, et al. *Nocardia asteroides* infections in patients with the acquired immunodeficiency syndrome (AIDS). Int Conf AIDS 1989; 5:255 (abstr MBP 204).
61. Recommendations of the CDC Advisory Committee on Immunization Practices (ACIP). Use of vaccines and immune globulins in persons with altered immunocompetence. MMWR 1993; 42(RR-4):1–15.
62. Huang K, Rubin FL, Rinaldo CR, Kingsley L, Lyter DW, Ho M. Antibody responses after influenza and pneumococcal immunization in HIV-infected homosexual men. JAMA 1987; 257:2047–2050.
63. Janoff EN, Douglas JM, Gabriel M, et al. Class-specific antibody response to pneumococcal capsular polysaccharides in men infected with human immunodeficiency virus type 1. J Infect Dis 1988; 158:983–990.
64. Klein RS, Selwyn PA, Maude D, Pollard C, Freeman K, Schiffman G. Response to pneumococcal vaccine among asymptomatic heterosexual partners of persons with AIDS and intravenous drug users infected with human immunodeficiency virus. J Infect Dis 1989; 160:826–831.
65. Glaser JB, Volpe S, Aguirre A, et al. Zidovudine improves response to pneumococcal vaccine among persons with AIDS and AIDS-related complex. J Infect Dis 1991; 164:761–764.
66. Rose DN, Schecter CB, Sacks HS. Influenza and pneumoccoccal vaccination of HIV-infected patients: a policy analysis. Am J Med 1993; 94:160–168.
67. Hardy WD, Feinberg J, Finkelstein DM, et al. A controlled trial of trimethoprim–sulfamethoxazole or aerosolized pentamidine for secondary prophylaxis of *Pneumocystis carinii* pneumonia in patients with the acquired immunodeficiency syndrome. N Engl J Med 1992; 327:1842-1848.

12

Pneumocystis carinii Pneumonia

JOHN D. STANSELL

University of California at San Francisco
San Francisco, California

I. Introduction

Since its discovery nearly a century ago (1), *Pneumocystis carinii* pneumonia (PCP) has been increasingly recognized as an opportunistic infection in immunocompromised persons. Because of its low virulence PCP poses no significant health threat to immunocompetent persons. However, persons with impaired host immunity because of malnutrition, neoplasia, organ transplant, or human immunodeficiency virus (HIV) infection are at risk of colonization, active infection, and possible death. Before the 1980s, only a few cases of PCP were diagnosed each year. Since 1981, however, the incidence of PCP has exploded, mirroring the rise of symptomatic HIV infection. Indeed, the recognition of *P. carinii* pneumonia in homosexual men and injection drug users in the early 1980s heralded the acquired immunodeficiency syndrome (AIDS) pandemic (23). Although accounting for nearly two-thirds of AIDS index diagnoses early in the epidemic (4), recent clinical experience suggests a subsiding incidence owing to prophylaxis and, possibly, preservation of immune function with antiretroviral therapy (5,6). Moreover, improved management of acute PCP and secondary prophylaxis have yielded better treatment outcomes and longer life expectancy for those persons at risk for the disease.

Although our knowledge about *P. carinii* is incomplete, much has been learned about susceptibility, prevention, and treatment of this disease during the AIDS epidemic. This chapter focuses on the current state of knowledge and emerging concepts about *P. carinii* pneumonia in HIV-infected persons.

II. Microbiology

The inability to culture *P. carinii* outside of immunocompromised animal models has severely limited our understanding of the organism. Furthermore, drug development and epidemiology are compromised by the inability to observe the organism's life cycle in vitro. Finally, the failure to identify a definitive environmental reservoir for the organism has led to much misunderstanding.

When first described by Chagas in 1909 in the lungs of trypanosome-infected guinea pigs, *P. carinii* was believed to be a new trypanosome (1). Although this error was quickly recognized, the misconception that *P. carinii* was a protozoan persisted for 80 years after its discovery. This misidentification was based on the organisms morphology, inability to grow on fungal media, and its susceptibility to antiprotozoal antibiotics. In 1970, ultrastructural studies began to cast doubt on the protozoal classification (7). The organism was noted to lack organelles characteristic of protozoa, while possessing features suggestive of fungi. In 1988, two independent groups presented evidence from 18S ribosomal RNA (rRNA) homology studies that strongly indicated the organism was a fungus (8,9). Since these first reports, a wide array of studies have confirmed the placement of *P. carinii* among the fungi. Sequence analysis of genes encoding dihydrofolate reductase (10), thymidylate synthase (11), actin (12) tubulin (13), ATPase (14), as well as mitochondrial gene sequences (15), all indicated that *P. carinii* is a fungus. Although the exact fungal lineage of *P. carinii* is indeterminate, recent reviews place it among the ascomycetes (16).

Pneumocystis carinii is a unicellular eukaryote that reproduces by both sexual and asexual means. Several distinct stages to the life cycle have been identified (17). The trophozoite, the predominant intrapulmonary form, is 3–5 μm in size and avidly adheres to type 1 pneumocytes. This adhesion may facilitate absorption of nutrients directly through the alveolocapillary membrane. Large trophozoites likely undergo asexual binary fission to produce small, haploid trophs, which subsequently mature to large, diploid trophozoites. The fusion of two haploid trophs, or gametic cells, may initiate the sexual reproduction of the organism, sporogenesis, or encystment. The parent cell, which resembles a large trophozoite, becomes round, smooth, and develops a thick cell wall. Within the mature cyst, eight haploid intracytoplasmic bodies or spores develop. These spores, which are indistinguishable from trophozoites, are released from a rupture in the cell wall. The collapsed cysts, which resemble crescents, are readily observed on silver-stained clinical specimens from *P. carinii*-infected persons (17).

III. Epidemiology and Transmission

Many mammalian species harbor *P. carinii* in their lungs—human, mouse, rat, ferret, pig, horse, and rabbit, to name a few. These organisms are morphologically indistinguishable. Thus, based on the widespread presence of the organism among commonly encountered animals, it might be attractive to consider human *P. carinii* infection a zoonosis. However, immunological and genetic studies clearly indicate that these organisms are not identical. DNA homology of highly conserved portions of the gene encoding mitochondrial RNA demonstrates significant divergence among all species (18,19). Examination of the chromosomes from each mammalian species reveals unique species karyotypes (20). The genetic divergence of the gene coding the major surface glycoprotein (MSG) of *P. carinii* suggests that organisms infecting different mammalian species are genetically distinct and that *P. carinii* is host-species-specific (21). This species specificity has been further documented in transmission studies. Although transmission of *P. carinii* can be achieved between animals of the same species (22), attempts to transmit *P. carinii* infection between separate, distinct species have failed (21). Thus, it is unlikely that animals are the environmental reservoir for *P. carinii* transmission to humans.

Transmission of *P. carinii* appears to require inhalation of air carrying the infectious unit. Immunocompromised germ-free rats maintained in sterile environments do not develop PCP (23). Similarly, immunocompromised animals maintained in isolators and fed unsterilized food and water or lung tissue from infected animals did not develop the disease (22). Conversely, even limited exposure of germ-free severe combined immunodeficiency (SCID) mice to ambient air or infected animals resulted in disease transmission (24). These studies attest to an airborne route of de novo infection. Moreover, air samples obtained from both laboratory and rural settings demonstrate human *Pneumocystis* genetic material when subjected to polymerase chain reaction (PCR) probes specific for *P. carinii* gene sequences (21,25).

Serological studies show that most humans develop an antibody response to specific *P. carinii* antigens by 4 years of age (26,27). This seroconversion occurs worldwide, attesting to the ubiquitous distribution of pneumocystis (28). It also indicates that primary infection in immunocompetent persons is asymptomatic, as no clinical syndrome can generally be associated with the humoral response. This widespread exposure and the seroconversion to *P. carinii* have been the basis of the theory that organisms lay dormant in the immunocompetent host and disease occurs as a result of reactivation at a time of progressive immunocompromise. However, studies using sensitive molecular probes fail to identify *P. carinii* genetic material in the lungs of immunocompetent persons. Peters et al. searched with PCR probes for *P. carinii* genetic material in the homogenized postmortem lungs of 15 immunocompetent persons, with negative results (29). Similarly, monoclonal antibody staining of fixed lung specimens from immunocompetent persons (30) and PCR probes of bronchoalveolar lavage (BAL) fluid fail to identify *P. carinii* (31). The situation is quite different in immunocompromised persons, however. *Pneumocystis* genetic material has been identified in the sputum and blood of persons with organ transplant or HIV infection (32–36). Despite the presence of *P. carinii* in body fluids of these immunocompromised individuals, many did not have clinical syndromes that would suggest pneumonia, nor did these patients progress to clinical PCP thereafter (32). Thus, long periods of asymptomatic colonization may precede recognizable respiratory disease in immunocompromised persons. Furthermore, the clearance of *Pneumocystis* organisms from the lungs of immunocompromised persons who have been treated for PCP may be slow or may not occur at all. Vargas et al. looked at the persistence of organisms in the lungs of steroid-treated rats after specific treatment for the infection and subsequent withdrawal of immunocompromising drugs. These investigators found persistence of the organisms for 1 year in a significant number of study animals (37). Certainly, it is conceivable that, in the face of progressive immunological decline and despite secondary prophylaxis, AIDS patients, even with clinical resolution of respiratory illness, may not completely eradicate *P. carinii* from their lungs. Thus, failure of secondary prophylaxis, either owing to breakthrough or noncompliance, inevitably will result in recurrent symptomatic respiratory disease with *P. carinii*.

These findings call into question whether *P. carinii* can be transmitted from person to person. Certainly, early reports of disease caused by *Pneumocystis* were clusters of pneumonia among malnourished children (38) or among children hospitalized for treatment of malignant disease (39,40). Moreover, ample documentation of animal-to-animal transmission by aerosols exists. Colonization with *P. carinii* in seemingly immunocompetent persons with exposure to pneumocystis-infected animals has been described (41); and moreover, two HIV-uninfected controls in a multicenter, observational study of the pulmonary complications of HIV disease, who had exposure to patients with PCP, harbored *P. carinii* in induced sputum and BAL. Neither of these participants was treated for *P. carinii* infection, and neither developed evidence of pulmonary disease during the course of the study (Stansell JD, unpublished data). Finally, serum titers of antibodies directed against *P. carinii* have been elevated among health care workers who care for AIDS patients (42). These results call into question whether infection control measures, especially respiratory isolation, are appropriate, particularly for persons infected with HIV. Recommendations await further research.

IV. Host Defenses

The host defenses that protect humans from *P. carinii* and modify the expression of disease are incompletely understood. Cell-mediated immunity appears to play the decisive role in protection from PCP, but studies indicate that humoral immunity is also important in the host's ability to avoid infection or to recover from active disease. Patients who, to all appearances, have isolated B- or T-lymphocyte dysfunction are at risk for developing PCP.

Early studies indicated that immunization and significant serum antibody titers against pneumocystis were inadequate to protect rats subjected to corticosteroid immunosuppression from PCP. A recent study, however, demonstrates near complete protection of mice immunized against PCP and subsequently administered intratracheal organisms, and then selectively CD4-depleted by administration of monoclonal antibodies directed against CD4 or Thy-1 epitopes (43). *P. carinii* were absent on microscopy at days 10 and 19 and were undetectable by a PCR probe. This study strongly indicates that humoral immunity plays a major role in protection from infection with *Pneumocystis*.

Passively administered antibodies to Pneumocystis can moderate the burden of organisms in immunodeficient animal models with PCP (44). Analagously, B cells, in addition to T cells, are necessary for resolution of PCP in immunodeficient rodents (45). Experiments using SCID mice, which spontaneously develop *P. carinii* infection, produce similar results (46). This study also demonstrated an improvement in survival by greater than threefold in mice treated with hyperimmune serum (46). How humoral immunity exerts its effect upon PCP is uncertain, but opsonization, complement-mediated organism lysis, and interference with cell adhesion, all have been postulated as possible mechanisms.

Cellular-mediated immunity occupies the pivotal role in preventing and controlling *P. carinii* infection. Coventional BALB/c rats could be made susceptible to PCP by administration of monoclonal antibodies directed against CD4 lymphocytes (47). SCID mice, which develop PCP spontaneously from their environment, can be protected from active disease by administration of CD4 lymphocytes from immunocompetent donors (48). Moreover, administration of anti-CD4 monoclonal antibody to these mice abolishes the protective effect. Similar studies in SCID mice have shown that $CD8^+$ cells do not exert similar control of pneumocystis (49). A recent study suggests a role for the major surface glycoprotein in eliciting the cellular immune response. $CD4^+$ cells incubated with the glycoprotein had a salutory effect upon PCP in rats (50). Although it is clear that CD4 lymphocytes are essential for the control of pneumocystis, the way these cells exert their effect and their interaction with other effector cells are largely unknown.

Two prospective, observational cohort studies have sought to define who is at risk for PCP. The Multicenter AIDS Cohort Study (MACS) was the first to demonstrate a markedly increased risk for PCP among subjects with CD4 lymphocyte counts of fewer than 200/μl and not receiving prophylaxis (51). These HIV-infected persons had a nearly fivefold higher risk of developing PCP compared with HIV-infected persons who had never had a CD4 cell of fewer than 200/μl. By multivariate analysis, fever and oral thrush also independently influence the risk of PCP. This study led to recommendations for the use of PCP prophylaxis in HIV-infected persons by the CDC in 1989 (52). However, the generalizability of the MACS study results is limited by the study design—the cohort was entirely composed of homosexual men; there was often a broad interval between CD4 determination and PCP diagnosis; and data were censored for any AIDS-defining illness. The Pulmonary Complications of HIV Infection Study (PCHIS) was designed to define the types and frequency of lung disorders and the course and outcomes of these disorders in a population that closely approximated the demographics of the AIDS epidemic in 1990 (53). The study cohort contained 775 homosexual or bisexual men, 253 injection drug users, and 54 women who acquired HIV infection through heterosexual contact. There were 968 HIV-seropositive men and 151 HIV-seropositive women enrolled in the study. Whites constituted 69% of the cohort, blacks 23%, and Hispanics and Asians 8%. The cohort was followed for a mean of 52 months and CD4 lymphocyte counts were tightly clustered around a *P. carinii* diagnosis. The median time from CD4 determination to diagnosis was 26 days. Data were censored only for first-episode PCP; other opportunistic infections or malignancies did not preclude follow-up. Ninety-five percent of PCP cases occurred in individuals with CD4 counts of fewer than 200/μl, and 79% of subjects had CD4 counts of fewer than 100/μl. The median CD4 cell count at the time of PCP diagnosis was 29/μl. The CD4/CD3 ratio did not add accuracy or predictability to the absolute CD4 count for assessing risk of PCP. Persons with baseline CD4 cell counts between 100 and 200 had a 5.95:100 person-years rate for developing PCP, irrespective of use of prophylaxis. The rate dramatically increased to 11.13:100 person-years for persons with baseline CD4 counts fewer than 100/μl (54).

Slightly over 5% of PCP cases occurred in cohort subjects who had never had a CD4 count of fewer than 200/μl. Univariate analysis revealed fever or nights sweats lasting longer than 2 weeks, and oral thrush or unintentional weight loss were related to a significant increase risk of PCP infection (54). Studies are underway to determine what other factors may have predisposed this seemingly immunologically intact subgroup to PCP.

V. Pathophysiology

Although *P. carinii* infection can be thought of as a systemic disease, the clinical expression of active infection is generally a pulmonary process. Once inhaled, the infective form of *P. carinii*, the precise identity of which is unknown, establishes residence in the alveolus. There the organism attaches itself to type 1 pneumocytes by bridges of cellular fibronectin and surface glycoproteins (55,56). Although the organism tightly interdigitates with the pulmonary type 1 cell, there is no fusion of the cellular membranes. Attachment may enable nutrient access directly from the capillary bed and appears necessary for its replication. The prolonged immunosuppression required to induce PCP in animal models and the indolent onset of respiratory symptoms in AIDS patients indicates that *P. carinii* replicates at a relatively slow pace. Inevitably, however, large numbers of organisms begin to fill the alveoli, and alveolocapillary permeability is abnormally increased. Microscopic examination of lung tissue at this time will reveal alveoli filled with foamy, vaculated, eosinophic exudates. This exudate consists of *P. carinii* organisms, degenerative cell membranes, surfactant, and host proteins (57,58). Few inflammatory cells are present. Production of surfactant by the type II pneumocytes is disrupted (58). Rarely, organisms invade the interstitium, and interstitial fibrosis follows treatment of severe cases. In time, the alvelolar epithelial surface degenerates. Subepithelial blebs form, filled with fluid that has traversed the alveolocapillary membrane because of disrupted permeability. Ultimately, the epithelial cells are lost with denudation of the basement membrane. This presents a clinical picture similar to the diffuse alveolar damage seen with adult respiratory distress syndrome. Lung volumes, lung compliance, and the diffusing capacity for carbon monoxide ($D_L$co) are severely reduced. The resulting functional abnormality in patients with PCP is impairment of gas exchange. Poor distribution of inspired air into alveoli that are partially or completely filled with PCP and inflammatory debris leads to ventilation–perfusion mismatch or frank right-to-left shunt. The result is progressive dyspnea and hypoxemia and, ultimately, respiratory failure.

VI. Clinical Presentation

Pulmonary Complications of HIV Infection Study clearly demonstrated that PCP rarely presents without respiratory symptoms. Cohort participants underwent physical examination; laboratory testing, including lymphocyte subsets; chest radiography; and pulmonary function testing at 3-to 6-month intervals designed to identify subclinical opportunistic infections (53). No diagnoses were established in asymptomatic subjects (59,60). The study also showed that respiratory illnesses, including PCP pneumonia, were preceded by respiratory symptoms—cough or shortness of breath. Nonspecific constitutional symptoms such as fever or weight loss, although associated with increased risk for developing PCP, were not associated with identifiable lung diseases in the absence of respiratory symptoms.

The greatest risk for PCP is in HIV-infected adults with CD4 counts of fewer than 100/μl. Unlike persons immunocompromised by conditions other than AIDS, HIV-infected adults usually have a prolonged prodromal illness associated with *P. carinii* infection. Kovacs and colleagues found nearly 1 month of constitutional symptoms before presentation in most HIV-infected patients (61). However, the tempo of the illness varies greatly from one patient to the next. Moreover, in assessing the HIV-infected patient with respiratory complaints, it is important to know the patient's baseline status. In the Pulmonary Complications of HIV Infection Study, 90% of participants had respiratory complaints at some time during the investigation, and over two-thirds complained of cough during a study visit. Clearly then, an understanding of the patients underlying functional status and symptom is invaluable in assessing for the presence of a possible opportunistic infection. Thus, the astute clinician may be able to dismiss the cough of a 60-pack/year smoker, while choosing to vigorously workup the aerobics instructor who has new dyspnea after only 45 min of exercise.

Pneumocystis carinii pneumonia commonly presents with fever, night sweats, and slowly progressive dyspnea on exertion. This protracted prodrome is frequently followed by the onset of nonproductive cough. Profound fatigue may be a hallmark of opportunistic infection, but in PCP usually presents in concert with respiratory symptoms. Rapid-onset spiking fevers or rigors are uncommon and can be used to distinguish *P. carinii* from pyogenic infection. Pleuritic chest pain can accompany either PCP or pyogenic pneumonia. Cough productive of purulent sputum usually indicates a bacterial infection, although coinfection with PCP is not uncommon. Persons presenting with purulent sputum should receive several days of antibacterial coverage and then be reassessed. If a high suspicion of opportunistic infection remains despite treatment for pyogenic infection, a workup for *P. carinii* should be undertaken. On physical examination, a temperature higher than 38.5°C and the stigmata of immunosuppression are frequently encountered. Physical examination of the chest of patients with PCP may be normal, but tachypnea, small respiratory volumes, and tachycardia may be present. Fine basilar rales may be encountered on auscultation. Associated physical findings, such as thrush, hairy leukoplakia, onychomycoses, or Kaposi's sarcoma, may be useful in directing the clinician toward a diagnosis of opportunistic infection in patients without a prior AIDS diagnosis or with unknown HIV status.

As with the physical examination, laboratory studies tend to show nonspecific abnormalities, simply reflecting the underlying HIV infection, rather than any specific opportunistic infection. Serum LDH levels are elevated in patients with PCP, the LDH concentration is elevated much less frequently in patients with other types of pulmonary infection, and increases or decreases in serum concentrations reflect worsening or improvement in the severity of infection (62). In evaluating the sensitivity of LDH elevations, it must be remembered that most of the studies of PCP and LDH arose early during the AIDS epidemic when prophylaxis was not employed and patients often presented with more severe disease. This having been said, a fall in LDH is usually a indicator of positive response to anti-PCP therapy.

The chest radiograph is virtually always abnormal in AIDS patients with PCP; however, virtually every possible radiographic abnormality has been described in association with this disease. Suffice it to say that any chest radiographic presentation is possible with PCP, but diffuse, symmetrical interstitial infiltrates are certainly the most common finding. Focal infiltrates, lobar consolidation, or nodules, with or without cavitation, are occasionally encountered (63). Apical disease or "fibrocavitary" PCP, mimicking tuberculosis, has been associated with aerosolized pentamidine prophylaxis (64,65), although a similar presentation has been encountered in patients receiving other forms of prophylaxis or no preventive therapy. Pneumatoceles are increasingly common and seem to be associated with prolonged, indolent disease and, perhaps, choice of prophylaxis. Pneumatoceles can be quite large (>10 cm) and may predispose to pneumothorax. However, pneumothorax may occur spontaneously in patients with PCP, even in the absence of demonstrable pneumatoceles, blebs, or bullae (66). Lymphadenopathy and pleural effusion have both been reported in AIDS patients with PCP, but are extremely rare and suggest alternative diagnoses.

Although treatment is discussed later in this chapter, little is written about the resolution or diminution of respiratory signs and symptoms of adequately treated PCP. Just as onset may be indolent, resolution of the disease may be slow. Fever and oxygen requirements may not diminish for several days to a week or more, even in the face of successful therapy. Often the first indication of therapeutic success is the subjective feelings of patients that they are recovering, or the observation that they can take a deeper breath. The pace of weaning from supplemental oxygen is dependent on the severity of disease (i.e., the degree of pulmonary inflammation and tissue destruction) and the antecedent pulmonary function. Persons with severe PCP superimposed on chronic lung disease, will experience a protracted requirement for supplemental oxygen.

Chest radiographs often worsen during the first week of treatment, despite clinical improvement. Severe inflammation with resulting fibrosis occasionally results in a clinical and radiographic picture not unlike that seen with advanced cystic fibrosis: markedly reduced lung volumes and compliance, severe reductions in the D_Lco on pulmonary function testing, and diffuse scarring on chest radiograph. These individuals may remain pulmonary cripples throughout the remainder of their course with HIV disease. Usually, however, chest radiographs and pulmonary function tests improve over the course of several weeks. Nonetheless, chest radiographs frequently show persistent interstitial changes weeks to months after the successful treatment of pneumonia. Similarly, the D_Lco typically improves to a plateau after several weeks, but rarely returns to predisease values. Serial chest radiographs and pulmonary function testing frequently document a stepwise deterioration in lung function with each episode of PCP. Exercise tolerance improves over the course of weeks to months. Unfortunately, further immunosuppression and infectious or malignant complications make long-term survival after PCP unlikely.

VII. Complications

A. Hypoxia and Respiratory Failure

Moderate to severe PCP is characterized by disruption of the alveolar epithelial surface and pertubation of the forces that govern the movement of gases and fluids across the alveolocapillary interface. Cellular debris sloughed from the alveolar wall and fluid leaked across the denuded alveolocapillary membrane accumulate in the alveolar space as a consequence of *P. carinii* infection. Gas exchange is impaired, pulmonary shunt fraction increases, and hypoxemia results. In severe cases this pathophysiological process has been likened to adult respiratory distress syndrome. Even less fulminant cases of PCP are frequently accompanied by a "treatment effect." In these patients, the initiation of antipneumocystis therapy is accompanied by a deterioration in gas exchange and worsening hypoxemia at 3–5 days into therapy. This has been likened to the Jarisch–Herxheimer reaction seen in treatment of secondary syphilis. It is hypothesized that the dead or dying *P. carinii* elicit an inflammatory reaction that hastens the injury of the pulmonary alveolocapillary membrane. In patients with moderate to severe disease, this deterioration may be sufficient to push them into frank respiratory failure and need for ventilatory assistance. The routine use of adjuvent corticosteroids in moderate to severe disease has significantly ameliorated the need for mechanical ventilation. The exact mechanism by which corticosteroids protect the lung from this treatment effect is not clearly understood. However, it is hypothesized that steroids may blunt the inflammatory reaction associated with initiation of treatment and, thereby, protect the pulmonary parenchyma from accelerated injury.

The recognition of impairment of hydrostatic forces across the alveolocapillary membrane by active *P. carinii* infection has prompted a reexamination of fluid therapy in patients with moderate–severe PCP. The parsimonious use of colloids and crystalloids reduces the risk of overhydration and alveolar flooding. In patients who require ventilatory assistance, the judicious use of positive end-expiratory pressure may significantly improve oxygenation; however, the risks of ventilator barotrauma are always present. The risk of pneumothorax and bronchopleural fistula formation versus potential for improvement in oxygenation and survival must always be weighed. Alternative ventilation techniques, such as high-frequency ventilation, have not improved survival.

The prognosis for patients requiring mechanical ventilation has seen improvement and deterioration over the course of the epidemic. Early in the epidemic, less than one in six persons with PCP survived ventilatory support at San Francisco General Hospital (67). By 1988 survival had improved to nearly 40% (68). The explanations for the improvement in survival are not entirely obvious. A learning effect likely played a role as house staff and attendants became more skilled in managing this previously obscure disease. In addition, more patients received adjunctive corticosteroids than during the previous era. Finally, more rigorous screening of candidates for ventilatory support may have been a factor.

A recent report suggests that the prognosis for severely ill PCP patients requiring mechanical ventilation has again deteriorated (69): the overall survival for 37 patients admitted to San Francisco General Hospital intensive care units for ventilatory support for severe PCP from 1989 to 1991 was 24%. Predictors of poor outcome were low CD4 count and pneumothorax. Indeed, to my knowledge, no patient with a pneumothorax who subsequently required mechanical ventilation has survived to leave the hospital. Similarly, no patient receiving mechanical ventilation who developed a noniatrogenic pneumothorax has survived the intensive care admission.

B. Pneumothorax

The emergence of cavitary disease and spontaneous pneumothorax demonstrates the tissue-destructive potential of *P. carinii*. As inflammation persists and tissue necrosis proceeds, airspaces may enlarge to form frank bullae. These bullae possess an active margin of inflammation that serves as the growth front for the enlarging airspace. As the bullae enlarges, they may impinge on the subpleural space and visceral pleura. Further tissue destruction or air-trapping may result in the bullae rupturing into the pleural cavity. Small pneumothoraces, frequently seen in the apices of the thorax on chest radiographs, may not require tube thoracostomy and may resolve without active intervention. However, careful observation is always warranted, for progressive enlargement of small pneumothoraces is common. Unfortunately, I have seen several life-threatening or fatal tension pneumothoraces owing to failure to vent seemingly clinically insignificant air leaks. Certainly, immediate venting is required for all pneumothoraces that impair hemodynamic or respiratory function.

Pneumothorax may be one of the most frustrating dilemmas confronting the clinician caring for an AIDS patient. Several factors converge to make resolution of pneumothorax a vexing problem. The PCP may reduce the lungs to a tissue paper consistency. Immunosuppression by HIV, debilitation associated with AIDS, and active opportunistic infection impair the tissue reparative process. The use of adjuvent corticosteroids may further impair tissue healing. Finally, the need for ventilatory support and increased airway pressures may make closure of an air leak impossible.

The goal of chest tube suction is full expansion of the lung. However, this may not be attainable, depending on how long the lung has been collapsed or the degree of loss of tissue compliance. Frequently, the use of tube thoracostomy to reduce intrapleural pressure will entrain a constant flow of air through a bronchopleural fistula (BPF). Various interventions have been used to produce closure of bronchopleural fistulas. Most have been unqualified failures. At San Francisco General Hospital we generally take a conservative approach toward management of BPF. Treatment of underlying infection, withdrawal, if possible, of iatrogenic complications (i.e., steroids or ventilation), and patience are the hallmarks of BPF management. If the lungs remain expanded for brief periods off suction, sclerosis may be attempted. The installation of tetracycline, bleomycin, or talc into the pleural space incites pleural inflammation and, subsequently, adhesion of the pleural surfaces. If successful, sclerosis may prevent further pneumothoraces. Moreover, if only partially successful, the partially adherent pleural surfaces may prevent tension pneumothorax. Thoracoscopy with stapling has been performed with success for rare patients in whom no alternatives existed. However, availability of this procedure is limited to those patients who can tolerate it and have single bronchopleural fistulas amenable to surgical closure. As a last resort, a patient may be discharged with a chest tube in place connected to a one-way valve. Unfortunately, my experience with the Heimlich valve has been disappointing. Blockage by pleural secretions, tension pneumothorax, and infection are frequent complications seen with one-way valve therapy.

C. Chronic Airway Disease

Much as we were slow to note the tissue destructive effects of PCP, we have been slow to appreciate the airway disease that develops as its consequence. Patients successfully treated for PCP may display symptoms suggestive of chronic bronchitis (i.e., chronic, often debilitating, cough productive of clear sputum). These unfortunate patients frequently become colonized with hospital- acquired bacterial pathogens that are difficult or impossible to eradicate, and pyogenic infections are common. In time, the cycles of infection and progressive airway disease may produce frank bronchiectasis. The vicious cycle of infection, treatment with broad-spectrum antibiotics, selection of increasingly resistant organisms, particularly *Pseudomonas* spp., and recurrent pneumonia is a common scenario among patients with advanced HIV disease and a history of PCP. Chronic, rotating antibiotics or adjuvant immunoglobulin therapy have not altered the natural history of these recurrent pneumonias.

D. Extrapulmonary Disease

Virtually all cases of *P. carinii* infection involve only the lungs, although its ability to disseminate in rare patients is widely recognized. Recent advances in detection of the organism by substrate amplification have affirmed the presence of organisms in the blood (33). Disseminated *P. carinii* infection has been related to inhaled chemoprophylaxis with aerosolized pentamidine. Extrapulmonary disease is generally not seen in patients receiving systemic chemoprophylaxis with trimethoprim–sulfamethoxazole or dapsone (70). Reported sites of dissemination include the lymph nodes, spleen, liver, bone marrow, skin, thyroid, choroid of the eye, adrenal gland, ear, peritoneum, intestine, meninges, and pancreas (70). Although the relation between aerosolized pentamidine and extrapulmonary pneumocytosis has not been proved, the association is compelling. At San Francisco General Hospital (SFGH), extrapulmonary PCP has virtually disappeared with the shift to systemic PCP prophylaxis. However, clinicians should always consider extrapulmonary PCP in the differential diagnosis of any febrile HIV-infected patient receiving aerosolized pentamidine or other, inadequate prophylaxis.

VIII. Diagnosis

Since HIV infection and PCP emerged as a clinical problem, we at SFGH have used a diagnostic algorithm to evaluate patients with respiratory complaints and immune compromise (Fig. 1). The cornerstone of this algorithm is the chest radiograph. Although it is true that PCP may present with virtually any radiographic presentation, including focal consolidation, pneumatoceles, "fibrocavitary" upper lobe disease, or asymmetrical reticulonodular infiltrates, most cases have more typical findings. A recent evaluation (Huang L, et al., unpublished data) of Pulmonary Complications of HIV Infection Study participants presenting with respiratory symptoms found that the typical diffuse interstitial infiltrates on a chest radiograph, conferred a 30-fold increased chance of PCP compared with persons not having such chest radiographic changes. Obviously, the radiographic presentation is

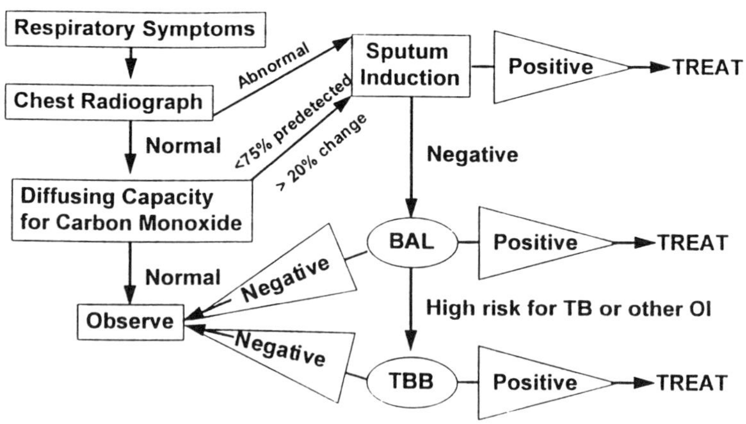

Figure 1 Diagnostic algorithm for *Pneumocystis carinii* pneumonia.

influenced by the stage of disease. Persons with mild symptoms may have a normal radiograph, whereas those with the most severe disease are likely to have chest films indistinguishable from any form of acute respiratory distress syndrome.

Persons with interstitial infiltrates on chest radiograph and a consistent clinical presentation should immediately undergo testing for microbiological confirmation of *P. carinii* infection. However, diagnostic difficulty arises for those persons with normal chest radiographs and persistent respiratory and constitutional symptoms. At SFGH, these persons have undergone pulmonary function testing. Persons with PCP often display restrictive pulmonary physiology, with abnormally small lung volumes and rapid airflows. However, these findings may be found inconsistently with early disease. A more sensitive indicator of alveolar–capillary block (71) and, hence, PCP, is a reduction in the D_Lco. Recent data confirms a near 90% sensitivity of a reduced diffusing capacity ($<$ 75% predicted) at detecting PCP among symptomatic persons with normal chest radiographs (Huang L, unpublished data). Moreover, a normal D_Lco, together with a normal chest radiograph, virtually rules out the possibility of PCP (72).

Gruden and colleages (unpublished data) have advocated the use of high-resolution computed tomography (HRCT) of the chest as a follow-up diagnostic test for HIV-infected persons with normal chest radiographs and respiratory symptoms. Preliminary studies suggest findings charcteristic of *Pneumocystis* infection: patchy areas of ground-glass attenuation through which vessels can be seen and a background of interlobular septal thickening. Whether HRCT will supplant the diffusing capacity assessment in the diagnostic algorithm for *Pneumocystis* infection awaits further data about the cost-effectiveness of the modality.

Gallium scanning is a highly sensitive, but poorly specific test for *P. carinii* infection. Although traditionally included in the algorithm for diagnosing PCP, the test suffers from relatively high cost, time delays in obtaining the imaging, and the baseline mild to moderate uptake of gallium into the lungs of HIV-infected persons without active pulmonary infection. These factors combine to render the test rarely useful in the pursuit of pulmonary opportunistic infections.

Once the decision to pursue a microbiological diagnosis has been made, pulmonary secretions must be examined for the presence of *Pneumocystis* organisms. Although cough productive of clear-white sputum is a frequent presenting complaint in patients with suspected PCP, expectorated sputum is rarely suitable for diagnostic evaluation. Similarly, a purulent sputum, whether spontaneously produced or induced, is inadequate for PCP examination. Cells and cellular debris in such specimens makes identification of *Pneumocystis* organisms impossible. If a purulent sputum is obtained in a patient with a high suspicion of PCP, the patient should be treated with a course of antibacterial antibiotics and antipneumocystis medications and a repeat sputum induction obtained after the respiratory secretions have cleared. A short course of antipneumocystis therapy does not adversely influence the sensitivity of definitive microbiological evaluation, inasmuch as weeks are required to clear *P. carinii* organisms from pulmonary secretions (73).

Induction of nonpurulent sputum is a simple, inexpensive, and effective means of diagnosis of PCP (74). After the patient cleanses the oral cavity with a soft brush and normal saline, a deep sputum specimen is induced by the inhalation of hypertonic (3%) saline. The sample is then digested, centrifuged, plated, and stained (75). Modified Giemsa, toluidine blue O, or Gomori methanimine silver stain may be used to identify the organisms. Newer direct and indirect fluorescent antibody techniques have improved the yield for induced sputums, especially among those institutions with a low volume of examinations (76,77). At San Francisco General Hospital, the yield of microscopic examination of these specimens has been consistently between 70 and 85% for persons with a diagnosis of PCP for the past 5 years. Unfortunately, neither the sensitivity nor the specificity of sputum induction is high enough to confidently exclude a diagnosis of PCP if a negative result is obtained.

In face of suspicion of PCP and a negative sputum examination, a fiberoptic bronchoscopy with bronchoalveolar lavage (BAL) or transbronchial biopsy (TBB) should be performed. Both BAL and TBB are sensitive and specific (78,79), and together, these procedures guarantee a nearly 100% sensitivity and specificity. However, BAL is the initial procedure of choice owing to the increased likelihood of hemorrhage or pneumothorax from TBB and, alone, BAL closely approximates the sensitivity and specificity of the combined procedures (72,79).

A review of nearly 800 HIV-infected patients at San Francisco General Hospital with suspected PCP who underwent BAL with negative results and were not treated with antipneumocystis therapy failed to identify a single missed episode of PCP occurring within 60 days of the procedure (72). Thus, a negative BAL may obviate the need for more invasive procedures to make the diagnosis of PCP. However, in populations of HIV-infected persons with a high-background incidence of *M. tuberculosis* infection, diagnosis of tuberculosis may be enhanced by use of transbronchial biopsy, and the routine use of this procedure may be considered when evaluating HIV-infected patients with respiratory symptoms and abnormal chest radiographs.

Do we know enough about the clinical presentation and course of PCP to make empiric diagnosis and treatment a viable option (80,81)? Certainly, there are a host of pressures on clinicians today demanding efficiency and cost-effectiveness in diagnosis and treatment. However, a variety of pathogens and neoplastic processes can mimic the presentation of PCP. Moreover, empiric treatment of PCP places the patient at potential risk of adverse drug reaction or interaction from unnecessary therapy, while allowing an untreated process to progress (72,82). This having been said, however, empiric therapy may be a suitable alternative to invasive procedures in highly selected patients (Table 1; 83).

IX. Treatment

At the time the first cases of AIDS-related *P. carinii* infection were identified, two drugs, trimethoprim–sulfamethoxazole and pentamidine isethionate, were available for treatment. Indeed, it was the sudden increase in requests for pentamidine that alerted the CDC of a possible new epidemic. Unfortunately, both drugs show a high frequency of adverse reactions and poor patient tolerance (84,85). Accordingly, a concerted effort has been made to identify and develop new single-agent or combination drugs that are free of serious side effects or that do not have overlapping toxicity. These efforts have met with mixed success. Currently, several choices are available for treatment of *P. carinii* infection (Tables 2 and 3).

A. Trimethoprim–Sulfamethoxazole

Trimethoprim-sulfamethoxazole (TMP–SMX) is the drug of choice for the treatment of PCP. No other drug or drug combination has been shown

Table 1 Criteria for Empiric Therapy of PCP

Patient at risk for PCP
HIV+, prior PCP, CD4 lymphocytes fewer than 200
No use of PCP prophylaxis (especially TMP–SMX)
Consistent clinical picture
Fever, sweats, dyspnea
Cough not productive of purulent sputum
Chest radiograph with typical bilateral interstitial infiltrates
Mild hypoxemia
$Po_2 > 70$, $D(A\text{–}a)o_2 < 35$
Compliant patient
No history of adverse drug reaction to medications
Low risk for other opportunistic infections or TB
Diagnostic test unavailable or of low sensitivity
Rapid and accessible follow-up

Table 2 Treatment Options for Mild or Moderate PCP

Regimen	Dose, route, frequency	Side effects
Trimethoprim (TMP)–Sulfamethoxazole (SMX)	15 mg/kg/day po divided every 8 hr	Rash, ↑ LFTs N/V, cytopenias
Clindamycin + primaquine	1800 mg po divided every 8 hr 15–30 mg (base) po once daily	Rash, N/V, diarrhea ↑ methemoglobin
Trimethoprim + dapsone	15 mg/kg/day po divided every 8 hr 100 mg po every day	Rash, N/V ↑ methemoglobin
Atovaquone	750 mg po twice daily	Rash, N/V (should not be used in patients with diarrhea)
Pentamidine isethionate	4 mg/kg IV given over at least 1 hr once daily	Renal dysfunction, ↑k^+, pancreatitis (islet cell destruction, diabetes mellitus)
Trimetrexate + Leucovorin + dapsone	45 mg/m^2 once daily IV 20 mg/m^2 IV or po every 6 hr 100 mg po once daily	LFTs, cytopenias Rash, ↑ methemoglobin

Table 3 Treatment Options for Moderate to Severe PCP

Regimen	Dose, route, frequency	Side effects
Trimethoprim (TMP)–sulfa-	15 mg/kg/day (TMP) IV divided	Rash, ↑ LFTs N/V, cytopenias
Pentamidine isethionate	4 mg/kg IV given over at least 1 hr once daily	Renal dysfunction, ↑k^+, pancreatitis (islet cell destruction, diabetes mellitus)
Trimetrexate + Leukovorin with/without dapsone	45 mg/m^2 once daily IV	LFTs, cytopenias
	20 mg/m^2 IV or po every 6 hr	
	100 mg po once daily	Rash, ↑ methemoglobin
Clindamycin + primaquine	1800 mg IV divided every 8 hr	Rash, N/V, diarrhea, ↑ methemoglobin
	15–30 mg (base) po once daily	

superior to TMP–SMX in efficacy (86–92). Trimethoprim and sulfamethoxazole both act to inhibit key enzymatic steps in folate metabolism. Trimethoprim inhibits dihydrofolate reductase (DHFR), preventing the synthesis of tetrahydrofolate from dihydrofolate, whereas sulfamethoxazole acts on dihydropteroate synthase (DHPS) to prevent the conversion of *p*-aminobenzoate to dihydrofolic acid. Although trimethoprim alone has no demonstrable antipneumocystic activity, together these compounds produce a synergistic inhibition of *P. carinii*. Significantly, neither of these two agents is the most avid enzyme inhibitor in their class. Pyrimethamine, trimetrexate, and methotrexate are orders of magnitude more inhibitory for DHFR, whereas many sulfones and sulfonamides show greater inhibition of DHPS. However, TMP–SMX benefits from the availability of a single-combination medication, excellent bioavailability, similar half-lives, and two decades of clinical experience. Moreover, with the rat model, Hughes and colleagues have recently demonstrated the combination of TMP and SMX to be the most potent inhibitor of PCP among commonly used medications when used in combination (93).

Hughes and colleagues documented the efficacy of TMP–SMX against PCP in children with cancer and established the dose at 20 mg/kg per day of the trimethoprim component in 1978 (94). Subsequent studies in AIDS patients sought to match this established dose in comparative trials. Wharton and colleagues studied 40 patients with moderate–severe disease in a prospective, randomized trial of TMP–SMX (20 mg/kg per day) versus pentamidine (4 mg/kg per day) (86). Of patients treated with TMP–SMX, 75% survived, but 50% of them had major adverse drug reactions necessitating discontinuation of the drug. Similarly, Klein and colleagues studied 163 patients with moderate–severe disease in a prospective, randomized trial of TMP–SMX (20 mg/kg per day) versus pentamidine (4 mg/kg per day) and found only 24% of patients assigned to TMP–SMX were successfully treated. Of those failing TMP–SMX therapy, 42% failed owing to disease progression, whereas 34% required alternative therapy because of drug toxicity (90). Finally, Sattler and colleagues studied 215 patients with moderate–severe disease, in a prospective, randomized trial of trimetrexate (45 mg/m^2 per day) versus TMP–SMX (20 mg/kg per day). Among those treated with TMP–SMX, 80% survived off respiratory support at day 21 of therapy, whereas 28% required discontinuation of study drug due to toxicity. All of these studies antedated the routine use of adjunctive corticosteroids.

In 1988, Sattler and colleages published the results of a prospective, noncrossover trial of TMP–SMX versus pentamidine in 70 patients (87). Rather than using a fixed dose of TMP–SMX, dosing was adjusted to maintain a blood level of 5–8 μg/mL TMP. The average dose received by those assigned to TMP–SMX was 12 mg/kg per day. Despite this dose reduction, 86% of TMP-SMX patients survived and were free of respiratory support at the end of the trial. As a consequence of this study, 15 mg/kg per day of the TMP component has become the widely accepted dose for TMP–SMX. Unfortunately, few trials have used this reduced dose in comparing therapies for moderate to severe PCP. A randomized trial of TMP–SMX versus clinidamycin–primaquine had a mixed population of mild and severe disease, oral and intravenous therapy, and inconsistent steroid use. However, dosing TMP–SMX at 15–20 mg/kg per day resulted in successful outcomes in 91% and dose-limiting toxicity in only 20% (95–97).

The best current insight into efficacy and tolerability of TMP–SMX comes from trials of oral therapy for mild or moderate disease (D[A–a]o_2 < 30 torr). In these studies, 320 mg TMP and 1600 mg SMX (two Septra DS) given three times daily approximates the 15 mg/kg per day dosing schedule. In a randomized, comparative trial of TMP–SMX, 320 mg TMP tid versus atovaquone 750 mg tid in 322 patients with histologically confirmed PCP, 64% of persons assigned to the TMP–SMX arm had a successful outcome (88). Among the 36% with unsuccessful outcomes, 7% had lack of therapeutic efficacy, 20% had treatment-limiting adverse reactions, and 9% could not be evaluated. Similar results were obtained in the recently completed AIDS Clinical Trials Group (ACTG) study (92). ACTG 108 examined the efficacy and safety of three orally available combinations for the treatment of mild or moderate PCP: TMP–SMX 320:1600 mg versus dapsone 100 mg/day with TMP 300 mg tid versus clindamycin 600 mg tid with primaquine base 30 mg/day. Overall, 53.6% of participants completed therapy on the assigned drug; 50% of participants randomized to TMP–SMX completed 3 weeks of therapy. Of persons not completing therapy with TMP–SMX 9.4% experienced clinical disease progression on or before day 21, necessitating alternative therapy and 35.9% had dose-limiting toxicity.

The commonly encountered toxicities associated with TMP–SMX include nausea, vomiting, rash, liver function abnormalities, hyperkalemia, drug fever, and myelosuppression, particularly neutropenia (84,87–90,92). Typically, these toxicities manifest within the first 8–12 days of therapy, but may develop at any point in treatment. The ACTG 108 study documented adverse drug reactions caused by TMP–SMX occurring well into the third week of PCP treatment (92). Adverse drug events often can be attributed to elevated drug levels of trimethoprim, sulfamethoxazole, or both (87,88), suggesting that monitoring drug levels or dose-reducing medications may ameliorate toxicity in persons with known sensitivity.

Over the course of the HIV epidemic, clinicians have grown increasingly comfortable with managing non-life–threatening drug toxicity caused by TMP–SMX without changing medications. The routine use of antihistamines to treat rash and antiemetics to treat the gastrointestinal complaints has decreased the need for alternative therapy. The use of granulocyte colony-stimulating factor (G-CSF) and erythropoetin may influence the course of drug-induced cytopenias; however, the adjunctive role these expensive modalities will play has yet to be determined. Attempts to ameliorate toxicity of TMP–SMX with coadministration of folinic acid have failed to define any beneficial effect. To the contrary, results would indicate a deleterious effect on outcome of PCP treatment and, perhaps, a worsening of mortality among persons receiving such adjunctive therapy (98).

B. Pentamidine

Traditionally, pentamidine has been the second-line agent for the treatment of PCP. Typically, clinicians turn to this agent when patients become intolerant of or fail to respond to TMP–SMX. Unfortunately, pentamidine is associated with frequent, severe and, oftentimes, permanent toxicities. Today, alternatives to pentamidine are available for the treatment of patients intolerant or unresponsive to TMP–SMX, and the strategy of turning to pentamidine as a second-line agent must be reexamined.

Pentamidine isethionate is an aromatic diamine of uncertain mechanism of action against *P. carinii*. Despite its long use in the treatment of PCP, relatively little is known about the pharmacokinetics and pharmacodynamics of this drug. Studies would indicate a large volume of distribution and a long elimination half-life (99). The drug appears to be preferentially concentrated in certain major organs, particularly the kidneys, and probably requires several days to reach a therapeutic concentration in the lungs (100).

Several major clinical trials have examined the efficacy and toxicity of pentamidine (4 mg/kg per day) compared with TMP–SMX. In a small early trial by Wharton (86), involving 40 patients with severe disease, 95% of those treated with pentamidine survived to day 21 of therapy. However, only 9 of the 20 patients actually completed therapy on pentamidine. In a study of 163 patients with severe disease, Klein (90) found 40% (27) of the pentamidine treatment group experienced progressive disease and an additional 25% (17) required alternative therapy owing to drug toxicity. Neither of these studies found any significant difference between pentamidine and TMP–SMX.

In a randomized, noncrossover trial involving 70 patients with severe disease, Sattler (87) found pentamidine considerably less effective than

TMP–SMX. Only 61% of persons assigned to treatment with pentamidine (4 mg/kg per day) survived off respiratory support to day 21 of therapy, compared with 86% of the TMP–SMX treatment arm ($p = 0.03$). Although the dose of pentamidine was adjusted 30–50% for rising serum creatinine, nephrotoxicity occurred in 64%, hypotension in 27%, and hypoglycemia in 21%. Finally, a small trial to evaluate an attenuated dose (3.2 ± 0.9 mg/kg per day) of pentamidine in the treatment of mild to moderate PCP found successful outcomes in 81%, with major adverse drug reactions occurring in 14%, and minor reactions in 38% (101).

The major toxicities related to pentamidine administration are nephrotoxicity and hypoglycemia. The exact mechanism of renal toxicity is incompletely understood. However, special caution must be exercised not to administer pentamidine with other potentially nephrotoxic drugs: aminoglycosides, nonsteroidal anti-inflammatory agents, foscarnet, or amphotericin B. Hypoglycemia results from direct toxicity to pancreatic islet cells and may presage frank diabetes mellitus or pancreatitis. These toxicities, occurring an average of 8 days into therapy appear to be dependent on the cumulative dose. O'Brien examined the incidence of pentamidine-related adverse drug reactions at SFGH in a 5-year retrospective review. To be evaluated patients had to receive at least 5 days of pentamidine therapy. This evaluation of over 100 cases of PCP documented a 72% incidence of treatment-limiting toxicity. Renal toxicity occurred in 49%, hypoglycemia in 24%, and pancreatitis in 9% of pentamidine-treated patients (102).

C. Clindamycin–Primaquine

The combination of the lincosamide antibiotic clindamycin (600–900 mg every 6–8 hr) with the dihydrofolate reductase inhibitor primaquine (15–30 mg/day) has gained widespread acceptance and use against all degrees of severity of PCP. Neither drug, by itself, has activity against *P. carinii*, but animal models confirm the activity of the combination (103). Unfortunately, rigorous, standardized trials using this drug combination are largely lacking. Various doses, dosing schedules, disease severity, and drug formulations have been investigated. Black and colleagues found a 92% rate of successful treatment and a 13% incidence of dose-limiting toxicities with clindamycin (900 mg every 8 hr IV or 450 mg every 6 hr PO)–primaquine (30 mg/day base) in 38 patients in a noncomparative, open-label study (104). Toma and colleagues reported a randomized, blinded trial in 74 patients with PCP (96,105). With 15 mg/day primaquine Toma found virtually identical efficacy compared with trimethoprim–sulfamethoxazole. Rash was the most common side effect, occurring in 60% of patients, whereas gastrointestinal upset was the most common side effect seen with TMP–

SMX. A recent update confirmed the foregoing findings in a cohort of over 100 patients (97).

The recently completed ACTG 108 trial offers the best insight into the use of oral clindamycin 600 mg every 8 hr and primaquine 30 mg/day versus TMP–SMX or TMP–dapsone. Sixty-four HIV-infected subjects with mild to moderate PCP were randomized to the clindamycin–primaquine arm of this three-arm treatment trial. Of persons assigned to clindamycin–primaquine, 52% completed 21 days of therapy with the study drug combination; 6.9% experienced therapeutic failure of the combination on or before day 21 of therapy; and 33% of the participants receiving clinidamycin–primaquine required alternative therapy owing to dose-limiting toxicity. This study was inadequately powered to find a difference in efficacy, but was powered to detect a 25% difference in adverse drug events. No statistical differences in efficacy or toxicity were found among any of the three treatment arms. Virtually all of the adverse drug events caused by clindamycin–primaquine occurred during the first 2 weeks of therapy. Among persons receiving clindamycin–primaquine, rash was the most frequently encountered dose-limiting toxicity, occurring in 21%. Cytopenias occurred in 12%, gastrointestinal intolerance in 3.4%, and elevations in liver enzymes in 1.7%. Drug fever accounted for less than 2% of dose-limiting drug reactions in the clindamycin–primaquine group.

Similar to dapsone, primaquine and clindamycin are strong oxidants and relatively contraindicated in persons with glucose-6-phosphate dehydrogenase deficiency. Also similar to dapsone, methemoglobinemia is a potential dose-limiting toxicity; although modest levels of methemoglobin ($<15\%$) can be found in most primaquine or dapsone-treated patients, few will require treatment with reducing agents or alternative therapy.

D. Trimetrexate

Trimetrexate is a highly lipophilic folate antagonist, structurally related to methotrexate. The drug readily diffuses across cell membranes and inhibits DHFR 1500 times more potently than trimethoprim (106). In fact, the avidity of trimetrexate for DHFR and the potential for interruption of folate metabolism is so great that folinic acid must be given with trimetrexate. Herein lies the mechanism of action of trimetrexate–folinic acid. Folinic acid, a hydrophilic compound, requires active transport across cell membranes. Mammalian cells possess such an active transport system, whereas *P. carinii* apparently lacks such a system. Therefore, human cells are protected from the antifolate effects of trimetrexate by the coadministration of folinic acid, whereas *P. carinii* cannot accumulate folinic acid and, therefore, is fully susceptible to the folate inhibitory effects of the drug. The long half-life of the drug (8–10 hr) permits once-a-day dosing. The drug is principally metabolized by the liver, and the glucuronide or sulfate salt is excreted by the kidney.

Allegra and colleagues performed an open-label, nonrandomized trial of trimetrexate (TMTX; 30 mg/m^2 per day)–folinic acid (20 mg/kg every 6 hr) alone or in combination with sulfadiazine (1 g every 6 hr); 49 patients were enrolled and stratified by intolerance to or disease progression on TMP–SMX. Eighty-eight percent of the patients treated with TMTX–folinic acid alone as initial treatment were alive and receiving no respiratory support 2 weeks after completion of therapy. In those treated with TMTX–folinic acid for disease progression while receiving TMP–SMX, 69% survived. Among those initially treated with TMTX–folinic acid plus sulfadiazine, 77% survived. Initial enthusiasm was somewhat tempered by a 60% relapse rate in the 3 months following completion of therapy in the group receiving TMTX–folinic acid as initial therapy. The relapse rate was 6% among those receiving TMTX–folinic acid–sulfadiazine, and 0% among those receiving TMTX–folinic acid for salvage. However, this study was performed before the routine use of secondary prophylaxis. But even the lack of secondary prophylaxis cannot explain the lack of relapse among those with the most severe disease, the salvage group. Trimetrexate was well tolerated, with neutropenia and thrombocytopenia being the most common dose-limiting toxicity (106). Sattler later established a trimetrexate dose of 45 mg/m^2 once daily, with folinic acid 80 mg/m^2 per day as the optimum dose for treatment of PCP (107).

The clearest insight into monotherapy with trimetrexate–folinic acid for PCP is ACTG 031. ACTG 031 was a randomized, double-blind multicenter trial comparing TMTX (45 mg/m^3 per day) and folinic acid (20 mg/m^2 every 6 hr) with TMP–SMX (20 mg/kg per day) in patients with confirmed moderate to severe PCP. Inasmuch as this trial began patient accrual before the National Institutes of Health (NIH) Consensus Panel recommendations for steroid use in PCP, use of adjunctive corticosteroids was not permitted. Study endpoints were mortality at day 21 of therapy and clinical response at days 10 and 21:215 patients were enrolled and maintained in the double-blind portion of the trial until day 10. At that point, patients were assessed as "responders" or "failures." Responders progressed into the open-label phase of the trial comparing oral TMP–SMX with continued intravenous TMTX–folinic acid, whereas failures were offered alternative therapy. By day 10 of therapy there was a 16% overall failure rate, with 16% of TMP–SMX and 27% of TMTX–folinic acid-treated patients requiring alternative therapy. By day 21, 20% of TMP–SMX patients and 38% of TMTX–folinic acid patients were clinical failures (p = 0.008). Similarly, there was a trend toward improved survival at day 21 with TMP–

SMX compared with TMTX–folinic acid. These differences in mortality were significant by day 49 of therapy, 16 versus 31% ($p = 0.028$). Relapse occurred in 13% of the TMTX treatment group and none of the TMP–SMX treatment group during days 21–49. Dose-limiting toxicity was much more common in the TMP–SMX treatment group, with 29% experiencing toxicity-related discontinuations. Only 10% of TMTX–folinic acid patients had similar dose-limiting toxicity. The most common side effects encountered were hepatitis (12.6 vs. 3.7%), gastrointestinal intolerance (7.2 vs. 0.9%), and cytopenias (12.6 vs. 3.7%). These results confirmed that although effective in the treatment of *P. carinii* infection, TMTX–folinic acid as monotherapy is not as effective as TMP–SMX. Similar results were obtained when single-agent dapsone was evaluated for treatment of PCP (108). However, both of these agents have activity against *P. carinii* and would be an attractive combination owing to efficacy and toxicity profiles. A small, phase 1 trial of TMTX (45 mg/m^2 per day), folinic acid (80 mg/m^2 per day) with dapsone (100 mg/day), compared with TMP–SMX (15 mg/kg per day) in moderate to severe PCP has been completed (109). All patients received adjunctive corticosteroids at recommended doses. Fifteen patients were randomized to TMTX–folinic acid–dapsone and 5 patients to TMP–SMX. Twelve of 15 TMTX–folinic acid–dapsone patients and 3 of 5 TMP–SMX patients were responders at day 21. There were two episodes of grade III/IV toxicity among the TMTX treated and 4 episodes among the TMP–SMX treatment group. No patient successfully completing either therapy relapsed during the month following therapy. These data suggest that TMTX–folinic acid plus dapsone may be of clinical usefulness against PCP. Just where the combination fits in the armamentarium awaits further large-scale clinical trials.

E. Trimethoprim–Dapsone

Because of the poor patient tolerability of oral TMP–SMX, alternative oral combinations have been sought for the treatment of mild PCP. One of the first combinations to receive widespread attention was trimethoprim plus the sulfone antibiotic dapsone. Dapsone is a powerful DHPS inhibitor that has been used successfully to treat murine PCP (110). Although dapsone had an unacceptably high rate of treatment failure when used alone (108), the combination of dapsone–trimethoprim (dapsone 100 mg/day with trimethoprim 20 mg/kg per day) was effective PCP treatment in an open-label, pilot study of 15 patients at San Francisco General Hospital (111). Two of 15 patients in this small trial experienced dose-limiting toxicity. A subsequent prospective, randomized clinical trial compared the safety and efficacy of trimethoprim (20 mg/kg per day) plus dapsone (100 mg/day) with TMP–SMX (20 mg/kg per day) in 60 patients with mild to moderate PCP (91). Disease progression occurred in 2 of 30 patients assigned to TMP–dapsone, compared with 3 of 30 assigned to the TMP–SMX treatment arm. Of the TMP–SMX-treated patients, 57% encountered dose-limiting toxicity, compared with 30% of the TMP–dapsone-treated group ($p < 0.025$). The major toxicities with TMP–dapsone were rash and gastrointestinal complaints compared with transaminitis and neutropenia with TMP–SMX.

ACTG 108 examined oral TMP–dapsone in a comparative trial with oral TMP–SMX and clindamycin–primaquine (C–P). Fifty-nine patients with mild to moderate PCP were randomized to trimethoprim (300 mg tid) plus dapsone (100 mg/day): 59.3% of patients on TMP–dapsone completed 21 days on assigned therapy; 11.9% of TMP–dapsone treated patients experienced disease progression on or before day 21 of therapy, compared with 9.4% of TMP–SMX and 6.9% of C–P treated patients ($p = 0.7$). There were no differences in death at day 81 between the treatment arms. Of patients assigned to TMP–dapsone, 23.7% experienced dose-limiting toxicity, compared with 35.9% of TMP–SMX-treated patients, and 32.8% of C–P treated patients. The most frequent dose-limiting adverse drug reactions were rash (10.2%), nausea and vomiting (8.5%), neutropenia (3.4%), and diarrhea (3.4%). Finally, a quality of life instrument indicated a trend toward better quality of life outcomes with TMP–dapsone compared with the other two study arms at completion of therapy. This study, as in earlier studies, demonstrates that TMP–dapsone is an effective and well-tolerated treatment for mild to moderate PCP. In light of this accumulated evidence, I believe that trimethoprim–dapsone should be first choice for treatment of mild pneumonia caused by *P. carinii* when oral therapy is appropriate.

F. Atovaquone

Atovaquone, an oral hydroxynaphthoquinone, inhibits electron transport in the mitochondrial oxidation–reduction pathway of *P. carinii*. Poor bioavailability complicates the use of this medication, particularly when coupled with chronic diarrhea, although the introduction of a suspension product has somewhat ameliorated concern about achieving adequate serum drug levels. The medication has been evaluated for the treatment of mild to moderate PCP in both open-label and randomized comparison clinical trials. Falloon and colleagues treated 34 patients with mild disease (mean room air P_aO_2 = 78 torr) with several dosages of single-agent atovaquone (112). Treatment was discontinued in 4 patients for toxicity (2 rash, 2 drug fever) and 5 for disease progression. Seven of the 27(26%) successfully treated patients experienced recurrent PCP within 6 months, despite secondary prophylaxis. Outcomes did not appear to be dose related. Hughes and colleagues have reported a randomized, double-blind clinical trial comparing oral atovaquone (750 mg every 8 hr) with oral TMP (320 mg)–SMX(1600 mg) every 8 hr (88). In this study of 322 patients with histologically confirmed mild ($D[A-a]o_2 < 35$) to moderate ($D[A-a]o_2 = 35–45$) PCP, 20% of the atovaquone-treated group experienced clinical treatment failure compared with 7% of the TMP–SMX-treated group ($p = 0.002$). However, atovaquone was much better tolerated than TMP–SMX: 7% of the atovaquone group required alternative therapy because of toxicity, compared with 20% of the TMP–SMX-treated group. The most common treatment-limiting adverse effects seen in the atovaquone group were rash (4%) and liver dysfunction (3%). Rash (8%), liver dysfunction (7%), vomiting (7%), fever (6%), nausea (5%), and neutropenia (3%) were the most common dose-limiting toxicities seen in the TMP–SMX arm. There were 11 deaths in the atovaquone arm, compared with a single death in the TMP–SMX arm within 4 weeks of completion of therapy ($p = 0.003$). These deaths and therapeutic failures on the atovaquone arm were highly correlated with the presence of diarrhea at entry into the study. A similar randomized, open-label trial has compared atovaquone (750 mg every 8 hr) with parenteral pentamidine (4 mg/kg per day) in patients with a history of intolerance to TMP–SMX (113). Similar to the previous study, atovaquone was less effective (29% disease progression for atovaquone vs. 17% for pentamidine), but better tolerated (4% dose-limiting toxicity compared with 36% for pentamidine). The mortality rate was similar in both groups, but is generally believed to be unacceptably high compared with other treatment regimens. These studies and continued concerns about the adequacy of drug levels achieved in AIDS patients lends uncertainty about the role of single-agent atovaquone in the treatment of HIV-associated PCP. Certainly, this medication cannot be viewed as a first- or second-line agent.

G. Aerosolized Pentamidine

Two small, open-label trials and a large, double-blind comparative trial with TMP–SMX (15 mg/kg per day) have shown that inhaled pentamidine is an inferior treatment for PCP. Conte (101) found significantly higher rates of recrudescence of symptoms and relapse of PCP in patients treated with inhaled pentamidine (600 mg/day) compared with those receiving parenteral pentamidine (3 mg/kg per day). Similarly, Soo Hoo (114) reported a significantly higher incidence of treatment failure (55%) with inhaled pentamidine than with parenteral pentamidine (4 mg/kg per day; 0%). ACTG 040 (115) examined the efficacy of aerosolized pentamidine (600 mg/day) versus TMP–SMX (15 mg/kg per day) in 367 patients with $D[A\text{–}a]o_2 <$ 55. This study documented a significantly higher rate of treatment failure, more protracted recovery, and more frequent relapse among the aerosolized pentamidine-treated group. These studies overwhelmingly affirm the limited, if any, role for aerosolized pentamidine in the treatment of PCP.

H. Adjuvant Corticosteroid Therapy

Despite the availability of effective antipneumocystis drugs, the mortality rate of PCP remains appreciable. Most of these deaths are caused by progressive lung disease that culminates in intractable hypoxemic respiratory failure. A frequent clinical observation is that worsening often takes place suddenly 3–5 days after beginning antipneumocystis therapy, even in patients whose disease had been slowly progressive. Several trials have now documented the usefulness of adjunctive corticosteroids in mitigating the sudden deterioration in gas exchange seen several days into standard treatment. Since early in the epidemic, there has been no shortage of anecdotal and retrospective reports on the benefits of corticosteroids in the management of severe PCP; four clinical trials now support the use of steroids in moderate to severe PCP. Montaner and colleagues (116) found 8 of 19 placebo-treated patients compared with 1 of 18 steroid-treated patients experienced an early deterioration in oxygen saturation. In the largest study, Bozzette et al. (117) showed that corticosteroids significantly decreased the early deterioration in gas exchange. These investigators further demonstrated that the most benefit was derived by patients with the most severe disease. In the most severely ill cohort studied, Gagnon and colleagues (118) found adjunctive corticosteroids significantly ameliorated respiratory failure and death. Given these conclusive studies, the NIH–University of California (UC) Expert Panel for Corticosteroids as Adjunctive Therapy for Pneumocystis Pneumonia (1990) concluded that such therapy "can clearly reduce the likelihood of death, respiratory failure, or deterioration of oxygenation in patients with moderate-to-severe pneumocystis pneumonia (119). The panel further recommended that adjunctive corticosteroids be used in adults or adolescents (children younger than 13 years old) with documented or suspected PCP if they are hypoxic, as defined by an arterial Po_2 of less than 70 mmHg or an alveolar–arterial Po_2 difference of 35 mmHg. Adjunctive corticosteroid therapy, either oral prednisone or intravenous methylprednisolone, should be started when specific antipneumocystis treatment is begun; a delay in the administration of corticosteroids may nullify their effectiveness. There is no reason why these drugs cannot be used along with antipneumocystis treatment in patients who meet the indications while diagnostic efforts are underway. But if no diagnosis or some other diagnosis is made, the need for corticosteroids must be carefully reevaluated.

X. Prophylaxis

The elaboration of when an HIV-infected person is at significant risk for developing PCP and the validation of effective preventive therapies have done more to improve the life of AIDS patients than any other intervention. Multiple studies convincingly document the benefit of prophylaxis over placebo in preventing PCP and extending life (120–123). The risk of developing first-episode PCP increases with declining CD4 lymphocyte count or the advent of constitutional symptoms (51,54). HIV-infected persons whose CD4 lymphocyte counts decline to fewer than 100/μl have nearly an order of magnitude greater risk of developing PCP compared with persons with CD4 cell counts between 200 and 400/μm. Even among those with fewer than 100 CD4 lymphocytes per microliter, the risk significantly increases as the CD4 count declines to zero. HIV-infected persons who have experienced an episode of PCP risk a 35% chance of recurrent disease at 6 months and a 60% chance of recurrence at 1 year if prophylaxis is not provided.

Trimethoprim–sulfamethoxazole, dapsone with or without pyrimethamine, and aerosolized pentamidine are the three agents most commonly used to prevent PCP (Table 4) Many studies have compared these drugs at different dosages and dosing intervals for primary and secondary prophylaxis. These studies document that all of these drugs and combinations have advantages and disadvantages; but, no single medication or combination of agents has been superior to trimethoprim–sulfamethoxazole for prevention of PCP. This is best illustrated by two large studies: one of primary prophylaxis and one of secondary prophylaxis.

ACTG 081 was a open-label, randomized trial that evaluated the effectiveness of three treatment strategies in preventing first-episode PCP in HIV-infected persons with CD4 lymphocyte counts of fewer than 200/μm (124). The study arms were TMP–SMX (one double-strength tablet bid), dapsone (50 mg bid), or aerosolized pentamidine (300 mg once per month). Subjects experiencing drug intolerance were assigned to an alternative therapy in a prescribed manner: 842 patients were studied for a median follow-up of 39 months. There were 137 reported cases of PCP during the follow-up period. The estimated 36-month risk of PCP was 18%, 17%, and 21% (p = NS), respectively for TMP–SMX, dapsone, and aerosolized pentamidine. For persons with fewer than 100 CD4 cells per microliter, the risk was 33% for aerosolized pentamidine, compared with 19% with TMP–

Table 4 PCP Prophylaxis Strategies

Regimen	Dose, route, frequency	Comments
TMP–SMX	Double-strength tablet every day or three times weekly Single-strength once daily	Effective against toxoplasma and bacterial pathogens
Dapsone with/without pyrimethamine	100 mg every day 25 mg every other day	Combination effective against toxoplasmosis
Aerosolized pentamidine	300 mg by nebulizer every month	Does not protect against systemic disease
Atovaquone	750 mg po every day or twice daily	Under investigation
Clarithromycin–azithromycin plus pyrimethamine	?	In vitro and animal model activity, untested in human

SMX and 22% with dapsone ($p = 0.04$). Moreover, an "as treated" analysis further manifests, the differences in treatment arms. Only 4 of the 34 patients in the TMP–SMX arm who, developed PCP did so while actually receiving the drug, whereas 37 of the 38 treatment failures occurring within the aerosolized pentamidine group occurred "on therapy." Twenty-one of the 34 treatment failures in the dapsone group occurred during actual drug delivery. Twenty-one percent of the TMP–SMX group and 25% of the dapsone group completed the study on their originally assigned drug regimen, compared with 88% of the aerosolized pentamidine treatment group. Twenty-eight percent of the TMP–SMX group and 33% of the dapsone group required dose reduction only, during the course of the study. This study clearly demonstrates the advantage of systemic therapy, particularly TMP–SMX, over inhalation therapy in preventing PCP. Other studies have found similar benefits to TMP–SMX prophylaxis strategies at either attenuated doses (125) or different dosing intervals (126 127). The bottom line is that TMP–SMX at any dose from 80 to 320 mg TMP per day, given at least three times weekly is the first-line choice for primary PCP prophylaxis for the markedly immunocompromised patient. Alternatives include other systemic therapies, usually dapsone, with or without pyrimethamine, but also including primaquine–clindamycin, pyrimethamine–clindamycin, and combinations with the extended spectrum macrolides, azithromycin and clarithromycin (93,128). Recent studies by Hughes suggest most of the prophylactic benefit from TMP–SMX can be achieved by using sulfamethoxazole alone (129). Aerosolized pentamidine should be considered for possible use in the less immunocompromised, but it clearly lacks the efficacy of systemic therapy in persons with fewer than 100 CD4 cell per microliter, and it probably should not be used in persons with a history of airway or lung disease. Trials comparing the efficacy of atovaquone suspension versus dapsone and aerosolized pentamidine in TMP–SMX-intolerant patients are underway.

Similar findings documented the superiority of TMP–SMX for the secondary prophylaxis (maintenance therapy) of AIDS patients after an initial of PCP. Hardy and colleages studied 310 AIDS patients who had recently recovered from PCP. Patients were randomized to receive either TMP–SMX double-strength tablet per day or aerosolized pentamidine 300 mg via nebulizer once per month. All patients received zidovudine, and the median follow-up was 17.4 months. There were 14 (11.4%) PCP recurrences among 154 patients assigned to the TMP–SMX arm versus 36 (27.6%) recurrences among the pentamidine-treated group ($p < 0.001$). By intent-to-treat analysis the risk of recurrence was 3.25 times higher for the pentamidine treatment group. In fact, only four of the participants who received TMP–SMX for more than 3 weeks and tolerated the drug actually developed recurrent disease. In contrast, all of the PCP recurrences in the aerosolized pentamidine treatment group occurred while the patients were receiving the drug. As expected, aerosolized pentamidine was the better-tolerated of the two regimens. Only 4% of the pentamidine treatment group required crossover, compared with 27% of the TMP–SMX group. These data establish the primacy of TMP–SMX for secondary PCP prophylaxis in AIDS patients. Unfortunately, there are few data on the role of other systemic antibiotics in secondary PCP prophylaxis. What information exists suggests activity of weekly dapsone or dapsone–pyrimethamine comparable with that of aerosolized pentamidine (130–132). No study has looked at dapsone, with or without pyrimethamine, given daily for the prevention of recurrent PCP. Certainly, the first choice to prevent recurrent PCP, as with primary prophylaxis, should always be systemic antibiotics. Aerosolized pentamidine should be considered only in those patients intolerant to all systemic options.

References

1. Chagas C. Nova tripanomiazaea humana. Ueber eine neve trypanosomiasis de menschen. Mem Inst Oswaldo Cruz 1909; 1:159–218.
2. Gottlieb M, Schroff R, Schanker H, et al. *Pneumocystis carinii* pneumonia and mucosal candidiasis in previously healthy homosexual men. Evidence of a new acquired cellular immunodeficiency. N Engl J Med 1981; 305:1425-1431.
3. Masur H, Michelis M, Green J, et al. An outbreak of community-acquired *Pneumocystis carinii* pneumonia. N Engl J Med 1981; 305:1431-1438.
4. Murray J, Felton C, Garay S, et al. Pulmonary complications of the acquired immunodeficiency syndrome: report of a National Heart, Lung and Blood Institute Workshop. N Engl J Med 1984; 310:1682.
5. Centers for Disease Control and Prevention. HIV/AIDS surveillance report, No 5, 1994.
6. Centers for Disease Control and Prevention. HIV/AIDS surveillance Report, No 6, 1994.
7. Vavra J, Kucera K. *Pneumocystis carinii*: its ultrastructure and ultrastructural affinities. J Protozool 1970; 17:463–483.
8. Edman J, Kovacs J, Masur H, Santi D, Elwood H, Sogin M. Ribosomal RNA sequence shows *Pneumocystis carinii* to be a member of the fungi. Nature 1988; 334:519–522.
9. Stringer SL, Stringer JR, Blase MA, et al. *Pneumocystis carinii*: sequence from ribosomal RNA implies a close relationship with fungi. Exp Parasitol 1989; 68:450–461.
10. Edman JC, Edman U, Cao M, et al. Isolation and expression of the *Pneumocystis carinii* dihydrofolate reductase gene. Pro Natl Acad Sci USA 1989; 86:8625–8629.

11. Edman U, Edman JC, Lundgren B, Santi DV. Isolation and expression of *Pneumocystis carinii* thymidylate synthase gene. Pro Natl Acad Sci USA 1989; 86:6503–6507.
12. Fletcher LD, McDowell JM, Tidwell RR, et al. Structure, expression and phylogenetic analysis of the gene encoding actin I in *Pneumosystis carinii*. Genetics 1994; 137:743–750.
13. Dyer M, Volpe F, Delves CJ, et al. Cloning and sequence of a β-tubulin cDNA from *Pneumocystis carinii*: possible implications for drug therapy. Mol Microbiol 1992; 6:991–1001.
14. Meade JC, Stringer JR. Cloning and characterization of an ATPase gene from *Pneumocystis carinii* which closely resembles fungal ATPases. J Eukaryotic Microbiol 1995; 42:298–307.
15. Pixley FJ, Wakefield AE, Banerji S, Hopkin JM. Mitochondrial gene sequences show fungal homology for *Pneumocystis carinii*. Mol Microbiol 1991; 5:1347–1351.
16. Edman JC, Sogin ML. Molecular phylogeny of *Pneumocystis carinii*. In: Waltzer PD, ed. *Pneumocystis carinii* Pneumonia, vol. 69. New York: Marcel Dekker, 1994:91–105.
17. Ruffolo JJ. *Pneumocystis carinii* cell structure. In: Walzer PD, ed. *Pneumocystis carinii* Pneumonia, vol 69. New York: Marcel Dekker, 1994:25–43.
18. Sinclair K, Wakefield AE, Banerji S, Hopkin JM. *Pneumocystis carinii* organisms derived from rat and human hosts are genetically distinct. Mol Biochem Parasitol 1991; 45:183–184.
19. Wakefield AE, Peters SE, Banerji S, et al. *Pneumocystis carinii* shows DNA homology with the ustomycetous red yeast fungi. Mol Microbiol 1992; 6:1903–1911.
20. Weinberg GA, Durant PJ. Genetic diversity of *Pneumocystis carinii* derived from infected rats, mice, ferrets and cell cultures. J Eukaryotic Microbiol 1994; 41:223–228.
21. Wakefield AE. Re-examination of epidemiological concepts. In: Sattler FR, Walzer PD, eds. *Pneumocystis carinii*, vol 2. London: Bailliere Tindall, 1995:431–448.
22. Hughes WT, Batley DL, Smith B. A natural source of infection due to *Pneumocystis carinii*. J Infect Dis 1983; 147:842–848.
23. Hughes WT. Natural mode of acquisition for de novo infection with *Pneumocystis carinii*. J Infect Dis 1982; 145:842–848.
24. Soulez B, Palluault F, Cesbron J-Y, Dei-Cas E, Capron A, Camus D. Introduction of *Pneumocystis carinii* in a colony of SCID mice. J Protozool 1991; 38:123S–125S.
25. Wakefield AE, Fritscher CC, Malin AS, et al. Genetic diversity of human-derived *Pneumocystis carinii* isolated from four geographical locations: analysis of mitochondrial ribosomal RNA gene sequences. J Clin Microbiol 1994; 32:2959–2961.
26. Meuwissen J, Tauber I, Leeuwenberg A, Beckers P, Sieben M. Parasitologic and serologic observations of infection with *Pneumocystis* in humans. J Infect Dis 1977; 136:43–49.

27. Pifer L, Hughes W, Stagno S, Woods D. *Pneumocystis carinii* Infection: evidence for a high prevalence in normal and immunosuppressed children. Pediatrics 1978; 61:35–41.
28. Smulian AG, Sullivan DW, Linke MJ, et al. Geographic variation in humoral responses to *Pneumocystis carinii*. J Infect Dis 1993; 167:1243–1247.
29. Peters SE, Wakefield AE, Sinclair K, Millard PR, Hopkin JM. A search for *Pneumocystis carinii* in post mortem lungs by DNA amplification. J Pathol 1992; 166:195–198.
30. Millard PR, Heryet AR. Observations favouring *Pneumocystis carinii* pneumonia as a primary infection: a monoclonal antibody study on paraffin sections. J Pathol 1988; 154:365–370.
31. Wakefield AS, Pixley FJ, Banerji S, Sinclair K, Miller RF, Hopkin JM. Detection of *Pneumocystis carinii* with DNA amplification. Lancet 1990; 336:451–453.
32. Leigh TR, Wakefield AE, Peters SE, Hopkin JM, Collins JV. Comparisons of DNA amplification and immunofluorescence for detecting *Pneumocystis carinii* in patients receiving immunosuppressive therapy. Transplantation 1992; 54:468–470.
33. Lipschik GY, Gill VJ, Lundgren JD, et al. Improved diagnosis of *Pneumocystis carinii* infection by polymerase chain reaction on induced sputum and blood. Lancet 1992; 340:203–206.
34. Evans R, Joss AW, Pennington TH, Ho-Yen DO. The use of polymerase chain reaction for detecting *Pneumocystis carinii* from lung and blood in rat and human infection. J Med Microbiol 1995; 42:209–213.
35. Eisen D, Ross BC, Fairbairn J, et al. Comparison of *Pneumocystis carinii* detection by toluidine blue O staining, direct immunofluorescence and DNA amplification in sputum specimens from HIV positive patients. Pathology 1994; 26:198–200.
36. Tamburrini E, Mencarini, DeLuca A, et al. Diagnosis of *Pneumocystis carinii* pneumonia: specificity and sensitivity of polymerase chain reaction in comparison with immunofluorescence in bronchoalveolar lavage specimens. J Med Microbiol 1993; 38:449–453.
37. Vargas SL, Hughes WT, Wakefield AE, Oz HS. Limited persistence and subsequent elimination of *Pneumocystis carinii* from the lungs after *P. carinii* pneumonia. J Infect Dis 1995; 172:506–510.
38. Gajdusek D. *Pneumocystis carinii*—etiologic agent of interstitial plasma cell pneumonia of premature and young infants. Pediatrics 1957; 19:543–565.
39. Perera DR, Western KA, Johnson HD, Johnson WW, Schultz MG, Ahers PV. *Pneumocystis carinii* pneumonia in a hospital for children. JAMA 1970; 214:1074–1078.
40. Ruebush TK, Weinstein RA, Baehner RL, et al. An outbreak of *Pneumocystis* pneumonia in children with acute lymphocytic leukemia. Am J Dis Child 1978; 132:143–148.
41. Stiller RA, Paradis IL, Dauber JH. Subclinical pneumonitis due to *Pneumocystis carinii* in a young adult with elevated antibody titers to Epstein–Barr virus. J Infect Dis 1992; 166:926–930.

42. Leigh TR, Millett MJ, Jameson B, Collins JV. Serum titres of *Pneumocystis carinii* antibody in health care workers caring for patients with AIDS. Thorax 1993; 48:619–621.
43. Harmsen AG, Chen W, Gigliotti F. Active immunity to *Pneumocystis carinii* reinfection in T-cell depleted mice. Infect Immun 1995; 63:2391–2395.
44. Gigliotti F, Hughes W. Passive immunoprophylaxis with specific monoclonal antibody confers partial protection against *Pneumocystis carinii* pneumonitis in animal models. J Clin Invest 1988; 81:1666.
45. Harmsen AG, Stankiewicz M. T cells are not sufficient for resistance to *Pneumocystis carinii* pneumonia in mice. J Parasitol 1991; 38:44S–45S.
46. Roths JB, Sidman CL. Single and combined humoral and cell mediated immunotherapy of *Pneumocystis carinii* pneumonia immunodeficient SCID mice. Infect Immun 1993; 61:1641–1649.
47. Shellito J, Suzara VV, Blumenfeld W, et al. A new model of *Pneumocystis carinii* infection in mice selectively depleted of helper T lymphocytes. J Clin Invest 1990; 85:1686–1693.
48. Harmsen AG, Stankiewicz M. Requirement for $CD4^+$ cells in resistance to *Pneumocystis carinii* pneumonia in mice. J Exp Med 1990; 172:937–945.
49. Roths JB, Sidman CL. Both immunity and hyperresponsiveness to *Pneumocystis carinii* result from transfer of CD4 but not CD8 T-cells into severe combined immunodeficiency mice. J Clin Invest 1992; 90:673–678.
50. Theus SA, Andrews RP, Steele P, Walzer PD. Adoptive transfer of lymphocytes sensitized to major surface glycoprotein of *Pneumocystis carinii* confers protection in the rat. J Clin Invest 1995:2587–2593.
51. Phair J, Munoz A, Detels R, et al. The risk of *Pneumocystis carinii* pneumonia among men infected with human immunodeficiency virus type 1. N Engl J Med 1990; 322:161–165.
52. Centers for Disease Control. Guidelines for prophylaxis against *Pneumocystis carinii* pneumonia for persons with human immunodeficiency virus infection. MMWR 1989; 38:1–8.
53. Group PCoHS. Design of a prospective study of the pulmonary complications of human immunodeficiency virus infection. J Clin Epidemiol 1990; 46:497–507.
54. Stansell JD, Osmond DH, Charlebois E, et al. Predictors of *Pneumocystis carinii* pneumonia in HIV-infected persons. Pulmonary Complications of HIV Infection Study Group. Am J Respir Crit Care Med. 1997; 155(1):60–66.
55. Pottratz ST, Martin WJ. Role of fibronectin in *Pneumocystis carinii* attachment to cultured lung cells. J Clin Invest 1990; 85:391–396.
56. Pottratz ST, Paulsrud J, Smith JS, Martin WJ. *Pneumocystis carinii* attachment to cultured lung cells by pneumocystis gp120, a fibronectin binding protein. J Clin Invest 1991; 88:403–407.
57. Yoneda K, Walzer PD. Attachment of *Pneumocystis carinii* to type I alveolar cells: study by freeze fracture electron microscopy. Infect Immun 1983; 40:812–815.
58. Walzer PD. Pathogenic mechanisms. In: Walzer PD, ed. *Pneumocystis carinii* Pneumonia. New York: Marcel Dekker, 1994:251–265.

59. Kvale P, Rosen M, Hopewell PC, et al. A decline in pulmonary diffusing capacity does not indicate opportunistic lung disease in asymptomatic persons infected with human immunodeficiency virus. Am Rev Respir Dis 1993; 148:390–395.
60. Kvale P, Hansen N, Markowitz N, et al. Routine analysis of induced sputum is not an effective strategy for screening persons infected with human immunodeficiency virus for *Mycobacterium tuberculosis* or *Pneumocystis carinii*. Clin Infect Dis 1994; 19:410–416.
61. Kovacs J, Hiemenz J, Macher A, et al. *Pneumocystis carinii* pneumonia: a comparison between patients with the acquired immunodeficiency syndrome and patients with other immunodeficiencies. Ann Intern Med 1984; 100:663–71.
62. Medina I, Mills J, Wofsy C. Serum lactate dehydrogenase levels in *Pneumocystis carinii* pneumonia in AIDS: possible indicator and predictor of disease activity (abstr). Third International Conference on AIDS, Washington, DC, 1987.
63. Goodman P. *Pneumocystis carinii* pneumonia. J Thorac Imaging 1991; 6:16–21.
64. Chaffey M, Klein J, Gamsu G, et al.Radiographic distribution of *Pneumocystis carinii* pneumonia in patients with AIDS treated with prophylactic inhaled pentamidine. Radiology 1990; 175:715–719.
65. Jules-Elysee K, Stover D, Zamen et al. Aerosolized pentamidine: effect on diagnosis and presentation of *Pneumocystis carinii* pneumonia. Ann Intern Med 1990; 112:750–757.
66. Goodman P, Daley C, Minagi H. Spontaneous pneumothorax in AIDS patients with *Pneumocystis carinii* pneumonia. AJR 1986; 147:697–702.
67. Wachter R, Luce J, Turner J. Intensive care of patients with the acquired immunodeficiency syndrome: outcome and changing patterns of utilization. Am Rev Respir Dis 1986; 134:891.
68. Wachter R, Russi M, Bloch D, et al. *Pneumocystis carinii* pneumonia with respiratory failure in AIDS: improved outcomes and increased use of intensive care units. Am Rev Respir Dis 1991; 143:251–256.
69. Wachter RM, Luce JM, Safrin S, et al. Cost and outcome of intensive care for patients with AIDS. *Pneumocystis carinii* pneumonia and severe respiratory failure. JAMA 1995; 273:23–235.
70. Northfelt D, Clement M, Safrin S. Extrapulmonary pneumocystosis: clinical features in human immunodeficiency virus infection. Medicine 1990; 69:392–398.
71. Sankary R, Turner J, Lipavsky A, et al. Alveolar–capillary block in patients with AIDS and *Pneumocystis carinii* pneumonia. Am Rev Respir Dis 1988; 137:443–449.
72. Huang L, Hecht FM, Stansell JD, et al. Suspected *Pneumocystis carinii* pneumonia with a negative induced sputum examination. Is early bronchoscopy useful? Am J Respir Crit Care Med 1995; 151:1866–1871.
73. Epstein LJ, Meyer RD, Antonson S, et al. Persistence of *Pneumocystis carinii* in patients with AIDS receiving chemoprophylaxis. Am J Respir Crit Care Med 1994; 150:1456–1459.
74. Bigby T, Margolskee D, Curtis J, et al. The usefulness of induced sputum in the

diagnosis of *Pneumocystis carinii* pneumonia in patients with the acquired immunodeficiency syndrome. Am Rev Respir Dis 1986; 133:515–518.
75. Ng V, Gartner I, Weymouth et al. The use of mucolysed induced sputum for the identification of pulmonary pathogens associated with human immunodeficiency virus infection. Arch Pathol Lab Med 1989; 113:488–493.
76. Ng V, Yajko D, McPhaul L. Evaluation of an indirect fluorescent-antibody stain for detection of *Pneumocystis carinii* in respiratory specimens. J Clin Microbiol 1990; 28:975–979.
77. Kovacs JA, Ng VL, Masur H, et al. Diagnosis of *Pneumocystis carinii* pneumonia: improved detection in sputum with use of mitochondrial antibodies. N Engl J Med 1988; 318:589.
78. Broaddus V, Dake M, Stulbarg M, et al. Bronchoalveolar lavage and transbronchial biopsy for the diagnosis of pulmonary infections in the acquired immunodeficiency syndrome. Ann Intern Med 1985; 102:747–752.
79. Golden JA, Hollander H, Stulbarg MS, et al. Bronchoalveolar lavage as the exlusive diagnostic modality for *Pneumocystis carinii* pneumonia. Chest 1986; 90:18.
80. Miller RF, Millar AB, Weller JVD, Semple JSG. Empirical treatment without bronchoscopy for *Pneumocystis carinii* pneumonia in the acquired immunodeficiency syndrome. Thorax 1989; 44:559.
81. Tu JV, Biem HJ, Detsky AS. Bronchscopy versus empirical therapy in HIV-infected patients with presumptive *Pneumocystis carinii* pneumonia: a decision analysis. Am Rev Respir Dis 1993; 148:370–377.
82. Bennett CL, Horner RD, Weinstein RA, et al. Empirically treated *Pneumocystis carinii* pneumonia in Los Angeles, Chicago and Miami: 1987–1990. J Infect Dis 1995; 172:312–315.
83. Masur H. Empiric outpatient management of HIV-related pneumonia: economical or unwise? Ann Intern Med 1996.
84. Gordin F, Simon G, Wofsy C, Mills J. Adverse reactions to timethoprim–sulfamethoxazole in patients with the acquired immunodeficiency syndrome. Ann Intern Med 1984; 100:495.
85. Masur H, Lane C, Kovacs J, et al. *Pneumocystis pneumonia*: from bench to bedside. Ann Intern Med 1989; 111:8813–8826.
86. Wharton J, Coleman D, Wofsy C, et al. Trimethoprim–sulfamethoxazole or pentamidine for *Pneumocystis carinii* pneumonia in the acquired immunodeficiency syndrome: a prospective randomized trial. Ann Intern Med 1986; 105:37–44.
87. Sattler F, Cowan R, Nielsen D, Ruskin J. Trimethoprim–sulfamethoxazole compared with pentamidine for treatment of *Pneumocystis carinii* pneumonia in the acquired immunodeficiency syndrome: a prospective, noncrossover study. Ann Intern Med 1988; 109:280–287.
88. Hughes WT, Leoung G, Kramer R, et al. Comparison of atovaquone (566C80) with trimethoprim–sulfamethoxazole to treat *Pneumocystis carinii* pneuomnia in patients with AIDS. N Engl J Med 1993; 328:1521–1527.
89. Sattler FR, Frame P, Davis R, et al. Comparison of trimethrexate with leuco-

vorin versus trimethoprim–sulfamethoxazole for moderate to severe episodes of *Pneumocystis carinii* pneumonia in patients with AIDS. Infect Dis 1994; 170:165–172.
90. Klein N, Duncanson F, Lenox T, et al. Trimethoprim–sulfamethoxazole versus pentamidine for *Pneumocystis carinii* pneumonia in AIDS patients: results of a large prospective randomized treatment trial. AIDS 1992; 6:301–305.
91. Medina I, Mills J, Leoung G, et al. Oral therapy for *Pneumocystis carinii* pneumonia in the acquired immunodeficiency syndrome: a controlled trial of trimethoprim–sulfamethoxazole versus trimethoprim–dapsone. N Engl J Med 1990; 323:776–782.
92. Safrin S, Finkelstein DM, Feinberg J, et al. Comparison of three regimens for treatment of mild to moderate *Pneumocystis carinii* pneumonia in patients with AIDS. A double-blind, randomized trial of trimethoprim–sulfamethoxazole, dapsone–trimethoprim and clindamycin–primaquine. ACTG 108 Study Group. Ann Intern Med 1996; 124(9):792–802.
93. Hughes WT, Killmar JT, Oz HS. Relative potency of 10 drugs with anti-*Pneumocystis carinii* activity in the animal model. J Infect Dis 1994; 170:906–911.
94. Hughes WT, Feldman S, Chaudhary SC, et al. Comparison of pentamidine isethionate and trimethoprim–sulfamethoxazole in the treatment of *Pneumocystis carinii* pneumonia. J Pediatr 1978; 92:436–440.
95. Toma E, Poisson M, Phaneuf D, et al. Clindamycin with primaquine for *Pneumocystis carinii* pneumonia. Lancet 1989; 13:1046–1048.
96. Toma E, Fournier S, Dumont M, et al. Clindamycin/primaquine versus trimethoprim–sulfamethoxazole as primary therapy for *Pneumocystis carinii* pneumonia in AIDS: a randomized, double-blind pilot trial. Clin Infect Dis 1993; 17:178–184.
97. Toma E, Raboud J, Thorne A, Singer J, et al. Clindamycin–primaquine versus trimethoprim–sulfamethoxazole for PCP in AIDS. 35th Interscience Conference on Antimicrobial Agents and Chemotherapy (ICAAC), San Francisco, CA: American Society for Microbiology, 1995.
98. Safrin S, Lee BL, Sande MA. Adjunctive folinic acid with trimethoprim–sulfamethoxazole for *Pneumocystis carinii* pneumonia in AIDS patients is associated with an increased risk of therapeutic failure and death. J Infect Dis 1994; 170:912–917.
99. Conte JE. Pharmacokinetics of intravenous pentamidine in patients with normal renal function or receiving hemodialysis. J Infect Dis 1991; 163:169–175.
100. Stein DS, Stevens RC. Treatment-associated toxicities: incidence and mechanisms. In: Sattler FR, Walzer PD, eds. *Pneumocystis carinii*. London: Bailliere Tindall, 1995:505–530.
101. Conte J, Chernoff D, Feigal D, Joseph P, McDonald C, Golder J. Intravenous or inhaled pentamidine for treating *Pneumocystis carinii* pneumonia in AIDS: a randomized trial. Ann Intern Med 1990; 113:203–209.
102. O'Brien JG, Dong BJ, Coleman RL, et al. Five year retrospective review of the risk factors associated with adverse drug reactions in patients with HIV treated

with intravenous pentamidine for *Pneumocystis carinii* pneumonia (abstr). ICAAC, San Francisco, CA: American Society for Microbiology 1995.
103. Queener SF, Bartlett MS, Richardson JD, et al. Activity of clinidamycin with primaquine against *Pneumocystis carinii* in vitro and in vivo. Antimicrob Agents Chemother 1988; 32:807–813.
104. Black J, Feinberg J, Murphy R, et al. Clindamycin and primaquine as primary treatment for mild and moderately severe *Pneumocystis carinii* pneumonia in patients with AIDS. Eur J Clin Microbiol Infect Dis 1991; 10:204–207.
105. Toma E. Clindamycin/primaquine vs. TMP/SMX. Eighth International Conference on AIDS, Amsterdam, Netherlands, 1992.
106. Allegra C, Chabner B, Tuazon C, et al. Trimetrexate for the treatment of *Pneumocystis carinii* pneumonia in patients with acquired immunodeficiency syndrome. N Engl J Med 1987; 317:978.
107. Sattler FR, Allegra CJ, Verdegem TD, et al. Trimetrexate–leucovorin dosage evaluation study for treatment of *Pneumocystis carinii* pneumonia. J Infect Dis 1990; 161:91–96.
108. Safrin S, Sattler F, Lee B, et al. Dapsone as a single agent is suboptimal therapy for *Pneumocystis carinii* pneumonia. J Acquir Immune Defic Syndr 1991; 4:244–249.
109. Stansell JD, Dube M, Sattler FR. A randomized, double blind comparison of trimetrexate 45 mg/m^2 and folinic acid 80 mg/m^2/day plus dapsone 100 mg/day compared with trimethoprim/sulfamethoxazole 15 mg/kg/day for moderate to severe *Pneumocystis carinii* pneumonia in AIDS patients. (manuscript in preparation) 1997
110. Hughes WT, Smith BL. Efficacy of diaminophenylsulfone and other drugs in murine *Pneumocystis carinii* pneumonitis. Antimicrob Agents Chemother 1984; 26:436–440.
111. Leoung GS, Mills J, Hopewell PC, et al. Dapsone–trimethoprim for *Pneumocystis carinii* pneumonia in the acquired immunodeficiency syndrome. Ann Intern Med 1986; 105:45–48.
112. Falloon J, Kovacs J, Hughes W. A preliminary evaluation of 566c80 for the treatment of *Pneumocystis carinii* pneumonia in patients with the acquired immunodeficiency syndrome. N Engl J Med 1991; 325:1534.
113. Dohn MN, Weinberg WG, Torres RA, et al. Oral atovaquone compared with intravenous pentamidine for *Pneumocystis carinii* pneumonia in patients with AIDS. Ann Intern Med 1994; 121:174–180.
114. Soo Hoo G, Mohsenifar Z, Meyer R. Inhaled or intravenous pentamidine therapy for *Pneumocystis carinii* pneumonia in AIDS: a randomized trial. Ann Intern Med 1990; 113:195–202.
115. Montgomery AB, Feigal DW, Sattler FR, et al. Pentamidine aerosol versus trimethoprm–sulfamethoxazole for *Pneumocystis carinii* in acquired immune deficiency syndrome. Am J Respir Crit Care Med 1995; 151:1068–1074.
116. Montaner J, Lawson L, Levitt N, et al. Corticosteroids prevent early deterioration in patients with moderately severe *Pneumocystis carinii* pneumonia and the acquired immunodeficiency syndrome (AIDS). Ann Intern Med 1990; 113:14–20.

117. Bozzette S, Sattler F, Chiu J, et al. A controlled trial of early adjunctive treatment with cortifcosteroids for *Pneumocystis carinii* pneumonia in the acquired immunodeficiency syndrome. N Engl J Med 1990; 323:1451.
118. Gagnon S, Boota A, Fischl M, et al. Corticosteroids as adjunctive therapy for severe *Pneumocystis carinii* pneumonia in the acquired immunodeficiency syndrome. N Engl J Med 1990; 323:1444.
119. Panel NIH–UoCE. Concensus statement on the use of corticosteroids as adjunctive therapy for severe *Pneumocystis carinii* pneumonia in the acquired immunodeficiency syndrome. N Engl J Med 1990; 323:1500–1504.
120. Fischl M, Dickinson G, LaVoie L. Safety and efficacy of sulfamethoxazole and trimethoprim chemoprophylaxis for *Pneumocystis carinii* pneumonia in AIDS. JAMA 1988; 259:1185–1189.
121. Hirschel B, Lazzarin KA, Chopard P, et al. A controlled study of inhaled pentamidine for primary prevention of *Pneumocystis carinii* pneumonia. N Engl J Med 1991; 324:1079–1083.
122. Girard PM, Landman R, Gaudebout C. Prevention of *Pneumocystis carinii* pneumonia relapse by pentamidine aerosol in zidovudine-treated AIDS patients. Lancet 1989; 1348–1353.
123. Montaner J, Lawson L, Gervais A, et al. Aerosol pentamidine for secondary prophylaxis of AIDS-related *Pneumocystis carinii* pneumonia: a randomized, placebo-controlled study. Ann Intern Med 1991; 114:948–953.
124. Bozzette SA, Finkelstein DM, Spector SA, et al. A randomized trial of three antipneumocystis agents in patients with advanced human immunodeficiency virus infection. N Engl J Med 1995; 332:93–699.
125. Schneider MME, Hoepelman AIM, Eeftinck-Schattenkerk J, et al. A controlled trial of aerosolized pentamidine or trimthoprim–sulfamethoxazole as primary prophylaxis against *Pneumocystis carinii* penumonia in patients with human immunodeficiency virus infection. N Engl J Med 1992; 327:1836–1841.
126. Mallolas J, Zamore L, Gatell JM, et al. Primary prophylaxis for *Pneumocystis carinii* pneumonia: a randomized trial comparing TMP–SMX, aerosolized pentamidine and dapsone plus pyrimethamine. AIDS 1993; 7:59–64.
127. Podzamczer D, Santin M, Jimenez J, et al. Thrice-weekly TMP–SMX is better than weekly dapsone–pyrimethamine for the primary prevention of *Pneumocystis carinii* pneumonia in HIV-infected persons. AIDS 1993; 7:501–506.
128. Heald A, Flepp M, Chave J-P, et al. Treatment for cerebral toxoplasmosis protects against *Pneumocystis carinii* pneumonia in patients with AIDS. Ann Intern Med 1991; 115:760–763.
129. Hughes WT, Killmar J. Efficacy of sulfonamides alone in prophylaxis for *Pneumocystis carinii* pneumonia (abstr). Third Conference on Retroviruses and Opportunistic Infections, Washington, DC: Infectious Diseases Society of America, 1996.
130. Slavin MA, Hoy JF, Stewart K, et al. Oral dapsone versus nebulized pentamidine for *Pneumocystis carinii* pneumonia prophylaxis: an open randomized prospective trial to assess efficacy and haematological toxicity. AIDS 1992; 6:1169–1174.

131. Opravil M, Hirschel B, Lazzarin A, et al. Once-weekly administration of dapsone/pyrimethamine vs. aerosolized pentamidine as combined prophylaxis for *Pneumocystis carinii* pneumonia and toxoplasmic encephalitis in human immunodeficiency virus-infected patients. Clin Infect Dis 1995; 20:531–541.
132. Torres RA, Barr M, Thorn M, et al. Randomized trial of dapsone and aerosolized pentamidine for the prophylaxis of *Pneumocystis carinii* pneumonia and toxoplasmic encephalitis. Am J Med 1993; 95:573–583.

13

HIV and Tuberculosis

BONITA T. MANGURA and LEE B. REICHMAN

University of Medicine and Dentistry of New Jersey–New Jersey Medical School
and New Jersey Medical School National Tuberculosis Center
Newark, New Jersey

I. Introduction

There are approximately 14 million human immunodeficiency virus (HIV) infected persons in the world today, and there are 1.7 billion persons infected with tuberculosis. The number who are coinfected with HIV and tuberculosis is estimated to be 5.6 million (1). Tuberculosis is the primary disease associated with HIV infection in the developing world (2). In the United States, HIV and the acquired immunodeficiency syndrome (AIDS) are largely, but not exclusively, responsible for the resurgence of tuberculosis. In the United States, there are at least 15 million people infected with tuberculosis and close to 1 million infected with the HIV; approximately 100,000 persons are infected with both diseases.

Risks for development of tuberculosis include injection drug use, birth in a country where heterosexual transmission of HIV is common, and homosexual sex (3). The preponderance of cases of tuberculosis is seen in those US cities where persons at risk of both HIV and tuberculosis are present (4). Drug dependency has been previously recognized as a risk factor for *Mycobacterium tuberculosis* infection and disease even before the AIDS epidemic (5). Inner cities with a high-background level of latent tuberculosis, in combination with the congregation of the drug-dependent population among the urban poor, have also been suggested as causes for the association of HIV and tuberculosis in the United States (6). For example, in specific groups, such as users of "crack" cocaine and injectable drugs, deliberate obstruction of windows to obscure or avoid detection by authorities may enhance the transmission of tuberculosis to cohorts at risk (7). The recent increase in immigration to the United States from countries with high prevalence of tuberculosis in the 1980s coincided with the resurgence of this infection (4).

In the United States, aside from the concurrent problem of injection drug use and rise in immigration from countries with high rates of tuberculosis, a major factor of perpetuation of transmission and resurgence of the disease is the breakdown of the health care infrastructure (8). Social factors in the United States in the 1980s, such as homelessness, substance abuse, and dismantling of the health care infrastructure for tuberculosis treatment, all have played a role in the resurgence of this infection (8). The health care infrastructure in the United States is the primary and first source of services for outcomes of social disenfranchisement ("medicalization" of social ills; 9).

The coexistence of HIV and tuberculosis is ominous, because of all the infectious lung complications of HIV, tuberculosis is the most transmissible, regardless of serological HIV status. Air travel and international field assignments have shrunk the world to make tuberculosis not only a developing nation's problem but a global problem.

II. Epidemiology

The clinical course after initial infection proceeds in three ways: (1) progression of primary infection; (2) reactivation of latent infection; and (3) reinfection with a new strain. The risk of an immunocompetent individual progressing to active tuberculosis is 10% over a lifetime, the first 5% within 2 years of the time of infection. However, HIV infection increases the risk of developing active tuberculosis. Nearly 90% of cases are thought to develop from reactivation disease in the previously infected; progression of primary infection occurs in the 10% who are newly infected. Information derived from restriction fragment length polymorphism (RFLP) DNA fingerprinting analysis and case–contact investigation indicate that infections with new strains also occur among the HIV-infected population, as in an outbreak of tuberculosis that occurred in an AIDS residential facility in San Francisco that was traced to a single strain and source (10). The secondary cases occurred within 20–60 days after the index case. The risk of progression to active tuberculosis in a newly infected person with HIV infection was calculated at 37% risk within 3 months. This risk of developing active disease is much greater than the prospective estimate of 7–9% a year for HIV-*M. tuberculosis* coinfected reactors (11).

Immunosuppression underlies many conditions that predispose to the development of opportunistic infections in the HIV-infected person. Other conditions associated with a high risk for developing tuberculosis are also associated with immunosuppression. These include prolonged therapy with corticosteroids, immunosuppressive therapy, hematological and reticuloendothelial disease, intestinal bypass, gastrectomy, chronic malabsorption syndromes, carcinomas of the oropharynx and upper gastrointestinal tract, malnutrition, and silicosis. Low body mass index in association with poor nutrition and a high-stress environment make additional sources of immunosuppression that may compound HIV effects on tuberculosis (12).

III. Clinical Manifestations

A. Clinical Presentation

Up to 80% of patients with tuberculosis present with fever, cough, and weight loss (13). The paucity of descriptions of pulmonary disease in the US literature may be biased by the early surveillance classification of AIDS in 1987, which did not include pulmonary tuberculosis as an AIDS-defining condition (14). Moreover, tuberculosis presented in a protean manner; even before the AIDS epidemic, tuberculosis was known as a "masquerader" of infectious diseases, accounting for its common underdiagnosis. In the early reports of tuberculosis in AIDS, symptoms were nonspecific, and included nonproductive cough, fever, shortness of breath, and chest pain (15–17). As part of the "protean" manifestations of tuberculosis, it may be considered in the differential diagnoses of "atypical pneumonias" (18,19). In drug-dependent patients with HIV infection, constitutional presentations can represent symptoms of drug abuse, because night sweats, malaise, and fever can be caused by withdrawal from abused drugs (6). A low index of suspicion for tuberculosis has commonly led to misdiagnosis and delayed diagnosis of tuberculosis, even in the absence of high prevalence of HIV (20). In some instances, delay in diagnosis led to serious morbidity, prolonged infectivity, and spread to close contacts (21).

In early descriptions of HIV and AIDS, pulmonary tuberculosis was relatively unusual, whereas extrapulmonary presentations were common (15). A more recent review of both AIDS and tuberculosis registries in San Francisco (from 1981–1988) show that there were slightly more pulmonary tuberculosis cases than extrapulmonary (38 compared with 30% of 132) cases (22). Pulmonary and extrapulmonary disease occurred together in 32%.

B. Chest Radiographs

The radiograph may provide valuable clues to the diagnosis of tuberculosis. Pleural effusions, thoracic lymphadenopathy, middle lobe disease, and miliary patterns should raise the suspicion of tuberculosis in HIV-infected persons (Figs. 1–3). However, the diagnosis should be considered in all patients with HIV infection who have undiagnosed pulmonary disease. The available descriptions of radiographic findings in tuberculosis in HIV-infected persons come from retrospective studies, during which diagnostic

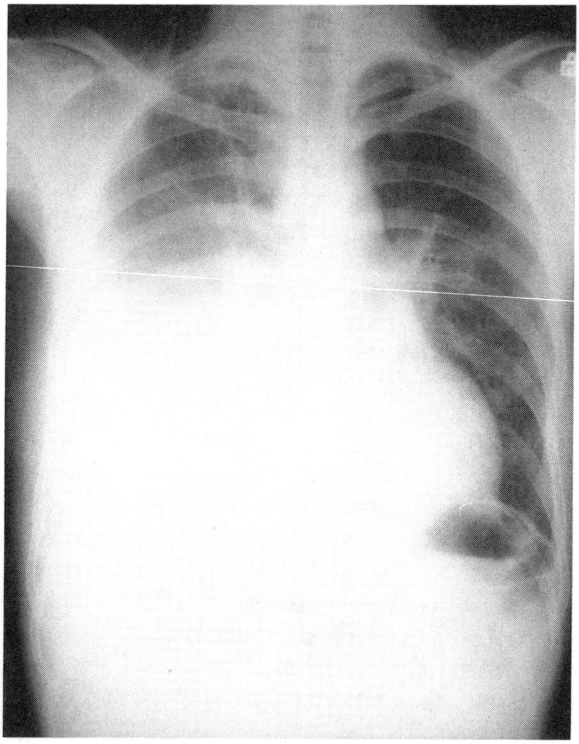

Figure 1 Chest radiograph of a patient with a tuberculous pleural effusion. The diagnosis was established by a pleural biopsy that showed poorly formed granulomas, with positive smear and culture of sputum.

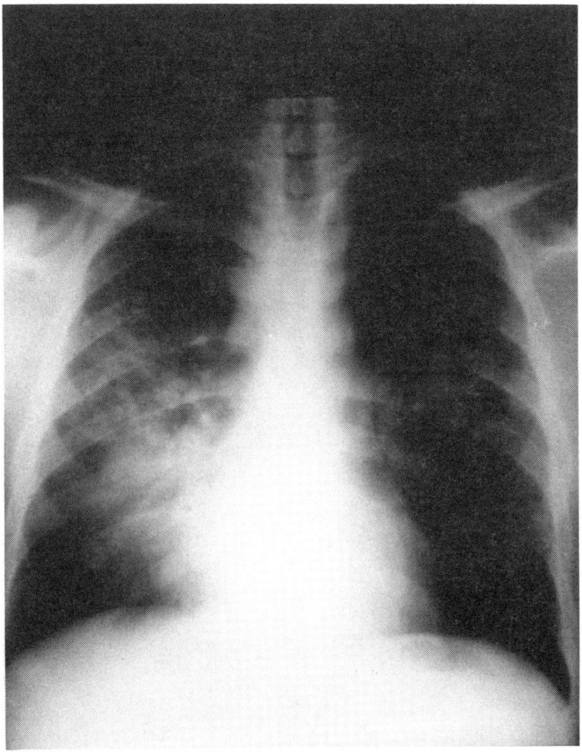

Figure 2 Mediastinal lymphadenopathy and localized areas of consolidation in a patient with HIV infection and *M. tuberculosis*.

procedures were performed based on the differential diagnosis suggested by radiologic findings, and specimens obtained by invasive techniques added very little to the information, even when multiple sites were sampled. For example, the following distribution of radiologic findings were observed in 23 cases of tuberculosis by Sunderam et al.: 6 had apical infiltrates, 4 had miliary infiltrates, 5 had cavitary disease (2 with air–fluid levels), 6 had hilar adenopathy, 4 had mediastinal adenopathy, 1 had paratracheal adenopathy, and 5 had pleural effusions (15). Although the pulmonary findings were not the predominant presentation, these findings occurred at some time during their disease. Rather, extrapulmonary sites, including the pericardium, bone, rectum, and the central nervous system, were prominent. These radiologic presentations were comparable with the findings of other cohorts in the United States (16,17,23).

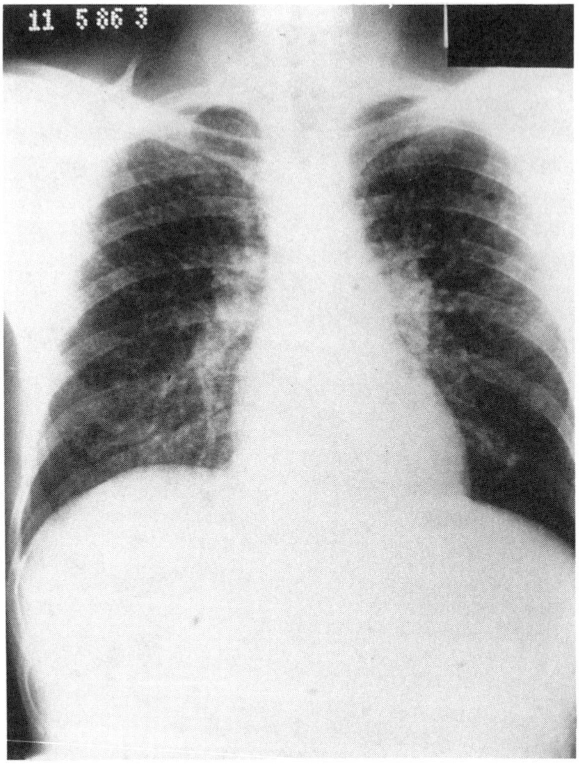

Figure 3 Miliary pattern in a patient with tuberculosis. The diagnosis was established by bronchoalveolar lavage.

In patients with abnormal chest radiographs, bacterial pneumonias and *Pneumocystis carinii* pneumonia (PCP) are considered in the differential diagnosis, especially in patients with diffuse parenchymal disease. However, in a retrospective review of 105 cases of pleuropulmonary tuberculosis, only 4 patients had radiographs that resembled those of typical PCP (23). The clinical presentation, sputum smears, and radiographic findings were all important in the initial diagnosis of tuberculosis. Clinical features such as CD4+ cell counts of more than 500/μl and lymphadenopathy were unlikely to accompany PCP. Other suggestive findings were an acid-fast smear of a clinical sample (including stool), and pleural effusion, predominant upper lobe infiltrate, cavitation, mediastinal adenopathy, or a miliary pattern.

Patients with pulmonary tuberculosis may present with no apparent parenchymal abnormality on chest radiograph. Normal-appearing lung fields, with and without adenopathy, have been observed in several HIV cohorts with pulmonary tuberculosis (15–17,24,25). These patients present a difficult challenge to the clinician, and the diagnosis of tuberculosis may be delayed, especially when mediastinal adenopathy is subtle or absent. However, many HIV-infected persons with tuberculosis have intrathoracic lymphadenopathy, even when the lung fields appear clear. In one series, one-third of the cases had pleural effusions (23). More importantly, pleural effusions and adenopathy are usually associated with early or "primary progressive tuberculosis," suggesting recent transmission or reactivation pleuritis (26). Therefore, tuberculosis should be suspected in all HIV-infected patients with undiagnosed lung disease. In a retrospective review of 88 HIV-infected patients with pulmonary tuberculosis, 6 of 18 patients with normal chest films had positive acid-fast bacteria (AFB) smears of their sputum (27). This study suggests that even in the absence of parenchymal radiographic changes, the sputum examination is still useful. Screening asymptomatic HIV-infected persons for tuberculosis with chest radiographs was investigated in the Pulmonary Complications of HIV Infection Study, and was not found to be useful (see Chap. 10) (28).

IV. Microbiological Diagnosis

In one of the first papers on AIDS and tuberculosis, Sunderam et. al reported that most patients with tuberculosis presented in a nonspecific manner, so that multiple specimens from different sites were required for diagnosis (15). Many patients presented with extrapulmonary disease, despite pulmonary involvement on the chest radiograph in 23 of the 29 cases. When pulmonary involvement was present, no respiratory specimens were readily accessible. Sputum examination for AFB is still the primary way to diagnose tuberculosis, including in HIV-infected persons. Although some investigators found a decreased frequency of sensitivity of sputum smears in culture-positive pulmonary tuberculosis in the HIV-infected population, most have reported yields similar to those in patients who do not have HIV infection., ranging from 66- to 83%-positive test rates (29,30).

Fiberoptic bronchoscopy is not generally employed as an initial diagnostic modality in the diagnosis of tuberculosis (31), but its use has increased with the AIDS epidemic. In this setting, bronchoscopy is usually employed in patients with undiagnosed pulmonary disorders after sputum smears are negative (32–34). The role of bronchoscopy in the diagnosis of tuberculosis is discussed in detail in Chapter 8. Bronchoscopists must practice appropriate respiratory precautions. In 1990, a higher tuberculin skin test conversion among pulmonary fellows than infectious disease fellows finishing training was reported in a national survey (35). The performance of a bronchoscopy examination, an aerosol-generating procedure, was implicated as the differentiating factor influencing the increased rates of tuberculin conversion among pulmonary fellows during training. The bronchoscopist must be alert to the possibility of endobronchial involvement with *M. tuberculosis*, which has been described in HIV-infected persons (36,37). In cases of endobronchial tuberculosis, the chest film may be nonspecific, different from "classic" reactivation tuberculosis, or it may simulate a neoplastic pulmonary disorder (38,39). Bronchoscopic findings of endobronchial tuberculosis include raised ulcerative, friable, and occlusive endobronchial masses similar to endobronchial lesions from a neoplasm. Bronchoscopy with bronchoalveolar lavage (BAL) is associated with increased morbidity in some cases, including extension and parenchymal spread to the corresponding segment or lobe (40). In cases of suspected endobronchial tuberculosis, we brush for a direct AFB smear on a glass slide, and take a biopsy specimen from the lesion for culture and tissue staining.

In patients with suspected tuberculosis who have negative sputum smears and nondiagnostic bronchoscopic studies, other sites may be sampled, including bone marrow, liver, or lymph nodes.

Over the last decade, newer techniques of rapid detection of *M. tuberculosis* in sputum samples have been developed. Direct amplification tests (DAT) that identify *M. tuberculosis* RNA or DNA were recently approved by the US Food and Drug Administration (FDA) (41–43). These tests are significantly more sensitive than the AFB smear, and the results are available much faster than culture. However, the clinical usefulness of the polymerase chain reaction (PCR) varies with institution, follow-up, and case definition (42,43). It is not useful in distinguishing active from prior infection, and has not yet been reported helpful in diagnosing extrapulmonary tuberculosis. In addition, a study of sensitivity and specificity on PCR of blinded standardized samples from seven experienced laboratories revealed varying results (44). In 1997, an American Thoracic Society workshop recommended that there is currently insufficient information on these assays to be useful in the clinical and public health setting (41). When the AFB smear and DAT are both positive, the diagnosis of tuberculosis can be considered to be established. Likewise, when both are negative, it is unlikely that a culture will be positive, although this by no means rules out the diagnosis. When the smear and DAT are discordant, the physician must rely on the clinical picture, pending the results of cultures and repeat studies. Finally, the workshop recommended that DATs always be performed in conjunction with smears and cultures. Further refinement in its general applicability and practicality is needed.

V. Tuberculin Skin Testing

The tuberculin test is a screening as well as diagnostic tool in the investigation of tuberculous infection. An individual's positive response is based on a delayed-type hypersensitivity (DTH) reaction (type IV) to the tuberculoprotein, which is seen 48–72 hr after an intradermal injection of 0.1 mL of 5 TU (tuberculin units) of purified protein derivative (PPD; Mantoux test).

The recommended interpretation of a positive response for the HIV-infected person is a 5-mm induration (45). With higher $CD4^+$ counts, patients with tuberculous and HIV infection generally respond to a tuberculin test. However, at lower $CD4^+$ levels (fewer than 200/mL), it is increasingly more difficult to interpret the Mantoux test. In addition, depending on immune status, DTH varies from a positive response to negative, and vice versa, in the same individual over time (46). The Pulmonary Complications of HIV Infection Study confirmed that a 5-mm cutoff for a positive test is clinically appropriate; after 5 years of follow-up, no cases of tuberculosis were identified in a large cohort who had a tuberculin reaction of 4 mm or smaller (7,47). An earlier report had suggested a lower cutoff (smaller than 5 mm) for the HIV-infected patient to allow for the deficient response to T-cell–mediated hypersensitivity, but this has not been borne out (48).

In clinical practice, anergy testing may be used to determine whether a negative tuberculin test is a "true" negative, or a false negative in the setting of nonspecific lack of reactivity to injected antigens. Anergy testing in patients with HIV infection is unreliable for this use. In the Pulmonary Complications of HIV Infection Study, the results of anergy testing were variable for many patients. Thirty percent of subjects initially classified as being anergic had positive reactions to mumps or candida skin tests 1 year later, and 39% of patients with documented false-negative tuberculin tests still reacted to mumps antigen (49). The authors suggested that the results of anergy testing should not be used to make clinical decisions on individual patients. Caiaffa et al. confirmed that the finding of DTH anergy was unstable in a group of injection drug users, but that it is more reliable when persistent over time, and unnecessary in persons with $CD4^+$ cell counts of more than 500/μl (50).

VI. Treatment

The treatment of tuberculosis is important not only to eradicate the infection, but it may also improve the course of a patient's HIV infection, because active tuberculosis increases HIV replication and viral load. The treatment of tuberculosis in these HIV-infected persons who adhere to their medication regimens is effective (53). Sterilization of sputum is achieved after an average of 10 weeks of treatment using isoniazid, rifampin, pyrazinamide, and ethambutol. Current recommendations for the treatment of both pulmonary and extrapulmonary tuberculosis in HIV-infected persons is 6 months, using four drugs daily for the first 2 months, and isoniazid and rifampin for the last 4 months. In Zaire, extending 6 months of therapy to a 12-month course reduced the relapse rate, but did not improve survival among a group of 260 HIV-infected and 186 HIV-seronegative patients (54). Because the major deterrent to success of treatment is adherence, strong consideration should be given to encouraging adherence by the use of directly observed therapy (DOT) as the standard of care. Susceptibility testing should be performed on all initial specimens, and extending treatment for longer than 6 months should be considered for patients with slow or suboptimal response to treatment, such as slower conversion of sputum smears from positive to negative.

A. Interactions with Protease Inhibitors

Protease inhibitors (PI) interfere with HIV maturation and replication by inhibition of HIV protease. They are the most potent antiretroviral agents available to treat patients with HIV disease, but they interact with rifamycin derivatives, notably rifampin. Rifamycins accelerate the metabolism of PI, resulting in subtherapeutic levels of PI, and PIs retard the metabolism of rifamycins, resulting in increased drug toxicity. Avoidance of rifampin in the regimen is undesirable, for it is the mainstay of a short-course tuberculosis treatment regimen. The risks and complications associated with tuberculosis regimens without rifampin include (1) prolonged treatment of at least 18–24 months, (2) increased likelihood of treatment failure and mortality, (3) patients remain infectious longer because of slower bacteriological conversion of sputum culture, and (4) tuberculosis disease accelerates progression of HIV infection.

There are no good studies involving patients taking protease inhibitors who have tuberculosis; until large clinical trials can support a formal recommendation, three options were presented by the Centers for Disease Control and Prevention (CDC) as *interim* guidelines (Table 1; 55).

B. Multidrug-Resistant Tuberculosis

The factors that fuel the increase in tuberculosis, namely, injection drug use, homelessness, and poor social support and public health systems, are each partly responsible for patient noncompliance with medical regimens.

Table 1 CDC Interim Guidelines for the Use of Protease Inhibitors and Rifampin in Patients with Tuberculosis and HIV Infection

Option 1: Discontinue PI therapy while undergoing rifampin-containing tuberculosis regimen. Complete short-course (6-month) therapy with the rifampin-containing regimen. PI therapy may be resumed when treatment with rifampin regimen is completed.

Option 2: Use four-drug tuberculosis regimen that includes rifampin (isoniazid, pyrazinamide, and ethambutol or streptomycin) for a minimum of 2 months (induction therapy) until bacteriological response and drug susceptibility are documented. Treatment modification of continuation phase to *16 months* consisting of isoniazid 15 mg/kg and ethambutol 50 mg/kg twice a week. The PI can be reintroduced in this phase. An additional third drug, streptomycin, has been suggested during this phase. Option 2 cannot be recommended for treatment of isoniazid-resistant strains.

Option 3: Continue PI therapy with indinavir (800 mg po every 8 hr) and use a four-drug, 9-month tuberculosis treatment regimen using daily rifabutin (150 mg/d) instead of rifampin. Careful monitoring, including serum levels of rifabutin, is required when using this option. Use of rifabutin is based on limited pharmacokinetic data. In the United States, rifabutin is FDA-approved for prevention of MAC, but not for prevention or treatment of tuberculosis.

For options 2 and 3, clinicians are advised:

1. At the start of therapy, perform frequent bacteriological evaluations to document bacteriological conversion to negative status, and after culture conversion to detect any possible treatment failures.
2. Extend duration of treatment to at least 18 months for option 2, or 9 months for option 3.
3. Use only indinavir with option 3.
4. Carefully monitor for drug toxicity.
5. Use directly observed therapy throughout.
6. Reevaluate periodically during the first 2 years after completion of therapy, including assessment of bacteriological status at 6-month intervals.
7. Instruct patients to report promptly any symptoms compatible with relapse of tuberculosis disease.

Source: Ref. 55.

In turn, this has led to a dramatic increase in tuberculosis resistant to conventional drugs. Multidrug-resistant tuberculosis (MDR-TB) may occur not only sporadically in patients who tend to be nonadherent to their medication regimen, but also in outbreaks in several congregate settings, including health care facilities (56). Patients who are immunosuppressed are most likely to develop active disease, which carries a very high mortality rate.

Over 350 cases were reported from a New York City multi-institutional outbreak between 1990 and 1993 involving MDR-TB strain W, including active disease in five health care workers (57). In this outbreak, 80% of the cases were HIV-infected, and more than two-thirds acquired MDR-TB nosocomially. Furthermore, this strain was accounted for nearly one-fourth of the cases of MDR-TB in the United States during a 43-month period. Institutional breach of published recommendations for prevention of nosocomial transmission of disease was often found.

There is no evidence to suggest that MDR-TB is any less transmissible than treatment-susceptible tuberculosis. A short exposure to MDR-TB, such as air travel has been reported (58). However, no transmission was demonstrated despite the MDR-TB source case being (4+ AFB) strongly positive and considered highly infectious.

VII. Preventive Therapy

An HIV infection increases the risk of developing active tuberculosis in patients with both infections. Persons without HIV infection who are tuberculin skin test positive have a 10% lifetime risk of developing active tuberculosis. In contrast, Selwyn et al. described a cohort of HIV-infected injection drug users, in whom the risk of developing active tuberculosis was 14% over 2 years, or 7.9 cases per 100 person-years (11). There was a high rate of skin test conversions among injection drug users, but only the HIV-seropositive individuals developed active tuberculosis, and none of the 13 seropositive patients who received tuberculosis prophylaxis with isoniazid developed tuberculosis. Injection drug use alone is an independent risk factor for developing tuberculosis (5). Among anergic injection drug users in New York City, the risk of developing active tuberculosis is high, and a decision analysis supports the use of universal tuberculosis prophylaxis (except for black women) in areas where the prevalence of tuberculosis is high (59,60).

In a sample of 118 predominantly female tuberculin-positive persons with HIV infection in Haiti, isoniazid offered protection against developing tuberculosis, and also increased the time to development of symptomatic HIV disease and AIDS (61). The patients were from a developing country, and the study did not have an adequate control population of tuberculin-negative patients to detect whether prophylaxis was beneficial to all patients from areas with high prevalence of tuberculosis who were HIV-positive.

Daley's investigation of tuberculosis cases among susceptible HIV-infected convalescent residents exposed to an infectious case showed a very rapid course of tuberculosis among the residents (10). The estimated risk of developing tuberculosis within 6 months clearly points to benefits of chemoprophylaxis. However, some suggest that lifetime prophylaxis may be indicated, for reinfection is a potential event among the HIV-infected population.

The CDC recommends preventive therapy for HIV-infected persons who have tuberculin skin tests with 5-mm or larger induration, a prior positive tuberculin test without treatment, or close contact with a person with active infection (62). Unless there is a high probability of exposure to a person with isoniazid-resistant infection, the recommended treatment is isoniazid, 300 mg daily plus pyridoxine 50 mg daily, for 12 months. In patients infected with suspected isoniazid-resistant strains, rifampin, 600 mg daily, is recommended, although the efficacy of this alternative is not as well established.

Adherence to preventive therapy among the dually infected persons (and especially injection drug users) is problematic (63). Preventive therapy is directed against a disease that the patient does not have, and drug interactions with agents used to treat HIV infection and prevent other opportunistic infections makes antituberculous prophylaxis a lower priority. To improve adherence, short-course chemoprophylaxis regimens are under investigation.

References

1. Raviglione M, Snider D, Kochi A. Global epidemiology of tuberculosis. JAMA 1995; 273:220–226.
2. DeCock K, Ekpini E, Gnaore E, Kadio A, Gayle H. The public health implications of AIDS research in Africa. JAMA 1994; 272:481–486.
3. Centers for Disease Control and Prevention (CDC). Acquired immunodeficiency syndrome—Dade County, Florida, 1981–1990. MMWR 1991; 40:489–493.
4. Centers for Disease Control and Prevention. Tuberculosis, 1985. MMWR 1986; 35:699–703.
5. Reichman L, Felton C, Edsall J. Drug dependence, a possible new risk factor for tuberculosis disease. Arch Intern Med 1979; 139:337–339.
6. O'Connor P, Selwyn P, Schottenfeld R. Medical care for injection-drug users with human immunodeficiency virus infection. N Engl J Med 1994; 331:450–459.
7. Crane C, Wise F, Reardon F, Brunner W, Dorfman B, Coulter S, Rutherford G. Crack cocaine use among persons with tuberculosis, Contra Costa County, California 1987–1990. MMWR 1991; 40:485–489.
8. Brudney K, Dobkin J. Resurgent tuberculosis in New York City, human immunodeficiency virus, homelessness and the decline of tuberculosis control programs. Am Rev Respir Dis 1991; 144:745–749.
9. Hurowitz J. Toward a social policy for health. N Engl J Med 1993; 329:130–133.
10. Daley C, Small P, Schecter G, et al. An outbreak of tuberculosis with accelerated progression among persons with the human immunodeficiency virus: an analy-

sis using restriction-fragment-length polymorphisms. N Engl J Med 1992; 326:231–235.
11. Selwyn P, Hartel D, Lewis VA, Schoenbaum E, Vermund SH, Klein RS, Walker AT, Friedland GH. A prospective study of the risk of tuberculosis among intravenous drug users with human immunodeficiency virus infection. N Engl J Med 1989; 320:545–550.
12. Lindan C, Allen S, Serufilira A, Lifson AR, Van de Perre P, Rundle AC, Batungwanayo J, Nsengumuremyi F, Bogaerts J, Hulley S. Predictors of mortality among HIV-infected women in Kigali, Rwanda. Ann Intern Med 1992; 116:320–328.
13. Chaisson R, Slutkin G. Tuberculosis and HIV infection. J Infect Dis 1989; 159:96–100.
14. Centers for Disease Control and Prevention. Revision of the CDC surveillance case definition for acquired immununodeficiency syndrome. MMWR 1987; 36:3–13.
15. Sunderam G, McDonald R, Maniatis T, Oleske J, Kapila R, Reichman L. Tuberculosis as a manifestation of the acquired immunodeficiency syndrome (AIDS). JAMA 1986; 256:362–366.
16. Pitchenik A, Rubinson H. The radiographic appearance of tuberculosis in patients with the acquired immune deficiency syndrome (AIDS). Am Rev Respir Dis 1985; 131:93–96.
17. Chaisson R, Schecter G, Theuer C, Rutherford G, Echenberg D, Hopewell P. Tuberculosis in patients with the acquired immunodeficiency syndrome: clinical features, response to therapy and survival. Am Rev Respir Dis 1987; 136:570–574.
18. Case record of the Massachusetts General Hospital. weekly clinico-pathologic exercises: case 15-1977. N Engl J Med 1977; 287:1390–1397.
19. Mangura B, Mangura C, Reichman L. Tuberculosis and the atypical pneumonia syndrome. Clin Chest Med 1991; 12:349–425.
20. Counsell S, Tan J, Dittus R. Unsuspected pulmonary tuberculosis in a community teaching hospital. Arch Intern Med 1989; 149:1274–1278.
21. Kissner D. Tuberculosis: missed opportunities. Arch Intern Med 1987; 147:2037–2040.
22. Small P, Schecter G, Goodman PC, Sande MA, Chaisson RE, Hopewell PC. Treatment of tuberculosis in patients with advanced human immunodeficiency virus infection. N Engl J Med 1991; 324:289–294.
23. Barnes P, Steele N, Young S, Vachol L. Tuberculosis in patients with human immunodeficiency virus infection: how often does it mimic *Pneumocystis carinii* pneumonia? Chest 1992; 102:428–432.
24. Pedro-Botet J, Gutierrez J, Miralles R, Coll J, Rubies-Prat J. Pulmonary tuberculosis in HIV-infected patients with normal chest radiographs. AIDS 1992; 6:91–93.
25. Henderson J, Conway D. Active intrathoracic tuberculosis with clear lung fields. Chest 1992; 101:1677–1758.
26. Anatoniskis D, Amin K, Barnes P. Pleuritis as a manifestation of reactivation tuberculosis. Am J Med 1990; 89:449–450.

27. Smith R, Yew K, Berkowitz K, Aranda C. Factors affecting the yield of acid fast sputum smears in patients with HIV and tuberculosis. Chest 1994; 106:684–686.
28. Schneider R, Hansen N, Rosen MJ, Kvale PA, Fulkerson WJ, Goodman P, Meiselman L, Glassroth J, Reichman LB, Wallace JM, Hopewell PC and the Pulmonary Complications of HIV Infection Study Group. Lack of usefulness of radiographic screening for pulmonary disease in asymptomatic HIV-infected adults. Arch Intern Med 1996; 156:191–195.
29. Long R, Salcini M, Manfreda J, Jean-Baptiste M, Hershfield E. The impact of HIV on the usefulness of sputum smears for the diagnosis of tuberculosis. Am J Public Health 1991; 81:1326–1328.
30. Modilevsky T, Sattler F, Barnes P. Mycobacterial disease in patients with human immunodeficiency virus infection. Arch Intern Med. 1989; 149:2201–2205.
31. Kvale P, Johnson M, Wroblewski D. Diagnosis of tuberculosis: routine cultures of bronchial washings are not indicated. Chest 1979; 76:140–142.
32. Stover D, White D, Romano P, Gellene R. Diagnosis of pulmonary disease in acquired immune deficiency syndrome (AIDS). Role of bronchoscopy and bronchoalveolar lavage. Am Rev Respir Dis 1984; 130:659–662.
33. Miro A, Gibilara E, Powell S, Kamholz S. The role of fiberoptic bronchoscopy for diagnosis of pulmonary tuberculosis in patients at risk for AIDS. Chest 1992; 101: 1211–1214.
34. Kramer F, Modilevsky T, Waliany A, Leedom J, Barnes P. Delayed diagnosis of tuberculosis in patients with human immunodeficiency virus infection. Am J Med 1990; 89:451–456.
35. Malasky C, Jordan T, Potulsky F, Reichman L. Occupational tuberculous infection among pulmonary physicians in training. Am Rev Respir Dis 1990; 142:505–507.
36. Judson M, Sahn S. Endobronchial lesions in HIV-infected individuals. Chest 1994; 105:1314–1324.
37. Wasser L, Shaw G, Talavera W. Endobronchial tuberculosis in the acquired immunodeficiency syndrome. Chest 1988; 94:1240–1243.
38. Macguire G, DeLorenzo L, Brown R, Davidian M. Case report. Endobronchial tuberculosis simulating carcinoma in a patient with the acquired immunodeficiency syndrome. Am J Med Sci 1987; 294:42–44.
39. Van Den Brande P, Lambrechts M, Tack J, Demedts M. Endobronchial tuberculosis mimicking lung cancer in elderly patients. Respir Med 1991; 85:107–109.
40. Rimmer J, Gibson P, Bryant D. Extension of pulmonary tuberculosis after fiberoptic bronchoscopy. Tubercle 1988; 69:57–61.
41. Catanzaro A. Rapid diagnostic tests for tuberculosis: what is the appropriate use? Am J Respir Crit Care Med 1997; 155:1804–1814.
42. Schluger N, Kinney D, Harkin T, Rom W. Clinical utility of the polymerase chain reaction in the diagnosis of infections due to *Mycobacterium tuberculosis*. Chest 1994; 105:1116–1121.
43. Chin D, Yajko D, Hadley W, Sanders C, Nassos P, Madej J, Hopewell P. Clinical utility of a commercial test based on the polymerase chain reaction for detect-

ing *Mycobacterium tuberculosis* in respiratory specimens. Am J Respir Crit Care Med 1995; 151:1872–1877.
44. Noordhoek G, Kolk A, Bjune G, Catty D, Dale JW, Fine PE, Godfrey-Fausesett P, Cho SN, Shinnick T, Svenson SB, Wilson S, van Embden J. Sensitivity and specificity of PCR for detection of *Mycobacterium tuberculosis*: a blind comparison study among seven laboratories. J Clin Microbiol 1994; 32:277–284.
45. Centers for Disease Control and Prevention. Purified protein derivative tuberculin anergy and HIV infection. Guidelines for anergy testing and management of anergic persons at risk of tuberculosis. MMWR 1994; 40:27.
46. Markowitz N, Hansen N, Wilcosky TC, Hopewell PC, Glassroth J, Kvale PA, Mangura BT, Osmond D, Wallace JM, Rosen MJ, Reichman LB for the Pulmonary Complications of HIV Infection Study Group. Tuberculin and anergy testing among HIV-seropositive and HIV seronegative persons. Ann Intern Med 1993; 119:185–193.
47. Markowitz N, Hansen NI, Hopewell PC, Glassroth J, Kvale PA, Mangura BT, Wilcosky TC, Wallace JM, Rosen MJ, Reichman LB, and the Pulmonary Complications of HIV Infection Study Group. The incidence of tuberculosis in the United States among HIV-infected persons. Ann Intern Med 1997; 126:123–132.
48. Graham N, Nelson K, Solomon L, Bonds M, Rizzo RT, Scavotto J, Astemborski J, Vlahov D. Prevalence of tuberculin positivity and skin test anergy in HIV-1 seropositive and seronegative intravenous drug users. JAMA 1992; 267:369–373.
49. Chin D, Osmond D, Page-Shafer K, Glassroth J, Rosen MJ, Reichman LB, Kvale PA, Wallace JM, Poole K, Hopewell PC and the Pulmonary Complications of HIV Infection Study Group. Reliability of anergy skin testing in persons with HIV infection. Am J Respir Crit Care Med 1996; 153:1982–1984.
50. Caiffa W, Graham N, Galai N, Rizzo R, Nelson K, Vlahov D. Instability of delayed-type hypersensitivity skin test anergy in human immunodeficiency virus infection. Arch Intern Med 1995; 155:2111–2117.
51. Whalen C, Horsburgh C, Hom D, Lahart C, Simberkoff M, Ellner J. Accelerated course of human immunodeficiency virus infection after tuberculosis. Am J Respir Crit Care Med 1995; 151:129–135.
52. Goletti D, Weissman D, Jackson R, Graham NMH, Vlahov D, Klein RS, Munisiff SS, Ortona L, Cauda R, Fauci AS. Effect of *Mycobacterium tuberculosis* on HIV replication: role of immune activation. J. Immunol 1996; 157:1271–1278.
53. American Thoracic Society, Centers for Disease Control and Prevention. Treatment of tuberculosis and tuberculosis infection in adults and children. Am J Respir Crit Care Med 1994; 149:1359–1374.
54. Perriens JH, St Louis M, Mukadi YB, Brown C, Prignot J, Pouthier F, Portaels F, Williame JC, Mandala JK, Kaboto M, Ryder RW, Roscigno G, Piot P. Pulmonary tuberculosis in HIV-infected patients in Zaire. A controlled trial of treatment for either six or twelve months. N Engl J Med 1995; 332:779–784.
55. Centers for Disease Control and Prevention. Clinical update: impact of HIV protease inhibitors on the treatment of HIV infected tuberculosis patients with rifampin. MMWR 1996; 45:921–925.

56. Centers for Disease Control and Prevention. Nosocomial transmission of multidrug-resistant tuberculosis among HIV infected persons—Florida and New York, 1988–1991. MMWR 1991; 40:585–591.
57. Frieden T, Sherman, L, Maw KL, Fujiwara PI, Crawford JT, Nivin B, Sharp V, Hewlett D, Brudeny K, Alland D, Kreiswirth BN. A multi-institutional outbreak of highly drug-resistant tuberculosis. Epidemiology and clinical outcomes. JAMA 1996; 276:1229–1235.
58. McFarland J, Hickman C, Osterholm M, MacDonald K.Exposure to *Mycobacterium tuberculosis* during air travel. Lancet 1993; 342:112–113.
59. Selwyn P, Sckell B, Alcabes P, Friedland G, Klein R, Schoenbaum E. High risk of active tuberculosis in HIV infected drug users with cutaneous anergy. JAMA 1992; 268:504–509.
60. Jordan T, Lewitt E, Montgomery R, Reichman L. Isoniazid as preventive therapy in HIV-infected intravenous drug abusers. A decision analysis. JAMA 1991; 265:2987–2991.
61. Pape J, Jean S, Ho J, Hafner A, Johnson W. Effect of isoniazid prophylaxis on incidence of active tuberculosis and progression of HIV infection. Lancet 1993; 342:268–272.
62. Centers for Disease Control and Prevention. USPHS/IDSA guidelines for the prevention of opportunistic infections in persons infected with human immunodeficiency virus: a summary. MMWR 1995; 44:
63. Sumartojo E. When tuberculosis treatment fails. Am Rev Respir Dis 1993; 147:1311–1320.

14

Viral Infections of the Lung in HIV Infection

JEANNE MARIE WALLACE

Olive View–UCLA Medical Center at Los Angeles
Sylmar, California

I. Introduction

Secondary viral infections frequently complicate human immunodeficiency virus (HIV) disease (1,2). In the lung, secondary viral infection is common, particularly during the later stages of HIV infection (1), but the extent to which viruses cause clinically significant pulmonary disease in HIV-infected persons has not always been clear. This uncertainty has been partly due to limitations in diagnosis and partly to difficulty in assessing the clinical significance once a viral agent has been identified.

The types of viruses that have been identified in lung tissue are listed in Table 1. Surveys of viruses identified in bronchoalveolar lavage (BAL) fluid and postmortem tissue indicate that, although cytomegalovirus (CMV) is the most frequently isolated, a variety of other viruses, including herpes simplex virus (HSV), adenovirus. influenza–parainfluenza viruses, rhinovirus. and respiratory syncytial virus (RSV), may also be present in the lower respiratory tract (3,4) of HIV-infected individuals. Because specific antiviral therapy is available for several of these infections, their recognition has become increasingly important.

Table 1 Viral Infections of the Lung in HIV Disease

Herpesviruses
Cytomegalovirus
Herpes simplex virus
Varicella–zoster virus
Epstein–Barr virus
Influenza viruses
Respiratory syncytial virus
Measles virus
Adenoviruses
Rhinovirus
Human immunodeficiency virus (primary)

II. Herpesvirus Infections

As with other immunodeficient conditions, secondary herpesvirus infections are a significant source of morbidity and mortality in acquired immunodeficiency syndrome (AIDS; 5). This family of viruses have in common a high frequency of asymptomatic infection during childhood and the ability to persist in a latent form in host tissue for many years after the initial infection. Intact cell-mediated immunity is of major importance for the constant containment of latent herpesvirus infection. With the progression of HIV infection, the development of altered cellular immunity allows reactivation and replication of herpes viruses, which may proceed to clinically apparent disease. Although CMV has been the most frequently demonstrated in lung tissue, all four of the herpesviruses have been implicated as direct or indirect causes of pneumonitis in persons with HIV disease.

A. Cytomegalovirus

Infection with CMV is a well-recognized complication of HIV disease. Autopsy studies have demonstrated active CMV infection in up to 90% of AIDS patients (6), and several have found CMV to be the most prevalent pathogen (6–8). The lung is frequently involved, and it may be the only site of CMV infection (7). Although pneumocystosis has been the most common clinically apparent pulmonary complication during life, CMV pneumonitis has been the most frequently noted at autopsy (7,8). In most cases. the presence of CMV lung infection was undetected during life (6–8), and in many, disease caused by CMV when evaluated at autopsy was considered insignificant (7). CMV disease or CMV pneumonitis has been specified as a primary cause of death in 14% of autopsy cases (8,9). The death rate owing to CMV infection appears to have declined slightly since the beginning of the AIDS epidemic (9).

The clinical manifestations of CMV pneumonitis have ranged from subclinical infection, to severe disease, causing respiratory failure. In patients with AIDS, most cases of CMV pneumonitis occur simultaneously with one or more additional pathological processes, such as *Pneumocystis* pneumonia or Kaposi's sarcoma. The clinical presentation is essentially the same as that of several other pulmonary opportunistic infections that affect patients with AIDS. Fever, dyspnea, and nonproductive cough are common. The rapidly fulminant course seen in bone marrow transplant patients seldom occurs in patients with HIV disease. Usually, the role of CMV in causing symptoms is difficult to assess because of the frequent coinfection with other agents.

Mechanisms of CMV Infection

Cytomegalovirus is ubiquitous in the environment. Although infection with CMV is common, clinical illness caused by the infection is rare in persons with normal immune status. The initial or primary infection usually occurs during childhood or early adulthood and is often asymptomatic. Subsequently, there may be a prolonged latent stage, during which the virus or viral genome resides in certain cells without actively replicating or causing detectable damage. During this period, CMV may persist in peripheral blood leukocytes, and in various organ sites, such as the colon, spleen, salivary glands, prostate, and testes (10).

Latent CMV may be reactivated after years of inapparent infection. Reactivation may be subclinical, evident only by the ability to culture the virus from body fluids; or it may cause significant disease. Several factors may lead to reactivation of latent CMV infection, but immunosuppression, particularly of cell-mediated immune mechanisms, appears to be the most important. Individuals seropositive for CMV may be reinfected by a different strain of virus from an exogenous source (11).

Latent CMV infection is common among groups of individuals at risk for HIV infection. Seroprevalence studies have shown that nearly 100% of asymptomatic homosexual men are infected, and more than half actively shed the virus in urine and semen (12). Accordingly, CMV infection has been demonstrated by viral culture or serological testing in most HIV-seropositive persons (13). It has been suggested that CMV infection may be associated with more rapid progression of HIV disease (13,14). As with other immunocompromised hosts, CMV infection is often widely disseminated in HIV-infected persons. The most common sites of organ involvement include lung, adrenal, colon, liver, retina, and central nervous system (CNS). The CMV infection may be particularly fulminant in the brain (15), where CMV-infected areas may be surrounded by dense collections of HIV-infected macrophages, and coinfection of the same cell by CMV and HIV has been demonstrated (16). suggesting synergistic interaction between the two viruses (13).

Pathogenesis of CMV Pneumonitis

Alveolar macrophages are extremely permissive to CMV replication (17). Thus, in patients with advanced HIV disease, the high prevalence of CMV pulmonary infection might be expected owing to the combination of reactivation of latent CMV infection and support of local replication in the lung.

The exact role of CMV in the pathogenesis of pneumonitis is not entirely clear. Lung tissue from patients with CMV pneumonitis has shown various degrees of interstitial pneumonitis, with focal or diffuse mononuclear infiltration, interstitial edema and fibrosis, and diffusely distributed cytomegalic cells. Severe cases have been associated with diffuse alveolar damage. These findings suggest that tissue destruction is due to cell infection and death, as well as to lung injury caused by a local inflammatory response. In bone marrow transplant patients, CMV pneumonitis usually occurs with graft-versus-host disease, and the lung injury may be due to an immunopathological process in which T-cell cytotoxicity is directed against viral antigens expressed on infected cells (17). In advanced HIV disease, cytotoxic responses are impaired (18), suggesting that any lung damage from CMV pneumonitis might be a direct effect of CMV infection and replication. However, severe CMV pneumonitis has been reported in a few patients with less-advanced HIV disease (18).

In addition to any direct effects, it is well-recognized that CMV infection itself may cause immunosuppression. CMV infection has been associated with elevated levels of $CD8^+$ cells and inverted CD4/CD8 cell ratios, as well as with impaired lymphocytic blastogenesis to mitogens and viral antigens (19,20). These phenomena suggest that CMV further impairs cell-mediated immune mechanisms. At a local level, this could be another factor contributing to the frequent respiratory coinfection with other infectious agents.

Clinical Significance

In contrast to patients with organ transplantation, in whom CMV pneumonitis is a major cause of morbidity and mortality, the clinical significance of CMV pneumonitis in HIV-infected patients has been difficult to assess. A major source of difficulty has arisen from the tendency for CMV to coexist with other pulmonary infections. Because there are a few cases in which

CMV has been the only pathogenic agent isolated, it is now accepted that CMV can cause significant lung disease and even death of respiratory failure (2,7). It is less clear what, if any, pathogenic role CMV plays when it it is one of multiple organisms infecting the lung. In HIV-infected patients with *Pneumocystis carinii* pneumonia, conflicting studies have suggested that coinfection with CMV results in a poorer outcome (21), or with a less severe course, possibly owing to decreased inflammatory response (22). Another source of confusion over the significance of CMV pneumonitis has been a lack of agreement in the definition. There has been a tendency to look at the consequences of detection of CMV in respiratory specimens, rather than documented CMV infection of the lung. Thus although several studies have shown that detection of CMV in respiratory specimens is not predictive of death or poorer outcome (23–25), it has not been clear if many of the patients included had CMV infection of the lower respiratory tract, or contamination of respiratory secretions by upper respiratory tract secretions.

A spectrum of pathological findings, ranging from relatively mild interstitial pneumonitis to severe lung injury, with diffuse alveolar damage, have been reported in lung tissue from patients dying of advanced HIV disease and CMV pneumonitis (Figs. 1 and 2). It is possible that mild fo-

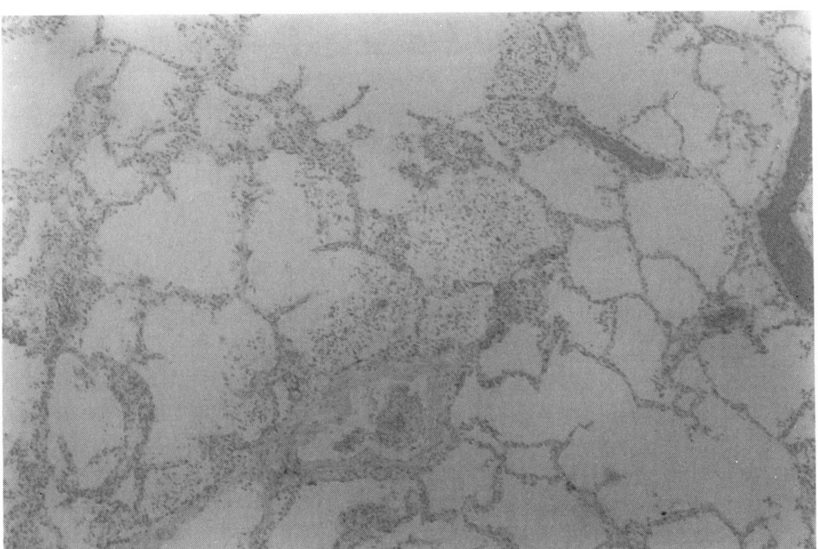

Figure 1 Mild CMV pneumonitis with minimal alveolar damage (hematoxylin–eosin [H&E] stain; original magnification ×100).

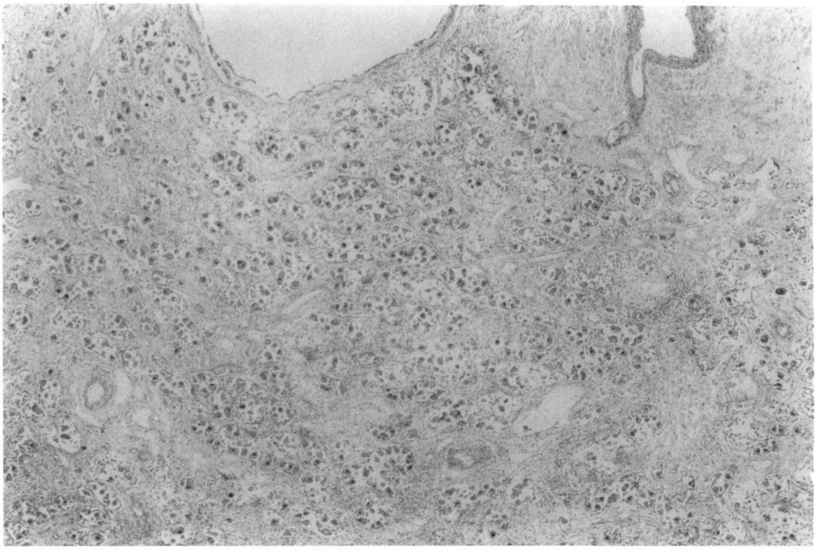

Figure 2 Severe CMV pneumonitis with diffuse alveolar damage (H & E stain; original magnification ×100).

cal interstitial pneumonitis represents early disease, which may occasionally progress to cause more severe pathology with time. Even the mild form of CMV infection could have important consequences. In addition to direct effects, CMV-related alterations of local immune and effector cells could predispose to more frequent and severe infection with other organisms, or to delayed treatment response.

Diagnosis

It is important to distinguish between CMV infection and CMV pneumonitis. Because the salivary glands are a frequent site of subclinical infection in patients with HIV disease, CMV may be constantly secreted in saliva so that the virus may be isolated from respiratory secretions in the absence of histopathological evidence of lung involvement. As a diagnostic test for CMV pneumonitis, conventional culture has been reported to have a positive predictive power of 57, compared with 100 for demonstration of CMV cells with inclusion bodies by cytological techniques (26). When considering the high prevalence of CMV infection in patients with HIV disease, there could be little diagnostic significance of CMV detection in respiratory specimens subject to contamination by upper airway secretions. Histological or cytological evidence of infected lung cells is a necessary criterion for the diagnosis of CMV pneumonitis.

Demonstration of pathognomonic cells with intranuclear or intracytoplasmic inclusion bodies in lung tissue or cytological specimens has been the most widely available means of demonstrating CMV pneumonitis in patients with HIV disease. Unfortunately, the CMV cells may be sparsely distributed even in individuals with significant disease; consequently, they may not be detected in the specimen obtained. With this conventional indicator, the diagnostic yield of all pulmonary procedures has been low (7).

The potential for diagnosis of CMV pneumonitis by procedures less invasive than open-lung biopsy could be influenced by progress in two areas: (1) better sampling of the lung by bronchoalveolar lavage (BAL); and (2) more sensitive techniques of detecting CMV-infected cells.

Because of the propensity for CMV to be unevenly, and sometimes sparsely, distributed in affected tissue, adequate sampling is essential to provide a diagnosis. Large tissue specimens obtained by open-lung biopsy or autopsy have been required. More recently, BAL has emerged as a means to obtain lower respiratory tract cells and to sample representative portions of the lung. BAL would appear to be an effective means of providing a diagnosis of CMV pneumonitis because the cells most often noted to contain the characteristic inclusions have been alveolar macrophages and alveolar epithelial cells, both of which are present in the specimens obtained. Yet, although cytological examination of BAL has a high specificity, it has had limited value owing to the low sensitivity, which has ranged from 20–30% (26–28). Nevertheless, because BAL is safe, relatively noninvasive, and widely available, it should be the first procedure performed if CMV pneumonitis is suspected.

The use of CMV-specific DNA probes and monoclonal antibodies (MAbs) has shown promise in detecting CMV-infected cells, and these methods have the potential for improving the sensitivity of BAL specimens (Fig. 3). Several reports have characterized in situ hybridization with DNA probes as being a rapid, sensitive, and specific method for diagnosing CMV infection in tissue and BAL specimens (29–31). This technique detects CMV DNA not only in cytomegalic inclusion cells, but also in histologically normal cells; therefore, it provides a higher diagnostic yield than conventional histopathological and cytological stains. Detection of virus by in situ hybridization does not require the presence of intact or replicating viruses. Therefore, care must be taken in interpreting positive results as an independent indication of active viral disease. The numbers of positive cells, as well as correlation with viral cultures and the patient's clinical status must also be considered when determining the presence of active CMV pneumonitis.

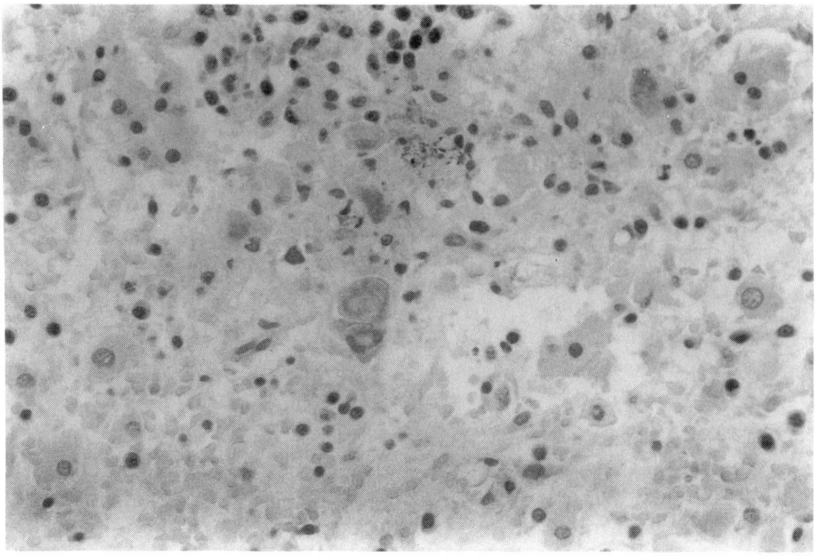

Figure 3 Lung tissue containing CMV cells stained with monoclonal antibody preparation. The round dark bodies represent intranuclear and intracytoplasmic CMV (original magnification ×200).

Human or murine MAbs have been reported to be useful for detecting CMV-infected cells in BAL specimens (32). A significant proportion of positive cells, more than 0.5%, has been correlated with the presence of clinical features, the ability to culture the virus from lung tissue, and histopathological evidence of CMV pneumonitis in lung tissue during life and at autopsy. A low proportion of positive cells, less than 0.1%, was noted in some patients not considered to have primary lung disease caused by CMV.

Treatment

Treatment for CMV pneumonitis in patients with HIV disease should be considered if (1) a symptomatic patient has documented lung involvement with CMV as the sole pathogen; or (2) another infectious agent is present in addition to CMV, but the patient is deteriorating clinically despite adequate treatment of the copathogen. Two antiviral agents, ganciclovir and foscarnet are effective in the treatment of CMV infections.

Ganciclovir acts by inhibiting viral replication by CMV DNA polymerase. It should be administered intravenously as a constant infusion over approximately 1 hr at a dosage of 5 mg/kg twice daily, although higher doses may be required to produce a clinical response. Because ganciclovir is excreted by the kidneys, its dosage must be reduced according to creatinine clearance. The most frequent toxicity has been granulocytopenia and thrombocytopenia that, in most cases, has been reversible with withdrawal of the drug. Viral resistance has been observed, usually with prolonged administration, and it is possible that some patients may develop primary infection with resistant strains.

Foscarnet is an organic analogue of inorganic pyrophosphate that selectively inhibits virus-specific DNA polymerases. CMV strains resistant to ganciclovir may be sensitive to foscarnet. It should be given as an infusion at a dosage of 60 mg/kg every 8 hr. Similar to ganciclovir, the dosage must be adjusted for renal insufficiency. Renal impairment is the major toxicity of foscarnet, and occurs to some degree in most patients receiving the drug over time; hence, renal function must be monitored. Foscarnet also alters plasma electrolyte levels, resulting in seizures; therefore, serum electrolyte concentrations should also be monitored during administration.

B. Herpes Simplex Virus

Defective cellular immunity is a strong predisposing factor for severe herpes simplex virus (HSV) infection. In such circumstances, the virus can proceed from cell to cell without entering the extracellular environment in which antibody neutralization may take place. Infection with HSV has been documented in one-third of patients with advanced HIV disease, who have opportunistic infections, as oral or perirectal ulcers or by isolation in throat washings in the absence of oral ulcers (5). It usually appears to be a reactivation of latent infection. In general, severe HSV disease may occur in the immunocompromised host as one of three syndromes: (1) chronic, often extensive cutaneous or mucocutaneous disease; (2) involvement of one organ site, usually esophagus or lung; or (3) widespread dissemination. In HIV disease, HSV infection usually takes the form of local involvement of the genital or perianal region or oral cavity, dissemination being uncommon.

Pneumonitis caused by HSV-1 or HSV-2 occasionally complicates advanced HIV disease (3,33,34) and has been observed in 0.2–4% of autopsy cases (4,9). Although detailed descriptions of the clinical manifestations HSV pneumonitis in HIV disease have not appeared in the literature, it appears that they are similar to what has been observed in patients with other underlying disorders, including organ transplantation, cancer, alcoholism, burns, and renal failure. Pulmonary HSV infection may cause a focal necrotizing process or diffuse interstitial pneumonitis (35). When focal, it often occurs with necrotizing tracheobronchitis, and it appears to be due to contiguous spread. Diffuse interstitial pneumonia is likely to be a manifestation of hematogenous dissemination.

Making a diagnosis of HSV pneumonitis may not be straightforward. Because immunocompromised patients frequently have oral lesions or asymptomatic shedding of HSV in saliva, characteristic mucocutaneous lesions or positive upper respiratory tract cultures are suggestive, but not diagnostic. Diagnosis should be based on demonstration of HSV infection in lower respiratory tract specimens by culture and histopathology. HSV may be identified in lung tissue and cytological preparations by the presence of typical giant cells and, less commonly, by Cowdry type A intranuclear cell inclusions that may also be seen with CMV and varicella-zoster infections. In one autopsy series, premortem specimens, including open-lung biopsies; were often nondiagnostic in patients dying of HSV pneumonitis (35). Therefore, treatment may be indicated in critically ill patients suspected of having HSV pneumonitis, even if the infection is not documented in lower respiratory specimens.

The importance of recognizing HSV pneumonitis lies in the availability of potentially effective treatment with acyclovir. Patients with life-threatening HSV pneumonitis should receive high-dose IV acyclovir at a dose of 30 mg/kg in three divided doses. The dosage must be adjusted for renal impairment. The minimal course of treatment should be 10 days, but a longer duration may be necessary. Patients requiring a prolonged course of acyclovir may be switched to oral therapy (200 mg five times daily).

C. Varicella–Zoster Virus

Children who are infected with HIV and who develop varicella-zoster virus (VZV) infection have a variable course, although those with low CD4 counts tend to have a longer duration of disease and a higher rate of complications (36, 37). Pneumonitis has been one of the most frequent severe complications of VZV infection in HIV-infected children. and has been reported occasionally in adults. Most cases present with diffuse alveolar-interstitial pulmonary infiltration, with or without other sites of visceral involvement (37). Some VZV infections have led to respiratory failure and death; others have had a relatively benign course, responding to acyclovir therapy. Although reactivated VZV infection (shingles) has been complicated by VZV pneumonitis in patients with severe immunocompromise, this phenomenon has not been reported in patients with HIV disease (38).

Early institution of acyclovir therapy may significantly improve the outcome in patients with VZV pneumonia or disseminated disease. Acyclovir should be given IV, 30 mg/kg in three divided doses, for at least 10 days.

D. Epstein–Barr Virus

Approximately 90% of healthy adults have evidence of previous Epstein–Barr virus (EBV) infection, most acquired during childhood or adolescence in the form of infectious mononucleosis, or as an asymptomatic infection (39). The primary target is the B cell, which has specific surface receptors that bind EBV. Cellular infection with EBV usually results in transformation, rather than active viral replication. Productive infection may occur in the epithelial cells of the oropharynx or parotid glands. Infection with EBV may evoke a potent immune response in the form of polyclonal proliferation of B cells and activation of cytotoxic T cells and macrophages. The type and extent of immune response appears to be a major factor determining the outcome of EBV infection. In patients with HIV infection, EBV may be manifested as a Burkitt-like non-Hodgkin's lymphoma, oral hairy leukoplakia, or asymptomatic replication in the oral epithelium or parotid glands (39,40).

A possible role of EBV in causing lymphoid interstitial pneumonia (LIP) and pulmonary lymphoid hyperplasia in children with HIV disease has been suggested (41,42). In one study, EBV DNA was found in 80% of lung biopsy specimens from HIV-infected children with LIP, and corresponding evidence of the virus being absent was noted in tissue from children with pulmonary disease other than LIP (41). In these cases, LIP might have been a result of EBV replication within the lung, leading to infiltration of EBV-infected cells, as well as reactive lymphocytes and macrophages. Other reports have suggested that HIV infection of the lung may play a role in the development of LIP (43). Because EBV-infected B cells are more susceptible to infection by HIV in vitro, the pathogenesis of LIP could involve coinfection with EBV and HIV (44).

III. The Influenza Viruses

Currently, there is no evidence that symptomatic influenza occurs with greater frequency (34) or severity (45–47) in HIV-infected individuals, although properly designed studies have not directly addressed this possibility. Reports of small numbers of HIV- infected patients with virologically proved episodes of influenza have suggested that some may have prolongation of respiratory symptoms (45) or viral shedding from the respiratory tract (48). Primary influenza pneumonia has been reported rarely in HIV disease (45,49), consistent with the low estimated rate in patients with influenza (50). Studies in mice suggest that local immune responses may contribute to the pathogenesis of influenza pneumonia (51,52), raising the possibility that this complication may be less likely in individuals with HIV-associated immunodeficiency.

Controlled trials of the efficacy of inactivated influenza vaccine in HIV-infected adults have found it to be safe. but to elicit suboptimal antibody responses, even in many without HIV-associated symptoms (53,54). Furthermore, one trial found that a booster dose given 1 month later did not significantly increase the frequency or magnitude of antibody response (55). The possibility that many individuals with HIV disease may remain unprotected after immunization, along with the question of whether influenza causes increased morbidity has raised questions about the cost-effectiveness of influenza vaccine in this group (56). Nevertheless, annual influenza vaccine is recommended in HIV-infected persons because of the safety of the vaccine, achievement of protective antibody levels in some recipients, and the greater risk for pulmonary infection by bacterial pathogens that complicate influenza. None of the influenza vaccine trials have shown evidence of more rapid HIV disease progression after immunization, a theoretical consideration that has been of concern to some clinicians.

Although there are no data on efficacy in HIV-infected persons, chemoprophylaxis and early treatment with amantadine or rimantadine appears to be well tolerated (47). During influenza epidemics, use of these agents should be considered in HIV-seropositive individuals with exposure or abrupt symptoms even when they have received their annual vaccination. The usual adult dosage of amantadine and rimantadine is 100 mg twice daily. The dosage must be reduced in persons with renal insufficiency or an active seizure disorder.

IV. Respiratory Syncytial Virus

Respiratory syncytial virus (RSV) has been documented alone or as a copathogen with *P. carinii* or *Pseudomonas aeruginosa* in cases of HIV-related pneumonitis in infants, children, and adults (57–59). HIV-infected children have a higher incidence of pneumonia caused by RSV and may have prolonged viral shedding; even after treatment (57). Severe disease that may lead to respiratory failure has been reported in adults as well as children (58,59). Rapid diagnosis from upper respiratory tract secretions or BAL specimens can be made using fluorescein-conjugated MAbs or enzyme-linked immunosorbent (ELISA) techniques (60). The virus may also be detected by culture of respiratory specimens (59).

The importance of considering this infection as a cause of severe respiratory disease in patients with HIV disease lies in the availability of potentially effective treatment with inhaled ribavirin. Because both children and adults with advanced HIV disease are at risk for severe or complicated

RSV infection, treatment should be considered for documented lower respiratory tract infection. In children ribavirin is nebulized into an oxygen tent or mask 12–18 hr/day from a 20-mg/mL solution by a small-particle generator supplied by the manufacturer. Adults with severe RSV pneumonitis may be treated with ribavirin aerosol by the same route at a dose of 6 g/day (58). Ribavirin can be administered during mechanical ventilation. However, because technical difficulties can occur if proper precautions are not observed, delivery by this route does require special expertise.

V. Measles (Rubeola) Virus

Several reports document that measles in HIV-infected children is often severe, and may be fatal (61–62). Pneumonia is a frequent complication that may lead to death, and may occur without a rash (64). Measles pneumonia presents as a diffuse interstitial process, characterized histologically by the presence of giant cells. It may go unrecognized when it occurs in the absence of the usual manifestations of measles. Life-threatening measles pneumonia has also been reported occasionally in adults (65,66). One survey of measles antibody prevalence in HIV-seropositive adults found that 95% had humoral evidence of measles immunity, and that declining immunity caused by progressive HIV infection was not associated with lack of antibody (67), suggesting that only a small proportion of adults are at risk for measles infection.

Immunization of HIV-infected children with live attenuated measles vaccine is safe, and the anticipated complications of possible clinically severe infection caused by the vaccine virus or accelerated HIV disease progression caused by triggering of HIV replication were not observed (62). Unfortunately, however, the immunogenicity of the vaccine was low, with severe, in some cases fatal, measles occurring in some children with advanced disease despite previous immunization. Postexposure passive immunization has also failed to prevent measles in a few HIV-infected children (62–64). Nevertheless, because of the absence of adverse consequences thus far observed, vaccination is recommended for asymptomatic HIV-infected children, as is consideration of vaccination for symptomatic HIV-infected children. In addition, postexposure immunoglobulin prophylaxis is recommended for all HIV-infected children, regardless of vaccination status (62).

Measles in HIV-infected children and adults has been treated successfully with aerosolized ribavirin, with or without intravenous immunoglobulin (62,65,66). The dosage and method of administration was the same as that for treatment of severe RSV infection.

VI. Adenoviruses

Adenovirus is an infrequent, but potentially clinically significant cause of pneumonitis in patients with HIV infection. Routine viral culture surveillance has resulted in isolation of adenovirus from BAL specimens (3) and from autopsy lung tissue (4,68) in a few patients with HIV disease who had pneumonitis. In addition. the lung was a prominent site of involvement in HIV-infected patients with disseminated adenovirus infection (69). The serotypes have included 1, 2, 3, 7, and 32.

In immunocompromised patients, with or without HIV disease, adenoviral pneumonitis has presented with high fever, severe systemic complaints, cough, and respiratory distress (69–71). Most patients have had diffuse bilateral pulmonary infiltration, although the radiographic findings have been focal in some cases. Pleural effusions may also be present. The clinical course has varied from death within a few days, to progressive improvement over several months. The pathological findings have been distinctive in that there may be extensive, sometimes necrotizing, bronchitis and bronchiolitis (71). Adenoviruses also have tropism for alveolar lining cells and may cause interstitial pneumonia, with hyaline membrane formation and interstitial fibrosis. Adenovirus infection may be demonstrated in lung tissue by the presence of characteristic "smudge cells" containing nuclei filled with basophilic material that obscures the nuclear membrane and by cells displaying amphophilic or eosinophilic intranuclear inclusions. The origin of the infection in immunocompromised hosts remains speculative. Because adenoviruses are known to establish latent infections, it is likely that some are endogenous. There is currently no specific treatment for adenoviral infection.

VII. Rhinoviruses

In a survey of viruses isolated from BAL specimens, rhinoviruses were isolated from eight immunocompromised patients, one of whom had advanced HIV disease (3). Radiographic evidence of diffuse or focal pulmonary infiltration was present at time of bronchoscopy. None of the cases was fatal.

VIII. Pulmonary HIV Infection

The HIV has been detected in the lung during asymptomatic, as well as advanced disease (72–74). In addition to resident lymphocytes and alveolar macrophages, pulmonary fibroblasts are susceptible to HIV infection

(74,75). Several observations raise the possibility that HIV may cause clinically significant lung disease.

Lymphocytic alveolitis associated with accumulation of $CD8^+$ cells has been described in patients with symptomatic and early symptomatic HIV disease (76,77). It has been suggested that lymphocytic alveolitis may arise from immunological responses to HIV in the lung, including the action of cytotoxic cells that are directed against HIV antigen and the surface membranes of infected cells (78,79). In a series of patients infected with HIV who had lymphocytic alveolitis and no detectable pulmonary infection or neoplasm, more than half had respiratory symptoms, primarily dyspnea on exertion or cough, a third had chest radiographic abnormalities, described as "diffuse interstitial opacities," and a third had a decreased carbon monoxide diffusing capacity or increased alveolar–arterial difference after exercise (76). A recent report has suggested that lymphocytic alveolitis is associated with increased mortality in HIV disease (80).

The possibility that HIV may play a role in the development of HIV-related LIP or nonspecific interstitial pneumonitis (NIP) has been raised by several investigators. Retroviruses other than HIV are known to have a the capability to cause a pulmonary disease similar to LIP, including maedi/visna virus, a lentiretrovirus that causes pulmonary disease in sheep (81). HIV has been detected in BAL fluid from HIV-infected patients with LIP (82) and HIV RNA has been demonstrated by in situ hybridization in lung tissue. (83). In a recent report, HIV RNA was demonstrated by in situ hybridization in seven lung biopsy specimens from HIV-infected patients with LIP or NIP, whereas other viruses, including CMV and EBV, were not found in any. This prompted the suggestion that HIV played a significant role in the pathogenesis (84). Further studies of this possibility are needed, because confirmation of the occurrence of primary HIV lung disease would have practical clinical implications.

References

1. Nelson JA, Ghazal P, Wiley CA. Role of opportunistic viral infections in AIDS. AIDS 1990; 4:1–10.
2. McKenzie R, Travis WD, Dolan SA, et al. The causes of death in patients with human immunodeficiency virus infection: a clinical and pathological study with emphasis on the role of pulmonary disease. Medicine 1991; 60:326–343.
3. Connolly MG, Baughman RP, Dohn MN, Linnemann CC. Recovery of viruses other than cytomegalovirus from bronchoalveolar lavage fluid. Chest 1994; 105:175–181.
4. Pillay D, Lipman MC, Lee CA, et al. A clinico-pathological audit of opportunistic viral infections in HIV-infected patients. AIDS 1993; 7:969–974.

5. Quinnan GV, Masur H. Rook AH, et al. Herpesvirus infections in the acquired immunodeficiency syndrome. JAMA 1984; 252:72–77.
6. Reichert CM, O'Leary TJ, Levens DL, et al. Autopsy pathology in the acquired immunodeficiency syndrome. Am J Pathol 1983; 112:357-382.
7. Wallace JM, Hannah J. Cytomegalovirus pneumonitis in patients with AIDS: findings in an autopsy study. Chest 1987; 92:198–203.
8. McKenzie R, Travis WD, Dolan S, et al. The causes of death in patients with human immunodeficiency virus infection: a clinical and pathologic study with emphasis on the role of pulmonary diseases. Medicine 1991; 70:326–343.
9. Klatt EC, Nichols L, Noguchi TT. Evolving trends revealed by autopsies of patients with the acquired immunodeficiency syndrome. Arch Pathol Lab Med 1994; 118:884–890.
10. Jordan MC. Latent infection and the elusive cytomegalovirus. Rev Infect Dis 1983; 5:205–215.
11. Onorato IM, Morens DM, Martone WJ, et al. Epidemiology of cytomegalovirus infections: recommendations for prevention and control. Rev Infect Dis 1985; 7:479–497.
12. Mintz L, Drew WL, Miner RC, et al. Cytomegalovirus infections in homosexual men: an epidemiologic study. Ann Intern Med 1983; 98:326–329.
13. Nelson JA, Ghazal P, Wiley CA. Role of opportunistic viral infections in AIDS. AIDS 1990; 4:1–10.
14. Morgello S, Cho ES, Nielson S, et al. Cytomegalovirus encephalitis in patients with acquired immunodeficiency svndrome. Hum Pathol 1987; 18:289–297.
15. Nelson JA, Reynolds-Kohler C, Oldstone MBA, et al. HIV and HCMV coinfect brain cells in patients with AIDS. Virology 1988; 165:286–290.
16. Drew WL, Mintz L, Hoo R, et al. Growth of herpes simplex and cytomegalovirus in cultured alveolar macrophages. Am Rev Respir Dis 1979; 119:287–291.
17. Frank I, Friedman HM. Progress in the treatment of cytomegalovirus pneumonia. Ann Intern Med 1988; 109:769–771.
18. Rosenberg ZF, Fauci AS. Immunopathogenesis of HIV infection. In: De Vita VT, Hellman S, Rosenberg SA, AIDS: Etiology, Diagnosis and Treatment. Philadelphia: JB Lippincott, 1992: 61–63.
18. Squire SB, Lipman MCI, Bagdades EK, et al. Severe cytomegalic pneumonitis in HIV infected patients with higher than average CD4 counts. Thorax 1992; 47:301–304.
19. Drew WL, Mills J, Levy J, et al. Cytomegalovirus infection and abnormal T-lymphocyte subset ratios in homosexual men. Ann Intern Med 1985; 103:61–63.
20. Rinaldo CR, Ho M, Hamoudi WH, et al. Lymphocyte subsets and natural killer responses during cytomegalovirus mononucleosis. Infect Immun 1983; 40:472–477.
21. Stover DE, White DA, Romano PA, et al. Spectrum of pulmonary diseases associated with the acquired immunodeficiency syndrome. Am J Med 1985; 78:429–437.
22. Bozzette SA, Arcia J Bartok, AE, et al. Impact of *Pneumocystis carinii* and cytomegalovirus on the course and outcome of atypical pneumonia in advanced human immunodeficiency virus disease. Infect Dis 1992: 165:93–98.

23. Miles PR, Baughman RP, Linneman CC. Cytomegalovirus in the bronchoalveolar lavage of patients with AIDS. Chest 1990; 97:1072–1076.
24. Millar AB, Patou G, Miller RF, et al. Cytomegalovirus in the lungs of patients with AIDS: respiratory pathogen or passenger? Am Rev Respir Dis 1990; 141:1474–1477.
25. Bower M, Barton SE, Nelson MR, et al. The significance of the detecton of cytomegalovirus in the bronchoalveolar lavage fluid of AIDS patients with pneumonia. AIDS 1990: 4:317–320.
26. Woods GL, Thompson AB, Rennard SL, et al. Detection of cytomegalovirus in bronchoalveolar lavage specimens. Chest 1990; 98:568–575.
27. Crawford SW, Bowden RA, Hackman RC, et al. Rapid detection of cytomegalovirus by bronchoalveolar lavage and centrifugation culture. Ann Intern Med 1988; 108:180–185.
28. Paradis IL, Grgurich WF, Dummer JS, et al. Rapid detection of cytomegalovirus pneumonia from lung lavage cells. Am Rev Respir Dis 1988; 138:697–702.
29. Spector S, Spector DH. The use of DNA probes in studies of human cytomegaloviruses. Clin Chem 1985; 31:1514–1520.
30. Keh WC, Garber MA. In situ hybridization for cytomegalovirus DNA in AIDS patients. Am J Pathol 1988: 131:490–496.
31. Hilborne LH, Nieberg RK, Cheng L, et al. Direct in situ hybridization for rapid detection of cytomegalovirus in bronchoalveolar lavage. Am J Clin Pathol 1987; 87:766–769.
32. Emanuel D, Peppard J, Stover D, et al. Rapid immunodiagnosis of cytomegalovirus pneumonia by bronchoalveolar lavage using human and murine monoclonal antibodies. Ann Intern Med 1986; 104:476–481.
33. Murray JF, Felton CP, Garay SM, et al. Pulmonary complications of the acquired immunodeficiency syndrome: Report of a National Heart, Lung and Blood Institute Workshop. N Engl J Med 1984; 310:1682–1688.
34. Wallace JM, Rao AV, Glassroth J, et al. Respiratory illness in persons with human immunodeficiency virus infection. Am Rev Respir Dis 1993; 148:1523–1529.
35. Ramsey PG, Fife KH, Hackman RC, et al. Herpes simplex virus pneumonia. Ann Intern Med 1982; 97:813–820.
36. Leibovitz E, Cooper D, Giurgiutiu D, et al. Varicella–zoster infection in Romanian children infected with the human immunodeficiency virus. Pediatrics 1993; 92:838–842.
37. Jura E, Chadwick EG, Josephs SH, et al. Varicella-zoster virus infections in children infected with human immunodeficiency syndrome. Pediatr Infect Dis 1989; 8:586–590.
38. Cohen PR, Beltrani VP, Grossman ME. Disseminated herpes zoster in patients with human immunodeficiency virus infection. Am J Med 1988; 84:1076–1080.
39. Purtilo DT, Lipscomb H, Kruger G, et al. Role of Epstein–Barr virus in acquired immunodeficiency syndrome. Adv Exp Med Biol 1985; 187:53–65.
40. Loning T, Henke RP, Reichert P, et al. In situ hybridization to detect Epstein-Barr vitus DNA in oral tissues of HIV-infected patients. Virchows Arch A 1987; 412:127–133.

41. Andiman WA, Eastman R, Martin R, et al. Opportunistic lymphoproliferation associated with Epstein–Barr viral DNA in infants and children with AIDS. Lancet 1985; 2:1390–1393.
42. Rubinstein A, Moreki R, Silverman B, et al. Pulmonary disease in children with acquired imunodeficiency syndrome. J Pediatr1986; 108:498–503.
43. Resnick I, Pitchenik AE, Fisher E, et al. Detection of HTLV-III/LAV specific IgG and antigen in bronchoalveolar lavage fluid from two patients with lymphocytic interstitial pneumonia associated with AIDS-related complex. Am J Med 1987; 82:553–556.
44. Montagnier L, Gruest J, Charmaret D, et al. Adaptation of lymphadenopathy associated virus (LAV) to replication in EBV-transformed B lymphoblastoid cell lines. Science 1984; 225:63–66.
45. Safrin S, Rush JD, Mills J. Influenza in patients with human immunodeficiency virus infection. Chest 1990; 98:33–37.
46. Thurn JR, Henry K. Influenza A pneumonitis in a patient infected with the human immunodeficiency virus. Chest 1989; 95:807–809.
47. Cohen JP, Macauley C. Susceptibility to influenza A in HIV-positivie patients. JAMA 1989; 261:245.
48. Josephs S, Kim HW, Brandt CD, et al. Parainfluenza 3 virus and other common respiratory pathogens in children with human immunodeficiency virus infection. Pediatr Infect Dis J 1988; 7:207–209.
49. Malderelli F, McPhee J, Ellner P, et al. Influenza in HIV exposed adults [abstr]. Clin Res 1988; 36:800A.
50. Couch RB. Orthomyxoviruses—influenza. In: Stein J, ed. Internal Medicine. Boston, MA: Little, Brown, & Co. 1983: 1259–1265.
51. Sullivan JL, Mayner RE, Barry DW, et al. Influenza virus infection in nude mice. J Infect Dis 1976; 133:91–94.
52. Wyde PR, Couch RB, Mackler BF, et al. Effects of low- and high- passage influenza virus infection in normal and nude mice. Infect Immun 1977; 15:221–229.
53. Ragni MV, Ruben FI, Winkelstein A, et al. Antibody respsonse to immunization of patients with hemophilia with and without evidence of human immunodeficiency virus (human T lymphotrophic virus type III) infection. J Lab Clin Med 1987; 109:545–549.
54. Nelson KE, Clements ML, Miotti P, et al. The influence of human immunodeficiency virus (HIV) infection on antibody responses to influenza vaccine. Ann Intern Med 1988; 109:383–388.
55. Miotti PG, Nelson KE, D'Allabetta GA, et al. The influence of HIV infection on antibody responses to a two-dose regimen of influenza vaccine. JAMA 1989; 262:779–783.
56. Rose DN, Schechter CB, Sacks HS. Influenza and pneumoncoccal vaccination of HIV-infected patients: a policy analysis. Am J Med 1993; 94:160–168.
57. Chandwani S, Borkowsky W, Krasinski K, et al. Respiratory syncytial virus infection in human immunodeficiency virus-infected children. J Pediatr 1990; 117:251–254.

58. Sriskandan S, Shaunak S. Respiratory syncytial virus infection in an adult with AIDS. Clin Infect Dis 1993; 17:1065.
59. Murphy DM, Rose R. Respiratory syncytial virus pneumonia in a human inununodeficiencv virus-infected man. JAMA 1989; 261:1147.
60. Kaplan SL. Rapid diagnostic techniques. In: Feigin RD, Cherry JD, eds. Textbook of Pediatric Infectious Diseases, 2nd ed. Philadelphia: WB Saunders, 1987:2401–2409.
61. Centers for Disease Control. Measles in HIV-infected chldren—United States. MMWR 1988; 37:183–186.
62. Krasinski K, Borkowsky W. Measles and measles immunity in children infected with human immunodeficiency virus. JAMA 1989; 261:2512–2516.
63. Chandwani S, Kaul A, Dijohn D, et al. Measles infection and immunoprophylaxis failure in HIV-1 infected children. 31st Interscience Conference on Antimicrobial Agents and Chemotherapy. Chicago, September 1991: (abstr 469).
64. Markowitz LE, Chandler FW, Rolden EO, et al. Fatal measles pneumonia without rash in a child with AIDS. J Infect Dis 1988; 158:480–483.
65. Stogner SW, King JW, Black-Payne C, Bocchini J. Ribavirin and intravenous immune globulin therapy for measles pneumonia in HIV infection. South Med J 1993; 86:1415–1418.
66. Ross LA, Kim KS, Mason WH Jr., et al. Successful treatment of disseminated measles in a patient with acquired immunodeficiency syndrome: consideration of antiviral and passive immunotherapy. Am J Med 1990; 88:313.
67. Kemper CA, Zolopa AR, Hamilton J, et al. Prevalence of measles antibodies in adults with HIV infection: possible risk factors of measles seronegativity. AIDS 1992; 6:1321–1325.
68. Wallace JM, Hannah JB. Pulmonary disease at autopsy in patients with the acquired immunodeficiency syndrome. West J Med 1988; 149:167–171.
69. Krilov LR, Rubin LG, Frogel M, et al. Disseminated adenovirus infection with hepatic necrosis in patients with human immunodeficiency virus infecton and other immunodeficiency states. Rev Infect Dis 1990; 112:303–307.
70. Zahradnik JM, Spencer MJ, Porter DD. Adenovirus infection in the immunocompromised patient. Am J Med 1980; 68:725–732.
71. Becroft DMO. Histopathology of fatal adenovirus infection of the respiratory tract in young children. J Clin Pathol 1967; 20:561–564.
72. Clarke JR, Krishnan V, Bennet J, et al. Detection of HIV-1 in lung macrophages using the polymerase chain reaction. AIDS 1990; 4:1133–1136.
73. Rose RM, Krivine A, Pinkston P, et al. Frequent identification of HIV-1 DNA in bronchoalveolar cells obtained from individual with the acquired immunodeficiency syndrome. Am Rev Respir Dis 1991; 143:850–851.
74. Plata F, Garcia-Pons F, Ryter A, et al. HIV-1 infection of lung alveolar fibroblasts and macrophages in humans. AIDS Res Hum Retroviruses 1990, 6:979–986.
75. Dolei A, Serra C, Arca MV, et al. Acute HIV infection of $CD4^+$ human lung fibroblasts. AIDS 1992; 6:232–234.
76. Guillon JM. Autran B. Denis M, et al. Human immunodeficiency virus related lymphocytic alveolitis. Chest 1988; 94:1264–1270.

77. Autran B, Mayaud C, Raphael M, et al. Evidence for a cytotoxic T lymphocytic alveolitis in human immunodeficiency virus infected patients. AIDS 1988; 2:179–183.
78. Plata F, Autran B, Martins LP, et al. AIDS-virus specific cytotoxic T lymphocytes in lung disorders. Nature 1987; 328:348–351.
79. Autran B, Plata F, Guillon JM, et al. HIV specific cytotoxic lymphocytes directed against alveolar macrophages in HIV infected patients. Res Virol 1990; 141:13111–13136.
80. Agostini C, Zambello R, Trentin L, et al. Prognostic significance of the evaluation of bronchoalveolar lavage populations in patients with HIV-1 infection and pulmonary involvement. Chest 1991; 100:1601–1606.
81. Lairmore MD, Rosadro RH, DeMortini JC. Ovine lentivirus lymphoid interstitial pneumonia: rapid induction in neonatal lambs. Am J Pathol 1986; 125:173–181.
82. Resnick L, Pitchenik AE. Fisher E, et al. Detection of HTLV-III/LAV specific IgG and antigen in bronchoalveolar lavage fluid from two patients with lymphocytic interstitial pneumonia associated with AIDS-related complex. Am J Med 1987; 82:553–556.
83. Chayt KJ, Harper ME, Marselle LM, et al. Detection of HTLV-III RNA in lungs of patients with AIDS and pulmonar involvement. JAMA 1986; 2356–2359.
84. Travis WD, Fox CH, DeVaney KO, et al. Lymphoid pneumonitis in 50 adult patients infected with the human immunodeficiency virus: lymphocytic interstitial pneumonitis versus nonspecific interstitial pneumonitis. Hum Pathol 1992; 23:529–541.

15

Fungal Pneumonias Complicating HIV Infection

SCOTT F. DAVIES

University of Minnesota Medical School
and Hennepin County Medical Center
Minneapolis, Minnesota

GEORGE A. SAROSI

Roudebush VA Medical Center
and Indiana University School of Medicine
Indianapolis, Indiana

I. Introduction

It would be hard to overstate the effect that the advent of the human immunodeficiency virus (HIV) epidemic has had on the whole field of fungal infections. The acquired immunodeficiency syndrome (AIDS) has brought a new level of T-cell immunosuppression; beyond that of hematological malignancies; beyond that of cytotoxic and immunosuppressive therapies for malignant and nonmalignant disorders, including organ transplantation; and beyond that of high-dose glococorticoid therapy. The result has been an increase in the number of serious fungal infections and an increase in severity of those infections. However, there are also new concepts about fungal infections and new manifestations of fungal illness that are unique or almost unique to this population of patients.

The most striking example is the concept of induction therapy, followed by lifetime maintenance therapy. Admittedly some non-AIDS patients (particularly patients with Hodgkin's disease undergoing immunosuppressive chemotherapy) had increased likelihood of relapse after treatment for disseminated histoplasmosis, for example. And some forms of fungal infection, notably coccidioidomycotic meningitis and other chronic forms of disseminated coccidioidomycosis, have always been very chronic and difficult to eradicate. Yet the basic concept was always a course of therapy and an attempt to cure the patient. With AIDS, there is no cure. Treatment involves strategies for treatment of acute infections, and for long-term maintenance to prevent nearly inevitable recrudescence of symptoms if therapy is stopped. In some situations strategies for early detection and even for preemptive chemoprophylaxis at a certain level of immunosuppression are also being developed and tested. None of these concepts existed before AIDS.

Also, AIDS has served to emphasize the differences in host resistance against various fungi. Shaffner, in 1986, published an important study that showed that the resistance of fungi to nonimmune killing by polymorphonuclear phagocytes discriminated *pathogenic* fungi from *opportunistic* fungi (1). The former, including *Histoplasma capsulatum* and agents of the other endemic mycoses, cannot be killed by nonimmune phagocytes. For control of infection, the cellular immune system has to be specifically engaged. Antigen processing, development of a clone of immune lymphocytes, and the arming of macrophages to wall off the fungi within granulomas are all necessary steps in recovery from clinical illness. In contrast, the spores of opportunistic fungi, including *Aspergillus* and *Mucor* species, are readily killed by non-immune phagocytes. These fungi are ubiquitous in the environment, where they participate in the recycling of dead plants and other organic matter. Infection in a living host is likely only when neutrophil numbers are markedly reduced or when there is phagocyte dysfunction, most often from prolonged therapy with high-dose glucocorticoids. Candidiasis is truly an overlap disease, with features of both types of fungal illness. T cells are vital to control overgrowth on mucosal surfaces. This was appreciated even before AIDS because of a condition called chronic mucocutaneous candidiasis, in which T-cell–deficient children develop difficult candidal infections of skin and nails. These children have little tendency to develop invasive candidiasis. It appears that adequate neutrophil number and function are sufficient to protect them against deep-organ seeding with *Candida* organisms. On the other hand, candidiasis is an extremely important sytemic fungal infection in the setting of prolonged severe neutropenia; for example, during intensive induction chemotherapy for leukemia.

The experience in AIDS patients supports Shaffner's laboratory work and has helped clarify these relations. It is somewhat ironic that the most immunosuppressed patients ever known are at high risk from the "pathogenic" organisms, but are relatively resistant to the "opportunistic" organisms. But it has been known for decades that the endemic mycoses are opportunists in the right settings; namely, in organ transplantation and high-dose glucocorticoid therapy (which depresses T-cell function even more than phagocyte function). Thus, although the concepts are valid, the nomenclature has to shift. The pathogenic organisms have been labeled as such because normal persons become sick when they inhale the organisms. These same normal persons almost always have self-limited infection with full recovery once specific T-cell immunity is engaged. These agents are poised to exploit T-cell deficiency, as the experience in AIDS patients has shown so clearly. The term *T-cell opportunist* is perhaps a better label than pathogenic.

Although AIDS patients are immunologically naked against a wide range of microbes, neutrophil function and number are relatively well preserved (except in far-advanced disease when effects of the HIV virus on the bone marrow are often aggravated by antiretroviral drugs and by other potentially myelotoxic therapies, including ganciclovir, flucytosine, trimethoprim–sulfamethoxazole, other antimicrobial and chemotherapeutic agents). The result is that *Aspergillus* and *Mucor* species are rarely opportunists in AIDS patients, despite their profound immunosuppression. The term *phagocyte opportunist* is perhaps a better label than opportunist. Of course this classification is too simple—the immune system is highly integrated, and AIDS affects more than T cells (2,3). However, the defects in humoral immunity and phagocyte function are certainly less profound than the T-cell embarrassment. The simple division into T-cell opportunists and neutrophil opportunists is a clinically useful way to classify the fungi. Candidal infection is an overlap disease, with features of both, overgrowing mucosal surfaces in the absence of T-cell immunity, but deeply invading with depression of phagocyte number or function.

This classification allows better placement of cryptococcosis, which never fit well with either the pathogenic or the opportunistic fungal infections. Clearly, it is a T-cell opportunist, and cryptococcosis is the most important and most common fungal infection complicating AIDS. The endemic mycoses also fit here, including illness caused by *Penicillium marneffei*, a dimorphic fungus endemic in Southeast Asia that is as capable of exploiting T-cell deficiency as are *H. capsulatum* and *Coccidioides immitis* in their respective endemic areas. So also does sporotrichosis fit here, although with less certainty. Sporotrichosis is an inoculation illness that, before AIDS, rarely presented as a pulmonary or systemic infection. In patients with AIDS sporotrichosis can behave much the same as the endemic mycoses, presenting with widespread disseminated disease, including meningitis. Finally, *Candida* organisms, overgrowing on mucosal surfaces, are clearly taking advantage of T-cell deficiency.

The phagocyte opportunists are less problematic in AIDS. Disseminated candidiasis is remarkably uncommon. Elevated antibody levels against *Candida* spp. have been reported, but it is uncertain whether these add to the protection afforded by relatively intact phagocyte defense. Invasive *Aspergillus* infections are becoming more of a problem, often in late disease with depressed phagocyte number and function, but occasionally, early in the course of AIDS, which is somewhat harder to understand. Nevertheless, the total effect of an invasive *Aspergillus* infection is very small relative to the effect of cryptococcal infections and infections caused by the agents of the endemic mycoses. From May 1983 to June 1984, only 0.16% of 3170 AIDS cases reported to the Centers for Disease Control and Prevention (CDC) had *Aspergillus* infections, prompting the deletion of aspergillosis from the list of AIDS-defining illnesses (4).

The AIDS epidemic has also brought new manifestations of fungal illnesses that will be discussed more fully later in the discussions of the various specific infections. In general, the burden of organisms is higher than in non-AIDS patients, making diagnosis easier, but treatment more difficult. There are many differences in clinical presentation, results of diagnostic tests, and response to treatment. For example, in cryptococcal infection the disease is almost always systemic as well as meningeal. Cryptococcal antigen is almost always present in the serum, usually at higher titers than in simultaneously obtained cerebrospinal fluid. One uncommon manifestation of illness is diffuse papular lesions of the skin, resembling molluscum contagiosum. The illness almost always relapses if therapy is stopped, and lifetime maintenance is required. None of these features were part of crypococcal disease before AIDS.

Histoplasmosis in AIDS is almost always disseminated. Fever and weight loss with a normal chest radiograph is common. Splenomegaly is common. A chronic febrile diarrheal illness, resembling parasitic gastrointestinal illness, is fairly common. Up to half of patients have visible organisms on the peripheral blood smear. Histoplasma polysaccharide antigen (HPA) is found in the serum or urine in up to 95% of patients, providing a specific and very sensitive diagnostic test. The illness almost always relapses if therapy is stopped, and lifetime maintenance is required. None of these features were part of histoplasmosis before AIDS.

With coccidioidomycosis, half the patients present with diffuse macronodular infiltrates on a chest radiograph. Bronchoscopy reveals large endobronchial ulcers in 10–20% of patients. Bulky intrathoracic adenopathy is a regular feature. Half of the patients die within 3–4 months. The illness almost always relapses if therapy is stopped, and lifetime maintenance is required. None of these features were part of coccidioidal disease before AIDS.

In the remainder of this chapter, the individual fungal infections will be discussed, starting with cryptococcosis, the most important. The clinical manifestations, diagnostic strategies, and therapeutic approaches will be discussed, with emphasis on the unique features of the illnesses in AIDS patients. It should be emphasized that much of this information, particularly on treatment, is evolving. The results of treatment trials now underway may alter the specifics of treatment and prevention.

II. Diseases Caused by T-Cell Opportunists

A. Cryptoctoccosis

Introduction

Cryptoctoccosis is the most common and most important deep fungal infection complicating AIDS. The combination of the AIDS epidemic plus the development of an effective vaccine for *Haemophilus influenzae* type B has so altered the frequency of the various types of meningitis that cryptococcal meningitis has now become the most common form of meningitis in the United States, with upward of 5000 cases annually. In 1975, it was a rare infection, with estimates of 400–500 cases per year in the United States. Treatment trials at that time required cooperation from many centers to enroll enough patients. Today, the proportion of cases that occur in AIDS patients is so high that it is almost impossible to do new studies of therapy in a non-AIDS population.

Microbiology

Cryptococcus neoformans is the only encapsulated fungus that infects humans. The fungus exists in a yeast form, both in nature and in infected mammalian tissue. The capsule is a polysaccharide and may offer some protection against phagocytosis. The capsule can be identified on direct smears of biological material (by India ink preparation, which shows a distinct halo around the yeast) or in histopathological preparations (by mucicarmine staining), offering rapid presumptive diagnosis. The fungus grows rapidly (within days) on blood agar and other routine media. It is identified by biochemical characteristics (does not ferment glucose, does hydrolyze urea) and by morphology (absence of pseudohyphae, presence of carbohydrate capsule).

Epidemiology

Cryptococcus neoformans is distributed worldwide. Bird-droppings, decaying fruit, and soil support fungal growth. The disease is acquired by inhalation (probably of a smaller relatively capsule-deficient yeast) and primary disease is in the lung. The primary infection in the lung elicits little inflammatory response and is usually asymptomatic or barely symptomatic; hence, it is rarely diagnosed. For unknown reasons, there is a remarkable tropism for the central nervous system (CNS). Before AIDS, chronic meningitis was by far the most common form of the illness. Half of cases occurred in patients with T-cell–deficient conditions, but half occurred in patients without recognized immunosuppression. Before AIDS most patients had isolated CNS disease, with no evidence of systemic involvement at time of diagnosis. Most persons have inhaled this fungus, and antibody against it is fairly common (5). About 7% of all patients with AIDS develop cryptococcosis, with fairly striking differences in different populations (6,7). The incidence is high in Central Africa, but low in Denmark (8,9). Within the United States, the incidence is also variable. Patients from New Jersey have a high incidence of infection, and patients from cities in the center of the country have a lower incidence. The reason for variable incidence among different groups of AIDS patients is unknown, as is the reason that an even higher percentage of AIDS patients do not develop infections (similar to *Pneumocystis* infection, for which past exposure is also presumed to be very common).

Clinical Features

Cryptococcal infection may occur at any time point in the course of AIDS, but it is most common when the CD4 cell count is fewer than 200/dl. It is the first opportunistic infection in one-quarter to one-half of cases. It can present in concert with other opportunistic infections.

Onset is often slow, and symptoms are nonspecific (6,10,11,12). More than 80% of patients have fever, which can persist for weeks. Early on, fever may be the only finding, without other localizing symptoms. By diagnosis most patients also have headache, ranging in severity from mild to severe. Stiff neck, decreased mental status, photophobia, and focal neurological defects are each observed in perhaps one-quarter of patients. Not all cases are this subacute. Some patients have meningeal signs developing over hours or days.

Half of patients have respiratory symptoms, including cough, dyspnea, and chest pain. Sputum production is usually minimal. When AIDS patients with respiratory symptoms have fever and subacute headache, cryptococcal infection should be strongly considered; however, some patients present with fever and cough without headache or other neurological symptoms. This presentation is entirely non-specific and suggests *Pneumocystis* infection or other opportunistic pulmonary infection more strongly than cryptococcosis. Even the patients who present mainly with respiratory symptoms usually have subclinical or subtle meningitis.

Hepatosplenomegaly occurs in a significant minority of patients with disseminated disease. Unusual distant sites of involvement include the skin (one form of cutaneous involvement is widespread umbilicated papules resembling molluscum contagiosum), the eye, bone, and the gastrointestinal tract (sites include mouth, esophagus, stomach, and colon).

A chest radiograph may show diffuse interstitial infiltrates, similar to those often observed in *Pneumocystis* pneumonia. Other patterns include localized interstitial infiltrates, focal alveolar infiltrates, single or multiple nodules, and small pleural effusions. There is nothing specific about any of these findings.

Diagnosis

Testing for cryptococcal antigen is specific and highly sensitive. Serum is positive for antigen in 99% of cases of meningitis (70 of 71 cases in one series; 6). Serum, cerebrospinal fluid, and urine are almost always positive for cryptococcal antigen, with titers highest in the serum, intermediate in the cerebrospinal fluid, and lowest in urine. Serum cryptococcal antigen should be measured in all AIDS patients with fever and headache, and in all AIDS patients with a subacute febrile illness without obvious diagnosis. Negative serum cryptococcal antigen virtually excludes cryptococcal meningitis.

Other cerebrospinal fluid tests include positive cultures and positive India ink preparations in the great majority of patients. Markers of the inflammatory response are often subtle, with 20 or fewer white blood cells (fewer than 5 is not exceptional) and normal or near normal glucose and protein values. Blood culture results are often positive.

Bronchoalveolar lavage (BAL) often shows organisms on direct smears and by culture. Cryptococcal antigen can also be detected in lavage fluid, but simultaneous serum titers are almost always positive.

Findings on the skin are quite variable and nonspecific. A histopathological study and culture of unusual skin lesions sometimes give an unexpected diagnosis of cryptococcosis.

Treatment

The treatment of cryptococcal meningitis in patients with AIDS has been studied extensively, but the final answer is not available, and treatment is still evolving. One approach is to give primary induction therapy with amphotericin B (AMB) 0.7 mg/kg per day, with 100 (rather than 150) mg/kg per day of flucytosine (5-fluorocytosine—*not* the same as fluconazole) in four divided doses, with target blood levels of 80 μg/dl (rather than 100). The dose reductions for flucytosine reflect the considerable toxicity of that agent in patients with AIDS. Many patients will simply not tolerate the myelosuppressive effect of the drug, especially with advanced AIDS and in the face of concurrent therapy with antiretroviral agents, ganciclovir, trimethoprim–sulfmethoxazole, and other drugs. For these patients AMB alone is often as effective and is much less toxic. If the initial therapy induces a remission, then maintenance therapy with fluconazole is begun and continued for life.

Fluconazole is well absorbed, even in AIDS patients. Cerebrospinal fluid levels are at least 70% of serum levels. Because of these features, fluconazole may yet prove to be the ideal agent, even for initial therapy of stable patients with cryptococcal meningitis. In a large comparative study between AMB and fluconazole, both drugs had similar efficacy (13). However, there were some early deaths in both treatment groups, and the study was criticized because the daily dose of AMB (0.4 mg/kg) was quite low. Other work has shown faster sterilization of the cerebrospinal fluid with AMB and has suggested a decrease in early deaths with full-dose AMB, as compared with fluconazole (14). Until further studies are completed, AMB alone or with flucytosine is the best validated initial treatment and should be used for all seriously ill patients with altered mental status. Fluconazole from onset is an option for stable patients with normal mental status at presentation. If fluconazole from onset proves to be equal or better therapy for these stable patients, that will simplify treatment considerably. Treatment is evolving and will be slightly different in 2 or 3 years from what it is today.

Following successful induction treatment of cryptococcal meningitis, patients with AIDS require lifetime maintenance therapy to prevent relapse. Fluconazole suppressive therapy is the treatment of choice. In a large clinical study, fluconazole outperformed weekly AMB and should be used at a dose of 200–400 mg daily for life to prevent relapse (15,16).

Some patients with cryptococcal meningitis develop hydrocephalus, which further embarrasses their mental status. Recognition and early therapy for this complication is important (17). High-volume lumbar punctures can be used to reduce cerebrospinal fluid pressures. Formal shunting procedures are occasionally done. Glucocorticoid therapy may have a minor adjunctive role.

Prevention

Most infections occur in severely immunosuppressed individuals. One study of patients with fewer than 68 CD4 cells per deciliter showed a substantial decrease in cryptococcal infections when fluconazole treatment was given for primary prevention, when compared with historical controls (18). Such therapy has also decreased the incidence of histoplasmosis and controlled oral candidal infections. Conversely, it is also very likely that the widespread clinical use of fluconazole to control oral candidiasis has somewhat decreased the incidence of cryptococcal infection.

B. Histoplasmosis

Introduction

Histoplasmosis is a major endemic mycoses most common in the south-central United States along major river valleys. Because most of the early AIDS expansion was along the coasts (San Francisco, New York, Miami, Los Angeles), histoplasmosis was relatively unimportant. As disease activity spread to the central states, histoplasmosis became more important as a common opportunistic infection.

Microbiology

Histoplasma capsulatum is a thermal dimorphic fungus. In nature and in the laboratory at 23°C, it grows as a mycelium, with characteristic tuberculate (spiny) macroconidia. The hyphae also have nonspecific microconidia that are easily aerosolized and are probably the infectious particle. In the infected mammalian host and in the laboratory at 37°C, the fungus converts to the parasitic yeast phase. The yeasts are small (2–4 μm) and are often seen intracellularly within parasitized phagocytes. Growth in the laboratory often takes 1 or more weeks. Once a mycelial isolate is established, the organism can be identified by exoantigen testing that eliminates the need for conversion to the yeast phase, which formerly delayed final isolation by additional weeks.

Epidemiology

The organism grows in nitrogen-rich soil enriched by bird or bat droppings. It is found worldwide along river valleys in temperate climates. The central United States has much more disease activity than any other endemic area. Following inhalation of the infectious microconidia, the organisms convert to the yeast phase, and an area of pneumonitis develops. During the preimmune phase of illness, the organisms spread to regional lymph nodes and to reticuloendothelial organs throughout the body (benign fungemia). With advent of cell-mediated immunity, specifically armed macrophages attack the fungus. There is granuloma formation, with central necrosis and eventual fibrosis and calcification. The infection is almost always self-limited in normal hosts. With AIDS the infection cannot be controlled, and progressive dissemination occurs. Untreated, it is fatal.

Histoplasmosis complicating AIDS is most common within the endemic area. In Houston, Texas, on the fringes of the endemic area, about 5% of patients with AIDS develop progressive disseminated histoplasmosis (PDH; 19) The incidence is much higher, up to 25%, in AIDS patients in Kansas City, Memphis, Nashville, and Indianapolis, all in the heart of the endemic area (20,21). The disease is acquired by inhalation. Progression of a primary infection, while immunosuppressed, is one infection mechanism. However, other cases probably represent reactivation of remote infection. One line of evidence is the presence of calcified hilar and mediastinal lymph nodes, characteristic of remote histoplasmosis, in 36% of cases of PDH in AIDS patients from Indianapolis (22). Stronger evidence for endogenous reactivation comes from the uncommon cases of PDH that occur in AIDS patients far from the endemic area (23). Cases appearing in San Francisco have usually had long prior residence in the central United States. Cases appearing in New York City and Miami have usually had long prior residence in endemic Caribbean countries, especially Puerto Rico. DNA testing has shown that strains of *Histoplasma* recovered from immigrants from the Caribbean are similar to strains from that area, rather than strains from the Midwest cities of the United States (24). A normal chest radiograph is common at presentation of PDH, more consistent with endogenous reactivation of a systemic process than with unchecked progression of a new pulmonary infection.

Clinical Features

The onset of illness is often subacute, and symptoms are nonspecific (19,25). More than 75% of patients have fever, which can persist for weeks. Early on, fever and weight loss, also occurring in 75% of patients, may be the only findings. Some patients have rapid progression of illness over hours or days.

Few patients have respiratory symptoms early on. As the illness progresses, most untreated patients develop cough and dypsnea. Sputum production is usually minimal. The presentation is often nonspecific and equally compatible with many opportunistic infections. Some patients present with fever, weight loss, and diarrhea from gastrointestinal involvement, others with upper gastrointestinal bleeding from ulcerations of the stomach. Unusual distant sites of involvement include the skin and the CNS. Up to one-quarter of patients have hepatosplenomegaly. Patients with rapidly progressive illness can present with disseminated intravascular coagulation, which has negative prognostic impact.

A chest radiograph is normal at the time of first evaluation in up to half the patients. Other patients have diffuse nodular infiltrates. Most patients eventually develop diffuse infiltrates unless the diagnosis is made and treatment is started. Respiratory symptoms usually accompany radiographic abnormalities. Other uncommon radiographic patterns include diffuse interstitial infiltrate (mimicking *Pneumocystis* infection), focal infiltrates or nodules, and small pleural effusions. Hilar adenopathy can occur, but is not common.

Diagnosis

Testing for *Histoplasma* polysaccharide antigen (HPA) in serum and urine is specific and highly sensitive. In one series, the test was positive in urine of 70 of 72 AIDS patients with PDH (26). The test for HPA is now available in a kit form and should become nearly as useful in AIDS patients with histoplasmosis as is testing for cryptococcal antigen in AIDS patients with cryptococcosis. A negative urine test for HPA virtually excludes disseminated histoplasmosis in an AIDS patient with prolonged unexplained fever.

The burden of organisms is high, and many other tests may be helpful. The goal is rapid diagnosis and early initiation of lifesaving therapy. The organism can be seen in circulating phagocytes on a smear of the peripheral blood in up to half of the cases. The blood culture is positive in up to 90% of cases if the lysis centrifugation system is used. However waiting for the blood culture may delay treatment, and faster diagnostic tests are preferable. Direct examination of bone marrow biopsy sections offers rapid diagnosis. There are usually many organisms and little if any tendency to granuloma formation. However, testing for HPA is even faster, and increasing use of the test should reduce the need for bone marrow biopsies to diagnose PDH in AIDs patients.

Bronchoalveolar lavage often shows organisms on direct smears (within phagocytes) and by culture.

Treatment

Progressive disseminated histoplasmosis in AIDS cannot be cured. Following successful initial induction of remission, lifetime maintenance therapy must be given to prevent relapse. Amphotericin B should be used as primary therapy for all severely ill patients. In AIDS patients, the duration of AMB therapy can be limited to the minimum required for a good clinical response, usually 500–1000 mg cumulative dose. The maintenance therapy with itraconazole, 200 mg twice daily, can begin, which must be continued for life (27). Recent information suggests that stable patients can be treated safely with itraconazole as the primary therapy from onset (28).

Ketoconazole did not prove effective for preventing relapse. Weekly infusions of AMB are effective, but usually require a perminent indwelling catheter (29). Fluconazole also has some efficacy for preventing relapse, but is less effective than itraconazole.

Prevention

Most infections occur in severely immunosuppressed individuals. One study of patients with fewer CD4 cells than 68/dL showed a decrease in histoplasmal infections, compared with historical controls, when fluconazole treatment was given for primary prevention of cryptococcal infection (18). Such therapy also controlled oral candidal infections. Fluconazole given as long-term maintenance therapy for cryptococcal or candidal infections will probably somewhat reduce the likelihood of PDH.

C. Coccidioidomycosis

Introduction

Coccidioidomycosis is a major endemic mycoses most common in the desert regions of the Southwestern United States. It is becoming a very important opportunistic infection in AIDS patients living in highly endemic areas. Lacking T-cell immunity, patients with advanced AIDS have severe and often fatal illnesses. Response to therapy is poor.

Microbiology

Coccidioides immitis is a tissue dimorphic fungus. In nature it grows as a mycelium, with characteristic arthrospores. In the infected mammalian host, the fungus converts to the parasitic phase, with characteristic giant spherules containing many endospores. After rupture of the spherule, each endospore can develop into a new spherule. The organism is easy to grow on artificial media, but it is a biohazard, and culture should be attempted only by experienced laboratories. Cultural isolation takes one or more weeks.

Once a mycelial isolate is established, the organism can be identified by exoantigen testing, which reduces risk to laboratory personnel and speeds the final identification.

Epidemiology

Coccidioidomycosis occurs in the Southwest United States deserts, particularly in southern and central Arizona and in the central valley of California. Climactic conditions characterized as the lower Sonoran life zone are most favorable for fungal growth. The organism grows in the soil. Infection is acquired by inhalation. The infecting particle is the arthrospore, which can be carried long distances by the wind. Some disease activity extends as far east as Texas. Coccidioidomycosis also occurs in northern Mexico and in semiarid parts of South America, mainly in central Argentina. A large prospective study of the incidence of disease was conducted in Tucson and Phoenix (30). A total of 170 newly diagnosed patients were followed from the time their HIV infection was first documented. About 25% of patients developed coccidiodomycosis within 3.5 years. For most patients, the disease was the result of new infection while immunosuppressed. For at least two patients the disease seemed to be endogenous reactivation, because they had a positive skin test at study entry. However, exogenous reinfection may also have occurred as T-cell immunity waned, for the possibility for new exposures certainly existed. The length of residency within the endemic area did not correlate with the development of coccidioidomycosis. In other cities within the endemic area, the incidence of coccidioidomycosis in HIV-infected persons is much lower, less than 5%. Risk of disease increases when the CD4 cell count drops to fewer than 250/dL.

Clinical Features

Similar to histoplasmosis, coccidioidomycosis is usually a self-limited infection in persons with normal T-cell immunity. Even in patients with early AIDS and well-preserved T-cell number, the disease can be fairly mild. In patients with advanced AIDS, it is often deadly.

In the severely immunosuppressed patient, the illness is usually a progressive respiratory illness over days to weeks (31). Most patients have fever and cough, productive of mucopurulent sputum. Weight loss is also common. About a third of patients have meningitis when they present, with a range of symptoms, including headache, nausea, vomiting, and depressed mental status. Most patients with meningitis also have respiratory symptoms, but some have symptoms related to only their CNS infection. About 5% of patients have a variety of skin lesions, including papules, plaques, pustules, and nodules. Dissemination to almost any organ can occur, including lymph nodes, liver, kidneys, thyroid, and gastrointestinal tract.

The chest radiograph usually shows diffuse macronodular infiltrates that are quite characteristic. Another pattern is a diffuse interstitial infiltrates similar to *Pneumocystis* infection. Many patients also have bulky hilar and mediastinal adenopathy. Patients with milder degree of immunosuppression can present with focal infiltrates, nodules, and thin-walled cavities, similar to the radiographic findings in normal host who present with primary coccidioidomycosis. Although some patients present with meningitis or other distant disease having a normal chest radiograph, a normal chest radiograph is much less common than in AIDS patients with histoplasmosis. The disease usually presents as a respiratory infection, with or without meningeal or other distant findings, and not as a nonspecific febrile illness with no localizing features (a common scenario in histoplasmosis).

Diagnosis

Tests for specific fungal antigen (as for cryptococcosis and histoplasmosis) are not available. Serological testing for antibodies is important, but lacks the high sensitivity and specificity of antigen testing. Immunodiffusion for IgM and IgG antibodies is positive in perhaps 75% of cases. Antibody response may be absent in severely immunosuppressed patients, and a negative test does not exclude the diagnosis. The complement fixation test has similar diagnostic usefulness, and it can also be used to follow the progression of the illness and response to therapy. Rising titers are associated with disease progression and falling titers with treatment response. Antibody detection (by complement fixation or other assay) in cerebrospinal fluid is very useful to diagnose meningeal involvement.

Because serodiagnosis is imperfect, the mainstays of diagnosis are direct visualization of the fungus in respiratory secretions or cultural recovery from respiratory or other specimens. Spherules are seen on KOH-prepared sputum less than 20% of the time. Direct staining of bronchoalveolar lavage fluid (stained with the Papanicolau technique and other vital stains) is positive in about 40% of proved cases (32). Cultures of sputum and bronchoalveolar fluid are usually eventually positive, but the diagnostic delay is too long for seriously ill patients who need urgent treatment. Some patients at bronchoscopy have large, even dime-sized, endobronchial ulcers. Biopsies of these ulcers often show spherules. If the endobronchial biopsies are negative and coccidioidomycosis is suspected, transbronchial biopsies should be done (if possible) to improve diagnostic yield (32).

Some patients require thoracoscopic or traditional open-lung biopsy. If there are obvious sites of distant disease, especially skin lesions, biopsies of those sites can give a rapid and safe specific diagnosis. The burden of organisms is very high, and involved tissues usually show many organisms and little if any tendency to granuloma formation.

Treatment

Coccidioidomycosis in patients with AIDS is a particularly aggressive and lethal infection. Occasional HIV-infected patients with relatively intact T-cell immunity develop the same type of illnesses as nonimmunosuppressed patients. Stabilization can be accomplished with AMB or with fluconazole, followed by lifetime maintenance therapy with fluconazole. Unfortunately, most AIDS patients with coccidioidomycosis have very depressed T-cell function when they present. Diffuse nodular pulmonary infiltrates are very common, and many patients have extensive endobronchial disease. The tempo of the illness is very rapid, and intravenous AMB should be used as primary therapy. If the patient stabilizes with 1000–1500 mg of AMB, then fluconazole (at least 400 mg/day) can be used for continued suppressive therapy with good effect. Unfortunately, most of these patients die rapidly, even in the face of AMB therapy. The mean survival is only a few months. A few patients live 1 or several years with good control of their illness.

Fluconazole has some efficacy for treatment of coccidioidal meningitis (33). It can be used as primary therapy if the level of consciousness is not depressed. The disease can be suppressed with good symptom control, but it cannot be cured. Intravenous plus intrathecal AMB should be used for severe meningitis with depressed level of consciousness; the prognosis is very poor, regardless of the choice of therapy.

Prevention

Experience with different prevention strategies is being acquired in the Tucson and Phoenix areas. At present, preventive treatment based on a specific CD4 count is not recommended, even for patients with known prior skin test positivity. This may change. Extreme vigilance is required so that the few AIDS patients within the endemic areas who develop coccidioidomycosis are diagnosed early and treated as effectively as possible.

D. Blastomycosis

Introduction

Blastomycosis is coendemic with histoplasmosis over much of the central United States. It is much less common, with perhaps 10% as many recognized cases. To date, blastomycosis complicating AIDS has been very rare. However, enough experience has been accumulated to show that aggressive infection in the lung and rapid, wide dissemination can occur when T-cell function is severely impaired (34).

Microbiology

Blastomyces dermatitidis is a thermal dimorphic fungus. In nature and in the laboratory at 23°C, it grows as a mycelium. The hyphae have nonspecific microconidia that are easily aerosolized and are probably the infectious particle. In the infected mammalian host and in the laboratory at 37°C, the fungus converts to the parasitic yeast phase. The yeast are large (8–20 μm) and have characteristic single buds, with a wide neck of attachment to the parent cell. Growth in the laboratory often takes 1 or more weeks.

Once a mycelial isolate is established, the organism can be identified by exoantigen testing that eliminates the need for conversion to the yeast phase, which formerly delayed final isolation by additional weeks.

Epidemiology

The organism grows in nitrogen-rich soil (enriched by organic matter, including bird and animal excrement, or by decaying vegetation) along rivers and streams. It is coendemic with histoplasmosis over much of the central United States, but disease activity extends further north across northern Wisconsin and Minnesota and into adjacent areas of Canada. Following inhalation of the infectious microconidia, the organisms coverts to the yeast phase, and an area of pneumonitis develops. The tissue response to the fungus is a mixed pyogenic and granulomatous response. With AIDS, the infection cannot be controlled and progressive dissemination occurs. Most cases occur in severely immunosuppressed patients with fewer than 200 CD4 cells.

Blastomycosis complicating AIDS is rare, even within the endemic area. Occasional patients have been diagnosed far from the endemic area, but most of them had recent or remote exposure in endemic areas. It is likely that both progression of infection while immunosuppressed and also endogenous reactivation of remote infection may occur.

Clinical Features

Most patients have respiratory symptoms of cough and dyspnea. Most produce purulent sputum. Some patients have isolated pulmonary disease that may be subacute, but more commonly is rapidly progressive. About half the patients have widely disseminated disease. Meningeal involvement is common in patients with widely disseminated disease, and it is usually symptomatic. Skin, bone, and male genitourinary tract are also common sites of involvement. Most patients with widely disseminated disease have extensive pulmonary involvement. In the largest reported series, the illness was quite aggressive (34). Six of 15 patients died within 1 month, 2 of rapidly progressing pulmonary illness, and 4 of progression of widely disseminated disease.

The chest radiograph may show single or multiple large alveolar infiltrates. Some patients have typical lobar pneumonia mimicking bacterial pneumonia. Other patients have multiple nodules. Yet another radiographic pattern is diffuse interstitial infiltrates, mimicking *Pneumocystis* infection.

Diagnosis

There is, as yet, no test for fungal antigen. There is an immunodiffusion test, a complement fixation test, and an enzyme-linked immunosorbent assay

(ELISA) test that all detect serum antibodies. The first test is fairly specific, but lacks sensitivity. The last test lacks specificity and still has imperfect sensitivity (approximately 70%). Combining the poor operating characteristics of these tests with the usual delay in obtaining the results makes it easy to see why serodiagnosis plays little role in this disease.

The burden of organisms is high and many other tests may be helpful. The goal is rapid diagnosis, and early initiation of lifesaving therapy. Because most patients have purulent sputum and because the yeast form has a characteristic morphology, direct examination of respiratory specimens after KOH digestion or after staining with a variety of special stains (periodic acid–Schiff [PAS]-stained preparations, Papanicolau preparations, and silver stains) are all useful. Demonstration of the characteristic yeast forms in infected secretions provides a quick and highly specific diagnosis. Cultures are usually positive, but in practice become confirmatory tests because the results return later.

Bronchoalveolar lavage often shows characteristic organisms on direct smears and by culture. A biopsy of skin lesions is easy and usually productive, showing the organism on histopathological sections and by culture.

Treatment

Blastomycosis in AIDS cannot be cured. Amphotericin B should be used as primary therapy for all seriously ill patients and for all patients with meningitis. In AIDS patients, the cumulative total dose of AMB should be 1000–2000 mg. If the patient stabilizes, then maintenance therapy with itraconazole, 200 mg twice daily, should be started and continued for life. It is not known whether itraconazole is effective maintenance when there is meningeal involvement.

Prevention

The disease is rare, and there is no skin test to detect patients with remote infection. There is no way to target, or even study, preventive therapy. It is possible that oral azoles given for treatment or primary prevention of other fungal illness may well have some effect in preventing recrudescence of blastomycosis. This is speculation, however, for no evidence exists.

E. Paracoccidioidomycosis

Introduction

Paracoccidioidomycosis is an endemic mycosis of Central and South America. Paracoccidioidomycosis complicating AIDS is still very rare. However, enough experience has been accumulated to show that aggressive infection in the lung and rapid wide dissemination can occur when T-cell function is severely impaired.

Microbiology

Paracoccidioides brasiliensis is a thermal dimorphic fungus. In nature and in the laboratory at 23°C, it grows as a mycelium. The hyphae have nonspecific microconidia that are easily aerosolized and are probably the infectious particle. In the infected mammalian host, and in the laboratory at 37°C, the fungus converts to the parasitic yeast phase. The yeast are large (8–20 μm) and have characteristic multiple, thin-necked buds. Growth in the laboratory often takes 1 or more weeks. Once a mycelial isolate is established, the organism can be identified by exoantigen testing that eliminates the need for conversion to the yeast phase, which formerly delayed final isolation by additional weeks.

Epidemiology

Paracoccidioidomycosis is a granulomatous and suppurative infection, endemic in hot subtropical regions of Central and South America. The disease is most prevalent in Brazil (60% of all recorded cases), Colombia, and Venezuela. It does not occur in the United States.

The organism grows in the soil. Following inhalation of the infectious microconidia, the organism coverts to the yeast phase, and an area of pneumonitis develops. The tissue response to the fungus is a mixed pyogenic and granulomatous response. With AIDS, the infection cannot be controlled and progressive dissemination occurs.

It is unknown whether clinical cases in patients with AIDS result from progression of infection while immunosuppressed, from endogenous reactivation of remote infection, or from both of these mechanisms.

Clinical Features

Most patients have respiratory symptoms of cough and dyspnea. Most produce purulent sputum. Many patients have bulky cervical adenopathy, a feature not common to the other endemic mycoses. Some patients have isolated pulmonary disease that may be subacute, but more commonly is rapidly progressive. Many patients have widely disseminated disease. Meningeal involvement occurs in patients with widely disseminated disease, and it is usually symptomatic. Skin, lymph nodes, and bone are also common sites of involvement. Most patients with widely disseminated disease have extensive pulmonary involvement. The illness is often quite aggressive.

The chest radiograph may show nodules or single or multiple large alveolar infiltrates. Many patients also have large, bulky hilar and mediastinal adenopathy. Some patients have diffuse interstitial infiltrates, mimicking *Pneumocystis* infection.

Diagnosis

There is no test for fungal antigen. Testing for serum antibodies has some usefulness, but direct smears of respiratory secretions, histopathological studies of tissue specimens, and cultures of biological materials are the mainstays of diagnosis.

The burden of organisms is high, and many other tests may be helpful. The goal is rapid diagnosis and early initiation of lifesaving therapy. Most patients have purulent sputum; because the yeast form has a characteristic morphology, direct examination of respiratory specimens after KOH digestion or after staining with a variety of special stains (periodic acid–Schiff [PAS]-stained preparations, Papanicolau preparations, and silver stains) are all useful. Demonstration of the characteristic yeast forms in infected secretions provides a quick and highly specific diagnosis. Cultures are usually positive, but in practice become confirmatory tests because the results return later.

Bronchoalveolar lavage often shows characteristic organisms on direct smears and by culture. Biopsy of skin lesions is easy and usually productive, showing the organism on histopathological sections and by culture.

Treatment

Itraconazole has been used for paracoccidioidomycosis since 1982 (8 years before release in the United States). A daily dose of 100 mg for 6 months successfully treats about 93% of patients who are not immunosuppressed. Best therapy for paracoccidioidomycosis in patients with AIDS is not yet established. It seems prudent to give AMB to seriously ill patients, aiming for a total cumulative dose of 1000–1500 mg. If the patient stabilizes, treatment with itraconazole 200 mg daily should be started and continued for life. It is likely that some AIDS patients with milder illness can be treated with itraconazole from diagnosis.

Prevention

A skin test is available to detect patients with remote infection. It is unknown what the risk of developing paracoccidioidomycosis is for patients with known positive skin tests who develop AIDS. No recommendations for preventive therapy can be given.

F. Other Rare Diseases Caused by T-Cell Opportunists

Penicillium marneffei is a very important pathogen for HIV-infected patients in a restricted geographic area (35–37). Most reports of infection have been from Southeast Asia. Incidence seems to be highest in Thailand, but the disease has also been reported from Indonesia, Hong Kong, and China. The organism is dimorphic and probably acquired by inhalation. Similar to histoplasmosis, it can present as a high fever with few localizing symptoms. More commonly, patients have fever, cough, and generalized papular skin lesions. Most other *penicillium* species causing human infection resemble *Aspergillus* species (complicating profound neutropenia and maintaining mycelial form in nature and in infected humans). Not so this organism: *P. marneffei* converts to a yeast form in infected hosts and yeast-laden macrophages can be seen in the peripheral blood, in bone marrow aspirates, and in touch preparations and tissue sections of skin lesions and lymph nodes (quite similar to histoplasmosis, with similar high burden of organisms). The epidemiology of the organism is incompletely understood, including the important question of whether self-limited infections ever occur in normal hosts. Nevertheless, the prominence of the infection in HIV-infected persons and the clinical features of the illness suggest a T-cell opportunist. Treatment is suppressive, rather than curative. AMB and itraconazole have efficacy.

Sporotrichosis is an uncommon fungal infection. The disease is usually acquired by inoculation and presents with a characteristic distal ulcer accompanied by marked involvement of the draining lymphatics, with thickening of the lymphatics and nodules along their course. The lymphocutaneous form of sporotrichosis is well treated with itraconazole 200–400 mg daily.

Isolated pulmonary sporotrichosis is very rare. The most common presentation is a subacute or chronic infection smoldering in the diseased upper lobes of patients with severe underlying chronic obstructive lung disease. It resembles atypical tuberculosis, chronic cavitary histoplasmosis, and chronic necrotizing aspergillosis; all occur in similar patients with bullous lung disease. The pulmonary disease is presumably acquired by inhalation because there is usually no current or remote history of a skin ulcer. However, the illness is so rare that information about pathogenesis is speculative.

Sportrichosis in patients with HIV infection can present with diffuse cutaneous lesions, polyarthritis, and meningitis (38,39). Itraconazole may have some efficacy for therapy (40). As with other fungal infections, lifelong therapy is necessary. Disseminated sporotrichosis is so rare that immune mechanisms preventing systemic invasion are poorly understood. It is discussed here only because disseminated sporotrichosis is even rarer in patients with prolonged severe neutropenia than it is in HIV-infected persons.

III. Diseases Caused by Phagocyte Opportunists

A. Aspergillosis

Aspergillus species are found worldwide in decaying organic matter. Spores are inhaled regularly by all persons. There is remarkably little tendency for invasive disease unless phagocyte number and function are reduced.

Microbiology

Aspergillus species are mycelial organisms. They exist as septate hyphae both in nature and in infected mammalian tissue. The hyphae are 5–10 μm in diameter. Hyphae exhibit dichotomous acute-angle branching, often giving a finger-like appearance to the branching elements. *Aspergillus fumigatus* is the most common species found in human infections, but other species are also found. These fungi grow rapidly from clinical specimen, including respiratory secretions. The difficulty is in distinguishing colonization from deep tissue invasion. The positive predictive value of a sputum culture increases with increasing risk factors for invasive disease; namely, prolonged neutropenia and high-dose glucocorticoid therapy. Absolute proof of invasion requires histopathological confirmation of tissue invasion or culture from usually sterile body fluids or tissues.

Epidemiology

Aspergillus species are ubiquitous in the environment, and spores are regularly inhaled by all persons. Spores are cleared by mechanical lung defenses and are killed by nonimmune phagocytes. Invasive infection is extremely unlikely in normal hosts, although rarely invasive infections do follow huge exposures to compost materials, decaying wood chips, or other organic matter.

Invasive *Aspergillus* infection is uncommon in patients with AIDS, occurring in 0.1–0.5% of patients. Over half of infected patients have classic risk factors, including neutropenia from advanced HIV infection or, more likely, from therapy of HIV infection and complicating infections and neoplasms. High-dose glucocorticoid therapy is another risk factor, used for *Pneumocystis* infection and as part of therapy for some neoplasms. A few AIDS patients with invasive *Aspergillus* infection do not have these classic risk factors. Most have very advanced AIDS with CD4 cell counts of fewer than 50/dL. Some have exposures to larger numbers of spores, sometimes from smoking of marijuana. Other cases likely reflect the complex integration of the immune system and the eventual effect of progressive AIDS on all of its components.

Clinical Features

Most cases involve the lung (41–44). There are several patterns of illness, including two forms that are relatively specific to AIDS, suggesting that *Aspergillus* infection may well be a specific complication of AIDS and not always simply a reflection of the associated neutropenia and glucocorticoid therapy. Patients with pulmonary involvement present with fever, cough, dyspnea, and occasionally chest pain, all common to every pulmonary complication of AIDS. Patients with cavitary and endobronchial forms of the disease often have hemoptysis, which is rare in *Pneumocystis* pneumonia and many of the other pulmonary infections complicating AIDS.

Nondescript focal infiltrates resembling bacterial pneumonia occur in a quarter of patients. These infiltrates can be surprisingly indolent over weeks or even months, or may progress focally or spread to involve multiple areas of the lung.

Cavitary infiltrates are common, most often in upper lung zones. These cavities are often quite large, even up to 10 cm in size. There are often one or two large cavities, rather than the typical appearance of chronic cavitary aspergillosis in non-AIDS patients (usually complicating advanced chronic obstructive lung disease), which is a tuberculosis-like nodular and fibrocavitary disease. There may be less surrounding infiltrate than expected. In non-AIDS patients, extensive pleural thickening over the involved area is common. In AIDS patients, pleural thickening is less, but there is more tendency for free rupture into the pleural space, resulting in pneumothorax or pyopneumothorax. Patients with cavitary disease can present with serious and even fatal hemoptysis (5 of 13 such patients described in one review had fatal hemoptysis; 44).

Patchy bilateral alveolar infiltrates is another presentation. Some cases represent multifocal parenchymal lung involvement. In other cases the primary disease in endobronchial with distal obstruction and atelectasis causing the patchy infiltrates. Obstructing bronchial aspergillosis occurs fairly commonly in AIDS and is rare in other immunosuppressed patients (45). There are bronchial casts containing *Aspergillus* organisms, which are sometimes expectorated as plugs. The disease progresses to ulceration, pseudomembranes, and plaque-like lesions, which all can obstruct distal airways. Cough and hemoptysis are very common. In some cases the chest radiograph is normal. Similar endobronchial disease is sometimes seen in lung transplant recipients and, rarely, in other immunosuppressed patients. The relative high frequency of endobronchial disease seems to be an important feature of aspergillosis in patients with AIDS.

Diffuse bilateral alveolar or interstitial infiltrates is another presentation. The infiltrates mimic *Pneumocystis* pneumonia and other opportunistic pulmonary infections. The prognosis of diffuse pulmonary *Aspergillus* infection is, not surprisingly, very poor. Many of these patients develop widely disseminated disease involving the CNS, the skin, the kidneys, and the heart, often in combination.

Diagnosis

Many patients with AIDS have positive cultures of *Aspergillus* species from respiratory secretions. The incidence of invasive pulmonary disease in these patients is low. Nonetheless, positive cultures from sputum or from specimens obtained at bronchoscopy in AIDS patients with a compatible pulmonary illness, and no other recognizable infectious cause, should always raise suspicion of invasive aspergillosis and prompt further diagnostic tests.

Fiberoptic bronchoscopy is the best test for obstructing endobronchial aspergillosis. Endobronchial biopsies usually show mucosal and invasive disease. Positive cultures in a patient with typical endobronchial abnormalities on inspection are enough to make a presumptive diagnosis.

Diagnosis of parenchymal disease is more difficult. Many patients have far advanced AIDS and invasive procedures have morbidity. Transbronchial biopsies and transthoracic fine-needle aspiration are useful for selected patients. Open-lung biopsies are sometimes done for diagnosis, but thoracotomy is done more often for treatment (see below).

Cultures of pleural fluid and histopathological results of skin biopsies and other tissue biopsies offer specific diagnosis in patients with disease at these sites. Positive urine cultures nearly always imply metastatic abscesses in the kidney and are diagnostic of invasive aspergillosis.

Treatment

Overall the results of treatment are very poor, even with AMB. Localized lung disease can be indolent and can be suppressed with AMB or with itraconazole in some patients. There have also been some treatment responses in patients with obstructing endobronchial aspergillosis. Most patients with diffuse bilateral parenchymal disease (often with coexisting widespread dissemination) die quickly, despite therapy.

Management of massive hemoptysis is very difficult. Surgical resection of selected patients may be helpful (those with reasonable overall status and localized disease). Bronchial artery embolization can be tried for patients who are poor surgical candidates, but still have some chance of meaningful survival given control of bleeding. Thoracotomy has also been used for selected patients with cavitary disease who present with pneumothoraces and have persistent major air leaks. If the cavity can be resected, control of the pleural space and removal of the chest tube can sometimes be accomplished. Otherwise the patient is fated to long-term chest drainage, and often a poorly expanded lung and a chronically infected pleural space. Under these conditions quality of life is poor and survival is short.

At present, AMB is the best choice for initial treatment, with a switch to itraconazole for patients who stabilize. Itraconazole from onset may be appropriate for patients with relatively indolent disease, but further study is needed.

Prevention

Prevention of all exposure to *Aspergillus* spores is not possible. Common sense dictates that extremely immunosuppressed patients, including those with advanced HIV infection, should avoid activities that expose them to unusually high concentrations of spores, including working with compost material, wood chips, or other decaying vegetation, and working in or around barns, confinement buildings, and other sites with abundance of organic material. Smoking of marijuana should also be avoided.

B. Other Rare Diseases Caused by Phagocyte Opportunists

Zygomycosis is about one-tenth as common as aspergillosis in neutropenic patients and is the second most common infection in this class. Clinical forms of the illness include sino-orbital disease, pulmonary disease, and disseminated disease. Localized invasion of burned or otherwise injured skin can also occur. Sino-orbital disease usually complicates uncontrolled diabetic ketoacidosis. Pulmonary and systemic disease occurs in the same type of patients who contract invasive aspergillosis; namely, patients with neutropenia and patients receiving glucocorticoid and other immunosuppressive therapy, including organ transplant recipients. Pulmonary mucormycosis resembles invasive pulmonary aspergillosis, but is much less common. The disease is acquired by inhalation, is similarly angioinvasive, and can also spread through the bloodstream to skin, visceral organs, and the brain. Excision of all devitalized tissue, whenever practical, together with high-dose AMB is the best approach to therapy. Results are often poor, and few patients survive if extensive areas of necrotic tissue are present that cannot be surgically removed.

Mucormycosis has been reported in patients with HIV infections. Localized skin infections have been reported at injection sites in intravenous drug users (46). Isolated renal infection, invasive sinus infection, esophageal and gastric infection, and pulmonary infection, all have been reported, but are extremely rare (47,48).

Not surprisingly, patients with HIV infection who are debilitated, neutropenic from the illness and from cytotoxic therapy, and who are suffering other infectious or malignant complications of advanced HIV infections can, on rare occasions, become infected with a wide range of other fungi with little tendency to invade any intact host. These infections are best thought of as "aspergillus-like" infections, rather than given great weight as separate entities. Only occasionally are there important clinical features, such as resistance to AMB for *Pseudoallescheria boydii* and high frequency of positive blood cultures for *Fusarium* species. The range of the possible at the extremes of immunosuppression is very broad. Dermatophytes such as *Trichosporon beigelii*, can present as invasive disseminated infection (49). Chronic sinus disease from the mushroom *Schizophyllum commune* has been reported (50), as has disseminated infection including meningitis with the blue-green algae *Prototheca wickerhamii* (51). These infections are testament to the severity of the immunosuppression; rather than to any particular properties of the infecting organisms.

IV. An Overlap Disease (T-Cell Opportunist on Mucosal Surfaces but Phagocyte Opportunist for Deep Invasion)

A. Candidiasis

Epidemiology

Candidiasis is an extremely important systemic fungal infection complicating neutropenia (other risk factors include glucocorticoid therapy, indwelling vascular catheters, broad-spectrum antibiotics, hyperalimentation, and abdominal surgeries), but it is really a systemic and not a pulmonary infection. It is the only major deep fungal infection that is not acquired by inhalation. Rather *Candida* species are part of the normal bowel flora and skin flora. Under appropriate circumstances *Candida* organisms gain access to the bloodstream across the bowel wall or through damaged or instrumented skin. Without neutrophil defense there is potential for hematogenous spread throughout the body. Microabscesses are found in many organs, including the lung. Pulmonary symptoms and findings are few, and the chest roentgenogram is often normal, although it may become diffusely abnormal late in the course of illness.

T-cell immunity is important to control overgrowth of *Candida* on mucosal surfaces, but as long as phagocyte function is intact, deep invasion is unlikely. Thus, patients with HIV infection frequently have problems with candidal pharyngitis and esophagitis (and vulvovaginitis), but seldom develop disseminated disease. Oral candidiasis occurs in virtually all HIV-infected persons sometime during the course of their illness (52). Although not AIDS-defining, it occurs as T-cell immunity wanes and is a predictor of progression to AIDS. Esophageal candidiasis is a common AIDS-defining infection.

Clinical Features

Oral candidiasis can involve the tongue and the mucosa of the oral cavity and oropharynx. White exudative lesions are common with mild immunosuppression. As the HIV infection progresses, the diseased mucosa can look erythematous and atrophic. Esophageal candidiasis is usually accompanied by oral candidiasis (53). Many patients have dysphagia or odynophagia, but others are asymtomatic. Vulvovaginal candidiasis presents with local itching and irritation and vaginal discharge. As in the mouth, mucosal abnormalities range from white and exudative to red and atrophic. *Candida* can also involve the trachea and proximal bronchi.

Despite the common overgrowth of *Candida* on mucosal surface, disseminated candidiasis with deep organ involvement is extremely uncommon in AIDS, even with advanced immunosuppression. Candidemia in HIV-infected patients usually occurs in patients with other classic risk factors, including indwelling vascular catheters, multiple antibiotics, and neutropenia from bone marrow toxic therapy of intercurrent infections and neoplasms complicating HIV infection. Even in patients with these risks factors, candidemia and disseminated candidiasis are surprisingly uncommon. Even at autopsy, disseminated candidiasis is uncommon. Systemic candidiasis is very rare in AIDS because *Candida* are phagocyte opportunists for invasive infection. Other factors may also play a role. The question of a protective role for an antibody against a specific 47-kDa candidal antigen has been raised (54). This antibody is apparently more common in AIDS than in other immunosuppressed conditions.

Diagnosis

Oropharyngeal candidiasis can be suspected on physical examination and confirmed by direct examination and by culture of scrapings from the lesions. Candidal esophagitis is presumed if a patient with candidal pharyngitis also has dysphagia. A barium swallow, if done, often shows a "cobblestone" appearance. If the treatment response is poor, then endoscopy should be performed to visualize the lesions (again ranging from white and exudative to red and atrophic). Biopsies of the lesions should be performed to exclude herpes or cytomegalovirus infection, either as the sole cause of the esophagitis or as a coinfection with *Candida*. Biopsies confirming candidal infection show characteristic pseudohyphae.

The extremely rare AIDS patient with disseminated candidiasis is diagnosed by positive blood cultures or by culture or histopathological examination of tissue biopsies or usually sterile body fluids, including pleural fluid or peritoneal fluid. Candidal opthalmitis, with typical lesions on fundoscopic examination, is also diagnostic of disseminated candidiasis. The concept of benign or transient candidemia, perhaps curable by removing an intravenous catheter, is flawed and should be abandoned. Candidemia is a serious infection, and all patients with positive blood cultures should be treated. Positive urine cultures are more difficult to interpret. In patients with urinary catheters such cultures usually reflect colonization of the bladder, rather than hematogenous spread to the kidney and subsequent renal excretion. Positive urine specimens in patients with AIDS should be interpreted much as they are in non-HIV patients.

Treatment

Topical therapy for oral and vaginal infections is somewhat successful. For oral infections clotrimazole troches are perhaps more effective than nystatin suspensions, if only because of longer contact time with the mucosa. For more advanced disease, systemic therapy is more effective (55). Fluconazole, 100–200 mg daily, for 4–7 days usually controls the infections. Many patients need intermittent therapy every few weeks or even continuous therapy to prevent relapse of highly symptomatic infection. Women with vaginitis can be treated with clotrimazole troches or with oral fluconazole. For severe infections, systemic therapy may be better. The initial course is continued until the patient is free of symptoms and has a negative culture. Maintenance regimens to prevent relapse include clotrimazole troches every week or oral fluconazole, 100–200 mg once weekly (54). Some patients require continuous suppressive therapy.

The treatment of choice for candidemia and for all cases of disseminated candidiasis has been AMB, with a daily dose of 0.5–0.7 mg/kg and a total cumulative dose of 1000–2000 mg. In a recent study, fluconazole was compared prospectively with AMB in nonneutropenic patients with candidemia (57). Fluconazole had equal (yet imperfect) efficacy and because of lesser toxicity can now be considered the treatment of choice. Proof of equal efficacy in neutropenic patients is not available, and AMB remains first therapeutic choice there. AMB also remains treatment of choice for patients with candidal ophthalmitis, whether or not they have neutropenia.

Prevention

Patients who are being treated with fluconazole or itraconazole for maintenance therapy of other fungal infections or with fluconazole as primary prophylaxis against cryptococcosis do have a lower incidence of oropharyngeal, vaginal, and esophageal candidiasis. The use of these agents for primary prevention of mucosal candidal infections is not recommended, however, because of cost, the fear that resistant strains of *C. albicans* or non–*C. albicans* might increase in frequency, and the benign nature of the illness and relative ease and efficacy of treatment for those who develop it. There is virtually no chance that mucosal disease will become systemic and, thus, no need to prevent it for fear of more serious infection.

References

1. Schaffner A, Davis CE, Schaffner T, Markert M, Douglas H, Braude AI. In vitro susceptibility to killing by neutrophil granulocytes discriminates between primary pathogenicity and opportunism. J Clin Invest 1986; 78:511–524.
2. Fauci AS. Immunological abnormalities in the acquired immunodeficiency syndrome (AIDS). Clin Res 1984; 32:491–499.
3. Ellis M, Gupta S, Galant S, Hakim S, VandeVen C, Toy C, Cairo MS. Impaired neutrophil function in patients with AIDS or AIDS-related complex. A comprehensive evaluation. J Infect Dis 1988; 158:1268–1276.
4. Kapholz A, Salomon N, Perlman DC, Talavera W. Aspergillosis in the acquired immunodeficiency syndrome. Chest 1991; 100:614–618.
5. Newberry WM, Walter JE, Chandler JW, et al. Epidemiologic study of *Cryptococcus neoformans*. Ann Intern Med 1967; 67:724–732.
6. Chuck SL, Sande MA. Infections with *Cryptococcus neoformans* in the acquired immunodeficiency syndrome. N Engl J Med 1989; 321:794–799.
7. Eng RHK, Bishburg E, Smith SM, Kapila R. Cryptococcal infections in patients with acquired immunodeficiency syndrome. Am J Med 1986; 81:19–23.
8. DeSmet P, Kayembe KD, DeVroey C. The value of cryptococcal serum antigen screening among HIV positive /AIDS patients in Kinshasa, Zaire. AIDS 1989; 3:77–78.
9. Hoffman S, Stenerup J, Mathiesen LR. Low yield of screening for cryptococcal antigen by latex-agglutination assay on serum and cerebrospinal fluid from Danish patients with AIDS or ARC. Scand J Infect Dis 1991; 23:697–702.
10. Kovacs JA, Kovacs AA, Polis M, Wright WC, Gill VJ, Tuazon CU, Gelmann EP, Lane HC, Longfield R, Overturf G, et al. Cryptococcosis in acquired immunodeficiency syndrome. Ann Intern Med 1985; 103;533–538.
11. Zuger A, Louie E, Holzman RS, Simberkoff MS, Rahal JJ. Cryptococcal disease in patients with the acquired immunodeficiency syndrome. Ann Intern Med 1986; 104:234–240.
12. White MH, Armstrong D. Cryptococcosis. Infect Dis Clin North Am 1994; 8:383–398.

13. Saag MS, Powderly WG, Cloud GA, Robinson P, Grieco MH, Sharkey PK, Thompson SE, Sugar AM, Tuazon CU, Fisher JF, et al. Comparison of amphotericin B with fluconazole in the treatment of acute AIDS-associated cryptococcal meningitis. N Engl J Med 1992; 326:83–89.
14. Larsen RA, Leal MA, Chan LS. Fluconazole compared with amphotericin B plus flucytosine for cryptococcal meningitis in AIDS. Ann Intern Med 1990; 113:183–187.
15. Powderly WG, Saag MS, Cloud GA, Robinson P, Meyer RD, Jacobson JM, Graybill JR, Sugar AM, McAuliffe VJ, Follansbee SE, et al. A controlled trial of fluconazole or amphotericin B to prevent relapse of cryptococcal meningitis in patients with the acquired immunodeficiency syndrome. N Engl J Med 1992; 326:793–798.
16. Bozzette BA, Larsen RA, Chiu J, Leal MA, Jacobsen J, Rofhman P, Robinson P, Gilbert G, McCutchan JA, Tilles J, et al. A placebo-controlled trial of maintenance therapy with fluconazole after treatment of cryptococcal meningits in the acquired immunodeficiency syndrome. N Engl J Med 1991; 580–584.
17. Denning DW, Armstrong RW, Lewis BH, Stevens DA. Elevated cerebrospinal fluid pressures in patients with cryptococcal meningitis and acquired immunodeficiency syndrome. Am J Med 1991; 91:267–272.
18. Nightengale SD, Cal SX, Peterson DM, Loss SD, Gamble BA, Watson DA, Manzone CP, Baker JE, Jockusch JD. Primary prophylaxis with fluconazole against systemic fungal infections in HIV-positive patients. AIDS 1992; 6:191–194.
19. Johnson PG, Hamill RJ, Sarosi GA. Clinical review: progressive disseminated histoplasmosis in the AIDS patient. Semin Respir Infect 1989; 4:139–146.
20. Wheat LJ, Slama TG, Zeckel MS. Histoplasmosis in the acquired immunodeficiency syndrome. Am J Med 1984; 144:2178-2181.
21. Wheat J. Histoplasmosis and coccidioidomycosis in individuals with AIDS. A clinical review. Infect Dis Clin North Am 1994; 8:467–482.
22. Conces DJ, Stockberger SM, Tarver RD, Wheat LJ. Disseminated histoplasmosis in AIDS: findings on chest radiographs. AJR 1993; 160:15–19.
23. Salzman SH, Smith RL, Aranda CP. Histoplasmosis in patients at risk for the acquired immunodeficiency syndrome in a non-endemic setting. Chest 1988; 93:916–921.
24. Keath EJ, Kobayashi GS, Medofff G. Typing of *Histoplasma capsulatum* by restriction fragment length polymorphisms in a nuclear gene. J Clin Microbiol 1992; 30:2104-2107.
25. Wheat LJ, Connolly-Stringfield PA, Baker RL, Curfman MF, Eads ME, Israel KS, Norris SA, Webb DH, Zeckel ML. Disseminated histoplasmosis in the acquired immune deficiency syndrome: clinical findings, diagnosis, and a review of the literature. Medicine 1990; 69:361–374.
26. Wheat LJ, Connolly-Stringfield PA, Kohler RB, Frame PT, Gupta, MR. *Histoplasma capsulatum* polysaccharide antigen detection in diagnosis and management of disseminated histoplasmosis in patients with acquired immunodeficiency syndrome. Am J Med 1989; 87:396–400.

27. Wheat J, Hafner R, Wulfsohn M, Spencer P, Squires K, Powderly W, Wong B, Rinaldi M, Saag M, Hamill R, et al. Prevention of relapse of histoplasmosis with itraconazole in patients with the acquired immunodeficiency syndrome. Ann Intern Med 1993; 118:610–616.
28. Como JA, Dismukes WE. Oral azole drugs as systemic antifungal therapy. N Engl J Med 1994; 330:263–272.
29. McKinsey DS, Gupta MR, Riddler SA, Driks MR, Smith DL, Kurtin PJ. Long-term amphotericin B therapy for disseminated histoplasmosis in patients with the acquired immunodeficiency syndrome. Am J Med 1988; 85:152–158.
30. Ampel NM, Dols CL, Galgiani JN. Coccidioidomycosis during human immunodeficiency virus infection: results of a prospective study in a coccidioidal endemic area. Am J Med 1993; 94:235–240.
31. Fish DG, Ampel NM, Galgiani JN, Dols CL, Kelly PC, Johnson CH, Pappagianis D, Edwards JE, Wasserman RB, Clark RJ, et al. Coccidioidomycosis during human immunodeficiency virus infection. A review of 77 patients. Medicine 1990; 69:384–391.
32. DiTomasso JP, Ampel NM, Sobonya RE, Bloom JW. Bronchoscopic diagnosis of pulmonary coccididiodomycosis. Comparison of cytology, culture, and transbronchial biopsy. Diagn Microbiol Infect Dis 1994;18:83–87.
33. Tucker RN, Galgiani JN, Denning DW, Hanson LH, Graybill JR, Sharkey K, Eckman MR, Salemi C, Libke R, Klein RA, et al. Treatment of coccidioidal meningitis with fluconazole. Rev Infect Dis 1990; 12(3 suppl):S380–S389.
34. Pappas PG, Pottage JC, Powderly WG, Fraser VJ, Stratton CW, McKenzie S, Tapper ML, Chmel H, Bonebrake FC, Blum R, et al. Blastomycosis in patients with the acquired immunodeficiency syndrome. Ann Intern Med 1992; 116:847–853.
35. Supparatpinyo K, Khamwan C, Baosoung V, Nelson KE, Sirisanthana T. Disseminted *Penicillium marneffe*i infection in Southeast Asia. Lancet 1994; 344:110–113.
36. Supparatpinyo K, Nelson KE, Merz WG, Breslin BJ, Cooper CR Jr., Kamwan C, Sirisanthana T. Response to antifungal therapy by human immunodeficiency virus infected patients with disseminated *Penicillium marneffei* infections and in vitro susceptibilities of isolates from clinical specimens. Antimicrob Agents Chemother 1993; 37:2407–2411.
37. Supparatpinyo K, Chiewchanvit S, Hirunsri P, Uthammachai C, Nelson KE, Sirisanthana T. *Penicillium marneffei* infection in patients infected with human immunodeficiency virus. Clin Infect Dis 1992; 14:871–874.
38. Heller HM, Fuhrer J. Disseminated sporotrichosis in patients with AIDS: case report and review of the literature. AIDS 1991; 5:1243–1246.
39. Donabedian H, O'Donnell E, Olszeewski C, MacArthur RD, Budd N. Disseminated cutaneous and meningeal sporotrichosis in an AIDS patient. Diagn Microbiol Infect Dis 1994; 18:111–115.
40. Sharkey-Mathis PK, Kauffman CA, Graybill JR, Stevens DA, Hostetler JS, Cloud G, Dismukes WE. Treatment of sporotrichosis with itraconazole: NIAID Mycoses Study Group. Am J Med 1993; 95:279–285.
41. Denning DW, Follansbee SE, Scolaro M, Norris S, Edelstein H, Stevens DA.

Pulmonary aspergillosis in the acquired immunodeficiency syndrome. N Engl J Med 1991; 324:654–662.

42. Minamato GY, Barlam TF, Vander ELS NJ. Invasive aspergillosis in patients with AIDS. Clin Infect Dis 1992; 14:66–74.
43. Lorholary O, Meyohas MC, Dupont B, Cadranel J, Salmon-Ceron D, Peyramond D, Simonin D. Invasive aspergillosis in patients with acquired immunodeficiency syndrome: report of 33 cases. Am J Med 1993; 95:177–187.
44. Miller WT Jr, Sais GJ, Frank I, Gefter WB, Arondrick JM, Miller WT. Pulmonary aspergillosis in patients with AIDS: clinical and radiographic correlations. Chest 1994; 105:37–44.
45. Kemper CA, Hostetler JS, Follansbee SE, Ruane P, Covington D, Leong SS, Deresinski SC, Stevens DA. Ulcerative and plaque-like tracheobronchitis due to infection with *Aspergillus* in patients with AIDS. Clin Infect Dis 1993; 17:344–352.
46. Sanchez MR, Ponge-Wilson I, Moy JA, Rosenthal S. Zygomycosis and HIV infection. J Am Acad Dermatol 1994; 30:904–908.
47. Santos J, Espagado P, Romero C, Andreu J, Rivero A, Pineda JA. Isolated renal mucormycosis in two AIDS patients. Eur J Clin Mircobiol Infect Dis 1994; 13:430–432.
48. Margolis PS, Epstein A. Mucormycosis esophagitis in a patient with the acquired immunodeficiency syndrome. Am J Gastroenterol 1994; 89:1900–1902.
49. Rosenthal J, Katz R, DuBois DB, Morrissey A, Machicao A. Chronic maxillary sinusitis associated with the mushroom *Schizophyllum commune* in a patient with AIDS. Clin Infect Dis 1992; 14:46–48.
50. Nahass GT, Rosengerg SP, Leonardi CL, Penneys NS. Disseminated infection with *Trichosporon beigelli*. Report of a case and review of the cutaneous and histologic manifestations. Arch Dermatol 1993; 129:1020–1023.
51. Kaminski ZC, Kapila R, Sharer LR, Kloser P, Kaufman L. Meningitis due to *Prototheca wickerhamii* in a patient with AIDS. Clin Infect Dis 1992; 15:704–706.
52. Phelen J, Saltzman B, Friedland G, Klein RS. Oral findings with acquired immunodeficiency syndrome. Oral Surg Oral Med Oral Pathol 1987; 64:50–56.
53. Porro GB, Parente F, Cernuschi M. The diagnosis of esophageal candidiasis in patients with acquired immunodeficiency syndrome: is endoscopy always necessary? Am J Gasroenterol 1989; 84:143–146.
54. Matthews R, Burnie J, Smith D, Clark I, Midgley J, Conolly M, Gazzard B. *Candida* and AIDS: evidence for protective antibody [review]. Lancet 1988; 2:263–266.
55. Greenspan D. Treatment of oropharyngeal candidiasis in HIV-positive patients. J Am Acad Dermatol 1994; 31:S51–S55.
56. Sobel JD. Controversial aspects in the management of vulvovaginal candidiasis. J Am Acad Dermatol 1994; 31:S10–S13.
57. Rex JH, Bennett JE, Sugar AM, Pappas PG, van der Horst CM, Edwards JE, Washburn RG, Scheld WM, Karchmer AW, Dine AP, et al. A randomized trial comparing fluconazole with amphotericin B for the treatment of candidemia in patients with neutropenia. N Engl J Med 1994; 331:1325–1330.

16

Pulmonary Toxoplasmosis

FRANK L. ACERRA

Beth Israel Medical Center
New York, New York

I. Introduction

Toxoplasma gondii is an intracellular protozoan that occurs in three forms: the oocyst, the tachyzoite, and the tissue cyst. Toxoplasmal infection may be defined as an asymptomatic carrier state caused by persistence of *T. gondii* in the tissue cyst form. It is the tachyzoite form that causes the clinical disease toxoplasmosis, usually as a reactivation phenomenon in persons who are immunocompromised (1).

Humans are infected through ingestion of undercooked meats that contain tissue cysts, or through congenital acquisition from mother to fetus. The organism multiplies within nucleated cells, including gray and white matter brain cells, retinal cells, skeletal muscle of the heart, and alveolar lining cells (2).

After initial exposure, the organism proliferates for a time, dependent on the host's native immunity. This is followed by a reduction in the protozoan population, and a chronic latent infection state that is asymptomatic in immunocompetent persons (3).

II. Toxoplasmosis in AIDS

In the normal host, toxoplasmosis is a self-limited disease. However, when cell-mediated immunity fails, the infection may become fulminant and lead to death. In the United States, 30–50% of patients with AIDS have been infected with *T. gondii*, as evidenced by the presence of antibodies (4). The incidence of toxoplasmosis in the HIV-infected population is lower in the United States than in Western Europe, where seropositivity can reach 96% (5,6). Reactivation toxoplasmosis usually occurs when CD4 lymphocyte counts fall below 100/μl in up to one-third of IgG-positive patients with HIV (7).

Encephalitis is the most common manifestation of *T. gondii* illness in patients with HIV infection. In the past 10 years, the number of reported cases of toxoplasmic pneumonia has increased, making it the second most common site of infection with this pathogen (5). However, *T. gondii* accounts for less than 1% of all cases of pulmonary disease in patients with HIV infection (8).

In the early descriptions of HIV-infected patients with toxoplasmic pneumonitis, most patients had concurrent CNS infection (8–12). More recent studies described patients with toxoplasmic pneumonitis without CNS involvement (6,13). Based on diagnostic studies of bronchoalveolar lavage and autopsy results, the overall prevalence of pulmonary toxoplasmosis in patients with lung disease ranges from less than 1 to 5% (8,14–16).

III. Pathogenesis

As in toxoplasmic encephalitis, pulmonary toxoplasmosis appears to be due to reactivation of latent infection (6,13). In the United States, less than 1% of patients with AIDS produce IgM antibodies to *Toxoplasma* spp., which would denote acute infection (17). In three studies that reviewed pulmonary toxoplasmosis in AIDS, 24 of 27 patients with available immunological data had evidence of past infection (5,6,13). It is unknown whether pulmonary involvement occurs from local cyst rupture or from hematogenous spread of tachyzoites from distant sites of reactivation. Given the diffuse pattern of pneumonitis and extrapulmonary involvement in up to one-half of patients, the latter seem more likely (6).

Mice with chronic toxoplasmic infection that are gradually depleted of CD4 lymphocytes develop a clinical syndrome resembling the disease in humans, in that reactivation occurs primarily in the central nervous system (18,19). Conversely, new infection with toxoplasma in mice with CD4 lymphopenia results in overwhelming systemic infection, with pulmonary disease and only mild CNS involvement (18).

IV. Clinical Presentation

Most patients with toxoplasmic pneumonia present with a febrile prodromal illness indistinguishable from *Pneumocystis carinii* pneumonia (PCP), but the onset may be more rapid (6). Dyspnea and nonproductive cough are the most common symptoms, and fever is the most common sign (5). Examination of the chest is usually unremarkable, but may reveal crackles, or rarely, findings consistent with pleural effusion (2,5,13). Lymphadenopathy and hepatosplenomegaly are uncommon (5). Coexistent encephalitis may provide a clue to the diagnosis of toxoplasmic pulmonary infection, but neurological abnormalities are by no means always present, and they may develop after the onset of pneumonia (20).

A recent national survey of extracerebral toxoplasmosis in France identified 52 cases of pulmonary infection (16). Cough was present in all cases, and dyspnea in 25%. Fever was seen in 83% of cases of extracerebral toxoplasmosis. Other reports described toxoplasmosis presenting as adult respiratory distress syndrome and septic shock (18,19).

Hypoxemia is a common presenting laboratory abnormality (6). Oksenhendler et al. found all patients in their study to be hypoxemic, with a mean Pao_2 at entry of 47 ± 12 mmHg (6). Expectorated and induced sputum analyses both have low diagnostic yields (13). Elevations of aspartate transaminase (AST), alanine transaminase (ALT), and lactate dehydrogenase (LDH) are also common. In fact, very high levels of LDH may be a clue to the diagnosis of toxoplasmosis, possibly related to infection of skeletal and cardiac muscle (21).

Chest radiographs are abnormal in up to 53% of patients with pulmonary toxoplasmosis (16). The most common patterns are bilateral interstitial infiltrates or coarse nodular infiltrates (Fig 1; 2,5). In one series of patients, 22% had pleural effusions (2). Bilateral lower lobe consolidation, cavitary infiltrates, and solitary pulmonary nodules have also been described (11,22).

V. Diagnosis

A definitive diagnosis of toxoplasmosis requires the demonstration of the tachyzoite form of the parasite (23). With hematoxylin and eosin (H & E)

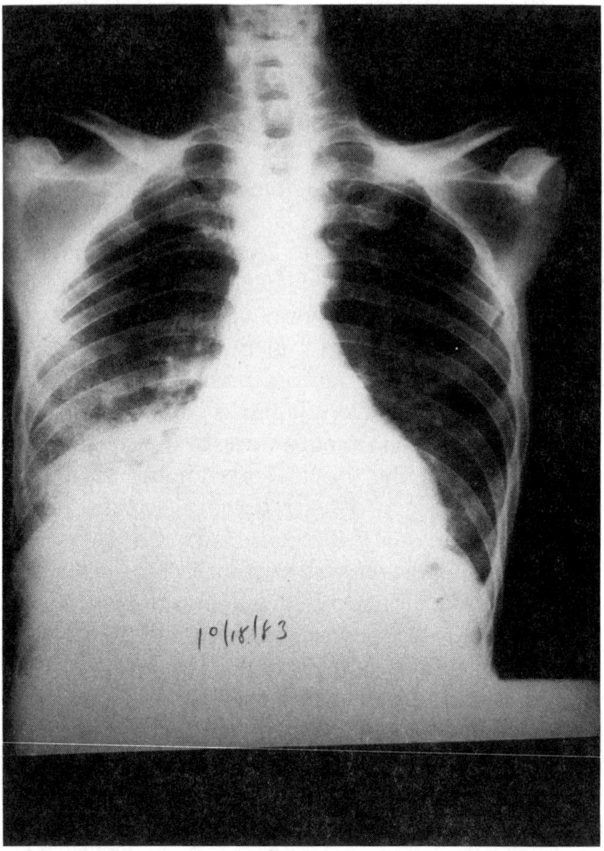

Figure 1 Chest radiograph of a patient with toxoplasmic pneumonia.

or Giemsa staining, tachyzoites can be seen in alveolar lining cells (5). The best results have been reported with the use of eosin–methylene blue fast staining (5,24) or Giemsa staining (5,24,25) of bronchoalveolar lavage fluid (BAL). In one series, BAL was diagnostic in 88% of patients with pulmonary toxoplasmosis (16). In the study by Oksenhendler et al., BAL was diagnostic in 10 of 11 patients (6). However, the yield of BAL may be lower with infection that is not severe. Derouin et al. recently proposed that tissue culture on human embryonic fibroblast cell line MRC5 (Bio Merieux, Lyon, France) provided evidence of infection within 2 days of inoculation in patients in whom diagnosis was not made by stained smears (24). In another series, the diagnosis was also made by observation of parasites in transbronchial biopsy specimens, pleural fluid, and open-lung biopsy (2).

The usefulness of polymerase chain reaction (PCR) for the diagnosis of toxoplasmic pneumonia has not been established, for PCR would detect tissue cyst present in dormant infection as well as the tachyzoite causing pneumonia (5).

VI. Treatment and Outcomes

Antimicrobial therapy must be tailored to the severity of the disease and the immune status of the patient (Table 1; 26,27). To date, there are no controlled trials that evaluate treatment regimens specifically for toxoplasmic pneumonia. The current recommendations for treatment are the same as those for toxoplasmic encephalitis, which includes acute (primary) treatment, maintenance treatment (secondary prophylaxis), and primary prophylaxis (1). Patients with AIDS and toxoplasmosis require lifelong maintenance therapy to prevent recurrence of infection, because relapse can occur in up to 80% of cases after treatment is discontinued (5,26,28).

In one large series, the overall clinical response to therapy for toxoplasmic pneumonia was 52% (16). However, pyrimethamine with sulfadiazine therapy is now considered the treatment of choice, and is associated with a response in up to 95% of patients (29). In one study, all eight patients with pulmonary toxoplasmosis who were treated with these agents recovered (6). Clindamycin is an effective alternative to sulfadiazine (30). Immediate therapy should be continued for 3–6 weeks, followed by maintenance therapy (1,31). Pyrimethamine and sulfadiazine have also shown the best results for maintenance when lower doses are used (32).

Recently, low-dose trimethoprim–sulfamethoxazole (TMP–SMX), pyrimethamine–dapsone, roxithromycin, and pyrimethamine–sulfadioxine (Fansidar) all have been effective as primary prophylaxis against toxoplasmosis (33–36). Thus, patients taking TMP–SMX to prevent PCP are also receiving effective prophylaxis against toxoplasmosis.

Despite the availability of maintenance therapy, pulmonary toxoplasmosis is associated with a high mortality rate. In one study, the median survival after a diagnosis of extracerebral toxoplasmosis was 150 days (16). Fifty-six percent died of other AIDS-related diagnoses, 34% from extracerebral toxoplasmosis, and 10% from cerebral toxoplasmosis.

VII. Summary

Although an uncommon disorder in AIDS, pulmonary toxoplasmosis should be considered in immunocompromised hosts who present with signs and

Table 1 *Toxoplasma gondii* in AIDS

Immediate therapy	Pyrimethamine 200 mg loading dose on day 1, then 50–75 mg daily po plus folinic acid 10 mg po daily plus sulfadiazine 4–8 g po or iv daily for 3–6 weeks	Alternate: substitute clindamycin 600 mg po or iv every 6 hr for sulfadiazine
Maintenance therapy	Pyrimethamine 50 mg po daily plus folinic acid 10 mg po daily plus sulfadiazine 1.0–1.5 g po every 6 hr	Alternate: substitute clindamycin 300 mg po every 6 hr for sulfadiazine
Prophylaxis (as for PCP recommendations)	Trimethoprim–sulfamethoxazole 1 double-strength tablet po daily or three times weekly	Pyrimethamine 50 mg po weekly plus dapsone 50 mg po daily, or pyrimethamine 25 mg po plus dapsone 100 mg po two times weekly (plus) folinic acid 25 mg weekly

Source: Refs. 37 and 38.

symptoms of pneumonia and abnormal radiographs, especially in the setting of encephalitis or with other neurological manifestations consistent with toxoplasmic encephalitis. The diagnostic algorithm used to diagnose *P. carinii* pneumonia will usually lead to this diagnosis. Hematoxylin and eosin or Giemsa staining of bronchoalveolar lavage fluid, and perhaps tissue culture, are the diagnostic methods for choice. Treatment strategies for toxoplasmic encephalitis are also effective for pulmonary toxoplasmosis, but mortality rates are still as high as 60% with even with early diagnosis and treatment.

References

1. Beaman M, McCabe R, Wong S, Remington J. *Toxoplasma gondii*. In: Mandell G, Dolin R, Bennett J, eds. Principles and Practices of Infectious Diseases, 4th ed. New York: Churchill-Livingston, 1995:2455–2474.
2. Goodman PC, Schnapp L. Pulmonary toxoplasmosis in AIDS. Radiology 1992; 184:791–793.
3. Remington JS, Jacobs L, Kaufman H. Toxoplasmosis in the adult. N Engl J Med 1960; 262:237–241.
4. Grant IH, Gold JW, Rosenblum M, Niedzwiecki D, Armstrong D, *Toxoplasma gondii* serology in HIV infected patients: The development of central nervous system toxoplasmosis in AIDS. AIDS. 1990; 4:519–521.
5. Pomeroy C, Filice G. Pulmonary toxoplasmosis: a review. Clin Infect Dis 1992; 14:863–870.
6. Oksenhendler E, Cadranel J, Sarfati C, Katlama C, Datry A, Marche C, Wolf M, Roux P, Derouin F, Clauvel JP. *Toxoplasma gondii* pneumonia in patients with the acquired immunodeficiency syndrome. Am J Med 1990; 88:18–21.
7. Porter SB, Sande MA. Toxoplasmosis of the central nervous system in the acquired immunodeficiency syndrome. N Engl J Med 1992; 327:1643–1648.
8. Murray T, Felton C, Garay S, Gottlieb M, Hopewell P, Stover D, Teirstein A. Pulmonary complications of the acquired immunodeficiency syndrome: report of a National Heart, Lung and Blood Institute workshop. N Engl J Med 1984; 310:1682–1688.
9. Tourani JM, Israel-Biet D, Venet A, Andrieu JM. Unusual pulmonary infection in a puzzling presentation of AIDS. Lancet 1985; 1:989.
10. Touboul JL, Salmon D, Lancastre F, Mayaud C, Fermand JP, Fouret P, Akoun G. Pneumopathie a *Tosoplasma gondii* chez un patient atteint du syndrome d'immunodipression acquis: mise en evidence du parasite par lavage bronchiolo alveolaire. Rev Pneumol Clin 1986; 42:150–152.
11. Tawney S, Masci J, Berger HW, Subietas A. Pulmonary toxoplasmosis: an unusual radiographic pattern in a patient with AIDS. Mt Sinai J Med 1986; 53:683–686.
12. Mendelson MH, Finkel JL, Meyers BR, Lieberman JP, Hirschman SZ. Pulmonary toxoxplasmosis in AIDS. Scand J Infect Dis 1987; 19:703–706.

13. Schnapp L, Geaghan S, Campagna A, Fahy J, Steiger D, Ng V, Hadley WK, Hopewell PC, Stansell JD. *Toxoplasma gondii* pneumonitis in patients infected with the human immunodeficiency virus. Arch Intern Med 1992; 152:1073–1077.
14. Derouin F, Sarfati C, Beauvais B, Garin YJ, Lariviere M. Prevalence of pulmonary toxoplasmosis in HIV-infected patients. AIDS 1990; 4:1036.
15. Marche C, Wolff M, Mayorga R, Matherson S, Salmon D, Matthiessen L, Claude B. Toxoplamose pulmonaire au cours du SIDA. V International Conference on AIDS. Montreal, June 1989:abstr WBP 3.
16. Rabaud C, May T, Amiel C, Katlama C, Lepopt C, Ambriose-Thomas P, Canton P. Extracerebral toxoplasmosis in patients infected with HIV: a French national survey. Medicine 1994; 73:306–314.
17. Mills J. *Pneumocystis carinii* and *Toxoplasma gondii* infections in patients with AIDS. Rev Infect Dis 1986; 8:1001–1011.
18. Gandhi S, Lyubsky S, Jiminez-Lucho V. Adult respiratory distress syndrome associated with disseminated toxoplasmosis. Clin Infect Dis 1994; 19:169–171.
19. Lucet JC, Bailly MP, Bedos JP, Wolff M, Gachot B, Vachon F. Septic shock due to toxoplasmosis in patients infected with human immunodeficiency virus. Chest 1993; 104:1054–1058.
20. Catterall J, Hofflin J, Remington J. Pulmonary toxoplasmosis. Am Rev Respir Dis 1986; 133:704–705.
21. Pugin J, Vanhems P, Hirschel B, Chave J, Flepp M. Extreme elevations of serum lactic dehydrogenase differentiating pulmonary toxoplasmosis from *Pneumocystis carinii* pneumonia. N Engl J Med 1992; 326:1226.
22. Cohen BA, Pomeranz S, Rabinowitz JG, Rosen MJ, Train JS, Norton KI, Mendelson DS. Pulmonary complications of AIDS: radiologic features. AJR 1984; 143:115–122.
23. Weller P. Parasitic pneumonias. In: Pennington JE ed. Respiratory Infections. Diagnosis and Management, 2nd ed. New York: Raven Press, 1988:583–600.
24. Derouin F, Sarfati C, Beauvais B, Iliou MC, Dehen L, Lariviere M. Laboratory diagnosis of pulmonary toxoplasmosis in patients with acquired immunodeficiency syndrome. J Clin Microbiol 1989; 27:1661–1663.
25. Bottone EJ. Diagnosis of acute pulmonary toxoplasmosis by visualization of invasive and intracellular tachyzoites in Giemsa stained smears of bronchoalveolar lavage fluid. J Clin Microbiol 1991; 29:2626–2627.
26. McCabe RE, Remington JS. The diagnosis and treatment of toxoplasmosis. Eur J Clin Microbiol 1983; 2:95–104.
27. McCabe RE, Oster S. Current recommendations and future prospects in the treatment of toxoplasmosis. Drugs 1989; 38:973–987.
28. Cohn J, McMeeking A, Cohen W, Jacobs J, Holzman RS. Evaluation of the policy of empiric treatment of suspected toxoplasma encephalitis in patients with the acquired immunodeficiency syndrome. Am J Med 1989; 86:521–527.
29. Wong SY, Remington JS. Toxoplasmosis in the setting of AIDS. In: Broder S, Merigan TC Jr, Bolognesi D, eds. Medical Management of AIDS. Baltimore: Williams & Wilkins, 1994:223–258.

30. Danneman B, McCutchen JA, Israelski D, Antoniskis D, Lepopt C, Luft B, Nussbaum J, Clumeck N, Morlat P, Chiu J. Treatment of toxoplasmic encephalitis in patients with AIDS. A randomized trial comparing pyrimethamine plus clindamycin to pyrimethamine plus sulfadiazine. The California Collaborative Treatment Group. Ann Intern Med 1992; 116:33–43.
31. Luft BJ, Remington JS. Toxoplasma encephalitis in AIDS. Clin Infect Dis 1992; 15:211–222.
32. Pedrol E, Gonzales-Clemente JM, Gatell JM, Mallolas J, Miro JM, Graus F, Alvarez R, Mercader JM, Berenguer J, Jimenez de Anta MT. Central nervous system toxoplasmosis in AIDS patients. Efficacy of an intermittent maintenance therapy. AIDS 1990; 4:511–517.
33. Carr A, Tindall B, Brew BJ, Marriott DJ, Harkness JL, Penny R, Cooper DA. Low dose trimethoprim–sulfamethoxazole prophylaxis for toxoplasma encephalitis in patients with AIDS. Ann Intern Med 1992; 117:106–111.
34. Clotet B, Sirera G, Romen J, Gimeno JM, Jou A, Condom MJ, Tor J, Foz M. Twice weekly dapsone–pyrimethamine for preventing PCP and cerebral toxoplasmosis. AIDS 1991; 5:601–602.
35. Durant J, Hazime F, Bernard E, Carles M, Pechere JC, Dellamonica P. An open randomised study of roxthromycin efficacy and tolerance in the primary prevention of pneumocystosis and cerebral toxoplasmosis in 52 HIV positive patients. VIII International Conference on AIDS. Amsterdam, Netherlands, July 1992:abstr PoB 1216.
36. Partisani M, DeMantort E, Hassari N, Divine A, Fraisse P, Lang JM. Primary prophylaxis of cerebral toxoplasmosis with pyrimethamine-sulfadiazine in human immunodeficiency virus infected individuals seropositive to toxoplasma. VIII International Conference on AIDS. Amsterdam, Netherlands July 1992:abstr PoB 125.
37. Sanford JP, Gilbert DN, Sande MA. Recommended antiparasitic therapy, drugs, side effects. In: The Sanford Guide to Antimicrobial Therapy, 1996. Vienna, VA: Antimicrobial Therapy, 1996:88.
38. Behbahani R, Moshfeghi M, Baxter JD. Therapeutic approaches for AIDS-related toxoplasmosis. Ann Pharmacother 1995; 29:760–768.

17

Pulmonary Cryptosporidiosis

EMANUEL I. WURM

Beth Israel Medical Center
New York, New York

I. Introduction

The genus *Cryptosporidium* is an intracellular, extracytoplasmic protozoan parasite long known to exist (discovered in 1907 in mice), but not linked to gastrointestinal disease in animals (cows and turkeys) until 1976, when the first case of human infection was documented (1–3). In 1982, cryptosporidial infection of the gastrointestinal tract was associated with diarrhea in patients with AIDS (1,2). Although more than 20 species have been identified, *Cryptosporidium parvum* is responsible for most clinical illness in humans and other mammals.

II. Epidemiology and Life Cycle

The prevalence of cryptosporidial infection worldwide ranges from 1 to 3 percent in the industrialized countries (North America and Europe), to as high as 10% in less-developed countries, probably owing to a lack of clean water and proper sanitary conditions, crowded living conditions, and in some cases, animal reservoirs in close proximity to residences (1,2). Although ingestion of as few as 3000 oocysts can cause infection in immunocompetent persons, ingestion of as few as 10 oocysts can cause infection in immunocompromised hosts. The onset from ingestion to clinical symptoms is approximately 7–10 days in immunocompetent hosts and longer in immunocompromised persons (1,2). The infection shows a seasonal preference for the warmer months, such as the late summer and fall. Transmission of cryptosporidial infection results from person-to-person contact, animal-to-person contact, and through environmental, mostly waterborne transmission. The organism is resistant to chlorination or other standard disinfectants; it must be filtered for proper purification of water reservoirs (2). There have been cases of transmission, documented among animals, that appear to be due to inhalation of aerosolized cryptosporidia, presenting the possibility of this mode of transfer applying to the human host as well. Pulmonary infection is believed to be acquired through aspiration of the organism, or less likely by hematogenous spread of oocysts from the gastrointestinal tract (2,4,5). The parasite is known to reside in the epithelial cells of whatever organ system it has invaded, with resultant inflammatory changes, with lymphocytes, neutrophils, plasma cells, and macrophages. The life cycle of *Cryptosporidium* spp. is completed in a single host; from ingestion of oocysts, to excystation of four banana-shaped sporozoites that attach to the epithelial cell wall, to maturation into meronts, releasing merozoites intraluminally, some of which may reinvade the host cell, and others that may mature into oocysts to be excreted and possibly infect another organism.

III. Clinical Features

The immunocompetent patients presenting with a cryptosporidial illness presents with mild to moderate flu-like symptoms and diarrhea. These symptoms are usually self-limited and resolve within 2 weeks. In the immunocompromised patient, such as those with human immunodeficiency virus (HIV) infection, the patient often presents with weight loss, fever, fatigue, and anorexia, associated with a prolonged diarrheal illness with malabsorption (1,2,5). Cryptosporidia have also been found in the gallbladder, pancreas, and biliary tract. There has been one reported case of toxic megacolon associated with cryptosporidial infection. Patients with respiratory infection have a predominant airway disease with cough, which may be associated with copious thick sputum and shortness of breath (1,2,4). There are no classic radiographic findings associated with the diagnosis of pulmonary cryptosporidial infection. Leukocystosis is uncommon, although eosinophilia has been noted. Diagnosis is based on the identification of the organism, which may be found in the tracheal secretions, and in the ciliated borders of respiratory epithelium. Oocysts must be differentiated from *Pneumocystis carinii* and *Toxoplasma*, owing to their similar presentations (1,2).

IV. Diagnosis

The diagnosis of cryptosporidiosis is established by identifying the oocyst in stool or bronchial secretions. Cryptosporidia can easily be overlooked owing to their small size (4- to 5-μm oocysts) during routine stool examination for ova and parasites, or can easily be mistaken for yeast. Many stains have been employed to make the identification easier. Modified acid-fast stains stain the oocysts red, whereas yeasts will stain blue-green. A modified cold Kinyoun's stain gives a similar staining pattern (2,6). The modified Sheather's sugar flotation procedure is a concentration technique that increases the diagnostic sensitivity in nonliquid stool specimens. Immunological studies have shown that anticryptosporidium IgM, IgG, and IgA develop within 3 months of infection with *Cryptosporidium* spp., but may persist for various lengths of time; however, their presence does not clearly correspond to the severity of infection (2). Commercially available tests for use in research, such as a monoclonal antibody to the cryptosporidial oocyst wall, or an enzyme-linked immunosorbant assay (ELISA) with a soluble *Cryptosporidium*-specific antigen, have seen little diagnostic use in the clinical setting (1). The foregoing staining procedures have been used successfully in the examination of bronchial secretions in patients presenting with pulmonary symptoms, often in association with other pathogens, such as *P. carinii* and cytomegalovirus (6–8).

V. Treatment

Although many agents have been used to attempt treatment of the chronic diarrheal illness caused by the *Cryptosporidium* parasite, none thus far have proved curative. Interventions currently under investigation are azithromycin, octreotide acetate, diclazuril, and letrazuril (currently used with some success in treating infected poultry) and hyperimmune bovine colostrum (2). Mohri et al. reported a case of a patient with AIDS who presented with respiratory symptoms and was diagnosed with pulmonary as well as gastrointestinal cryptosporidiosis. This patient was treated with inhaled paromomycin therapy with success. Inhalation was attempted because of the aminoglycosides' poor systemic absorption from the gastrointestinal tract

(4). Although promising, further study is necessary to clearly establish its usefulness as a reliable treatment option (4,9,10).

References

1. Peterson C, Mills J, Parasitic infections. In: Murray, Nadel. eds. Textbook of Respiratory Medicine, 2nd ed. Philadelphia: WB Sanders, 1994:1221.
2. Ungar BLP. Cryptosoridium. In: Mandel G, Bennett J, Dolin R, eds. Principles and Practice of Infectious Disease, 4th ed. New York: Churchill–Livingstone, 1995:2500–2510.
3. Pitlik SD, Fainstein V, Garza D, Guarda L, Bolivar R, Rios A, Hopfer RL, Mansell PA. Human cryptosporidiosis: spectrum of disease. Arch Intern Med 1983; 143:2269–2275.
4. Mohri H, Fujita H, Asakura Y, Katoh K, Okamoto R, Tanabe J, Harano H, Naguchi T, Inayama Y, Amano T, et al. Case report: inhalation therapy of paromomycin is effective for respiratory infection and hypoxia by *Cryptosporidium* with AIDS. Am J Med Sci 1995; 309:60–62.
5. Brady EM, Margolis ML, Korzeniowski OM. Pulmonary cryptosporidiosis in acquired immune deficiency syndrome. JAMA 1984; 252:89–90.
6. Ma P, Villanueva TG, Kaufman D, Gillooley JF. Respiratory cryptosporidiosis in the acquired immune deficiency syndrome. JAMA 1984; 252:1298–1301.
7. Hojlyng N, Jensen BN. Respiratory cryptosporidiosis in HIV-positive patients. Lancet 1988; 1:590–591.
8. Jensen BN, Gerstoft J, Hojlyng N, Backer V, Paaske M, Gemme G, Skinhoj P. Pulmonary pathogens in HIV-infected patients. Scand J Infect Dis 1990; 22:413–420.
9. Armitage K, Flanigan T, Carey J, Frank I, MacGregor RR, Ross P, Goodgame R, Turner J. Treatment of cryptosporidiosis with paromomycin. Arch Intern Med 1992; 152:2497–2499.
10. Fichtenbaum CJ, Ritchie DJ, Powderly WG. Use of paromomycin for treatment of cryptosporidiosis in patients with AIDS. Clin Infect Dis 1993; 16:298–300.

18

Strongyloidiasis

JUAN CARLOS CELEDÓN

Harvard Medical School and
Brigham and Women's Hospital
Boston, Massachusetts

I. Introduction

Human infection with *Strongyloides stercoralis* is prevalent worldwide. Normal hosts who are chronically infected are often asymptomatic. In contrast, immunocompromised individuals, including those with HIV infection, may develop systemic strongyloidiasis, a potentially fatal condition characterized by rapid multiplication and migration of larvae throughout the body (1,2).

II. Epidemiology and Life Cycle

Although most prevalent in tropical and subtropical areas, *S. stercoralis* can be found throughout the world. Infection occurs in residents of, or visitors from, endemic areas, including developing countries, southern, eastern, and central Europe, and the Appalachians in the United States. Strongyloides infection may also be acquired in chronic care institutions. Although the usual mode of transmission is by skin contact with soil contaminated with feces containing infective larvae, transmission by fecal–oral and sexual contact may also occur (3).

Strongyloides stercoralis has a self-perpetuating cycle involving the soil and its host. After penetration of human skin, filariform larvae travel to the alveolar spaces of the lungs and then migrate up the tracheobronchial tree and are swallowed. In the small bowel, larvae mature into adult female worms. These produce ova that develop into rhabdoid larvae, which are excreted in the stools. The rhabdoid larvae may also molt into filariform larvae within the intestinal lumen. These infective larvae can then penetrate the bowel mucosa or the perianal skin and continue the autoinfection cycle that allows the parasite to persist almost indefinitely in the host (1,4).

In certain hosts, most frequently immunosuppressed, the uncontrolled multiplication of *S. stercoralis* leads to either the hyperinfection syndrome or disseminated strongyloidiasis. Whereas hyperinfection is characterized by an augmentation of the normal life cycle of the parasite, dissemination occurs when filariform larvae invade organs outside their usual migration pattern. Both conditions form part of the spectrum of systemic strongyloidiasis and lead to a high morbidity and mortality (1,2).

Because infection with the human immunodeficiency virus (HIV) causes profound abnormalities in the host immune response, a higher incidence of systemic strongyloidiasis can be expected among persons living in areas where both HIV disease and *S. stercoralis* are prevalent. However, autopsy series and clinical studies from Africa and South America (where both *S. stercoralis* and HIV infection are prevalent) revealed a low number of cases of systemic strongyloidiasis (5,6). In addition, although 3.9% of homosexual men attending a clinic for sexually transmitted diseases in 1981 were infected with *S. stercoralis*, only 5 cases of systemic strongyloidiasis were reported among the first 13,042 AIDS cases in the United States (7). To date, only 16 cases of systemic strongyloidiasis in HIV-infected patients have been reported in the English literature (8–10; Fig. 1). Fourteen were already diagnosed with AIDS, indicating an advanced stage of their HIV disease. As expected, most patients were born in or had traveled to an endemic area. Patients with systemic strongyloidiasis who are immunocompromised, both with and without HIV disease, have been preponderantly male (3,8).

III. Immunobiology

The immunobiology of strongyloidiasis is not well understood (11,12). Dissemination of the parasite can occur in individuals showing strong cellular and humoral immune responses to *S. stercoralis* infection (13,14).

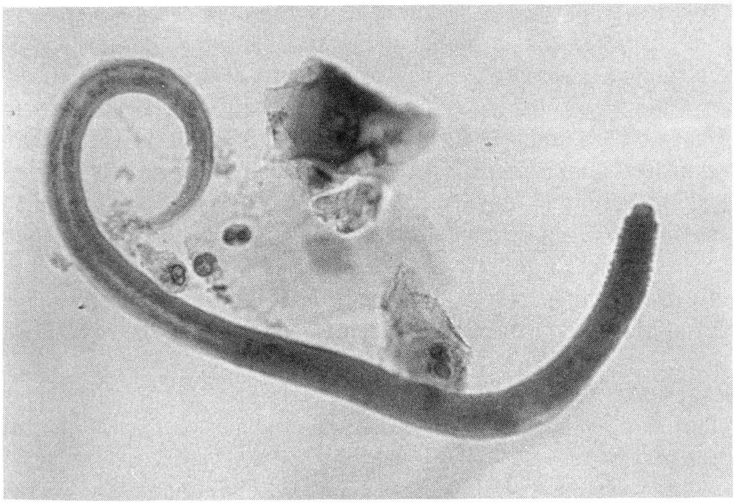

Figure 1 At autopsy, a larva of *S. stercoralis* and a mixed exudative reaction are seen in the alveolar spaces of a case (hematoxylin and eosin staining; original magnification × 200). (From Ref. 8.)

Various corticosteroid-responsive mechanisms of protective host response have been implicated in the control of strongyloidiasis. These include mucosal mast cells (15), eosinophil and IgE responses (12), and local intestinal immunity (16). Whether one or more aspects of the host immune response could be affected in HIV disease owing to AIDS, HIV enteropathy, AIDS gastropathy, or coexisting infection with the human T-cell leukemia virus type I (HTLV-I) is unknown at this time (8,17).

IV. Diagnosis

A. Chronic Strongyloidiasis

Patients with uncomplicated *S. stercoralis* infection may have mild gastrointestinal complaints or be asymptomatic (1). The stool examination is the most readily available laboratory test for the detection of the helminth. In chronic strongyloidiasis, the sensitivity of three or more fecal smears ranges from 33 to 60%, because larval output can be low and irregular (12). Thus, negative fecal smears are not absolute evidence against suspected infection with *S. stercoralis*, and more sensitive diagnostic methods should be pursued if the patient is at risk for dissemination, as in persons with HIV disease (8).

The formalin–ether concentration method, in which a large amount of stool is examined, has a higher diagnostic yield than direct fecal smears. However, larvae may not be easy to identify because they are killed by formalin (11). If the diagnosis is still suspected after negative results of serial fecal smears and the formalin–ether concentration technique, more sensitive procedures, such as stool culture or the Baermann concentration method (12), should be employed. These techniques have high diagnostic yields, but they are more complex and are not routinely performed in most clinical laboratories. Stool culture also carries a higher risk of laboratory-acquired infection than other methods (11,12). More invasive studies, such as duodenal fluid aspirate and the string test, may be helpful in selected cases (1,2).

Serological tests have been developed for the diagnosis of chronic strongyloidiasis. The enzyme-linked immunoabsorbent assay (ELISA) has a high sensitivity (85–90% in immunocompetent patients with proven infection with *S. stercoralis*) and specificity (higher than 90% with certain modifications; 11,18). ELISA may be especially helpful in the evaluation of travelers with unexplained eosinophilia (12). Furthermore, serial antibody titers may be followed to assess eradication of the parasite in patients treated for uncomplicated strongyloidiasis (11). However, the test is not widely available and may be unable to distinguish acute from past infection (11,12). In addition, the accuracy of ELISA testing has not been adequately evaluated in HIV-infected individuals with chronic or systemic strongyloidiasis (8).

B. Systemic Strongyloidiasis

Systemic strongyloidiasis commonly produces various combinations of gastrointestinal or respiratory symptoms, fever, anorexia, weight loss, and generalized malaise (1,8). The diagnosis is often difficult, because the protean manifestations of the disease may mimic other conditions commonly encountered in HIV-infected patients (8). Bacteremia and meningitis, often caused by enteric organisms, are found in up to 50% of cases and may be an important diagnostic clue (8). Eosinophilia, although common in immunocompetent individuals with chronic *S. stercoralis* infection, is frequently absent in systemic strongyloidiasis (2,8).

Chest roentgenograms are frequently abnormal in HIV-infected patients. The most common findings are bilateral infiltrates, in either an interstitial or alveolar pattern (8). However, unilateral involvement is occasionally present. Unfortunately, these radiographic patterns are nonspecific, and may be seen in other opportunistic diseases, such as *Pneumocystis carinii* pneumonia and tuberculosis (8).

The best study to diagnose systemic strongyloidiasis in HIV-infected individuals is serial stool examinations. The sensitivity of three direct fecal smears is very high, owing to the large parasitic burdens (8,12). In addition, sputum examination or bronchoscopy with bronchoalveolar lavage may disclose abundant filariform larvae (Fig. 2). Duodenal biopsy and cytological examination of spinal fluid are occasionally helpful (8).

V. Treatment

A. Chronic Strongyloidiasis

Thiabendazole, 25 mg/kg orally, twice daily for 2 or 3 days, is the agent of choice for the treatment of immunocompetent patients with chronic strongyloidiasis (19). Unfortunately, short-term side effects are common, and treatment is not always effective, thus requiring repeat therapeutic courses (20). An alternative in patients with persistent *S. stercoralis* infection after adequate treatment with thiabendazole is ivermectin (20). This medication, administered as a single oral dose of 200 μg/kg, achieves parasitological cures in over 80% of patients, with a low incidence of side effects (20,21). Regardless of the drug employed, follow-up stool examinations should be obtained to assess therapeutic efficacy.

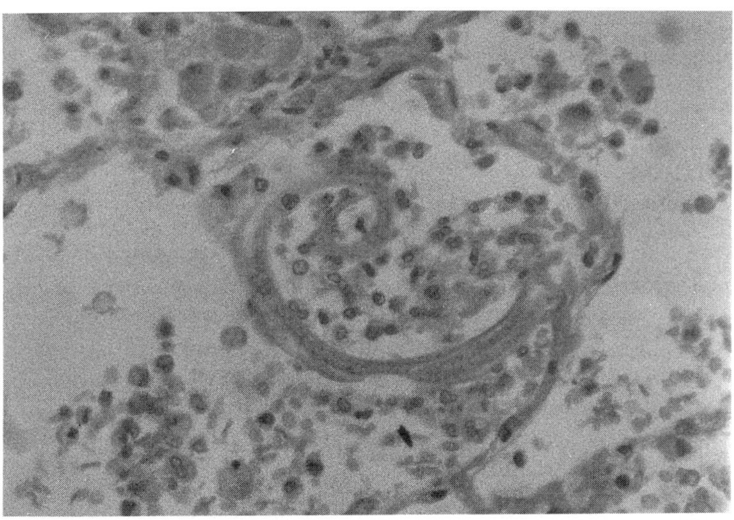

Figure 2 Cytologic examination of a sputum sample showing filariform larvae of *S. stercoralis* (Papanicolaou staining, original magnification × 400). (From Ref. 8.)

B. Systemic Strongyloidiasis

Prolonged courses of thiabendazole, from 5 to 14 days, are recommended for the treatment of systemic strongyloidiasis (2). The optimal duration of therapy, however, is unknown, and treatment failures are very common in HIV-infected persons (8). Thus, courses of at least 5 days of thiabendazole should be employed, followed by posttreatment stool examinations. If persistent *S. stercoralis* infection is present after the initial course, therapy should be continued for 2 weeks. If an adequate clinical response is then obtained, consideration should be given to monthly prophylactic therapy with 2- to 3-day courses of thiabendazole (8).

In patients who do not respond to thiabendazole, alternative therapies include ivermectin, albendazole, or a combination of both. Although ivermectin, a new anthelmintic drug, seems promising, controlled studies of its therapeutic efficacy in systemic strongyloidiasis are not yet available.

VI. Prognosis

Even though the number of cases of systemic strongyloidiasis in HIV-infected individuals is small, the rate of mortality is very high, with only 1 of 16 reported cases alive after a 6-month follow-up. Even if the parasitic infection is successfully treated, most patients with strongyloidiasis have advanced HIV disease, and a poor prognosis (8–10).

VII. Summary

Systemic strongyloidiasis is an unusual, but often fatal, complication of advanced HIV disease. A combination of gastrointestinal and respiratory symptoms in an HIV-infected patient who has been to an endemic area should prompt the clinician to examine serial stool and sputum specimens. Therapeutic failures are very common, and careful clinical follow-up is warranted, regardless of the mode of therapy employed.

References

1. Scowden EB, Schaffner W, Stone WJ. Overwhelming strongyloidiasis: an unappreciated opportunistic infection. Medicine 1978; 57:527–544.
2. Igra-Siegman Y, Kapila R, Sen P, Kaminski ZC, Louria DB. Syndrome of hyperinfection with *Strongyloides stercoralis*. Rev Infect Dis 1981; 3:397–407.
3. Genta RM. Global prevalence of strongyloidiasis: critical review with epidemiologic insights into the prevention of disseminated disease. Rev Infect Dis 1989; 11:755–67.

4. Pelletier LL Jr. Chronic strongyloidiasis in World War II Far East ex-prisoners of war. Am J Trop Med Hyg 1984; 33:55–61.
5. Neto VA, Pasternak J, Moreira AA, Duarte MI, Campos R, Braz LM. *Strongyloides stercoralis* hyperinfection in the acquired immunodeficiency syndrome [letter]. Am J Med 1989; 87:602–603.
6. Petithory JC, Derouin F. AIDS and strongyloidiasis in Africa [letter]. Lancet 1987; 1:921.
7. Maayan S, Wormser GP, Widerhorn J, Sy ER, Kim YH, Ernst JA. *Strongyloides stercoralis* hyperinfection in a patient with the acquired immunodeficiency syndrome. Am J Med 1987; 83:945–948.
8. Celedon JC, Mathur-Wagh U, Fox J, Garcia R, Wiest P. Systemic strongyloidiasis in patients infected with the human immunodeficiency virus. A report of three cases and review of the literature. Medicine 1994; 73:256–263.
9. Kao D, Murakawa GJ, Kerschmann R, Berger T. Disseminated strongyloidiasis in a patient with acquired immunodeficiency syndrome [letter]. Arch Dermatol 1996; 132:977–978.
10. Cahill KM, Shevchuk M. Fulminant, systemic strongyloidiasis in AIDS. Ann Trop Med Parasitol 1996; 90:313–318.
11. Neva FA. Biology and immunology of human strongyloidiasis. J Infect Dis 1986; 153:397–406.
12. Liu LX, Weller PF. Strongyloidiasis and other intestinal nematode infections. Infect Dis Clin North Am 1993; 7:655–672.
13. Genta RM, Douce RW, Walzer PD. Diagnostic implications of parasite-specific immune responses in immunocompromised patients with strongyloidiasis. J Clin Microbiol 1986; 23:1099–1103.
14. Genta RM, Lillibridge JP. Prominence of IgG4 antibodies in the human responses to *Strongyloides stercoralis* infection. J Infect Dis 1989; 160:692–699.
15. Barrett KE, Neva FA, Gam AA, Cicmanec J, London WT, Phillips JM, Metcalfe DD. The immune response to nematode parasites: modulation of mast cell numbers and function during *Strongyloides stercoralis* infection in nonhuman primates. Am J Trop Med Hyg 1988; 38:574–581.
16. Genta RM. Immunobiology of strongyloidiasis. Trop Geogr Med 1984; 36:223–229.
17. Newton RC, Limpuangthip P, Greenberg S, Gam A, Neva FA. *Strongyloides stercoralis* hyperinfection in a carrier of HTLV-I virus with evidence of selective immunosuppression. Am J Med 1992; 92:202–208.
18. Conway DJ, Atkins NS, Lillywhite JE, Bailey JW, Robinson RD, Lindo JF, Bundy DA, Bianco AE. Immunodiagnosis of *Strongyloides stercoralis* infection: a method for increasing the specificity of the indirect ELISA. Trans R Soc Trop Med Hyg 1993; 87:173–176.
19. De Vault GA Jr, King JW, Rohr MS, Landreneau MD, Brown ST 3d, McDonald JC. Opportunistic infections with *Strongyloides stercoralis* in renal transplantation. Rev Infect Dis 1990; 12:653–671.
20. Gann PH, Neva FA, Gam AA. A randomized trial of single- and two dose ivermectin versus thiabendazole for treatment of strongyloidiasis. J Infect Dis 1994; 169:1076–1079.

21. Datry A, Hilmarsdottir I, Mayorga-Sagastume R, Lyagoubi M, Gaxotte P, Biligui S, Chodakewitz J, Neu D, Danis M, Gentilini M. Treatment of *Strongyloides stercoralis* infection with ivermectin compared with albendazole: results of an open study of 60 cases. Trans R Soc Trop Med Hyg 1994; 88:344–345.

Part Five

NONINFECTIOUS PULMONARY DISORDERS

19

Neoplastic Diseases

DOROTHY A. WHITE

Memorial Sloan–Kettering Cancer Center
New York, New York

I. Introduction

There is an increased risk of development of malignancy associated with conditions of immunosuppression, whether they are secondary to cancer, congenital or acquired immunodeficiency syndromes, or immunosuppressive therapy given for organ transplants, autoimmune diseases, or other conditions (1–5). The cancers that occur are not the malignancies most commonly found in the general population, such as colon, breast, or lung cancer, but rather they are lymphoma and Kaposi's sarcoma (KS), which are unusual tumors in the general population. The reasons for the occurrence of cancer in a setting of immunosuppression are not fully elucidated, but it has been postulated that one cause may be activation of latent oncogenic viruses. One example is activation of Epstein–Barr virus (EBV), which has been associated with the development of lymphoma. A generalized decrease in tumor surveillance in a setting of immunosuppression and possibly direct mutagenic potential of immunosuppressive drugs have also been postulated as causes for the increased risk of cancer (5).

In those patients with the acquired immune deficiency syndrome (AIDS), it was apparent, soon after it was recognized, that there was a marked predisposition for patients to develop KS. This tumor occurred 20,000 times more frequently in those with AIDS, compared with the general population, and at a much higher frequency than in other immunosuppressed patients (6). Indeed, the exquisite susceptibility of HIV-infected patients to develop KS has provided, over the last decade, a unique opportunity to study the factors responsible for the pathogenesis of this previously rare neoplasm (7,8).

Other associations with malignancy were subsequently noted as the epidemic of AIDS expanded. Non-Hodgkin's lymphoma occurs 60 times more frequently in HIV-infected patients than in the general population, and the disease appears to follow a more aggressive course, with a poor prognosis (9). Additionally, Hodgkin's disease also presents at a more-advanced stage and follows a very aggressive course in those who are HIV-infected, although it remains unclear if the incidence of the disease is increased (10,11). Among HIV-infected women, studies have recently documented an increased prevalence of cervical dysplasia, a precursor of cervical cancer (12,13), and HIV infection has been noted to adversely affect the clinical course and treatment of both cervical dysplasia and cancer (14). Three cancers are now included as indicator conditions for the most recent definition of AIDS, as formulated by the Centers for Disease Control and Prevention (CDC): KS, non-Hodgkin's lymphoma, and cervical cancer (15).

There are also reports of possible increases in many other cancers in HIV-infected patients, including carcinoma of the skin, testes, breast, pancreas, anus, and lung, among others (16–20). Notable among these for its pulmonary manifestations is lung cancer. Epidemiological analysis of large groups of patients are needed to clarify whether there is a true increased prevalence or altered course of these cancers. It is likely that prophylaxis and treatment of opportunistic infections will reduce mortality in HIV-infected persons, and any associated malignancies may become more prevalent.

This review will focus on cancers for which a clear association to HIV has been documented, specifically KS and lymphoma, and pulmonary manifestations are a significant problem. Additionally, the data on lung cancer in HIV-infected patients will be critically reviewed because of its special relevance to the respiratory system.

II. Relation of HIV to Malignancy

Although HIV gene sequences have been found in many tissue specimens from infected patients, viral genomes have not been seen in KS lesions (21).

A role for HIV as an etiologic agent for KS, however, is supported by animal experiments. Tat, a transactivating protein release by HIV-infected T cells, produced KS-like skin lesions in some male mice after introduction into the germline (22). These lesions contained spindle-shaped cells (the KS cell), and slit-like vascular spaces, with and without red blood cells. When KS cells from AIDS patients were grown in culture, the Tat protein served as an extracellular growth factor, and cell proliferation was blocked by anti-Tat antibodies (23). Thus, the Tat protein induces and facilitates development of KS lesions (24).

Some investigators believe that KS may not be a true malignancy, but rather, a nonmalignant proliferative lesion of vascular endothelium that grows in response to disordered regulation and expression of growth factors (25). Inflammatory cytokines, such as interleukin-1 (IL-1), IL-6, tumor necrosis factor (TNF), oncostatin M, and interferon gamma (INF-γ), and angiogenic factors, such as β-fibroblast growth factor, promote growth of endothelial cells and fibroblasts and induce new blood vessel formation (8,25,26). These are actions vital to development of KS-like lesions. In HIV infection, increased cytokines are secreted by both activated T cells and HIV-infected T cells. Additionally, cell-free supernatants from KS cultures can induce a KS-like lesion in mice (27). Thus, KS when associated with HIV may develop as a hyperplastic focus of cells proliferating in response to a cascade of inflammatory and angiogenic factors elicited by HIV infection.

The etiology of lymphoma in HIV is probably similar to that in other immunosuppressed states, for the incidence of the malignancy is the same in both groups (9). In the immunosuppressed state, polyclonal B-cell proliferation is stimulated. The source of the B-cell stimulation is probably multifactorial and includes reactivation of EBV, increased cytokines [specifically B-cell growth factors (28,29), such as IL-6 and IL-10), and impaired T-cell surveillance. Proliferation of B cells leads to an increased risk of rearrangements or translocations that contributes to an increased frequency of malignancy.

In AIDS-associated lymphomas, both monoclonal and polyclonal tumors are seen, similar to other immunosuppression-related lymphomas. It has been suggested that the lymphostimulatory molecules come from outside the B- and T-cell compartment, possibly from HIV-infected macrophages (30). In some cases c-*myc* oncogene rearrangements are found, and this has been considered to be a marker of AIDS-associated malignancies (31). The AIDS-associated tumors also show evidence of EBV genomic integration in 38–68% of systemic AIDS lymphoma cases (32). The mechanism by which EBV genomic integration leads to B-cell immortalization is unknown.

III. Kaposi's Sarcoma

Kaposi's sarcoma was originally described in 1872 by the Hungarian physician Moricz Kaposi, and before the advent of AIDS was a rare tumor. It was found in three settings. Most cases in Europe and North America presented as indolent skin lesions affecting the skin of the lower extremities in elderly men of Jewish and Mediterranean ancestry. The course was slow, and visceral disease was unusual (33). A more aggressive form was found in equatorial Africa that also occurred predominantly in men, but frequently had visceral involvement (34). Finally, KS occurred as a second malignancy associated with tumors that affected immunity, such as lymphoma and leukemia (1,5). It was later noted in other immunosuppressive conditions, such as following organ transplants or associated with autoimmune diseases (2,3).

A. Epidemiology

It was initially thought that KS associated with AIDS might be occurring secondary to the presence of immunosuppression. However, KS in the setting of AIDS, does not increase in frequency as the underlying immunosuppression worsens. The tumor occurs in HIV-infected patients at a relatively constant rate, starting 1–2 years after initial infection (17), and many patients with profound immunosuppression do not develop KS. KS also does not occur in all risk groups, but rather, occurs predominantly in homosexual or bisexual men (7). In the United States, KS is ten times more common in homosexual men with AIDS than among patients from other HIV transmission groups (7). Some geographic variation has also been noted, with KS being noted more commonly in HIV-infected patients in all risk groups from California and New York, compared with those from other areas of the United States (6). A similar geographic trend has not been seen with other clinical manifestations of AIDS reported to the CDC. Blacks are also less likely than whites or Hispanics to develop KS (7).

Another striking epidemiological feature of AIDS KS is the overall decline in its occurrence in HIV-infected patients over time (20,35). It was an initial presenting feature in a third of patients at the beginning of the AIDS epidemic, but now the overall incidence of KS is only 6–20% in homosexual men (20,35,36). This observation is not completely explained by the broader definition of AIDS-defining conditions and the possibility of incomplete documentation of the presence of KS. Rather, these epidemiological observations strongly suggest that there is another factor, other than HIV infection itself or the level of immunosuppression, that determines KS development. It is widely believed that an unidentified infectious agent, which is sexually transmissible, is the likely cause of KS (6,7). Results of testing for known viruses, such as herpes simplex 1 and 2, polyomavirus, human herpes virus 6, among others, have been negative. Most evidence has pointed to cytomegalovirus (CMV), but extensive investigations have been inconclusive. Recently, human papillomavirus, type 16, has been considered as a candidate, but evidence is still very preliminary (37). Investigators have also recently reported evidence of DNA from a virus most likely from the herpes family in KS skin lesions, but this exciting development awaits confirmation and further study (38). It is postulated that changes in the environment or safe sexual practices have led to a decrease in this second transmissible agent and thus to fewer cases of KS.

B. Clinical Presentation

The clinical presentation of AIDS-associated KS varies from indolent skin disease to extensive visceral involvement. Cutaneous manifestations are most common and usually precede visceral disease. This may be by months to years, and the clinical course is protracted in many patients. Skin lesions appear as pink, red, or violet macules, papules, or nodules, which can often coalesce to form larger plaque-like lesions. Lesions may be small and single, or large, extensive, and quite disfiguring (39). In addition to the lesions themselves, lymphedema can be a major disfiguring and debilitating complication of more extensive KS (39). Commonly involved areas of skin are the face, especially the tip of the nose, periorbital and periauricular areas, the trunk, and the extremities. The mucous membranes of the oral pharynx, gingiva, tongue, and tonsils are also frequent sites of KS. Lymph nodes and visceral organ involvement, particularly of the liver, gastrointestinal tract, lungs, kidneys, adrenals, and spleen, usually develop in most patients with a long history of KS (39).

Although the prevalence of KS has been decreasing, its clinical significance has not. Because of effective prophylaxis and treatment of opportunistic infection, more patients are developing extensive debilitating visceral KS, and this malignancy is becoming a common cause of death in AIDS patients (36).

C. Pulmonary Kaposi's Sarcoma

The development of pulmonary KS usually causes severe symptoms and has a negative influence on mortality. Median survival of 2–6 months has been reported in patients with extensive pulmonary disease, although survival up to several years occurs in some patients (39–46). Features predictive of shortened survival are the presence of a pleural effusion, severe shortness of breath, and a CD4 cell count of fewer than 100 (46).

Pulmonary disease almost always accompanies cutaneous disease, although there have been occasional reports of lung involvement in the absence of other evidence of disease (40,43,47). Clinical studies have reported an incidence of pulmonary KS in up to a third of patients with cutaneous disease (40,43,47,48); at autopsy there is evidence of involvement in approximately 50% of KS patients (40,41,44,49).

D. Pathology

Gross examination at autopsy often reveals patchy areas of involvement of lung parenchyma, endobronchial lesions, and pleural disease. Multiple parenchymal hemorrhagic nodules are seen that can coalesce in some areas (41). Microscopically, the lesions are in a perivascular and peribronchial distribution. They are composed of spindle-shaped cells surrounding vascular slits containing erythrocytes and hemosiderin deposits. These vascular slits give the KS lesions their characteristic red hemorrhagic appearance (41,43). The architecture of spindle cells and accompanying vascular structures characteristic of KS may also proliferate along the interlobular septa of the lungs in an angiomatous fashion producing reticular, rather than nodular, involvement (41,43).

Endobronchial lesions are violaceous or bright red, irregularly shaped lesions that are flat or slightly raised (40,41,43,44,50). These lesions are found at branching points or carinas of the lower airways, but may occur anywhere in the bronchi or trachea (47,40). Histologically, these lesions are identical with the parenchymal nodules. Pleural disease is characterized by visceral plaques composed of a fibroblastic or neoplastic spindle cell proliferation and relatively large vascular spaces filled with erythrocytes (41). Associated effusions are variable in size, but are often large. The fluid may be clear or serosanguinous (40,51,52) and is usually an exudate; rarely, transudates and chylous effusions are found (51,53–55).

E. Clinical, Radiographic, Physiological Presentation

Dyspnea, nonproductive cough, and fever are the most common symptoms associated with pulmonary KS. These, unfortunately, are nonspecific symptoms and are found with many respiratory problems. Blood streaking of sputum is less frequent, but is slightly more suggestive of pulmonary involvement with KS (41–43). Gross hemoptysis is extremely rare, in spite of the vascular nature of these lesions and the extensive parenchymal involvement that occurs in some patients. Chest pain has also been reported only rarely, despite the relatively common occurrence of pleural disease (41,42). Some patients may be asymptomatic and pulmonary involvement is apparent only on chest radiography. The physical examination is non-contributing in most cases; occasionally, wheezing has been described (41,56). Significant upper airway obstruction, with stridor and respiratory distress, can rarely occur from endobronchial lesions of the trachea and larynx (41,44,56).

Two chest radiographic patterns are most characteristic of pulmonary KS. Interstitial infiltrates, which are usually homogeneous in appearance and have a perihilar predominance, are seen in approximately 60% of cases (44,51,57). On a chest computed tomography (CT) scan, ill-defined hilar densities are found, extending into the adjacent pulmonary parenchyma along perivascular and peribronchial pathways (58,59). Infiltrates may be localized (40,41,52,57), and focal areas of consolidation can occur (41,44). The second major pattern is that of nodular infiltrates, which occur in approximately one-quarter of patients. The nodules are ill-defined and of various sizes with coalescence in some areas. A small percentage of patients will have no abnormalities noted on chest radiograph (40,49,55).

Pleural effusions are found in up to 66% of patients with pulmonary KS (41,44,51,52,55,59). They may be unilateral or bilateral and are usually, (90% in one series) associated with concomitant parenchymal disease (40,51,60). The incidence of radiographically observed hilar and mediastinal lymphadenopathy is extremely variable, ranging from none to 63% (41,44,52,59,60). Intrathoracic nodes are compatible with the diagnosis of KS, but need to be distinguished from other conditions that can cause this finding.

Although no radiographic pattern is totally pathognomonic, findings of nodular or reticular opacities in a patient with known KS strongly suggest the presence of intrathoracic disease (57). A concomitant opportunistic infection in addition to KS, however, is often difficult to diagnose or exclude using the radiograph alone.

Pulmonary function tests (PFTs) in patients with pulmonary KS show a decreased diffusing capacity (ranging from 41 to 78% of predicted), and a low forced expiratory volume in 1 sec (FEV_1) to forced vital capacity (FVC) ratio (41,42,49,60). The airway obstruction reported often correlates with the presence of endobronchial KS (41,49,61,62) and may be a manifestation of extensive peribronchial involvement with tumor. Oxygenation may be normal or decreased, with a normal or increased A–a gradient, and the response to exercise is variable (41). The PFT abnormalities overlap those seen with other pulmonary entities in HIV-infected patients (42,62).

F. Diagnosis

The diagnosis of pulmonary KS is difficult to histologically confirm without an open biopsy. Practically, it is often made presumptively given clinical and radiographic findings and exclusion of other likely entities. The cytology and analysis of respiratory sputums are not helpful because the diagnosis of KS can be made only on biopsy when the architecture of spindle cells in association with vascular slits is seen. Unfortunately, with the small amount of tissue from either endobronchial, transbronchial, or pleural biopsies, the yield is low (40–42,51). Reported yields from transbronchial biopsies are generally less than 10%. Some investigators consider biopsy of KS lung lesions to be a high risk for potential bleeding complications, given the vascular nature of the lesions (39,47), but others have not found this to be so. The presence of typical endobronchial lesions is generally considered adequate to make a presumptive diagnosis of concomitant pulmonary parenchymal KS (41,55,63). One autopsy study confirmed the presence of parenchymal disease in 100% of patients with known endobronchial disease (41). Endobronchial disease, however, may be absent in many cases of parenchymal disease, and the diagnosis may need to be presumptive, given the clinical picture and exclusion of infectious causes. Open-lung biopsy gives the highest yield for KS, but is not 100% sensitive, given the focal nature of the disease (40,43).

Sequential nuclear scanning with thallium and gallium has been proposed as a way to noninvasively distinguish intrathoracic KS from other malignancies and infections (42,64). Gallium uptake is seen with some malignancies, such as lymphoma, and commonly with infections, but it rarely occurs in association with KS (42,61). An abnormal chest radiograph with a negative gallium scan in the proper setting is suggestive of KS and usually excludes concomitant infection. In contrast to *P. carinii* pneumonia (PCP), but KS and lymphoma are thallium avid (64). Thus, an absence of gallium uptake, but a positive thallium uptake, suggest KS, but further study is needed to confirm these findings in larger numbers of patients.

G. Prognosis and Treatment

Treatment for AIDS KS is palliative in almost all cases. Nevertheless, it is often indicated, because KS lesions, particularly large ones, can cause disfigurement, pain, edema, and bleeding, and visceral involvement often causes very significant morbidity (39,65). Modalities available to treat KS include biological modifiers, radiotherapy, and chemotherapy. Local therapy with laser or cryotherapy is also sometimes used (66). Interferon alfa was shown to have therapeutic potential in the treatment of KS early in the epidemic, but patients most likely to respond are those with CD4 T-cell counts of more than 200×10^6 and minimal symptomatology related to their HIV infection (65). Once pulmonary disease occurs, chemotherapy is almost always indicated, because pulmonary KS tends to progress rapidly and requires treatment that is quickly effective.

Kaposi's sarcoma responds to a variety of single agents, including vincristine, vinblastine, bleomycin, doxorubicin, and possibly epirubicin (24). Most responses, however, are partial and short-lived. Higher response rates can be obtained with combination chemotherapy, which leads to a longer disease-free interval and, in pulmonary KS, has also led to improved survival (46). In a retrospective review of patients with disseminated pulmonary KS treated with cytotoxic chemotherapy (doxorubicin, bleomycin, and vincristine), 80% had complete or partial remissions. Median survival for responding patients was 10 months versus 6 months for nonresponders (46). Hematological toxicity, however, is appreciable, and a high incidence of infectious problems can be expected (46). Regimens containing doxorubicin are most active, and the combination of doxorubicin, bleomycin, and vincristine is relatively well tolerated and frequently used (24). Liposomal daunorubicin, which may target KS cells, is an effective antitumor modality and has less toxicity than when the drug is given as conventional chemotherapy (67,68). In those with cytopenias, the marrow-sparing regimen of vincristine or vinblastine with bleomycin is commonly used (69).

Continuing antiretroviral therapy during chemotherapy is important. The myelosuppressive effects of zidovudine, however, have limited the ability to do this. The newer antiretroviral drugs didanosine (dideoxyinosine; ddI) or zalcitabine (dideoxycytidine; ddC), which do not cause myelosuppression, may be useful new approaches. Hematopoietic growth factors, such as granulocyte colony-stimulating factor (GCSF) and granulocyte–macrophage colony-stimulating factor (GMCSF) can also minimize hematological toxicity (70,71). Given the recent insights into the etiology of KS, new approaches are under consideration. These include the use of angiogenesis inhibitors, anti-Tat therapy, and cytokine antagonists (24).

Whole-lung radiation therapy has occasionally been used to palliate extensive pulmonary disease in patients unable to tolerate or unresponsive to chemotherapy (72–74). Although median survival is short, there was significant relief of dyspnea or hemoptysis (72,73). Symptomatic airway obstruction from KS has been successfully treated with localized radiotherapy (41,75). Management of pleural effusions remains difficult. Sclerosis has been successful in only a few cases (38).

IV. Non-Hodgkin's Lymphoma

The association between non-Hodgkin's lymphoma (NHL) and HIV infection was recognized by the CDC as an AIDS-defining condition only in 1985 (76). Since then, the number of cases of this malignancy appear to be increasing in the HIV-infected population, as opposed to KS, which is decreasing (77,78). It is projected that in the United States, up to a quarter of the lymphoma cases that present will be related to HIV. Prognosis is poor, and median survival is only 6.5 months (79). It is unusual for the respiratory effects of these lymphomas to result in significant morbidity or mortality, but this occasionally occurs (79).

A. Epidemiology

Epidemiological studies report a 2–5% incidence of NHL in AIDS patients, which is seen in all HIV transmission groups (9). However, it has been reported most commonly in homosexuals and hemophiliacs. Those with hemophilia have the highest relative risk (9). One study suggests that HIV-infected patients who survive longer and develop the most severe immunodeficiency have a higher likelihood of developing lymphoma, suggesting it is an "opportunistic" malignancy (77). If survival of HIV patients increases with treatment of other complications, this malignancy may become more common.

Nearly all NHL in HIV-infected patients are of B-cell origin. Diffuse, intermediate, and high-grade lymphomas of either small cell uncleaved or large cell immunoblastic type are seen in 82–98% of AIDS-associated NHL (11,79–82). Central nervous system (CNS) and Burkitt's lymphoma are less commonly seen (81). The systemic lymphomas tend to occur earlier in the course of HIV infection than the CNS lymphomas. In one report, the median CD4 cell count for those with systemic lymphoma was $139 \times 10^6/mm^3$, and it was the first AIDS indicator condition in approximately 60% of these patients. For CNS lymphoma patients, the CD4 cell count was a median of $30 \times 10^6/mm^3$, and lymphoma was the AIDS indicator condition in only one-third of patients (82).

B. Clinical and Radiographic Presentation

The most consistent clinical feature of AIDS-related NHL is presentation with widespread disease. There is an unusually high incidence of extranodal disease, commonly involving the CNS, gastrointestinal tract, bone marrow, and mucocutaneous tissues (10,11,83–88). Less than 20% of patients present with disease confined to the lymph nodes. The presence of "B" symptoms at the time of initial diagnosis is also common and is reported in up to 74% of patients (89).

Pulmonary disease is not usually a prominent presenting factor. There are rare cases in whom the lung is the initial or sole site of involvement (87,90–94), but more commonly, pulmonary involvement is found at presentation, in association with other clinical manifestations or is discovered during the staging process.

The frequency of pulmonary involvement in AIDS-related lymphomas ranges from 6 to 31% in various clinical reviews (11,82,87,90,94–97), although some studies report no pulmonary involvement. At autopsy, the incidence of pulmonary involvement is higher; in one study of 20 patients, pulmonary involvement was seen in 15% premortem and 40% at autopsy (98).

Within the thorax, endobronchial, parenchymal, and pleural disease are described (92,94,96,99). Intrathoracic lymph node involvement occurs, but not nearly as frequently as in the non-HIV population with lymphoma. Indeed, the most characteristic radiographic finding is the relative paucity of mediastinal and hilar adenopathy when compared with non-AIDS lymphoma (88,94,96,100).

Pleural disease in HIV-associated lymphoma is commonly noted and occurred in 8 of 11 patients (72%) in one study (96). Effusions are unilateral or bilateral and range in size from small to large. Effusions are regularly noted in the absence of parenchymal disease, unlike KS, in which they usually occur in association with pulmonary disease. Parenchymal involvement shows no predominant pattern. Alveolar or interstitial infiltrates and single or multiple nodules are all reported with or without associated adenopathy (90,94,96). Endobronchial lymphoma has been reported in a few cases of HIV-associated lymphoma (93,99). In these cases, tracheal involvement was seen and, in one patient, the endobronchial lesion originated from a mediastinal node that had eroded into the trachea.

C. Diagnosis

Thoracentesis and pleural biopsy have some diagnostic use in establishing the diagnosis of lymphoma, as opposed to the experience with Kaposi's sarcoma (10,90,92,96,101). In one study, thoracentesis and pleural biopsy were diagnostic in five of eight cases (96). Little data is available on the usefulness of various diagnostic techniques in establishing the diagnosis of lung parenchymal lymphoma. Generally, open-lung biopsy has been required (91,94,96). Bronchoscopy with transbronchial biopsy has a poor yield and was nondiagnostic in each of four patients in one report (96). There are, however, rare reports of positive biopsies with this technique (90,102). Needle aspirates of focal lesions have been useful, but experience is limited (96,103). Endobronchial biopsies may be positive when a lesion is present, but the use of a rigid bronchoscope was necessary in at least one case (99).

Nuclear scanning may play a role in differentiating lymphoma from other AIDS-related processes involving the chest, although only a few cases are reported (64). Whereas KS is generally thallium avid and PCP is gallium avid, lymphoma commonly shows avidity to both.

D. Treatment

The HIV-associated lymphomas are aggressive and difficult to treat. Therapy is similar to that administered to non-AIDS patients with systemic lymphoma, and consists of aggressive multiagent chemotherapeutic regimens (10,11,81,83,84,94). Factors associated with a poor response to therapy and decreased survival include a history of AIDS before the diagnosis of lymphoma, involvement of bone marrow, and a low Karnofsky performance status (81). In the absence of these factors, reports suggest a more favorable prognosis, with complete remission attained after therapy in up to 75% of patients, and a median survival of 11.3 months (81).

Complications of therapy are generally related to enhanced immunosuppression, potentially increasing the likelihood of bacterial and opportunistic infections, particularly *Aspergillus* pneumonia (56,97). The administration of growth factors, thereby reducing the periods of neutropenia, may help mitigate this toxicity (70). Continued antiretrovial therapy may also be important, and there is a report of regression of lymphoma following initiation of zidovudine therapy (104).

Radiation therapy has been used for well-circumscribed disease, but this modality is rarely effective alone, given the usual disseminated disease, and chemotherapy must also be used (103). Pleural effusions can be treated with systemic therapy; occasionally, sclerosis is necessary.

V. Lung Cancer

Many reports have suggested that lung cancer may be increased in incidence in HIV-infected patients, or may follow a more aggressive course (105–112). There is no theoretical reason for such an increase other than generalized decreased immune surveillance. Of note, this tumor has not increased in frequency in other immunosuppressed patients, and there is no correlation between the level of CD4 counts and the diagnosis of lung cancer in HIV-infected patients (113,114).

Only limited epidemiological studies in HIV are available, and their results are conflicting. One review of 6 cases of bronchogenic carcinoma from a population of 500 HIV seropositive patients, appeared to represent a 14-fold increase in the incidence of primary lung cancer, compared with the general population (106). Other studies, however, have found different results, including a retrospective review comparing the incidence of bronchogenic carcinoma within age-stratified groups in the pre- and post-AIDS eras. This showed no significant difference in the occurrence of lung cancer in the two groups (112).

The HIV-infected patients may present with a more advanced stage of disease and have a fulminant, rapidly declining course, when compared with control populations (108,112). The median survival for HIV patients was 4 weeks in one series and 3 months in another. These are significantly shorter time periods than those seen in the HIV-seronegative control populations in which median survival was reported as 25 weeks and 10 months, respectively (108,113). This data, however, is somewhat limited by the failure to account for concomitant illnesses, treatment given, and the lack of documentation of the cause of death (113–115).

The patients reported with lung cancer and HIV infection are all smokers and are young men in 86–100% of the cases (106,108,112,113). Although there are reports of primary lung cancer in patients from all HIV risk groups, most are intravenous (iv) drug users (108,112,113). These are all features that might be expected if the occurrence of lung cancer (and its association with smoking) occurred coincidentally with HIV infection (which occurs most frequently in young males; iv drug abuse is associated with smoking).

Although all histological subtypes of lung cancer are associated with HIV infection, adenocarcinoma is the most common type of malignancy, representing 44–100% of cases (18,106,108,113), but this does not differ from findings in the general population who develop lung cancer before the age of 40 (115). The clinical presentation of lung cancer is similar to that seen in other patients with the disease. Usual symptoms are cough, dyspnea, chest pain, and hemoptysis. The radiographic features are masses or infiltrates, as expected. The HIV-infected patients who do develop primary lung cancer all appear to have a poor prognosis.

In summary, HIV-infected patients who smoke are at risk for development of lung cancer. The magnitude of the risk compared with other smokers is unknown. This entity should be considered in the appropriate clinical setting, but unfortunately, it carries a grave prognosis.

References

1. Frizzera G, Rosai J, Dehner LP, Spector BD, Kersey JH. Lymphoreticular disorders in primary immunodeficiency: new findings based on an updated histologic classification of 35 cases. Cancer 1980; 46:692–699.
2. Holm LE, Blomgren H, Lowhagen T. Cancer risks in patients with chronic lymphocytic thyroiditis. N Engl J Med 1985; 312:601–604.

3. Penn I. Cancers complicating organ transplantation. N Engl J Med 1990; 323:1767–1769.
4. Klein MB, Pereira FA, Kantor I. Kaposi's sarcoma complicating systemic lupus erythematosus treated with immunosuppression. Arch Dermatol 1974; 110:602–604.
5. Penn I. Principles of tumor immunity: immunocompromised patients. AIDS Updates 1990; 3:1–4.
6. Beral V, Peterman TA, Berkelman RL, Jaffe HW. Kaposi's sarcoma among persons with AIDS: a sexually transmitted infection? Lancet 1990; 335:123–128.
7. Peterman TA, Harold WJ, Beral V. Epidemiologic clues to the etiology of Kaposi's sarcoma. AIDS 1993; 7:605–611.
8. Roth WK, Brandsetter H, Stürzl M. Cellular and molecular features of HIV-associated Kaposi's sarcoma. AIDS 1992; 6:895–913.
9. Beral V, Peterman T, Berkelman R, Jaffe H. AIDS-associated non-Hodgkin lymphoma. Lancet 1991; 337:805–809.
10. Knowles DM, Chamulak GA, Subar M, Burke JS, Dugan M, Wernz J, Slywotzky C, Pelicci P, Dalla-Favera R, Raphael B. Lymphoid neoplasia associated with the acquired immunodeficiency syndrome (AIDS). Ann Intern Med 1988; 108:744–753.
11. Lowenthal DA, Straus DJ, Campbell SW, Gold JWM, Clarkson BD, Koziner B. AIDS-related lymphoid neoplasia. The Memorial Hospital experience. Cancer 1988; 61:2325–2337.
12. Laga M, Icenogle JP, Marsella R, Manoka AT, Nzila N, Ryder RW, Vermund SH, Heyward WL, Nelson A, Reeves WC. Genital papillomavirus infection and cervical dysplasia—opportunistic complications of HIV infection. Int J Cancer 1992; 50:45–48.
13. Schafer A, Friedmann W, Mielke M, Schwartlander B, Koch MA. The increased frequency of cervical dysplasia-neoplasia in women infected with the human immunodeficiency virus is related to the degree of immunosuppression. Am J Obstet Gynecol 1991; 164:593–599.
14. Maiman M, Fruchter RG, Serur E, Remy JC, Feuer G, Boyce J. Human immunodeficiency virus infection and cervical neoplasia. Gynecol Oncol 1990; 38:377–382.
15. Centers for Disease Control and Prevention (CDC). 1993 revised classification system for HIV infection and expanded surveillance case definition for AIDS among adolescents and adults. MMWR 1992; 41:1–13.
16. Palefsky JM. Anal human papillomavirus infection and anal cancer in HIV-positive individuals: an emerging problem. AIDS 1994; 8:283–295.
17. Rabkin CS, Biggar RJ, Horm JW. Increasing incidence of cancers associated with the human immunodeficiency virus epidemic. Int J Cancer 1991; 47:692–696.
18. Monfardini S, Vaccher E, Pizzocaro G, Stellini R, Sinicco A, Sabbatani S, Marangolo M, Zagni R, Clerici M, Foa R, Tirelli U, Gavosto F. Unusual malignant tumours in 49 patients with HIV infection. AIDS 1989; 3:449–452.

19. Remick SC, Boguniewicz A, Wolf B. Solid tumors in HIV-infected patients other than AIDS-defining neoplasms. Adv Exp Med Biol 1993; 335:219–241.
20. Coté T, Howe H, Anderson S, Martin R, Evans B, Francis B. A systematic consideration of the neoplastic spectrum of AIDS: registry linkage. AIDS 1991; 5:49–53.
21. Jahan N, Razzaque A, Greenspan J, Conant MA, Josephs SF, Nakamura S, Rosenthal LJ. Analysis of human KS biopsies and cloned cell lines for cytomegalovirus, HIV-1, and other selected DNA virus sequences. AIDS Res Hum Retroviruses 1989; 5:225–231.
22. Vogel J, Hinrichs SH, Reynolds RK, Luciw PA, Jay G. The HIV *tat* gene induces dermal lesions resembling Kaposi's sarcoma in transgenic mice. Nature 1988; 335:66–71.
23. Ensoli B, Barillari G, Salahuddin SZ, Gallo RC, Wong-Staal F. Tat protein of HIV-1 stimulates growth of cells derived from Kaposi's sarcoma lesions of AIDS patients. Nature 1990; 345:84–86.
24. Lilenbaum RC, Ratner L. Systemic treatment of Kaposi's sarcoma: current status and future directions. AIDS 1994; 8:141–151.
25. Ensoli B, Barillari G, Gallo RC. Pathogenesis of AIDS-associated Kaposi's sarcoma. Hematol Oncol Clin North Am 1991; 5:281–295.
26. Miles SA, Martínez-Masa O, Rezai A, Magpantay L, Kishimoto T, Nakamura S, Radka SF, Linsley PS. Oncostatin M as a potent mitogen for AIDS-Kaposi's sarcoma derived cells. Science 1992; 255:1432–1434.
27. Albini A, Fontanini G, Masiello L, Tacchetti C, Bigni D, Luzzi P, Noonan DM, Stetler-Stevenson WG. Angiogenic potential in vivo by Kaposi's sarcoma cell-free supernatants and HIV-1 *tat* product: inhibition of KS-like lesions by tissue inhibitor of metalloproteinase-2. AIDS 1994, 8:1237–1244.
28. Benjamin D, Knobloch TJ, Dayton MA. Human B-cell interleukin-10: B-cell lines derived from patients with acquired immunodeficiency syndrome and Burkitt's lymphoma constitutively secrete large quantities of interleukin-10. Blood 1992; 880:1289–1298.
29. Emilie D, Coumbaras J, Raphael M, Devergne O, Delecluse HJ, Gisselbrecht C, Michiels JF, Van Damme J, Taga T, Kishimoto T. Interleukin-6 production in high-grade B lymphomas: correlation with the presence of malignant immunoblasts in acquired immunodeficiency syndrome and in human immunodeficiency virus-seronegative patients. Blood 1992; 80:498–504.
30. Herndier BG, Kaplan LD, McGrath MS. Pathogenesis of AIDS lymphomas. AIDS 1994; 8:1025–1049.
31. Pelicci PG, Knowles DM, Arlin ZA, Wieczorek R, Luciw P, Dina D, Basilico C, Dalla-Farera R. Multiple monoclonal B cell expansions and c-*myc* oncogene rearrangements in acquired immune deficiency syndrome-related lymphoproliferative disorders. Implications for lymphomagenesis. J Exp Med 1986; 164:2049–2076.
32. Hamilton-Dutoit SJ, Pallesen G, Karpov J, Skinhoj P, Franzmann MB, Pedersen C. Identification of EBV-DNA in tumour cells of AIDS-related lymphomas by in-situ hybridisation. Lancet 1989; 1:554–555.

33. Cox FH, Helwig EB. Kaposi's sarcoma. Cancer 1959; 12:289–298.
34. Taylor JF, Tempelton AC, Vogel CL, Ziegler JL, Kyalwazi SK. Kaposi's sarcoma in Uganda: a clinical–pathological study. Int J Cancer 1971; 8:122.
35. Rutherford GW, Kahn JO. The epidemiology of AIDS-related Kaposi sarcoma. J Acquir Immune Defic Syndr 1990; 3(suppl 1):S1–S55.
36. Peters BS, Beck EJ, Coleman DG, Wadsworth MJH, McGuinness O, Harris JRW, Pinching AJ. Changing disease patterns in patients with AIDS in a referral centre in the United Kingdom: the changing face of AIDS. Br Med J 1991; 302:203–207.
37. Huang YQ, Li JJ, Rush MG, Poiesz BJ, Nicolaides A, Jacobson M, Zhang WG, Coutaras E, Abbott MA, Fredman-Kien AE. HPV-16-related DNA sequences in Kaposi's sarcoma. Lancet 1992; 339:515–518.
38. Chang Y, Cesarman E, Pessin MS, Lee F, Culpepper J, Knowles DM, Moore PS. Identification of herpes-like DNA sequence in AIDS associated Kaposi's sarcoma. Science 1994; 266:1865–1869.
39. Krown S. AIDS-associated Kaposi's sarcoma: pathogenesis, clinical course and treatment. AIDS 1988; 2:71–80.
40. Garay S, Belenko M, Fazzini E, Schinella R. Pulmonary manifestations of Kaposi's sarcoma. Chest 1987; 91:39–43.
41. Meduri G, Stover D, Lee M, Myskowski P, Caravelli J, Zaman M. Pulmonary Kaposi's sarcoma in the acquired immune deficiency syndrome: clinical, radiographic, and pathologic manifestations. Am J Med 1986; 81:11–18.
42. Kaplan L, Hopewell P, Jaffe H, Goodman P, Bottles K, Volberding P. Kaposi's sarcoma involving the lung in patients with the acquired immunodeficiency syndrome. J Acquir Immune Defic Syndr 1988; 1:23–30.
43. Fouret P, Touboul J, Mayaud C, Akoun G, Roland J. Pulmonary Kaposi's sarcoma in patients with acquired immune deficiency syndrome: a clinicopathological study. Thorax 1987; 42:262–268.
44. Zibrak J, Silvestri R, Costello P, Marlink R, Jensen W, Robins A, Rose R. Bronchoscopic and radiologic features of Kaposi's sarcoma involving the respiratory system. Chest 1986; 90:476–479.
45. Gill P, Rarick M, McCutchan J, Slater L, Parker B, Muchmore E, Bernstein-Singer M, Akil B, Espina B, Krailo M, Levine A. Systemic treatment of AIDS-related Kaposi's sarcoma: results of a randomized trial. Am J Med 1991; 90:427–433.
46. Gill PS, Akil B, Colletti P, Rarick M, Loureiro C, Bernstein-Singer M, Krailo M, Levine AM. Pulmonary Kaposi's sarcoma: clinical findings and the results of therapy. Am J Med 1989; 87:57–61.
47. Kornfeld H, Axelrod JL. Pulmonary presentation of Kaposi's sarcoma in a homosexual patient. Am Rev Respir Dis 1983; 127:248–249.
48. Ognibene FP, Steis RG, Macher AM, Liotta L, Gelmann E, Pass HI, Lane C, Fauci AS, Parrillo JE, Masur H, Shelhamer JH. Kaposi's sarcoma causing pulmonary infiltrates and respiratory failure in the acquired immunodeficiency syndrome. Ann Intern Med 1985; 102:471–475.

49. Miller R, Tomlinson M, Cottril C, Donald J, Spittle M, Semple S. Bronchopulmonary Kaposi's sarcoma in patients with AIDS. Thorax 1992; 47:721–725.
50. Pitchenik A, Fischl M, Saldana M. Kaposi's sarcoma of the tracheobronchial tree. Chest 1985; 87:122–124.
51. O'Brien RF, Cohn DL. Serosanguineous pleural effusions in AIDS-associated Kaposi's sarcoma. Chest 1989; 96:460–466.
52. Sivit C, Schwartz A, Rockoff S. Kaposi's sarcoma of the lung in AIDS: radiologic–pathologic analysis. AJR 1987; 148:25–28.
53. Schulman L, Grimes M. Metastatic Kaposi's sarcoma and bilateral chylothorax. NY State J Med 1986; 205–206.
54. Panya K, Lal C, Tuckochmidt J, Boylen CT, Sharma OP. Bilateral chylothorax with pulmonary Kaposi's sarcoma. Chest 1988; 94:1316–1317.
55. White, DA, Matthay RA. Noninfectious pulmonary complications of infection with the human immunodeficiency virus. Am Rev Respir Dis 1989; 140:1763–1787.
56. Greenberg J, Fischl M, Berger J. Upper airway obstruction secondary to acquired immunodeficiency syndrome-related Kaposi's sarcoma. Chest 1985; 88:638–640.
57. Davis S, Henschke C, Chamides B, Westcott J. Intrathoracic Kaposi sarcoma in AIDS patients: radiographic–pathologic correlation. Radiology 1987; 163:495–500.
58. O'Brien RF. Pulmonary and pleural Kaposi's sarcoma in AIDS. Semin Respir Med 1989; 10:12–20.
59. Wolff SD, Kuhlman JE, Fishman EK. Thoracic Kaposi sarcoma in AIDS: CT findings. J Comput Assist Tomogr 1993; 17:60–62.
60. Naidich D, Tarras M, Garay S, Birnbaum B, Rybak B, Schinella R. Kaposi's sarcoma: CT–radiographic correlation. Chest 1989; 96:723–728.
61. Stover DE, White DA, Romano PA, Gellene RA, Robeson WA. Spectrum of pulmonary diseases associated with the acquired immune deficiency syndrome. Am J Med 1985; 78:429–437.
62. Gagliardi AJ, White DA, Meduri GU, Stover DE. Pulmonary function abnormalities in AIDS patients with respiratory illness (abstr). Am Rev Respir Dis 1985; 131:A75.
63. Vianna LA, Bronchoscopy in the diagnosis of pulmonary Kaposi's sarcoma in patients with AIDS. J Bronchol 1994; 1:9–14.
64. Lee V, Fuller J, O'Brien M, Parker D, Cooley T, Liebman H. Pulmonary Kaposi sarcoma in patients with AIDS: scintigraphic diagnosis with sequential thallium and gallium scanning. Radiology 1991; 180:409–412.
65. Krown S, Myskowski P, Paredes J. Kaposi's sarcoma. Med Clin North Am 1992; 76:235–252.
66. Nathan S, Vaghaiwalla R, Mohsenifar Z. Use of Nd:YAG laser in endobronchial Kaposi's sarcoma. Chest 1990; 98:1299–1300.
67. Presant C, Blayney D, Proffitt R, Turner A, Williams L, Nadel H, Kennedy P, Wiseman C, Gala K, Crossly R, Preiss S, Ksionski G, Presant S. Preliminary

report: imaging of Kaposi sarcoma and lymphoma in AIDS with indium-111-labelled liposomes. Lancet 1990; 335:1307–1309.
68. Presant C, Scolaro M, Kennedy P, Blayney D, Flanagan B, Lisak J, Presant J. Liposomal daunorubicin treatment of HIV-associated Kaposi's sarcoma. Lancet 1993; 341:1242–1243.
69. Gompels M, Hill A, Jenkins P, Peters B, Tomlinson D, Harris J, Stewart S, Pinching A. Kaposi's sarcoma in HIV infection treated with vincristine and bleomycin. AIDS 1992; 6:1175–1180.
70. Miles S. The use of hematopoietic growth factors in HIV infection and AIDS-related malignancies. Cancer Invest 1991; 9:229–238.
71. Gill PS, Bernstein-Singer M, Espina BM, Rarick M, Magy F, Montgomery T, Berry MS, Levine A. Adriamycin, bleomycin and vincristine chemotherapy with recombinant granulocyte–macrophage colony-stimulating factor in the treatment of AIDS-related Kaposi's sarcoma. AIDS 1992; 6:1477–1481.
72. Berson A, Quivey J, Harris J, Wara W. Radiation therapy for AIDS-related Kaposi's sarcoma. Int J Radiat Oncol Biol Phys 1990; 19:569–575.
73. Meyer JL. Whole-lung irradation for Kaposi's sarcoma. Am J Clin Oncol 1993; 16:372–376.
74. Doyle M, Johnstone PA, Watkins EB. Role of radiation therapy in management of pulmonary Kaposi's sarcoma. South Med J 1993; 86:285–288.
75. Windle-Taylor PC, Shah N. Oropharyngeal Kaposi's sarcoma: report of two cases and review of the literature. J Laryngol Otol 1983; 97:1065.
76. Centers for Disease Control. Revision of case definitions of acquired immunodeficiency syndrome for national reporting—United States. MMWR 1985; 34:373–375.
77. Pluda JM, Yarchoan R, Jaffe ES, Feuerstein IM, Solomon D, Steinberg SM, Wyvill KM, Raubitschek A, Katz D, Broder S. Development of non-Hodgkin lymphoma in a cohort of patients with severe human immunodeficiency virus (HIV) infection on long-term antiretroviral therapy. Ann Intern Med 1990; 113:276–282.
78. Moore RD, Kessler H, Richman DD, Flexner C, Chaisson RE. Non-Hodgkin's lymphoma in patients with advance HIV infection treated with zidovudine. JAMA 1991; 265:2208–2211.
79. Irwin DH, Kaplan LD. Pulmonary manifestations of acquired immunodeficiency syndrome-associated malignancies. Semin Respir Infect 1993; 8:139–148.
80. Levine AM, Gill PS, Meyer PR, Burkes RL, Ross R, Dworsky RD, Krailo M, Parker JW, Lukes RJ, Rasheed S. Retrovirus and malignant lymphoma in homosexual men. JAMA 1985; 254:1921–1925.
81. Levine AM, Sullivan-Halley J, Pike MC, Rarick MU, Loureiro C, Bernstein-Singer M, Willson E, Brynes R, Parker J, Rasheed S, Gill PS. Human immunodeficiency virus-related lymphoma. Cancer 1991; 68:2466–2472.
82. Levine AM, Sullivan-Halley J, Pike MC, Rarick MU, Loureiro C, Bernstein-Singer M, Byrnes R, Parker J, Rashud S. AIDS-related lymphoma: prognostic factors predictive of survival. Cancer 1991, 68:2466–2472.
83. Kaplan LD, Abrams DI, Feigal E, McGrath M, Kahn J, Neville P, Ziegler J,

Volberding PA. AIDS-associated non-Hodgkin's lymphoma in San Francisco. JAMA 1989; 261:719–724.
84. Ioachim HL, Cooper MC, Hellman GC. Lymphomas in men at high risk for acquired immune deficiency syndrome (AIDS). A study of 21 cases. Cancer 1985; 56:2831–2842.
85. Ziegler JL, Beckstead JA, Volberding PA, Abrams DI, Levine AM, Lukes RJ, Gill PS, Burkes RL, Meyer PR, Metroka CE, Mouradian J, Moore A, Riggs SA, Butler JJ, Cabanillas FC, Hersh E, Newell GR, Laubenstein LJ, Knowles D, Odajnyk C, Raphael B, Koziner B, Urmacher C, Clarkson BD. Non-Hodgkin's lymphoma in 90 homosexual men. Relation to generalized lymphadenopathy and the acquired immunodeficiency syndrome. N Engl J Med 1984; 311:656–570.
86. Levine AM, Meyer PR, Begandy MK, Parker JW, Taylor CR, Irwin L, Lukes RJ. Development of B-cell lymphoma in homosexual men. Ann Intern Med 1984; 100:7–13.
87. Kalter SP, Riggs SA, Cabanillas F, Butler JJ, Hagemeister FB, Mansell PW, Newell GR, Velasquez WS, Salvador P, Barlogie B, Rios A, Hersh EM. Aggressive non-Hodgkin's lymphomas in immunocompromised homosexual males. Blood 1985; 66:655–659.
88. Heitzman CR. Pulmonary neoplastic and lymphoroliferative disease in AIDS: a review. Radiol 1990; 177:347–351.
89. Levine A. AIDS-associated lymphoma. Med Clin North AM 1992; 57:809–843.
90. Dolly E, Naidich D, Rom W, Garay S. AIDS-related pulmonary lymphoma. Chest 1990; 98:51S.
91. Poelzleitner D, Huebsch P, Mayerhofer S, Chott A, Zielinski C. Primary pulmonary lymphoma in a patient with the acquired immune deficiency syndrome. Thorax 1989; 44:438–439.
92. Sider L, Horton ES. Pleural effusion as a presentation of AIDS-related lymphoma. Invest Radiol 1989; 24:150–153.
93. Chaouat A, Fraisse P, Kessler R, Lang JM, Weitzenbaum E. A life-threatening tracheal localization of lymphoma in a patient with AIDS. Chest 1993; 103:1297–1299.
94. Polish LB, Cohn DL, Ryder JW, Myers AM, O'Brien RF. Pulmonary non-Hodgkin's lymphoma in AIDS. Chest 1989; 96:1321–1326.
95. Bermudez MA, Grant KM, Rodvien R, Mendes F. Non-Hodgkin's lymphoma in a population with or at risk for acquired immunodeficiency syndrome: indications for intensive chemotherapy. Am J Med 1989; 86:71–76.
96. Sider L, Weiss AJ, Smith MD, VonRoenn JH, Glassroth J. Varied appearance of AIDS-related lymphoma in the chest. Radiology 1989; 171:629–632.
97. Sourour MS, Stover DE, Fels AOS. Pulmonary disease in AIDS patients with lymphoma (abstr). Am Rev Respir Dis 1987; 135:A168.
98. Loureiro C, Gill PS, Meyer PR, Rhodes R, Rarick MU, Levine AM. Autopsy findings in AIDS-related lymphoma. Cancer 1988; 62:735–739.
99. Judson MA, Sahn SA. Endobronchial lesions in HIV-infected individuals. Chest 1994; 105:1314–1323.

100. Naidich DP, McGuinness G. Pulmonary manifestations of AIDS: CT and radiographic correlations. Radiol Clin North Am 1991; 29:999–1017.
101. Alts AE, Shintaku IP, Said JW. Diagnosis of malignant lymphoma in effusions from patients with AIDS by gene rearrangement. Am J Clin Pathol 1990; 94:170–175.
102. Cechani V, Allam AA, Kamholtz SL. Pulmonary non-Hodgkin's lymphoma mimicking infection. Respir Med 1990; 84:401–405.
103. Ognibene FP. Evaluating pulmonary neoplasm associated with HIV infection. J Respir Dis 1993; 14:296–310.
104. Baselga J, Krown SE, Telzak EE, Filippa DA, Straus DJ. Acquired immune deficiency syndrome-related pulmonary non-Hodgkin's lymphoma regressing after zidovudine therapy. Cancer 1993; 71:2332–2334.
105. Chan T, Aranda C, Rom W. Bronchogenic carcinoma in young patients at risk for acquired immunodeficiency syndrome. Chest 1993; 103:862–64.
106. Braun M, Killam D, Remick S, Ruckdeschel J. Lung cancer in patients seropositive for human immunodeficiency virus. Radiology 1990; 175:341–343.
107. Cowan N, Salisbury J, Moxham J. Intrathoracic lymphadenopathy and HIV infection. Br J Radiol 1992; 65:940–942.
108. Karp J, Profeta G, Marantz P, Karpel J. Lung cancer in patients with immunodeficiency syndrome. Chest 1993; 103:410–413.
109. Moser R, Tenholder M, Ridenour R. Oat-cell carcinoma in transfusion-associated acquired immunodeficiency syndrome. Ann Intern Med 1985; 103:478.
110. Irwin L, Begandy M, Moore T. Adenosquamous carcinoma of the lung and the acquired immunodeficiency syndrome. Ann Intern Med 1984; 100:158.
111. Bagheri K, Connell R, Safirstein B. Lung cancer in a drug addict seropositive for human immunodeficiency virus. AJR 1992; 158:210.
112. Fraire A, Awe R. Lung cancer in association with human immunodeficiency virus infection. Cancer 1992; 70:432–436.
113. Sridhar K, Flores M, Raub W, Saldana M. Lung cancer in patients with human immunodeficiency virus infection compared with historic control subjects. Chest 1992; 102:1704–1708.
114. Remick S. Lung cancer: an HIV-related neoplasm or a coincidental finding? Chest 1992; 102:1643–1644.
115. Pemberton J, Nagorney D, Gilmore J, Taylor W, Bernatz P. Bronchogenic carcinoma in patients younger than 40 years. Ann Thorac Surg 1983; 36:509–515.

20

Inflammatory Disorders

Spectrum, Pathogenesis, and Pathology

WILLIAM D. TRAVIS

Armed Forces Institute of Pathology
Washington, D.C.

I. Introduction

Infectious pneumonia is the most common cause of lung inflammation in human immunodeficiency virus (HIV)-infected individuals. If one excludes the infectious pneumonias, there is a group of inflammatory lung disorders, the most common of which is lymphocytic interstitial pneumonia (1–5). Also included in this category of inflammatory lung conditions are pulmonary lymphoid hyperplasia and chronic interstitial pneumonitis (6,7). A few less common inflammatory lung conditions can occur, including bronchiectasis (8–10), bronchiolitis obliterans with organizing pneumonia (BOOP) (11,12), eosinophilic pneumonia (13,14). and sarcoidosis (Table 1;15–17). In this chapter we review the spectrum, pathogenesis, and pathological features of these inflammatory pulmonary lesions.

II. Spectrum of Lymphoid Lung Lesions in HIV Infection

Pulmonary lymphoid lesions in HIV-infected patients embrace a spectrum of interstitial inflammation, ranging from lymphocytic interstitial pneumoni-

Table 1 Inflammatory Pulmonary Complications of HIV Infection

Lymphoid lesions
Lymphocytic interstitial pneumonitis
Lymphoid hyperplasia (follicular bronchiolitis)
Chronic interstitial pneumonitis
Lymphocytic alveolitis
Diffuse infiltrative lymphocytosis syndrome
Diffuse alveolar damage
Bronchiolitis obliterans organizing pneumonia
Bronchiectasis
Eosinophilic pneumonia
Sarcoidosis

tis and lymphoid hyperplasia, to a mild chronic interstitial pneumonitis (5). A lymphocytic alveolitis (LA) is also frequently detected by bronchoalveolar lavage (BAL; 18–20) in HIV-infected patients. Some HIV-infected patients with lymphocytic interstitial pneumonitis develop a diffuse infiltrative lymphocytosis syndrome that resembles Sjogren's syndrome (21,22). Although these disorders probably represent a continuum of lymphoid proliferation in the lung, there are certain distinct clinicopathological differences that can be determined. The similarities and differences between lymphocytic interstitial pneumonitis–lymphoid hyperplasia and chronic interstitial pneumonitis are compared in Table 2.

A. Lymphocytic Interstitial Pneumonitis and Pulmonary Lymphoid Hyperplasia

Lymphocytic interstitial pneumonitis (LIP) is defined pathologically as a diffuse interstitial chronic inflammatory infiltrate (5,7). In addition to HIV infection, it occurs in a variety of other conditions, such as Sjogren's syndrome, systemic lupus erythematosus, and myasthenia gravis (5,23–25). Lymphocytic interstitial pneumonitis occurs in about 1% of adult and 30–50% of pediatric HIV-infected patients (4,5,26,27). It is more common in perinatally acquired HIV-infected children than in those who become infected by contaminated blood products (28). In children, it is one of the defining criteria for the acquired immunodeficiency syndrome (AIDS) proposed by the Centers for Disease Control and Prevention (29,30). The clinical features of lymphocytic interstitial pneumonitis are discussed in Chapter 21.

A diffuse interstitial and alveolar septal infiltrate of lymphocytes and plasma cells characterizes the histological appearance of lymphocytic in-

Table 2 Features That Distinguish Chronic Interstitial Pneumonitis from Lymphocytic Interstitial Pneumonitis

Distinguishing feature	CIP/NIP[a]	LIP[a]
Clinical		
Age	Common in adults; can occur in up to 33% of symptomatic patients. Frequency in children is unknown.	Rare in adults Common in children
Severity of symptoms	Mild; can occur in up to 48% of asymptomatic adults	Moderate to severe respiratory symptoms
Extrapulmonary involvement	Uncommon	Common both in children and adults; generalized lymphadenopathy in up to 94%; intrathoracic adenopathy in up to 25%; parotid enlargement; lymphocytic infiltration of kidney, liver, nasopharynx, bone marrow, and GI tract
Peripheral CD8 lymphocytosis	Not known	Common
Radiologic		
Normal chest radiograph	Common (up to 44%)	Uncharacteristic
Subtle increased perihilar markings	Common (up to 36%)	Uncharacteristic
Prominent nodular, interstitial, or alveolar infiltrates	Uncharacteristic (up to 6%)	Characteristic
Pleural effusion	Uncommon (up to 11%)	Common (up to 31%)
Pathological		
Severity of lymphoid infiltrate	Mild/moderate	Marked
Distribution along lymphatic routes: peribronchiolar, perivascular, pleural, interlobular septal	Characteristic	Characteristic
Alveolar septal infiltration	Uncharacteristic	Characteristic
Lymphoid aggregates (with or without germinal centers	Common	Common

[a]CIP, chronic interstitial pneumonitis; NIP, nonspecific intertitial pneumonitis; LIP, lymphocytic intersticial pneumonitis.
Source: Ref. 5.

terstitial pneumonitis (Fig. 1; 5). The severity of the infiltrate can vary from a moderate to a severe degree. The lymphocytes are small, without large atypical forms. Reactive type II pneumocyte hyperplasia may accompany the interstitial infiltrate. The majority of the lymphocytes are of T-cell origin (Fig. 2). Noncaseating granulomas are occasionally seen, but are usually inconspicuous (5). Perivascular lymphoid infiltrates may be seen, but vasculitis is typically absent. It is important to exclude an infectious pneumonia caused by organisms such as *Pneumocystis carinii* or *Mycobacterium avium–intracellulare*, which can be accompanied by prominent interstitial chronic inflammation resembling lymphocytic interstitial pneumonitis (7,31–33). In biopsies, when the diagnosis of lymphocytic interstitial pneumonitis is suspected, it is important to search carefully for alveolar exudates of *P. carinii* pneumonia and examine special stains for *P. carinii*, fungi, and acid-fast bacilli.

Lymphoid hyperplasia frequently accompanies lymphocytic interstitial pneumonitis (Fig. 3), but it may occur independently in the absence of alveolar septal lymphoid infiltration (Fig. 4). It consists of enlarged or hyperplastic lymphoid aggregates frequently situated adjacent to bronchioles (1,5). Follicular bronchiolitis is another term used, which is applied for hyperplastic lymphoid follicles situated adjacent to bronchioles (34).

A lung biopsy is the ultimate way to achieve a definitive diagnosis of lymphocytic interstitial pneumonitis–lymphoid hyperplasia. Open biopsies are more likely to achieve a diagnosis than transbronchial biopsies, which are more susceptible to sampling problems. The diagnosis can be established, based on a transbronchial biopsy, if the biopsy samples a piece of lung with extensive lymphoid interstitial infiltrates (Fig. 5). Since the mid-1980s, when lymphocytic interstitial pneumonitis–lymphoid hyperplasia was recognized to represent one of the most common pulmonary manifestations of pediatric HIV infection in children, there has been a reluctance to perform lung biopsies, and the diagnosis is often made based on clinical features (9). A presumptive diagnosis is sometimes made in patients with a reticulonodular pattern, with or without hilar and mediastinal lymphadenopathy that does not change after treatment with antibiotics for 2 months (28). Bronchoalveolar lavage can also be useful to confirm a lymphoid pulmonary process by demonstrating a lymphocytic alveolitis and to exclude certain infections such as with P. *carinii*.

Chronic Interstitial Pneumonitis

Lymphoid infiltrates may be mild or moderate, without alveolar septal infiltration, falling short of the criteria for lymphocytic interstitial pneumonitis. The term chronic interstitial pneumonitis (CIP) has been applied to these

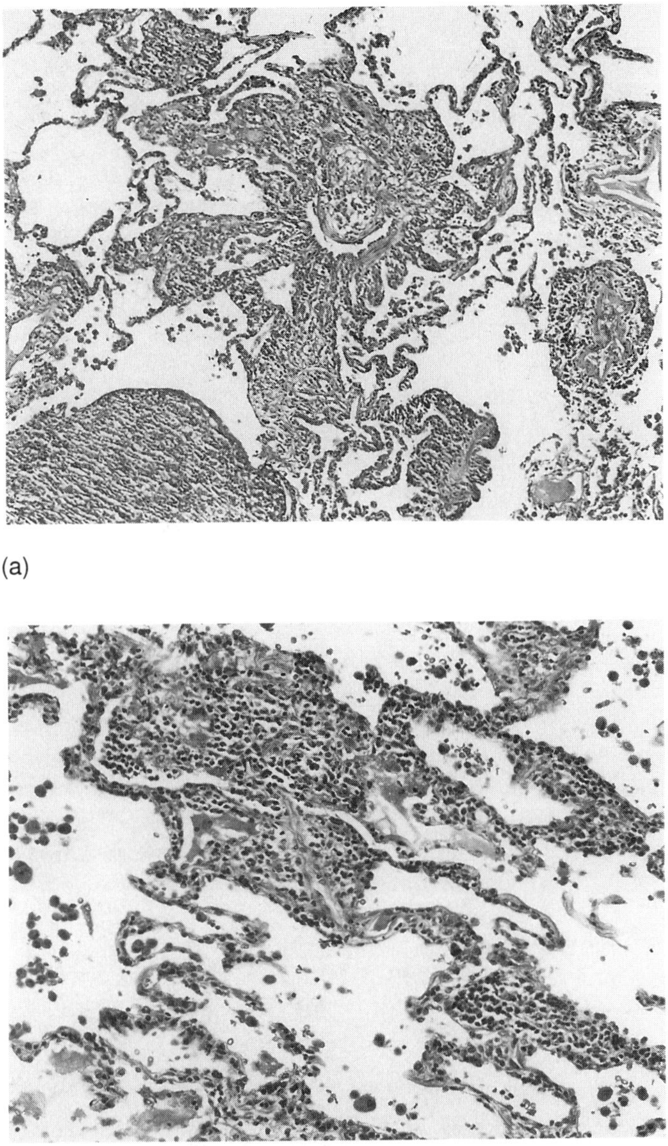

(a)

(b)

Figure 1 (a) Lymphocytic interstitial pneumonia: Open-lung biopsy from a patient with lymphocytic interstitial pneumonia shows an extensive interstitial chronic inflammatory infiltrate. The lymphoid cells are perivascular and peribronchiolar but they extend into the surrounding alveolar septa (hematoxylin and eosin [H & E]; × 100). (b) Extensive alveolar septal infiltration is present in other areas of this same biopsy (H & E; × 250). (From Ref. 5.)

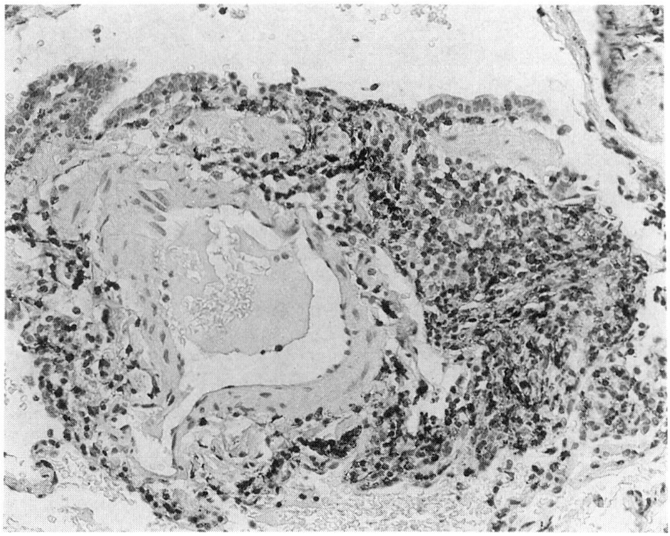

Figure 2 Lymphocytic interstitial pneumonia: Most of the lymphocytes in this example of lymphocytic interstitial pneumonitis are T cells (Immunohistochemistry for UCHL-1; × 250). (From Ref. 5.)

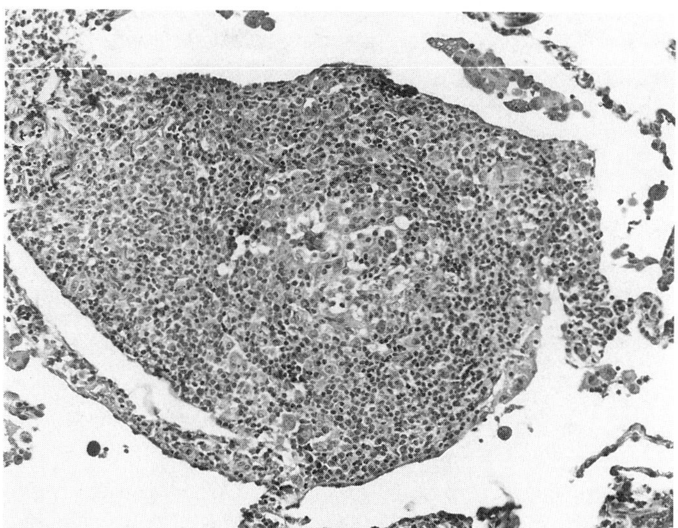

Figure 3 Lymphoid hyperplasia: This hyperplastic germinal center was present in a lung biopsy showing lymphocytic interstitial pneumonia (H & E; × 200). (From Ref. 5.)

cases (5). Lymphoid hyperplasia can occur in these cases as well as lymphocytic interstitial pneumonia (see Fig. 4). A case reported as lymphocytic bronchiolitis by Ettensohn et al. probably fits best into this group of lesions (35). In these cases, lung biopsies show mild to moderate interstitial chronic inflammation, frequently in a peribronchiolar or perivascular location (Figs. 6 and 7). The lymphoid infiltrate lacks the extensive alveolar septal infiltration seen in lymphocytic interstitial pneumonitis (see Figs. 4 and 7). Mild type 2 pneumocyte hyperplasia can be present (Fig. 8). Chronic interstitial pneumonitis represents a diagnosis of exclusion after the presence of an opportunistic infection has been ruled out by bronchoalveolar lavage or review of special stains for organisms on lung biopsies.

Chronic interstitial pneumonitis is found in lung biopsies from most patients who have the clinicopathological syndrome described as nonspecific interstitial pneumonitis in HIV-infected adults (36–38). The term nonspecific intersitial pneumonitis was proposed by Suffredini et al. to describe a subgroup of HIV-infected adults who had clinical evidence of pneumonitis in the absence of a detectable infectious agent after lung biopsy or bronchoalveolar lavage (38). Nonspecific interstitial pneumonitis was encountered in 38% of patients with AIDS and pulmonary symptoms (38). Some of these patients had Kaposi's sarcoma, prior *P. carinii* pneumonia, or previous drug therapy; but in a subset of cases, the patient had no other underlying condition or exposure other than HIV-infection. Subsequently, Ognibene et al.

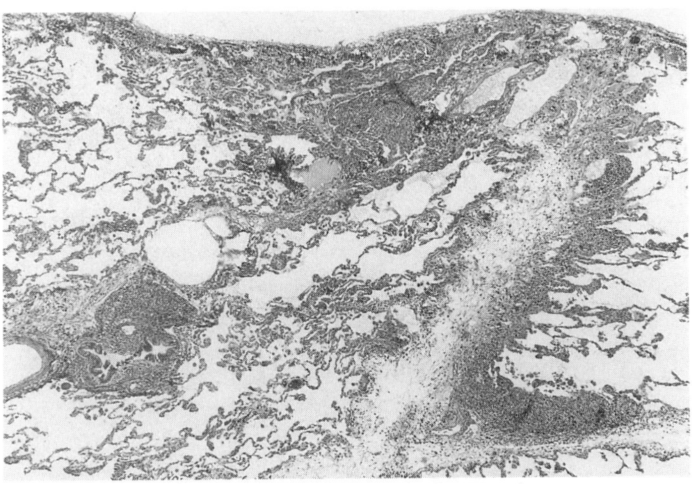

Figure 4 Lymphoid hyperplasia–chronic interstitial pneumonia: Lymphoid hyperplasia is the predominant finding in this open-lung biopsy. Alveolar septal infiltration is not present (H & E; × 42). (From Ref. 5.)

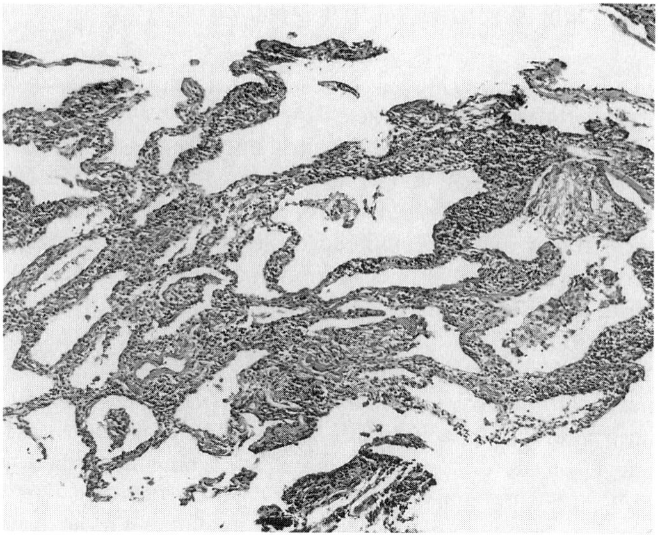

(a)

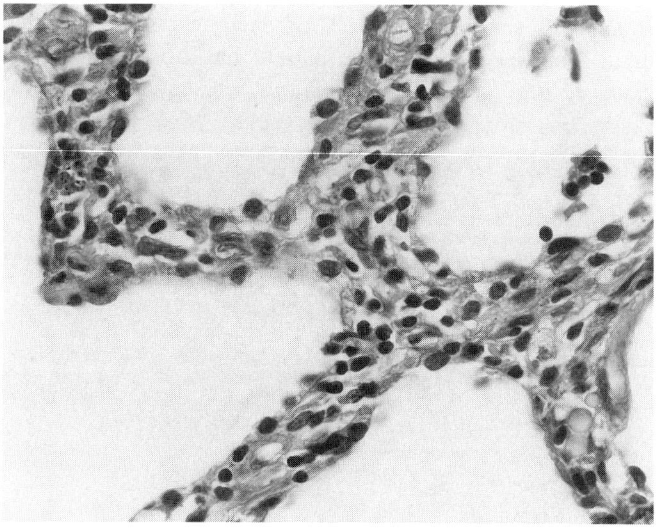

(b)

Figure 5 (a) Lymphocytic interstitial pneumonia: This transbronchial biopsy specimen shows extensive interstitial and alveolar septal infiltration by chronic inflammation. (b) These alveolar septa are infiltrated by lymphocytes. There are a few hyperplastic type 2 pneumocytes (H & E; × 630). (From Ref. 5.)

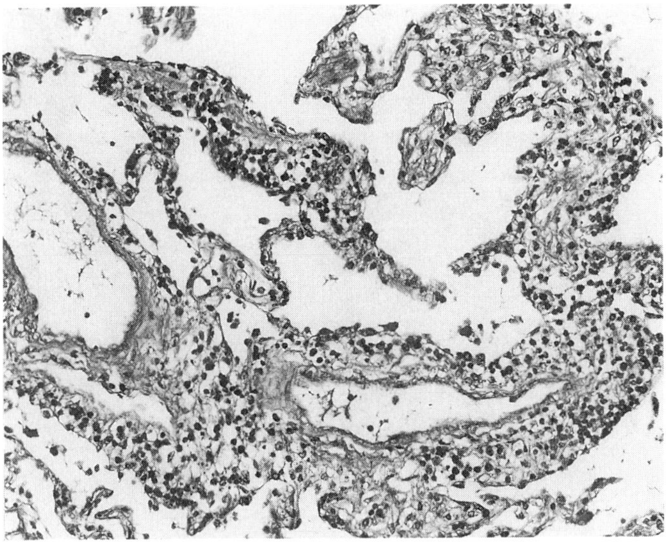

Figure 6 Chronic interstitial pneumonitis: This transbronchial biopsy specimen showed focal perivascular interstitial chronic inflammation (H & E; × 100). (From Ref. 5.)

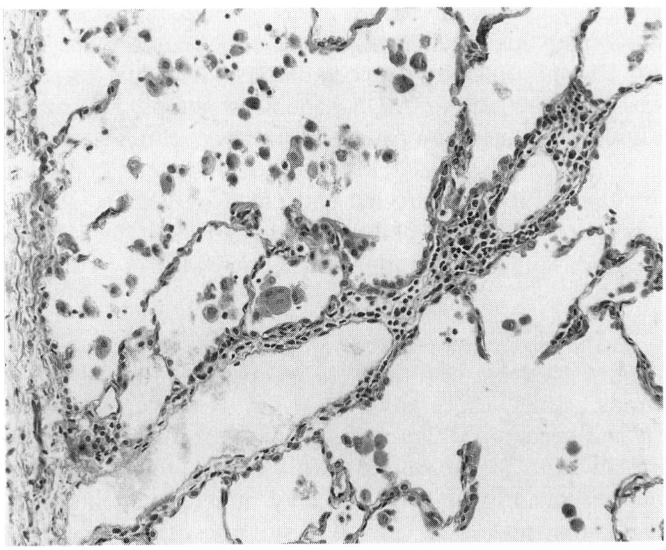

Figure 7 Chronic interstitial pneumonitis: This open-lung biopsy sample shows perivascular interstitial chronic inflammation and a few alveolar macrophages (H & E; × 42). (From Ref. 5.)

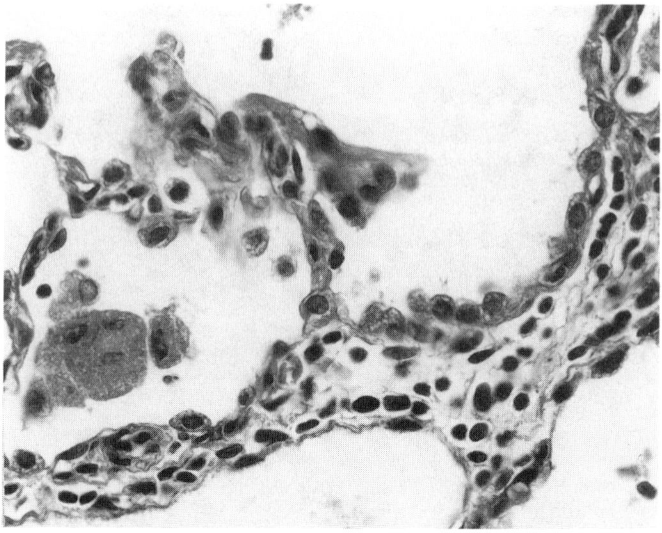

Figure 8 Chronic interstitial pneumonitis: Hyperplastic type 2 pneumocytes were prominent in this example of chronic interstitial pneumonitis (H & E; × 630). (From Ref. 5.)

found chronic interstitial pneumonitis in 48% of asymptomatic HIV-infected adults (36). Chronic interstitial pneumonitis–nonspecific interstitial pneumonitis was found in 13% of AIDS patients at autopsy, but it was not the primary cause of death in any patient (39). Thus, chronic interstitial pneumonitis represents a subclinical form of pneumonitis that goes unrecognized in many asymptomatic HIV-infected patients. Nonspecific interstitial pneumonitis is not well defined in children, although the term has been applied in several cases, without a detailed description (40).

Lymphocytic Alveolitis

In HIV-infected patients, bronchoalveolar lavage is a sensitive way to detect infectious agents, especially *P. carinii*. However, early in the HIV epidemic it was recognized that a significant percentage of patients have a lymphocytic alveolitis (19,20,41–46). Guillon et al. found a bronchoalveolar lavage lymphocytosis in 78% of 154 HIV-infected patients with lung infections or tumors, and in 72% of 122 patients without lung infections or tumors (19). Most of these broncoalveolar lavage lymphocytes were $CD8^+$ and $CD44^+$ (19). Autran et al. and Plata et al. demonstrated that the cytotoxic T lymphocytes from the bronchoalveolar lavage in HIV-infected patients have a cytolytic activity against HIV-infected alveolar macrophages and that this activity is restricted by class I histocompatibility (HLA) transplantation antigens (41,47). Agostini et al. reported that patients without opportunistic infections who had an increase in $CD3^+$ and $CD8^+$ bronchoalveolar lavage lymphocytes had a significantly increased mortality rate.

Open-lung biopsies from four of the patients reported by Guillon et al. without lung infections or tumors appeared to show histological features of chronic interstitial pneumonitis, and the lymphocytes were $CD8^+$ (19). Thus, chronic interstitial pneumonitis probably represents the histological counterpart to this CD8 lymphocytic alveolitis. It is not surprising that chronic interstitial pneumonitis–nonspecific interstitial pneumonitis and lymphocytic alveolitis are found in a similar percentage of asymptomatic HIV-infected patients, that is 48 (36) and 59%, respectively (19).

Diffuse Infiltrative Lymphocytosis Syndrome

Itescu et al. described a diffuse infiltrative lymphocytosis syndrome in HIV-infected patients who have a Sjogren's syndrome-like disorder (21). The similarities and differences between diffuse infiltrative lymphocyte syndrome and Sjogren's syndrome are summarized in Table 3. There is a bimodal age distribution, with a peak in children up to 14 years of age and in adults from 22 to 62 years of age (22). These patients have frequent bilateral parotid gland enlargement and xerostomia or xerophthalmia. In addition, most patients have generalized lymphadenopathy and lymphocytic interstitial pneumonitis, whereas a few may have neurological involvement or lymphocytic infiltration of the gastrointestinal tract (21). Polyclonal hypergammaglobulinemia is a consistent finding, and a small number of patients may have low-level positive rheumatoid factors (21). The infiltrating lymphocytes are $CD8^+$ T cells, with a memory phenotype (22). Salivary gland biopsies show inflammatory changes similar to those seen in Sjogren's syndrome (48).

The pathogenesis of this disorder is tied to an immunogenetic predisposition (21,22). Susceptibility to diffuse infiltrative lymphocyte syndrome in blacks is associated with HLA-DR5 and HLA-DR6, whereas in whites it is associated only with HLA-DR6 (21). This suggests that the occurrence of diffuse infiltrative lymphocyte syndrome in HIV-infection may be dependent on host immune characteristics (21). It is thought that both major histocompatibility complex (MHC) classes I and II are involved in the susceptibility to diffuse infiltrative lymphocyte syndrome. Studies in HIV-infected mother–child pairs suggest that the host immune response is more important than the viral strain of HIV in determining the risk for developing diffuse infiltrative lymphocyte syndrome (21).

Table 3 Diffuse Infiltrative Lymphocytosis Syndrome (DILS) in HIV Infection Versus Sjogren's Syndrome

Characteristic	Sjögren's syndrome	DILS
Glandular manifestations	Moderate parotid enlargement	Massive parotid enlargement
Extraglandular manifestations	*Infrequent*	*Prominent*
	May have pulmonary, gastrointestinal, renal, and neurological involvement	Pulmonary, gastrointestinal, renal, and neurological involvement
Infiltrative lymphocytic phenotype	CD4 predominant	CD8 predominant
Autoantibodies	*High frequency*	*Low frequency*
	Rheumatoid factor, ANA, anti-Ro/SSA, anti-LA/SSB	Rheumatoid factor, ANA, anti-Ro/SSA, anti-LA/SSB
HLA association	B8, DR2, DR3, DR4 (rheumatoid arthritis)	DR5, DR6 (blacks), DR6 (whites)

Source: Ref. 22.

B. Diffuse Alveolar Damage

Diffuse alveolar damage is the histological counterpart to the adult respiratory distress syndrome (38,49). In almost all cases when diffuse alveolar damage is encountered in lung biopsies from HIV-infected patients, there is an underlying infection. However, in a small percentage, a specific cause may not be detectable. This phenomenon was recognized by Ramaswamy et al., who described 12 AIDS patients with lung biopsies showing diffuse alveolar damage or interstitial fibrosis in the absence of detectable infection (49). Histological study of lung biopsies from a series of 46 adult HIV-infected patients with nonspecific interstitial pneumonitis, including those reported by Suffredini et al. (38) and Ognibene et al. (36), revealed features of diffuse alveolar damage in 6.5% of cases (5).

Histologically, diffuse alveolar damage consists of two phases: The acute or cellular phase of diffuse alveolar damage consists of alveolar and interstitial edema, hyaline membranes, and acute inflammation. The chronic or proliferative phase of diffuse alveolar damage shows interstitial organizing fibrosis, chronic inflammation, and prominent type II pneumocyte proliferation (Fig. 9; 50,51). This reaction is nonspecific and can result

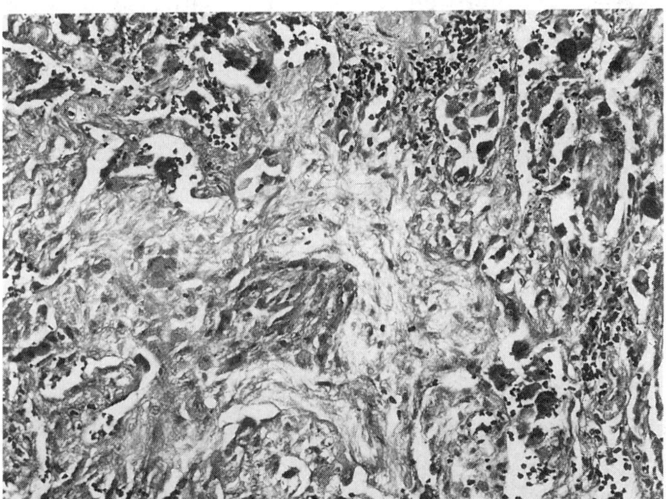

Figure 9 Diffuse alveolar damage: This transbronchial biopsy shows features of the organizing phase of diffuse alveolar damage, with prominent interstitial organizing loose fibrosis and type 2 pneumocyte proliferation. No viral inclusions or granulomas were seen and no organisms were seen on special stains (H & E; × 200). (From Ref. 5.)

from a variety of types of lung injury, including infection, drug toxicity, uremia, radiation, and collagen vascular disease. Outside the setting of HIV-infection the term acute interstitial pneumonia is sometimes applied for cases of idiopathic diffuse alveolar damage (52). If this pattern of lung injury is encountered in an HIV-infected patient, an infection should be suspected until proved otherwise. Infection should be excluded by careful examination of routine sections for viral inclusions and special stains for acid-fast organisms, fungi, bacteria, or *P. carinii* (6).

C. Bronchiolitis Obliterans Organizing Pneumonia

Several cases of bronchiolitis obliterans organizing pneumonia are reported in HIV-infected patients (11,12,53). Idiopathic bronchiolitis obliterans organizing pneumonia, also known as cryptogenic organizing pneumonia, is a form of interstitial lung disease that often presents following a 4- to 6-week history of a flu-like illness, with dry cough, dyspnea, and patchy nodular radiographic infiltrates (54,55). Lung biopsies show patchy nodules of organizing intraluminal fibrosis, with plugs of young connective tissue protruding into the lumens of alveoli and alveolar ducts (56). The lung architecture is preserved, and the connective tissue is of uniform age. Patients generally respond well to a course of corticosteroids. Separation from an organizing infectious pneumonia is important in HIV-infected patients, for this pattern of fibrosis is commonly seen as a response to infection. In particular, organizing *P. carinii* pneumonia can result in a histological reaction identical with that seen in bronchiolitis obliterans organizing pneumonia (32). The clinical details of bronchiolitis obliterans organizing pneumonia in HIV-infected patients are discussed in Chapter 22.

The cause of bronchiolitis obliterans organizing pneumonia in the few HIV-infected patients reported is unknown. This histological pattern of response could be due to an unrecognized infection, especially viral, or it could be truly idiopathic.

D. Bronchiectasis

A few cases of bronchiectasis have been reported, mostly in pediatric HIV-infected patients (8–10). In the study by Amorosa et al., bronchiectasis developed in 4 of 32 patients with lymphocytic interstitial pneumonitis (9). The etiology and pathogenesis of the bronchiectasis was unclear in these cases. None of the patients had recurring pulmonary infections or aspiration. However, each of the patients was a long-term survivor, living an average of 8 years. Holmes et al. reported bronchiectasis in seven patients without lymphocytic interstitial pneumonitis, six of whom had recurrent episodes of infection (10). Both Amorosa and Holmes suggested that bronchiectasis may be a long-term pulmonary complication of HIV-infection.

E. Eosinophilic Pneumonia

A few cases of eosinophilic pneumonia are reported in HIV-infected patients (13,14). Acute eosinophilic pneumonia of unknown cause was found in several cases (13,57). These patients presented with features of the syndrome acute eosinophilic pneumonia, described by Davis et al. in 1986, including fever, acute respiratory failure, diffuse alveolar or interstitial infiltrates, and bronchoalveolar lavage fluid eosinophilia, with or without peripheral eosinophilia (58). Steroid therapy resulted in a dramatic response without recurrence (13,57). Several cases occurred in association with exposure to medications, such as maloprim (59) or pentamidine (14). Llibre et al. found greater than 10% bronchoalveolar lavage eosinophilia in 5 of 91 (5%) of HIV-infected patients, 3 of whom had *P. carinii* pneumonia and 2 who appeared to have idiopathic acute eosinophilic pneumonia (57).

The pathogenesis of acute eosinophilic pneumonia is unknown. Potential causes include medications, IgE-mediated hypersensitivity to unrecognized antigens, or HIV-induced activation of $CD4^+$ eosinophils (13). Although several of the reported HIV-infected patients with eosinophilic pneumonia have been intravenous (iv) drug abusers, at the time of the pulmonary eosinophilia, iv drugs were not felt to be the cause (13).

F. Sarcoidosis

Sarcoidosis in HIV-infected patients is rare, with just a few case reports (15–17). There are similarities between the clinical picture of sarcoidosis and HIV-infection, but the lymphocyte populations may be quite different (15). Patients with both disorders can have fever, weight loss, fatigue, and pulmonary symptoms, as well as cutaneous anergy, peripheral lymphopenia, and elevated serum polyclonal gamma globulin levels (15). A lymphocytic alveolitis can be shown by bronchoalveolar lavage in both types of patients. However, sarcoidosis and HIV-infected patients differ in that the bronchoalveolar lavage lymphocytes consist predominantly of CD4 and CD8 lymphocytes, respectively.

The diagnosis of sarcoidosis requires clinicopathological correlation. Clinically, the most patients have systemic and respiratory symptoms, often with bilateral hilar adenopathy or pulmonary infiltrates (60). Histological confirmation of noncaseating granulomas is also required and is typically demonstrated in a biopsy of a lymph node or the lung (61). Infection is very important to exclude, because granulomas can occur in HIV-infected patients with fungal, mycobacterial, or *P. carinii* infection.

Treatment for patients with sarcoidosis and HIV-infection presents a dilemma, because the immunosuppressive effect of steroids may render a patient especially susceptible to infection. Three of seven patients reviewed by Lowery et al. were effectively treated with steroids, without complications (15). However, two patients had to be weaned from their steroids as the HIV-infection progressed. Another patient spontaneously improved as the HIV infection developed. Given these observations, it was suggested that sarcoidosis may stabilize or improve with HIV infection owing to progressive loss of activated CD4 lymphocytes. Steroids may be needed for HIV-infected patients with active sarcoid (15).

III. Pathogenesis of Lymphoid Lesions in HIV Infection

The pathogenesis of chronic interstitial pneumonitis, lymphoid hyperplasia, and lymphocytic interstitial pneumonitis in HIV infection is not completely understood (62). Evidence suggests that host genetic and immune characteristics may be important (21,22). There has been much speculation whether HIV is an innocent bystander or a true pathogen in the lung (62). Epstein–Barr virus has also been considered as a potential etiologic factor. Potentially these viral agents could cause lymphoid infiltration and hyperplasia in these lung disorders through mechanisms involving a variety of cytokines or growth factors. Adhesion of lymphocytes to high endothelial venules may be important in the migration of lymphocytes from the bloodstream into the lung (63,64). Thus, many factors are probably involved with the pathogenesis of inflammatory lung conditions in HIV infection.

The HIV was initially recovered from the lung of HIV-infected patients by Ziza et al. (65) and confirmed by multiple subsequent investigators (66–72). HIV infects alveolar macrophages, CD4 lymphocytes, and fibroblasts both in vivo and in vitro (62,67). The absence of opportunistic infections or other detectable etiologic agents for chronic interstitial pneumonitis, lymphocytic alveolitis, and many examples of lymphocytic interstitial pneumonitis–lymphoid hyperplasia, has led to speculation that HIV plays an important role in the pathogenesis of these lesions (65,73).

Few studies have demonstrated HIV directly in lung biopsy tissue. By in situ hybridization, HIV was shown to be concentrated in the germinal centers of one patient with lymphocytic interstitial pneumonitis (Fig. 10; 5). This correlates with data from lymphoid tissue that show that lymphoid germinal centers are reservoirs of HIV (74). A variety of cytokines

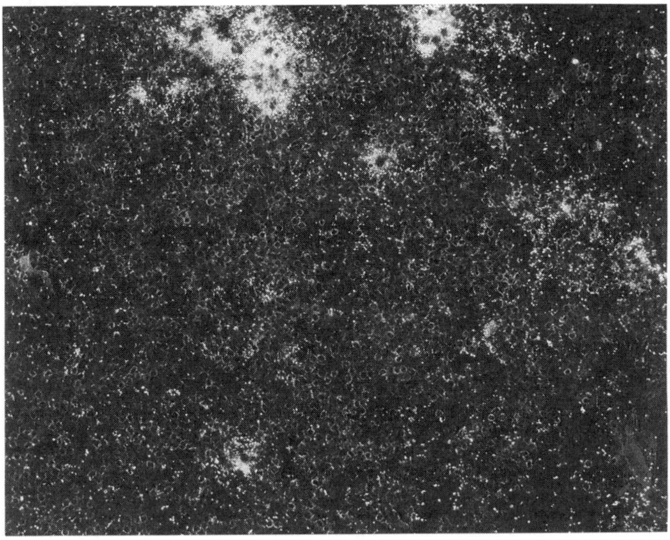

Figure 10 HIV RNA in germinal centers in a case of lymphocytic interstitial pneumonitis: In situ hybridization for HIV RNA shows concentration of virus within germinal centers. (In situ hybridization for HIV-RNA; × 250). (From Ref. 5.)

are abnormally expressed in vitro by HIV infected cells including IL-1, IL-2, IL-6, IL-8, IL-10, macrophage inflammatory protein-1α, TNF-α, and GM-CSF (62,75–77). Cytokines may be mediators influencing lung injury, inflammatory cell recruitment, or HIV replication (62). In addition, immune complexes have been shown in the bronchoalveolar lavage of HIV-infected children (78) and adults.

Data from animal studies are supportive of the concept that HIV may be important in the pathogenesis of lymphoid pulmonary lesions in HIV-infected patients. Interestingly, pulmonary lesions similar to nonspecific interstitial pneumonitis and lymphocytic interstitial pneumonitis can occur in sheep infected with ovine lentivirus (79,80). A mild inflammatory infiltrate similar to that seen in chronic interstitial pneumonitis is seen with nonlytic ovine lentivirus strains, and a marked inflammatory infiltrate similar to lymphocytic interstitial pneumonitis is seen with lytic strains (79). The lymphocytes in these cases are also mostly of T-cell origin. The similarity to the spectrum of HIV-associated lymphoid lesions in humans is significant because HIV is considered to be within the lentivirus group, owing to genome sequence homology, morphology, and replicative mechanisms (79). Lung inflammation with the pattern of nonspecific interstitial pneumonitis was seen in transgenic mice containing HIV proviral DNA (81).

The EBV has also been proposed to play a role in some, but not all, cases of lymphocytic interstitial pneumonitis associated with HIV-infection. Malamou-Mitsi et al. found EBV in three of six lung biopsies from HIV-infected patients with lymphocytic interstitial pneumonitis, suggesting that EBV plays a role in some, but not all, cases (82). In another study, EBV was not found in lung biopsy tissue from HIV-infected adults with lymphocytic interstitial pneumonitis (5). In several studies of lymphocytic interstitial pneumonitis in HIV-infected children, EBV has been recovered from lung biopsies (83,84).

Epstein–Barr virus has also been implicated in lymphoproliferative disorders involving the lung in children (85). It has been proposed that polyclonal B-cell lymphoproliferative disorders represent part of the spectrum of lymphoid disorders in HIV-infection (86) and that EBV may play a role in this, for AIDS patients have a defective regulation of EBV-infection (87).

Much needs to be learned about the pathogenesis of these inflammatory lung disorders in HIV-infected patients. One of the difficulties in studying this problem is the paucity of open-lung biopsy material because many of these patients are managed clinically, and few open biopsies are obtained. In addition, when open biopsies are performed, it is rare that a portion is frozen for research studies. Unfortunately, many of the molecular markers of interest cannot be studied based on sections cut from formalin-fixed and paraffin-embedded sections. Perhaps a registry of frozen and formalin-fixed lung tissue from these patients should be initiated to permit future studies to be performed.

References

1. Joshi VV, Oleske JM, Minnefor AB, et al. Pathologic pulmonary findings in children with the acquired immunodeficiency syndrome: a study of ten cases. Hum Pathol 1985; 16:241–246.
2. Grieco MH, Chinoy-Acharya P. Lymphocytic interstitial pneumonia associated with the acquired immune deficiency syndrome. Am Rev Respir Dis 1985; 131:952–955.
3. Kornstein MJ, Pietra GG, Hoxie JA, Conley ME. The pathology and treatment of interstitial pneumonitis in two infants with AIDS. Am Rev Respir Dis 1986; 133:1196–1198.
4. Pitt J. Lymphocytic interstitial pneumonia. Pediatr Clin North Am 1991; 38:89–95.
5. Travis WD, Fox CH, Devaney KO, et al. Lymphoid pneumonitis in 50 adult patients infected with the human immunodeficiency virus: lymphocytic intersti-

tial pneumonitis versus nonspecific interstitial pneumonitis. Hum Pathol 1992; 23:529–541.
6. Travis WD, Roth DB. Histopathologic evaluation of lung biopsy specimens. In: Shelhamer J, Pizzo PA, Parrillo JE, Masur H, ed. Respiratory Disease in the Immunosuppressed Host. Philadelphia: JB Lippincott, 1991; 182–217.
7. Travis WD, Lack EE, Ognibene FP, Suffredini AF, Shelhamer J. Lung biopsy interpretation in the acquired immunodeficiency syndrome: experience of the National Institutes of Health with literature review. Prog AIDS Pathol 1989; 1:51–84.
8. Berdon WE, Mellins RB, Abramson SJ, Ruzal-Shapiro C. Pediatric HIV infection in its second decade—the changing pattern of lung involvement. Clinical, plain film, and computed tomographic findings. Radiol Clin North Am 1993; 31:453–463.
9. Amorosa JK, Miller RW, Laraya-Cuasay L, et al. Bronchiectasis in children with lymphocytic interstitial pneumonia and acquired immune deficiency syndrome. Plain film and CT observations. Pediatr Radiol 1992; 22:603–606; discussion 606–607.
10. Holmes AH, Trotman-Dickenson B, Edwards A, Peto T, Luzzi GA. Bronchiectasis in HIV disease. Q J Med 192; 85:875–882.
11. Joseph J, Harley RA, Frye MD. Bronchiolitis obliterans with organizing pneumonia in AIDS [letter]. N Engl J Med 1995; 332:273.
12. Leo YS, Pitchon HE, Messler G, Meyer RD. Bronchiolitis obliterans organizing pneumonia in a patient with AIDS. Clin Infect Dis 1994; 18:921–924.
13. Mayo J, Collazos J, Martinez E, Diaz F. Acute eosinophilic pneumonia in a patient infected with the human immunodeficiency virus. Tuberc Lung Dis 1995; 76:77–79.
14. Dupon M, Malou M, Rogues AM, Lacut JY. Acute eosinophilic pneumonia induced by inhaled pentamidine isethionate. Br Med J 1993; 306:109.
15. Lowery WS, Whitlock WL, Dietrich RA, Fine JM. Sarcoidosis complicated by HIV infection: three case reports and a review of the literature. Am Rev Respir Dis 1990; 142:887–889.
16. Coots LE, Lazarus AA. Bronchoalveolar lavage in sarcoidosis and HIV infection [letter; comment]. Chest 1990; 98:517–518.
17. Gowda KS, Mayers I, Shafran SD. Concomitant sarcoidosis and HIV infection. Can Med Assoc J 1990; 142:136–137.
18. Agostini C, Zambello R, Trentin L, et al. Prognostic significance of the evaluation of bronchoalveolar lavage cell populations in patients with HIV-1 infection and pulmonary involvement. Chest 1991; 100:1601–1606.
19. Guillon JM, Autran B, Denis M, et al. Human immunodeficiency virus-related lymphocytic alveolitis. Chest 1988; 94:1264–1270.
20. Autran B, Sadat-Sowti B, Hadida F, et al. HIV-specific cytotoxic T lymphocytes against alveolar macrophages: specificities and downregulation. Res Virol 1991; 142:113–118.
21. Itescu S, Brancato LJ, Buxbaum J, et al. A diffuse infiltrative CD8 lymphocyto-

sis syndrome in human immunodeficiency virus (HIV) infection: a host immune response associated with HLA-DR5. Ann Intern Med 1990; 112:3–10.
22. Itescu S. Diffuse infiltrative lymphocytosis syndrome in children and adults infected with HIV-1: a model of rheumatic illness caused by acquired viral infection. Am J Reprod Immunol 1992; 28:247–250.
23. Koss MN, Hochholzer L, Langloss JM, Lazarus AA, Wehunt WD. Lymphoid interstitial pneumonitis: clinicopathologic and immunopathologic findings in 18 patients. Pathology 1987; 19:178–185.
24. Liebow AA, Carrington CB. Diffuse pulmonary lymphoreticular infiltrations associated with dysproteinemia. Med Clin North Am 1973; 57:809–843.
25. Jaffe ES, Travis WD. Lymphomatoid granulomatosis and lymphoproliferative disorders of the lung. In: Lynch JP, DeRemee RA, eds. Immunologically Mediated Pulmonary Diseases. Philadelphia: JB Lippincott, 1991:274–301.
26. Lin RY, Gruber PJ, Saunders R, Perla EN. Lymphocytic interstitial pneumonitis in adult HIV infection. NY State J Med 1988; 88:273–276.
27. Joshi VV, Oleske JM, Saad S, Connor EM, Rapkin RH, Minnefor AB. Pathology of opportunistic infections in children with acquired immune deficiency syndrome. Pediatr Pathol 1986; 6:145–150.
28. Grattan-Smith D, Harrison LF, Singleton EB. Radiology of AIDS in the pediatric patient. Curr Probl Diagn Radiol 1992; 21:79–109.
29. Centers for Disease Control. Classification system for human immunodeficiency virus (HIV) infection in children under 13 years of age. MMWR 1987; 36:225–230; 235–26.
30. Centers for Disease Control and Prevention. 1993 revised classification system for HIV infection and expanded surveillance case definition for AIDS among adolescents and adults. JAMA 1993; 269:729–730.
31. Murphy PM, Fox C, Travis WD, Koenig S, Fauci AS. Acquired immunodeficiency syndrome may present as severe restrictive lung disease. Am J Med 1989; 86:237–240.
32. Travis WD, Pittaluga S, Lipschik GY, et al. Atypical pathologic manifestations of *Pneumocystis carinii* pneumonia in the acquired immune deficiency syndrome. Review of 123 lung biopsies from 76 patients with emphasis on cysts, vascular invasion, vasculitis, and granulomas. Am J Surg Pathol 1990; 14:615–625.
33. Travis WD. Pathologic features. In: Walzer P, ed. *Pneumocystis carinii* Pneumonia. New York: Marcel Dekker, 1993:155–180.
34. Yousem SA, Colby TV, Carrington CB. Follicular bronchitis/bronchiolitis. Hum Pathol 1985; 16:700–706.
35. Ettensohn DB, Mayer KH, Kessimian N, Smith PS. Lymphocytic bronchiolitis associated with HIV infection. Chest 1988; 93:201–202.
36. Ognibene FP, Masur H, Rogers P, et al. Nonspecific interstitial pneumonitis without evidence of *Pneumocystis carinii* in asymptomatic patients with human immunodeficiency virus (HIV). Ann Intern Med 1988; 109:874–879.
37. Simmons JT, Suffredini AF, Lack EE, et al. Nonspecific interstitial pneumonitis in patients with AIDS: radiologic features. AJR 1987; 149:265–268.

38. Suffredini AF, Ognibene FP, Lack EE, et al. Nonspecific interstitial pneumonitis: a common cause of pulmonary disease in the acquired immunodeficiency syndrome. Ann Intern Med 1987; 107:7–13.
39. McKenzie R, Travis WD, Dolan SA, et al. The causes of death in patients with human immunodeficiency virus infection: a clinical and pathologic study with emphasis on the role of pulmonary diseases. Medicine 1991; 70:326–343.
40. Bye MR, Bernstein L, Shah K, Ellaurie M, Rubinstein A. Diagnostic bronchoalveolar lavage in children with AIDS. Pediatr Pulmonol 1987; 3:425–428.
41. Autran B, Mayaud CM, Raphael M, et al. Evidence for a cytotoxic T-lymphocyte alveolitis in human immunodeficiency virus-infected patients. AIDS 1988; 2:179–183.
42. Wallace JM, Barbers RG, Oishi JS, Prince H. Cellular and T-lymphocyte subpopulation profiles in bronchoalveolar lavage fluid from patients with acquired immunodeficiency syndrome and pneumonitis. Am Rev Respir Dis 1984; 130:786–790.
43. Venet A, Clavel F, Israël-Biet D, et al. Lung in acquired immune deficiency syndrome: infectious and immunological status assessed by bronchoalveolar lavage. Bull Eur Physiopathol Respir 1985; 21:535–543.
44. Palange P, Carlone S, Venditti M, et al. Alveolar cell population in HIV infected patients. Eur Respir J 1991; 4:639–642.
45. de Blic J, Blanche S, Danel C, Le Bourgeois M, Caniglia M, Scheinmann P. Bronchoalveolar lavage in HIV infected patients with interstitial pneumonitis. Arch Dis Child 1989; 64:1246–1250.
46. Plaza V, Jimënez P, Xaubet A, et al. Bronchoalveolar lavage cell analysis in patients with human immunodeficiency virus related diseases. Thorax 1989; 44:289–291.
47. Plata F, Autran B, Martins LP, et al. AIDS virus-specific cytotoxic T lymphocytes in lung disorders. Nature 1987; 328:348–351.
48. Atkinson JC, Travis WD, Pillemer SR, Bermudez D, Wolff A, Fox PC. Major salivary gland function in primary Sjögren's syndrome and its relationship to clinical features [see comments]. J Rheumatol 1990; 17:318–322.
49. Ramaswamy G, Jagadha V, Tchertkoff V. Diffuse alveolar damage and interstitial fibrosis in acquired immunodeficiency syndrome patients without concurrent pulmonary infection. Arch Pathol Lab Med 1985; 109:408–412.
50. Olson J, Colby TV, Elliott CG. Hamman-Rich syndrome revisited [see comments]. Mayo Clin Proc 1990; 65:1538–1548.
51. Katzenstein AL, Bloor CM, Leibow AA. Diffuse alveolar damage—the role of oxygen, shock, and related factors. A review. Am J Pathol 1976; 85:209–228.
52. Katzenstein AL, Myers JL, Mazur MT. Acute interstitial pneumonia. A clinicopathologic, ultrastructural, and cell kinetic study. Am J Surg Pathol 1986; 10:256–267.
53. Allen JN, Wewers MD. HIV-associated bronchiolitis obliterans organizing pneumonia. Chest 1989; 96:197–198.

54. Epler GR, Colby TV, McLoud TC, Carrington CB, Gaensler EA. Bronchiolitis obliterans organizing pneumonia. N Engl J Med 1985; 312:152–158.
55. Davison AG, Heard BE, McAllister WAC, Turner-Warwick ME. Cryptogenic organizing pneumonitis. Q J Med 1983; 207:382–394.
56. Colby TV, Myers JL. Clinical and histologic spectrum of bronchiolitis obliterans, including bronchiolitis obliterans organizing pneumonia. Semin Respir Med 1992; 13:119–133.
57. Allen JN, Pacht ER, Gadek JE, Davis WB. Acute eosinophilic pneumonia as a reversible cause of noninfectious respiratory failure [see comments]. N Engl J Med 1989; 321:569–574.
58. Davis WB, Wilson HE, Wall RL. Eosinophilic alveolitis in acute respiratory failure. A clinical marker for a non-infectious etiology. Chest 1986; 90:7–10.
59. Begbie S, Burgess KR. Maloprim-induced pulmonary eosinophilia. Chest 1993; 103:305–306.
60. Crystal RG, Bitterman PB, Rennard SI, Hance AJ, Keogh BA. Interstitial lung diseases of unknown cause. Disorders characterized by chronic inflammation of the lower respiratory tract [part 2 of 2]. N Engl J Med 1984; 310:235–244.
61. Carrington CB, Gaensler EA, Mikus JP, Schachter AW, Burke GW, Goff AM. Structure and function in sarcoidosis. Ann NY Acad Sci 1976; 278:265–283.
62. Mayaud CM, Cadranel J. HIV in the lung: guilty or not guilty? [editorial]. Thorax 1993; 48:1191–1195.
63. Berman JS. Lymphocytes in the lung: should we continue to exalt only BALT? Am J Respir Cell Mol Biol 1990; 3:101–102.
64. Berman JS, Beer DJ, Theodore AC, Kornfeld H, Bernardo J, Center DM. Lymphocyte recruitment to the lung. Am Rev Respir Dis 1990; 142:238–257.
65. Ziza JM, Brun-Veznet F, Venet A, et al. Lymphadenopathy-associated virus isolated from bronchoalveolar lavage fluid in AIDS-related complex with lymphoid interstitial pneumonitis [letter]. N Engl J Med 1985; 313:183.
66. Resnick L, Pitchenik AE, Fisher E, Croney R. Detection of HTLV-III/LAV-specific IgG and antigen in bronchoalveolar lavage fluid from two patients with lymphocytic interstitial pneumonitis associated with AIDS-related complex. Am J Med 1987; 82:553–556.
67. Plata F, Garcia-Pons F, Ryter A, et al. HIV-1 infection of lung alveolar fibroblasts and macrophages in humans. AIDS Res Hum Retroviruses 1990; 6:979–986.
68. Clarke JR, Mitchell D. Evidence for human immunodeficiency virus infection of the lung. Monaldi Arch Chest Dis 1993; 48:360–365.
69. Chayt KJ, Harper ME, Marselle LM, et al. Detection of HTLV-III RNA in lungs of patients with AIDS and pulmonary involvement [published erratum appears in JAMA 1987 Jan 16;257(3):317]. JAMA 1986; 256:2356–2359.
70. Dean NC, Golden JA, Evans LA, et al. Human immunodeficiency virus recovery from bronchoalveolar lavage fluid in patients with AIDS. Chest 1988; 93:1176–1179.
71. Linnemann CC Jr, Baughman RP, Frame PT, Floyd R. Recovery of human immunodeficiency virus and detection of p24 antigen in bronchoalveolar lavage fluid from adult patients with AIDS. Chest 1989; 96:64–67.

72. Rose RM, Krivine A, Pinkston P, Gillis JM, Huang A, Hammer SM. Frequent identification of HIV-1 DNA in bronchoalveolar lavage cells obtained from individuals with the acquired immunodeficiency syndrome. Am Rev Respir Dis 1991; 143:850–854.
73. Setoguchi Y, Takahashi S, Nukiwa T, Kira S. Detection of human T-cell lymphotropic virus type I-related antibodies in patients with lymphocytic interstitial pneumonia. Am Rev Respir Dis 1991; 144:1361–1365.
74. Fox CH, Tenner-Racz K, Racz P, Firpo A, Pizzo PA, Fauci AS. Lymphoid germinal centers are reservoirs of human immunodeficiency virus type 1 RNA [published erratum appears in J Infect Dis 1992 Jun;165(6):1161]. J Infect Dis 1991; 164:1051–1057.
75. Denis M, Ghadirian E. Alveolar macrophages from subjects infected with HIV-1 express macrophage inflammatory protein-1 alpha (MIP-1 alpha): contribution to the $CD8^+$ alveolitis. Clin Exp Immunol 1994; 96:187–192.
76. Denis M, Ghadirian E. Dysregulation of interleukin 8, interleukin 10, and interleukin 12 release by alveolar macrophages from HIV type 1-infected subjects. AIDS Res Hum Retroviruses 1994; 10:1619–1627.
77. Lairmore MD, Butera ST, Callahan GN, DeMartini JC. Spontaneous interferon production by pulmonary leukocytes is associated with lentivirus-induced lymphoid interstitial pneumonia. J Immunol 1988; 140:779–785.
78. Nowakowski M, Clarke ML, Amaro R, Pellegrino MG, Sierra MF, Steiner P. Characterization of cells, immunoglobulins, and immune complexes present in the bronchoalveolar lavage of pediatric AIDS patients. Regul Immunol 1992; 4:34–40.
79. Lairmore MD, Poulson JM, Adducci TA, DeMartini JC. Lentivirus-induced lymphoproliferative disease. Comparative pathogenicity of phenotypically distinct ovine lentivirus strains. Am J Pathol 1988; 130:80–90.
80. Lairmore MD, Rosadio RH, DeMartini JC. Ovine lentivirus lymphoid interstitial pneumonia. Rapid induction in neonatal lambs. Am J Pathol 1986; 125:173–181.
81. Leonard JM, Abramczuk JW, Pezen DS, et al. Development of disease and virus recovery in transgenic mice containing HIV proviral DNA. Science 1988; 242:1665–1670.
82. Malamou-Mitsi V, Tsai MM, Gal AA, Koss MN, O'Leary TJ. Lymphoid interstitial pneumonia not associated with HIV infection: role of Epstein–Barr virus. Mod Pathol 1992; 5:487–491.
83. Andiman WA, Eastman R, Martin K, et al. Opportunistic lymphoproliferations associated with Epstein–Barr viral DNA in infants and children with AIDS. Lancet 1985; 2:1390–1393.
84. Rubinstein A, Morecki R, Silverman B, et al. Pulmonary disease in children with acquired immune deficiency syndrome and AIDS-related complex. J Pediatr 1986; 108:498–503.
85. Beissner RS, Rappaport ES, Diaz JA. Fatal case of Epstein–Barr virus-induced lymphoproliferative disorder associated with a human immunodeficiency virus infection. Arch Pathol Lab Med 1987; 111:250–253.
86. Joshi VV, Kauffman S, Oleske JM, et al. Polyclonal polymorphic B-cell

lymphoproliferative disorder with prominent pulmonary involvement in children with acquired immune deficiency syndrome. Cancer 1987; 59:1455–1462.
87. Birx DL, Redfield RR, Tosato G. Defective regulation of Epstein–Barr virus infection in patients with acquired immunodeficiency syndrome (AIDS) or AIDS-related disorders. N Engl J Med 1986; 314:874–879.

21

Lymphocytic Interstitial Pneumonitis

DEBORAH M. USHKOW

Beth Israel Medical Center
New York, New York

ROSLYN F. SCHNEIDER

Albert Einstein College of Medicine and
Beth Israel Medical Center
New York, New York

I. Introduction

Interstitial lung diseases are frequently encountered in patients infected with human immunodeficiency virus (HIV). Most patients with HIV and diffuse lung disease have opportunistic infections or Kaposi's sarcoma (KS) involving the lung, but some have a syndrome of primary interstitial pneumonitis (1). Interstitial pneumonitis in HIV infection includes nonspecific, or chronic, intersitial pneumonitis (NIP/CIP) and lymphocytic interstitial pneumonitis (LIP) (1–4). NIP is seen in as many as half of symptomatic or asymptomatic persons with HIV infection who have lung biopsies (5,6). The clinical features of nonspecific pneumonitis in HIV infection are discussed in Chapters 20 and 22.

Lymphocytic interstitial pneumonitis is a rare disease of unknown etiology associated with a variety of autoimmune disorders (7). Besides HIV infection, the most common conditions associated with LIP include Sjogren's syndrome, myasthenia gravis, chronic active hepatitis, chronic thyroiditis, autoimmune hemolytic anemia, and systemic lupus erythematosus. The frequent occurrence of hypo- or hypergammaglobulinemia further suggests that disordered immune regulation plays a significant role. The mechanisms of development of nonspecific and lymphocytic pneumonitis are discussed in Chapter 22, along with a description of the pathological findings in these disorders.

II. Clinical Findings

Lymphocylic interstitial pneumonitis occurs in approximately 40% of infants and in children with HIV infection and lung disease. It is considered an AIDS-defining condition in persons younger than 13 years of age (8,9). LIP is uncommon in HIV-infected adults and is not an AIDS-defining disorder. The risk of developing LIP seems to be more common in blacks than in whites, and it is more common in injection drug users than in homosexual men. It may occur at any stage of HIV infection.

Clinically, LIP may resemble a pulmonary infection. Patients usually present insidiously with low-grade fever, nonproductive cough, dyspnea, weight loss, and generalized lymphadenopathy (4,10–12). Examination of the lungs may be normal or abnormal, with diffuse rales, predominantly at the bases (3,11). Clubbing, is reported in children, but not in adults (13,14). Chest roentgenograms range from normal to reticular or nodular opacities, or patchy consolidation (Fig. 1). Computed tomography (CT) scans of the chest typically reveal 2- to 4-mm nodules, with a peribronchial distribution, or a diffuse ground-glass appearance (Fig. 2; 15). Gallium-67 scanning may result in diffuse, intense bilateral uptake, but this finding is nonspecific, and the test has little role in the diagnostic evaluation (14). Pulmonary function testing shows varying degrees of restrictive dysfunction, hypoxemia, and a reduction of diffusing capacity. Laboratory data are generally not useful, but may demonstrate a slightly increased lactate dehydrogenase (LDH) and mild lymphocytosis. For these reasons, many presenting patients are presumed to have opportunistic infections including *Pneumocystis carinii* pneumonia (PCP).

Some patients with LIP have prominent extrapulmonary manifestations as part of a diffuse infiltrative lymphocytosis syndrome (DILS; 10). Patients may have lymphocytic infiltration of bone marrow, kidneys, liver, and the nasopharynx; this syndrome is strongly associated with the HLA-DR5 phenotype (3,10,11). LIP rarely occurs together with opportunistic infections, supporting the hypothesis that the development of this disorder is not a lung response to common infectious agents (1).

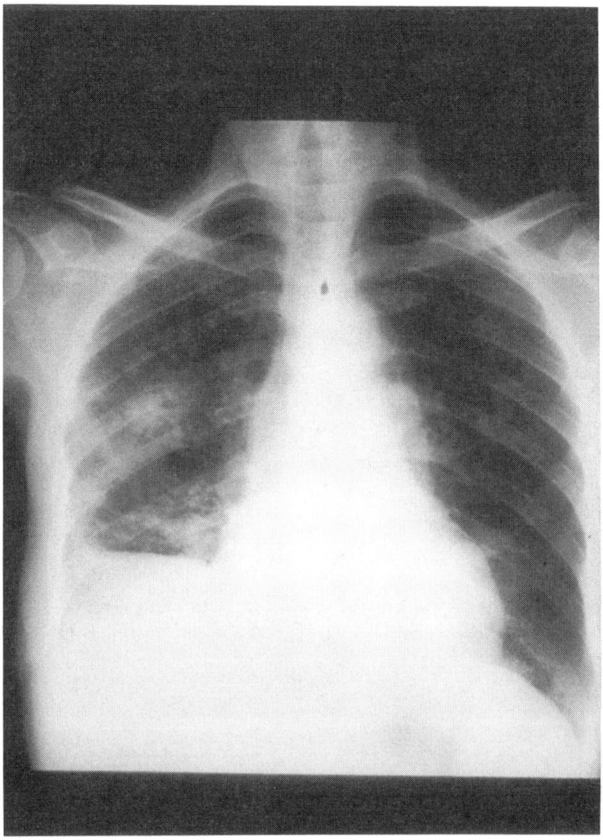

Figure 1 Chest radiograph of a patient with lymphocytic interstitial pneumonitis, showing ill-defined opacities, predominantly in the lower lobes.

III. Diagnosis

The diagnosis can be established only by lung biopsy, but some clinicians make a presumptive diagnosis in children based on the clinical picture. Although open-lung biopsy is most conclusive, transbronchial biopsy is sometimes sufficient (1,10). LIP is characterized by peribronchial, perivascular, paraseptal, and pleural infiltration by nonneoplastic mature lymphocytes and plasma cells (1,16). Septal infiltration is a prominent feature that differentiates LIP from NIP/CIP.

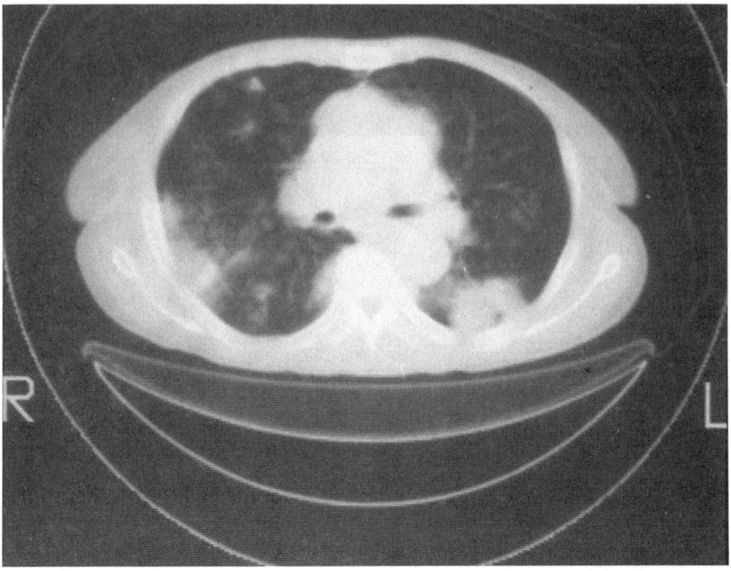

Figure 2 Computed axial tomogram of a patient with lymphocytic interstitial pneumonitis, showing nodules and confluent areas of consolidation.

IV. Treatment

The course of the disease is widely variable, ranging from spontaneous remission to respiratory failure and death. Therapy with corticosteroids may be helpful, and zidovudine was associated with improvement in two reported adult patients (3,4). Intravenous immunoglobulin has been used in children with variable results (8). There is no dose of corticosteroid that is recommended as optimal. Patients with mild disease may be observed, and patients who are more symptomatic should be treated with the lowest dose that alleviates the symptoms (16). Although some patients with LIP die of that disease, usually mortality is from unrelated HIV-associated illness (4,17).

References

1. Travis WD, Fox CH, Devaney KO, Weiss LM, O'Leary TJ, Ognibene FP, Suffredini AF, Rosen MJ, Cohen MB, Shelhamer J. Lymphoid pneumonitis in 50 adult patients infected with the human immunodeficiency virus: lymphocytic interstitial pneumonitis versus nonspecific interstitial pneumonitis. Hum Pathol 1992; 23:529–541.

2. Guillon J-M, Autran B, Denis M, Fouret P, Plate F, Maynaud CM, Akoyn GM. Human immunodeficiency virus-associated lymphocytic alveolitis. Chest 1988; 94:1264–1270.
3. Lin RY, Gruber PJ, Saunders R, Peria EN. Lymphocytic interstitial pneumonitis in adult HIV infection. NY State J Med 1988; 88:273–276.
4. Morris JC, Rosen MJ, Marchevsky A, Teirstein AS. Lymphocytic interstitial pneumonitis in patients at risk for the acquired immunodeficiency syndrome. Chest 1987; 91:63–67.
5. Ognibene FP, Masur H, Rogers P, Travis WD, Suffredini RF, Feuerstein I, Gill, W, Baird BF, Carrasquillo JA, Parillo JE. Nonspecific interstitial pneumonitis without evidence of *Pneumocystis carinii* in asymptomatic patients infected with human immunodeficiency virus (HIV). Ann Intern Med 1988; 109:874–879.
6. Suffredini AF, Ognibene FP, Lack EE, Simons JT, Brenner M, Gill VJ, Lane HC, Fauci AS, Parillo SE, Masur H. Nonspecific interstitial pneumonitis: a common cause of pulmonary disease in the acquired immune deficiency syndrome. Ann Intern Med 1987; 107:7–13.
7. Teirstein AS, Rosen MJ. Lymphocytic interstitial pneumonitis. Clin Chest Med 1988; 9:467–472.
8. Centers for Disease Control. Revision of case definitions of acquired immunodeficiency syndrome for national reporting—United States. MMWR 1985; 34:373–375.
9. Rubenstein A, Morecki R, Silveman B, Gregerson PK, Rizk CC, Croxon TS. Pulmonary disease in children with acquired immune deficiency syndrome and AIDs-related complex. J Pediatr 1986; 108:498–503.
10. Itescu S, Brancato LJ, Buxbaum J, Solomon GE. Winchester R. A diffuse infiltrative CD8 lymphocytosis syndrome in human immunodeficiency virus infection: a host immune response associated with HLA-DR5. Ann Intern Med 1990; 112:3–10.
11. Solal-Celigny P, Couderc J, Herman D, Herve P, Schaffar-Deshayes L, Brun-Vezinet F, Tricot G, Clauver JP. Lymphoid interstitial pneumonitis in acquired immunodeficiency syndrome-related complex. Am Rev Respir Dis 1985; 131:956–960.
12. White DA, Matthay RA. Noninfectious pulmonary complications of infection with the human immunodeficiency virus. Am Rev Respir Dis 1989; 140:1763–1787.
13. Rubenstein A, Morecki R, Goldman H. Pulmonary disease in infants and children. Clin Chest Med 1988; 9:507–517.
14. Schiff RG, Kabat L, Kamani N. Gallium scanning in lymphoid interstitial pneumonitis in children with AIDS, J Nucl Med 1987; 28:1915–1919.
15. Carignan S, Staples CA, Muller NL. Intrathoracic lymphoproliferative disorders in the immunocompromised patient: CT findings. Radiology 1995; 197:53–58.
16. Kornstein MJ, Pietra GG, Hoxie JA, Conley, ME. The pathology and treatment of interstitial pneumonitis is two infants with AIDS. Am Rev Respir Dis 1986; 133:1196–1198.
17. Grieco MH, Chinoy-Acharya P. Lymphocytic interstitial pneumonia associated with the acquired immune deficiency syndrome. Am Rev Respir Dis 1985; 131:952–955.

22

Nonspecific Interstitial Pneumonitis

FREDERICK P. OGNIBENE

Warren G. Magnuson Clinical Center
National Institutes of Health
Bethesda, Maryland

I. Introduction

Noninfectious pulmonary diseases are important causes of lung disorders in patients with human immunodeficiency virus (HIV) infection. An important class of such disorders is interstitial pneumonitis. The diagnosis of interstitial pneumonitis is further subclassified and characterized histopathologically as either lymphocytic interstitial pneumonitis (LIP) or nonspecific interstitial pneumonitis (NIP). Not only are there histopathological differences between the two types of interstitial pneumonia, but there are also etiologic, demographic, and clinical distinctions. This chapter will provide demographic, clinical, roentgenographic, histopathological, and therapeutic information about nonspecific interstitial pneumonitis.

II. Epidemiology

Nonspecific interstitial pneumonitis (NIP) is a common cause of pulmonary disease in adults with HIV infection (1). The exact frequency of its occurrence is not established; however, it has been documented histopathologically in up to approximately one-third of adult HIV-infected patients with clinical pulmonary disease (1,2). In some of these patients, prior *Pneumocystis carinii* pneumonia (PCP) or associated Kaposi's sarcoma (KS) may have produced the histopathological abnormalities. Of important note, is an additional report in which 11 of 23 (nearly 50%) HIV-infected adult patients with no pulmonary symptoms, a circulating CD4 cell count of fewer than 200/mm^3, no previous history of *P. carinii* pneumonia, and a normal chest roentgenogram, who were enrolled in a prospective bronchoscopy study employing transbronchial biopsy, were documented to have histopathological evidence of nonspecific interstitial pneumonitis (3).

Data from a large cohort of patients, consisting of both HIV-seropositive and HIV-seronegative subjects, in whom respiratory manifestations of HIV infection were prospectively assessed, indicated an incidence of nonspecific interstitial pneumonitis of less than 1% during the 18-month study period (4). However, the patient registry included subjects with a full range of CD4 counts. Of note, NIP was diagnosed only in the larger cohort of HIV-seropositive participants. Because this is an ongoing study, the authors concluded that as the observation period is extended and as immunological function declines in the HIV-seropositive cohort, the incidence of NIP in this subgroup will likely increase. Despite these reports in adult HIV-infected patients, there are minimal data on the incidence of nonspecific interstitial pneumonitis in the HIV-infected pediatric population.

III. Clinical Findings

There are no clinical symptoms unique to this form of interstitial pneumonitis. Therefore, it is difficult to distinguish it from other pulmonary diseases complicating HIV infection, based on only symptoms. Most patients complain of mild to moderate shortness of breath, have a cough, and may have a fever. On physical examination, the lungs are usually clear to auscultation; however, occasionally rales may be heard. There is usually evidence of a mild widening of the alveolar–arterial oxygen gradient (1,3). With exercise testing, patients with nonspecific interstitial pneumonitis may also manifest an increase in their alveolar–arterial oxygen gradients. In two series, pulmonary function tests also demonstrated a mild decrease in mean diffusing capacities (82–85%) compared with predicted values (2,3).

The chest roentgenogram is also not helpful diagnostically. The chest roentgenogram may be normal, despite histopathological evidence of the disease, or it may have a diffuse increase in interstitial markings (1,2,5,6). In one series, nearly half (44%) of chest roentgenograms in symptomatic patients with histopathological evidence of nonspecific interstitial pneumonitis were normal (6). When interstitial infiltrates are present, they may either be subtle in appearance or may appear coarser and almost reticulonodular. Pleural effusions have rarely been observed (6). Importantly, these roentgenographic abnormalities are indistinguishable from those of other infectious agents. ^{67}Gallium citrate scans are usually normal; however, mild to moderate pulmonary uptake of the isotope has been reported in a small percentage of patients (3,7).

IV. Diagnosis

The hallmark of the diagnosis is the abnormal pulmonary histopathology. However, because NIP was initially defined as a clinicopathological, rather than a histopathological entity, the pathological findings may be heterogeneous. The histopathology of nonspecific interstitial pneumonitis is typically characterized by "chronic" interstitial inflammation, with lymphocyte and plasma cell infiltration (1,8). In addition, with hematoxylin and eosin (H&E) staining one can observe edema, fibrin deposition, hyperplasia of the alveolar lining cells, and thickening of alveolar septa. These histopathological changes can be observed in varying degrees, ranging from mild to more fulminant abnormalities. Figure 1 is from a transbronchial biopsy specimen of a patient with NIP and demonstrates the perivascular and interstitial infiltrate typical of this process. In addition to these abnormali-

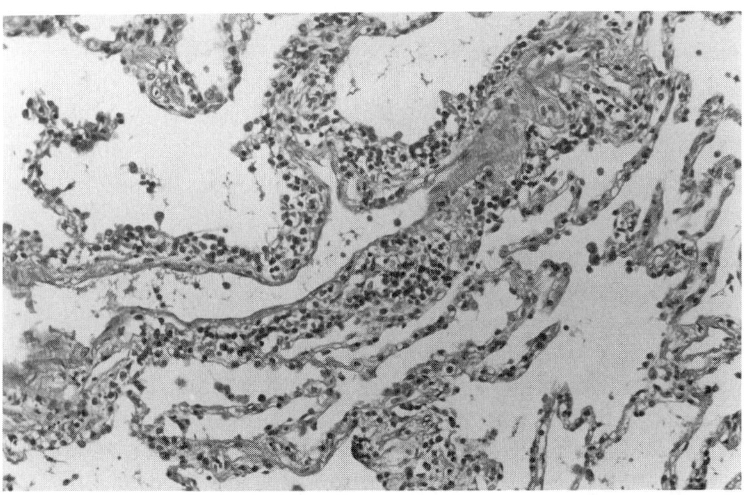

Figure 1 Transbronchial biopsy from a patient with NIP demonstrates a mild-to-moderate perivascular and interstitial lymphoid infiltrate (H & E; magnification × 220).

ties, there may be evidence of hyaline membrane formation consistent with damage to the pulmonary endothelium. In some patients, lymphoid aggregates, with or without germinal centers, may be noted in the pulmonary interstitium. In most asymptomatic patients who had histopathological evidence of NIP, the primary findings were perivascular and peribronchial lymphocytic infiltrates. Edema, alveolar macrophage hyperplasia, and hyaline membranes were rarely observed (3). In all cases, the diagnosis of NIP should be established only in the absence of an opportunistic infectious agent or HIV-related neoplasm, as evidenced by standard histopathological, cytological, and microbiological culture and staining techniques (1,3,8).

It is possible that NIP as a pathological entity may actually be underdiagnosed. It has been suggested that some pathologists may dismiss subtle interstitial lymphocytic interstitial infiltrates or lymphoid follicles as nondiagnostic findings in HIV-infected patients (8). However, Travis and colleagues remain convinced that the histopathological findings of NIP represent genuine pathological abnormalities capable of causing episodes of symptomatic and clinically significant findings in these patients.

In addition to the histopathological abnormalities, alterations may also be noted in the cellular constituents of bronchoalveolar lavage (BAL) in patients with NIP. In one series of 43 HIV-seropositive patients divided into three categories of pulmonary disease, all 19 patients with acute pulmonary symptoms caused by either opportunistic infection (n = 9) or NIP (n = 10) had evidence of an alveolar lymphocytosis, as well as a decrease in the number and percentage of alveolar macrophages (9). Other studies have also reported an alveolar lymphocytosis in HIV-seropositive patients, regardless of the stage of HIV disease or the presence of an opportunistic pulmonary pathogen (10). Thus, evidence of alveolar lymphocytosis in the absence of an identifiable pulmonary pathogen in the bronchoalveolar lavage may be an indicator of underlying NIP and may be indicative of the lymphocytic interstitial inflammation observed in this disorder.

V. Pathogenesis

The exact etiology of nonspecific interstitial pneumonitis has not been determined. Some have speculated that NIP may be due to prior pulmonary infections or to exposure to toxins in the form of recreational or therapeutic drugs (1,11). However, in other patients, no documentation of either prior pulmonary infection or toxin exposure has been documented, yet NIP has been histopathologically documented. Human immunodeficiency virus, Epstein–Barr virus (EBV), and cytomegalovirus (CMV), have been considered as possible infectious agents responsible for the pathogenesis of NIP. One recent series failed to document the presence of Epstein–Barr virus or cytomegalovirus by in situ hybridization studies, although Epstein–Barr virus was detected by polymerase chain reaction (PCR) in one patient (8). However, in that same series, there was evidence of HIV RNA expression in pulmonary mononuclear cells, resembling either macrophages or lymphocytes, obtained from patients with NIP (8). With this evidence, plus the knowledge that lentiviruses may cause lymphocytic pulmonary lesions, HIV may either be the primary causative agent or may play a significant role in the pathogenesis of NIP (8,12). However, it is possible that other viruses or other infectious agents (e.g., chlamydia) may also play a role in the pathogenesis of NIP.

Immunohistochemistry studies performed by Travis et al. indicated that, predominantly, the lymphocytes observed in NIP were of the T subclass (8). This is consistent with the results of other investigators, who have observed predominantly $CD8^+$ lymphocytes from open-lung biopsy specimens of patients with the lavage diagnosis of lymphocytic alveolitis (10). In addition, other investigators have observed the predominance of cytotoxic T lymphocytes in lavage specimens from HIV-infected individuals (13–15). Most of these series, however, did not include histopathological data and presented only cellular data from lavage. Most investigators concluded that the $CD8^+$ lymphocytes, which are cytotoxic, can actually induce local pulmonary inflammation, either directly or by interacting with HIV-infected alveolar macrophages, thereby leading to the histopathological abnormalities observed.

In addition to the direct viral or T-lymphocyte cytotoxic theories, other mechanisms have been proposed for the etiology of NIP. Lipschik and colleagues assessed the bronchoalveolar lavage of HIV-infected individuals with a variety of lung disorders for levels of leukotriene B_4, interleukin-8, and phospholipase A_2. They noted that lavage levels of all three compounds were elevated in patients with histopathological evidence of NIP (16). In addition, lavage neutrophil counts correlated with leukotriene B_4 and phospholipase A_2 levels. Because these compounds are involved in acute inflammatory processes, it was suggested that they may contribute to the pathogenesis of the lung injury observed in NIP. The authors also noted that the levels of the three inflammatory mediators were higher in NIP patients with symptoms, compared with the subgroup of NIP patients without pulmonary symptoms. Thus, there very well may be a dynamic environment in which antigenic stimulation, cellular constituents of the lung, and inflammatory mediators, all contribute to the pulmonary damage of NIP.

Another intriguing possibility for the etiology of pulmonary damage is the release of the superoxide anion by alveolar macrophages. In a series of HIV-seropositive individuals, with no pulmonary symptoms, who underwent bronchoalveolar lavage, there was evidence of more frequent expression of class II major histocompatibility complex (MHC) molecules, and they were also present in greater cell surface density on alveolar macrophages (17). In addition, there was a significantly higher increase in spontaneous release of the superoxide anion—the primary product of the NADPH-oxidase system used by phagocytes to kill microorganisms—by alveolar macrophages. The authors postulated that, in addition to its function in host defense mechanisms, the exaggerated release of the superoxide anion could also be responsible for some of the HIV-related pulmonary changes observed in NIP. Specifically, these extracellular oxidants could have the potential to damage surrounding cells. The authors noted that the levels of oxidant released by the alveolar macrophages in these asymptomatic HIV-infected individuals were comparable with the levels of oxidants released by the alveolar macrophages of cigarette smokers (17). Because cigarette smoking is known to cause some degree of chronic pulmonary damage by this mechanism, then it is conceivable that this degree of superoxide anion generation could lead to pulmonary tissue damage in HIV-seropositive patients.

VI. Treatment

The natural history of NIP is typically characterized by either a chronic or indolent course. Symptoms, as well as the histopathological abnormalities, may stabilize or actually resolve without any therapeutic intervention (1,2). Some patients may also be entirely asymptomatic, despite histopathological evidence of NIP (3). Typically, NIP does not progress to respiratory failure, and a role for immunosuppressive therapy has not been established, although data from some investigators on the inflammatory components in lavage would lead to the postulation that anti-inflammatory agents may provide some benefit (16). The major dilemma for the clinician is to demonstrate that a HIV-infected patient with pulmonary symptoms, with or without an abnormal chest roentgenogram, does not have an infection caused by an opportunistic pathogen or a HIV-related pulmonary neoplasm. Nonspecific interstitial pneumonitis is the diagnosis only if an infectious pulmonary process has been completely excluded.

VII. Summary

Pulmonary disease caused by nonspecific interstitial pneumonitis can occur, with variable incidences, in patients with HIV infection. From the data presented, plus that of others, HIV appears to be either primarily responsible or secondarily responsible, in the setting of cytokines or cellular factors, for its etiology (18,19). Accurate diagnosis is established based on characteristic histopathological abnormalities as well as the failure to demonstrate an opportunistic pathogen as the cause of the pneumonitis.

References

1. Suffredini AF, Ognibene FP, Lack EE, et al. Nonspecific interstitial pneumonitis: a common cause of pulmonary disease in the acquired immunodeficiency syndrome. Ann Intern Med 1987; 107:7–13.
2. Stover DE, White DA, Romano PA, Gellene R, Robeson WA. Spectrum of pulmonary diseases associated with the acquired immunodeficiency syndrome. Am J Med 1985; 78:429–437.
3. Ognibene FP, Masur H, Rogers P, et al. Nonspecific interstitial pneumonitis without evidence of *Pneumocystis carinii* in asymptomatic patients infected with human immunodeficiency virus (HIV). Ann Intern Med 1988; 109:874–879.
4. Wallace JH, Rao AV, Glassroth J, et al. Respiratory illness in persons with human immunodeficiency virus infection. Am Rev Respir Dis 1993; 148:1523–1529.
5. Conces DJ, Tarver RD. Noninfectious and nonmalignant pulmonary disease in AIDS. J Thorac Imaging 1991; 6:53–59.
6. Simmons JT, Suffredini AF, Lack EE, et al. Nonspecific interstitial pneumonitis in patients with AIDS: radiologic features. AJR 1987; 149:265–268.
7. Kramer EL, Sanger JH, Garay SM, et al. Gallium-67 scans of the chest in patients with acquired immunodeficiency syndrome. J Nucl Med 1987; 28:1107–1114.
8. Travis WD, Fox CH, Devaney KO, et al. Lymphoid pneumonitis in 50 adult HIV-infected patients: lymphocytic interstitial pneumonitis versus nonspecific interstitial pneumonitis. Hum Pathol 1992; 23:529–541.
9. Palange P, Carlone S, Venditti M, et al. Eur Respir J 1991; 4:639–642.
10. Guillon JM, Autran B, Denis M, et al. Human immunodeficiency virus-related lymphocytic alveolitis. Chest 1988; 94:1264–1270.
11. Ramaswamy G, Jagadha V, Tchertkoff V. Diffuse alveolar damage and interstitial fibrosis in acquired immunodeficiency syndrome patients without concurrent pulmonary infection. Arch Pathol Lab Med 1985; 109:408–412.
12. Lairmore MD, Poulson JH, Adducci TA, De Martini JC. Lentivirus-induced lymphoproliferative disease. Comparative pathogenicity of phenotypically distinct ovine lentivirus strains. Am J Pathol 1988; 130:80–90.
13. Wallace JM, Barbers RG, Oishi JS, Prince H. Cellular and T-lymphocyte subpopulation profiles in bronchoalveolar lavage fluid from patients with acquired immunodeficiency syndrome and pneumonitis. Am Rev Respir Dis 1984; 130:786–790.
14. Plata F, Autran B, Martins LP, et al. AIDS-virus specific cytotoxic T lymphocytes in lung disorders. Nature 1987; 328:348–351.

15. Autran B, Mayaud C, Raphaël M, et al. Evidence for a cytotoxic T lymphocyte alveolitis in HIV-infected patients. AIDS 1988; 2:179–183.
16. Lipschik GY, Doerfler ME, Kovacs JA, et al. Leukotriene B_4 and interleukin-8 in human immunodeficiency-virus related pulmonary disease. Chest 1993; 104:763–769.
17. Buhl R, Jaffe HA, Holroyd KJ, et al. Activation of alveolar macrophages in asymptomatic HIV-infected individuals. J Immunol 1993; 150:1019–1028.
18. Mayaud CM, Cadranel J. HIV in the lung: guilty or not guilty? Thorax 1993; 48:1191–1195.
19. Agostini C, Trentin L, Zambello R, Semenzato G. HIV-1 and the lung. Infectivity, pathogenic mechanisms, and cellular immune responses taking place in the lower respiratory tract. Am Rev Respir Dis 1993; 147:1038–1049.

23

Primary Pulmonary Hypertension and HIV Infection

JEFFREY I. KURITZKY

Beth Israel Medical Center
New York, New York

I. Introduction

Primary pulmonary hypertension (PPH) is a rare clinical syndrome characterized by sustained elevations of pulmonary artery pressure and pulmonary vascular resistance not attributable to underlying heart, lung, or other identifiable diseases (1). the estimated incidence of PPH in the general population is one to two cases per million (0.02%), and it occurs more commonly in females and blacks (1). Although the etiology of PPH is unknown, there is an increased incidence of persons with HIV infection, estimated to be high as 0.5% (2,3).

Human immunodeficiency virus (HIV) infection is associated with many other cardiopulmonary complications, including opportunistic infections, dilated cardiomyopathy, pleural and pericardial effusions, and neoplastic infiltration (4). Secondary forms of pulmonary hypertension in HIV-infected patients are not uncommon; generally occurring in the setting of active pulmonary infection with *Pneumocystis carinii* pneumonia (PCP) and cytomegalovirus (CMV), or in patients who injected crushed medication intended for oral use (4,5). Primary or idiopathic pulmonary hypertension is less common. Since Kim and Factor (6) first described an association between HIV infection and unexplained pulmonary hypertension in 1987, approximately 80 similar patients have been reported in the literature (5,7,8). Several recent studies of HIV-infected patents, who did not have known causes of pulmonary hypertension, have identified a small group with clinical, histological, and pathological features indistinguishable from those with classic PPH (5,7,8).

II. Pathophysiology

Factors resulting in increased pulmonary vascular resistance and pulmonary artery hypertension in patients diagnosed with PPH include vasoconstriction, vascular wall remodeling, and thrombosis in situ (2). Autopsies of these patients demonstrate specific features of pulmonary arteriopathy, including intimal fibrosis, medial hypertrophy, and aneurysmal dilations of pulmonary arterioles, known as plexiform lesions (2,5,7,8; Fig. 1). Weiss et al. (5) reviewed 23 patients with HIV infection and unexplained pulmonary hypertension for whom histological evaluation was available. With the exception of 1 patient who had evidence of pulmonary veno-occlusive disease, all had the typical findings of classic PPH described previously. Interestingly, there were no foreign body granulomas found in the intravenous drug users. This confirms another study reporting that patients with PPH did not have foreign body granulomas, unless crushed oral medications were injected (12). In fact, only 5% of drug abusers use drugs in this fashion (5,8,13).

Although the pathogenesis of PPH is unknown, several hypotheses have been proposed. Early investigators of HIV-infected patients with hemophilia speculated that factor VIII administration caused the pulmonary arterial disease (5,8). However, later reports of patients with PPH, who had had minimal or no exposure to factor VIII, directed investigators to search elsewhere (8). Several groups speculated on a direct viral cause of disease. However, methods such as electron microscopy, immunohistochemical stains, DNA in situ hybridization, and polymerase chain reaction (PCR) techniques, failed to identify HIV or evidence of other viral particles (9). Others suggested that pulmonary hypertension results from the production of specific growth factors, or is mediated through infected T cells, causing pulmonary endothelial cell proliferation (7,8). Aarons and Nye hypothesized that pulmonary arteriopathy is a result of endothelial damage inflicted by HIV, or possibly, by the release of inflammatory mediators not yet identified (11). Morse speculated on an autoimmune basis for the disease in susceptible patients with distinct immunogenetic profiles, because the fre-

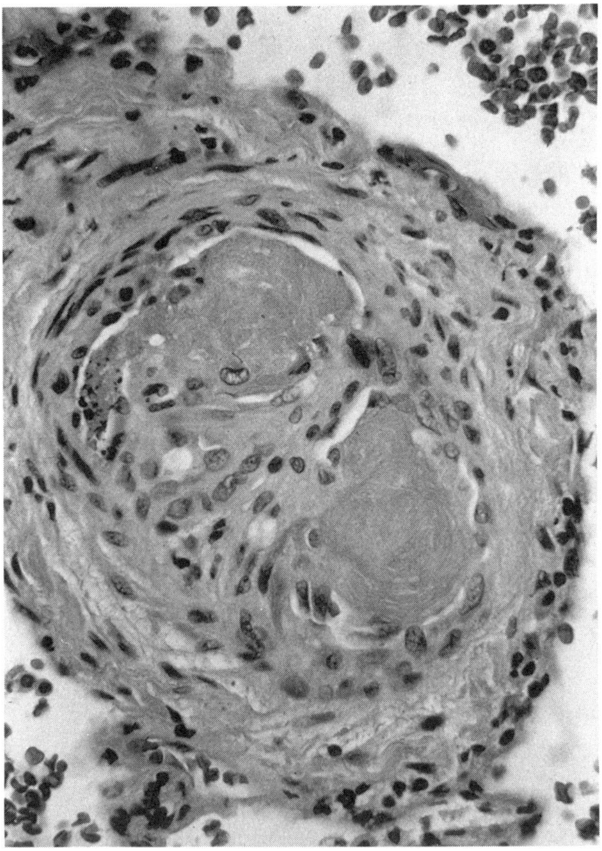

Figure 1 Open-lung biopsy of a patient with HIV infection and primary pulmonary hypertension showing arterial medial hypertrophy and intimal hyperplasia.

quency of HLA-DR6 and HLA-DR52 genotypes is increased in patients with PPH and HIV infection (10). HLA-DR6 was previously reported with increased frequency in HIV-positive patients who developed diffuse infiltrative lymphocytosis syndrome (DILS). This autoimmune syndrome closely resembles Sjogren's disease and was associated with prolonged survival (10); the association and its signifigance remain unclear.

The development of PPH is not related to the severity of immunodeficiency in HIV-infected persons. Only 33% of HIV-infected patients with PPH have the Centers for Disease Control and Prevention (CDC)-defined AIDS (8). Risk for contracting HIV and medications taken by this population of patients have also not been implicated.

III. Diagnosis

The symptoms associated with PPH are nonspecific, reflected in an average 2-year interval between the onset of symptoms and diagnosis (2). The clinical characteristics of patients with classic PPH and pulmonary hypertension associated with HIV disease are indistinguishable, with few exceptions. Petitpretz et al. (8) found that HIV-infected patients with PPH were, on average, 10 years younger at diagnosis (32 years old, compared with 42 years in HIV-negative patients), and had less severe disability and pulmonary hypertension. Fifty percent of HIV-positive patients were NYHA class III or IV, compared with 75% of HIV-negative patients in these classes. Also, in the HIV-infected patients, the diagnosis was arrived at more quickly once symptoms developed, probably owing to closer medical follow-up.

Most patients present with dyspnea on exertion (60%) and with angina or syncope when disease is more severe (2). The physical examination is frequently significant for a loud pulmonic component of the second heart sound and the midsystolic murmur of tricuspid regurgitation. The chest film classically demonstrates prominence of the main pulmonary artery and cardiomegaly (Fig. 2). The most common electrocardiographic manifestation is right axis deviation and right ventricular hypertrophy. Right heart catheterization remains the gold standard for diagnosis, but Doppler echocardiography is effective for screening and follow-up (3). The diagnosis is one of exclusion in patients who have pulmonary hypertension with no identifiable cause. Although open-lung biopsy reveals diagnostic histological findings, it is not necessary to make the diagnosis.

IV. Clinical Course

Primary pulmonary hypertension is a progressive disease for which there is no cure. Medical therapy currently consists of oxygen, anticoagulation to prevent in situ microthrombi, and vasodilators, such as calcium channel blockers, to attentuate vasoconstriction (2). Patients demonstrating a beneficial response to a sudden challenge with potent short-acting vasodilators, such as nitric oxide and adenosine, are considered for long-term therapy with oral agents. A positive response, defined as a decrease in pulmonary artery pressure and pulmonary vascular resistance, with maintenance of cardiac output and systemic blood pressure, is seen in 25–30% of patients (3). In a study by Petitpretz, hemodynamic changes during vasodilator trials using epoprostenol (prostacyclin) were similar in HIV-infected and control groups (8). Encouraging results have been reported

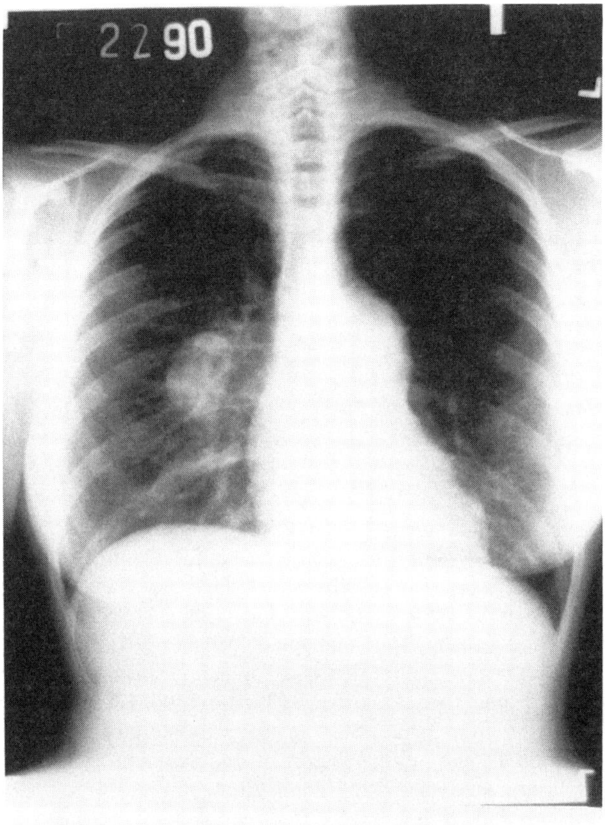

Figure 2 Chest radiograph of a patient with HIV infection and primary pulmonary hypertension showing enlarged pulmonary arteries and oligemia of the lung fields.

by Opravil, who observed a beneficial effect of antiretroviral therapy on hemodynamics, and recommended initiation of antiretroviral treatment in all HIV-infected patients with PPH, irrespective of CD4 count or viral load (3).

The prognosis for patients with PPH remains poor; PPH in HIV-infected patients is considered an independent risk factor for morbidity and mortality (3). The median period of survival after diagnosis is estimated to be 2 years, but many patients live longer with the use of anticoagulants and vasodilators. Most patients die of progressive right ventricular failure, but sudden death occurs in approximately 10% of fatalities (2).

Although controlled epidemiological studies are needed to confirm a cause-and-effect relationship between the two diseases, the indications are that HIV is a risk factor for the development of PPH. PPH should be included in the differential diagnosis of HIV-infected patients presenting with cardiopulmonary complaints. The screening of appropriate patients is recommended to identify patients who may benefit from currently available therapy, including antiretrovirals and, possibly, protease inhibitors. Furthermore, HIV testing is recommended in all patients presenting with PPH, even when they deny HIV risk behaviors.

References

1. Rich S, Dantzker DR, Ayres SM, Bergofsky EH, Brundage BH, Detre KM, Fishman AP, Goldring RM, Groves BM, Koerner SK, Levy PC, Reid LM, Vreim CE, Williams GW. Primary pulmonary hypertension: a national prospective study. Ann Intern Med 1987; 107:216–223.
2. Rubin LJ. Primary pulmonary hypertension. N Engl J Med 1997; 336:111–117.
3. Opravil M, Pechae M, Speich R, Jiler-Jemeika, HI, Jenni R, Russi EW, Hirschel B, Luthy R, the Swiss HIV Cohort Study. HIV-associated primary pulmonary hypertension. Am J Respir Crit Care Med. 1997; 115:990–995.
4. Himelman RB, Dohrmann M, Goodman P, Schiller NB, Starksen NF, Warnock M. Severe pulmonary hypertension and cor pulmonale in the acquired immunodeficiency syndrome. Am J Cardiol 1989; 64:1396–1399.
5. Weiss JR, Pietra GG, Scharf SM. Primary pulmonary hypertension and the human immunodeficiency virus. Report of two cases and a review of the literature. Arch Intern Med 1995; 155:2350–2354.
6. Kim KK, Factor SM. Membranoproliferative glomerulonephritis and plexogenic pulmonary arteriopathy in a homosexual man with acquired immunodeficiency syndrome. Hum Pathol 1987; 18:1293–1296.
7. Coplan NL, Shimony RY, Ioachim HL, Wilentz JR, Posner DH, Lipschitz A, Ruden RA, Bruno MS, Sherrid MV, Gaetz H, Englard A, Kukin M, Packer M. Primary pulmonary hypertension associated with human immunodeficiency viral infection. Am. J Med 1990; 89:96–99.
8. Petitpretz PF, Brenot R, Azarian F, Parent B, Rain P, Herve P, Simonneau G. Pulmonary hypertension in patients with human immunodeficiency virus infection: comparison with primary pulmonary hypertension. Circulation 1994; 89:2722–2727.
9. Mette SA, Palevsky HI, Pietra GG, Pietra GG, Williams TM, Bruder E, Prestipino AJ, Patrick AM, Wirth JA. Primary pulmonary hypertension in association with human immunodeficiency virus infection: a possible viral etiology for some forms of hypertensive pulmonary arteriopathy. Am Rev Respir Dis 1992; 145:1196–1200.

10. Morse JH, Banst RJ, Itescu S, Flaster ER, Sinha G, Zhang Y, Fotino M. Primary pulmonary hypertension in HIV infection. Am J Respir Crit Care Med 1996; 153:1299–1301.
11. Aarons EJ, Nye FJ. Primary pulmonary hypertension and HIV infection. AIDS 1991; 5:1276–1277.
12. Tomashefski JE, Hirsch CS. The pulmonary vascular lesions of intravenous drug abuse. Hum Pathol 1980: 11:133–145.
13. Hind CRK. Pulmonary complications of intravenous drug misuse: epidemiology and noninfective complications. Thorax 1990: 45:891–898.

Part Six

INFECTION CONTROL

24

Infection Control for the Pulmonary Specialist

BETH G. RAUCHER

Albert Einstein College of Medicine and
Beth Israel Medical Center
New York, New York

I. Introduction

Medical historians will no doubt look on the past decade as one in which the practice of medicine dramatically changed. Driven largely by the general public's nearly hysterical fear of "catching acquired immunodeficiency syndrome (AIDS)" from blood transfusions, needles, doctors or dentists, and health care workers (HCW) rational and irrational concerns of contracting human immunodeficiency virus (HIV) infection from patients, the "era of infection control" was hastily ushered in. Our recently expanded knowledge of the mechanisms and frequency of spread of blood-borne and other pathogens during many aspects of patient care has led to the increasing use of latex gloves, safer medical devices, as well as to assumptions about the potential infectiousness of every patient.

Besides the routine examination of patients, the pulmonary specialist may have significant exposure to respiratory infections and infectious body fluids, such as blood and pleural fluid. In addition, invasive procedures, bronchoscopy, and intensive care services often requiring the use of sharp devices (arterial, Swan-Ganz, and central line insertion) may place him or her at risk for acquiring agents such as hepatitis B or C virus (HBV, HCV), HIV, or *Mycobacterium tuberculosis* (TB). It is the purpose of this chapter to acquaint the pulmonologist with current knowledge of the transmission of blood-borne agents and *M. tuberculosis*, to review the precepts of universal precautions, and to focus on protection of the pulmonologist in the patient care setting.

II. Blood-Borne Pathogens

A. Hepatitis B: A Model of Blood-Borne Infection

Hepatitis B virus is transmitted in blood and most body fluids, and health care workers exposed to these fluids are at increased risk of contracting infection. Infection in a susceptible person usually presents as a self-limited hepatitis, frequently subclinical, that confers immunity following recovery. Two-thirds of affected individuals have few or no symptoms, whereas the remainder develop a severe illness characterized by jaundice, fatigue, anorexia, nausea, arthralgia, and fever. Approximately 20% of patients with these symptoms require hospitalization, and convalescence can take weeks to months. Death from HBV occurs in 2% of reported cases, and up to 10% of those infected become chronic carriers (1,2).

In the health care setting, the most common route of transmission is needle stick or puncture by other sharp instruments. In addition, transmission can occur when infectious materials come into contact with a health care worker's cuts, abrasions, lacerations, or other nonintact skin. Entry of the virus through mucosal surfaces, such as the mouth or eyes, is also well documented. Transmission of HBV is extremely efficient; only a small number of virus particles are required for infection to take place. Tiny volumes of blood may contain millions of infectious units. The risk of a susceptible health care worker acquiring HBV following a single percutaneous exposure (i.e., skin puncture by a sharp device contaminated with blood from a HBV-positive patient) may be as high as 30%. The Centers for Disease Control and Prevention (CDC) has estimated that 12,000 health care workers become infected with HBV annually, and of these, 700–1200 become permanent carriers; 250 will ultimately die of their infection (2). We eagerly await future reports revealing a marked decrease in occupationally acquired HBV as more health care workers roll up their sleeves for the hepatitis B vaccine.

B. Human Immunodeficiency Virus

The CDC has reported 401,749 cases of AIDS in the United States, as of June 1994. New York and California each reported over 70,000 cases, with

Florida, Texas, and New Jersey next in overall incidence. By now, no city, state, or town is isolated from cases of HIV infection. The rate of infection is growing fastest among children, women, and minorities (3). Health care workers must be most concerned with the thousands of HIV-infected individuals who are as yet unaware of their infection and may not present with any signs, symptoms, or recognizable risk factors for HIV infection. The incidence and seroprevalence of HIV in hospitalized patients is variable, but has been reported to be as high as 16% in trauma victims treated in a Baltimore emergency room (4).

Fortunately, unlike HBV, HIV is a difficult virus to transmit. A large inoculum or infectious dose is required to transmit the infection. Blood is the single most important source. Although the virus is contained in saliva, alveolar fluid, lung tissue, semen, spinal fluid, breast milk, and urine in small quantities, spread of infection to a health care worker by exposure to these fluids has not been reported. Occupational transmission of HIV has occurred under circumstances similar to those described by HBV; that is, primarily through percutaneous injury or, less frequently, through nonintact skin. Transmission by accidental exposure of mucous membranes (eyes, mouths) has not been reported.

As of June 30, 1994, 130 cases of occupational transmission of HIV to health care workers in the United States have been reported to the CDC. Exposure with documented seroconversion has occurred in 42 of these. Most exposures were to blood, although two health care workers were exposed to body fluid contaminated with blood, and two sustained an exposure in the laboratory with concentrated virus. percutaneous injury accounted for 87% of the exposures, with the rest being through nonintact skin. Fifteen of these infected workers have developed full-blown AIDS (3,5).

The remaining 88 workers also reported occupational exposure to HIV-infected blood and fluid; however, baseline HIV serology was not done and, therefore, seroconversion could not be documented. These persons deny nonoccupational risk factors for HIV (Table 1). In addition, surveys have documented that many injuries resulting in HIV exposure are never reported, especially by physicians, and thus, the full extent of occupational acquisition is most likely understated (6).

A health care worker's risk of acquiring an HIV infection after a percutaneous injury involving a needle or medical device contaminated with blood from an HIV-infected patient is estimated to be 0.3% (5,7). This transmission rate is markedly lower than the corresponding 30% rate for HBV infection. The rate of HIV transmission, calculated from surveillance of over 3000 exposed health care workers, has remained constant for several years. The greatest risk of acquiring HIV is from percutaneous injury

Table 1 Health Care Workers with Documented and Possible Occupationally Acquired AIDS/HIV Infection, by Occupation, Reported Through June 1994, United States[a]

Occupation	Documented occupational transmission[b] (No.)	Possible occupational transmission[c] (No.)
Dental worker, including dentist	—	7
Embalmer/morgue technician	—	3
Emergency medical technician/paramedic	—	9
Health aide/attendant	1	9
Housekeeper/maintenance worker	1	6
Laboratory technician, clinical	15	14
Laboratory technician, nonclinical	2	1
Nurse	13	19
Physician, nonsurgical	6	9
Physician, surgical	—	1
Respiratory therapist	1	2
Technician, dialysis	1	1
Technician, surgical	2	1
Technician/therapist, other than those listed above	—	4
Other health care occupations	—	2
Total	42	88

[a]*Health care workers* are defined as those persons, including students and trainees, who have worked in a health care, clinical, or HIV laboratory setting at any time since 1978 (see MMWR 1992; 41:823–825).

[b]Health care workers who had documented HIV seroconversion after occupational exposure or had other laboratory evidence of occupational infection; 36 had percutaneous exposure, 4 had mucocutaneous exposure, 1 had both percutaneous and mucocutaneous exposures, and 1 had an unknown route of exposure. Thirty-eight exposures were to blood from an HIV-infected person, 1 to visibly bloody fluid, 1 to an unspecific fluid, and 2 to concentrated virus in a laboratory. Fifteen of these health care workers developed AIDS.

[c]These health care workers have been investigated and are without identifiable behavioral or transfusion risks; each reported percutaneous or mucocutaneous occupational exposures to blood or body fluids, or laboratory solutions containing HIV, but HIV seroconversion specifically resulting from an occupational exposure was not documented.

Source: Ref. 3.

with a hollow-bore needle, owing to the larger volume of blood which is contained within the shaft (5).

C. Hepatitis C Virus

Hepatitis C virus is responsible for 80–90% of the cases of posttransfusion hepatitis and a large proportion of sporadic cases of non-A, non-B hepatitis. Similar to HBV, transmission of HCV has also been linked to percutaneous injury, injection drug use, and less frequently, to sexual contact, and vertically from mother to fetus. Surprisingly, HCV has generally not been found in body fluids not contaminated with blood (8). The spectrum of illness caused by HCV is similar to that of HBV, with most individuals remaining asymptomatic after infection. However, chronic liver disease will develop in 60% or more of individuals infected with HCV. Progressive liver disease and cirrhosis may develop insidiously. Although morbidity may be significant, life expectancy of patients infected with HCV may not be decreased (9).

Two percent of all acute HCV infections occur in health care workers (10). The potential risk to these workers is obvious: the incidence of HCV in all patients treated in an inner-city emergency room was 18%, and as high as 51% in certain defined populations (11). A single percutaneous exposure to HCV-infected blood may result in transmission of the virus in up to 3–10% of cases (12). Health care workers may have increased rates of chronic HCV infection compared with the general population (10).

D. Transmission of HIV from Health Care Worker to the Patient

The theoretical risk of an HIV-infected health care worker transmitting his or her infection to a patient is real; however, documented cases are scarce. One case, widely publicized by the media in 1990, involved a young woman who claimed to have become infected with HIV by her dentist during a routine procedure. An investigation by the local health department and the CDC identified five additional patients who were infected, presumably while receiving care from the dentist. According to investigators, the six patients had no other risk factors for acquiring HIV, and their viral strains were closely related to the strain isolated from the dentist. The investigation never conclusively proved the mechanism of transmission, in part, because the office records were incomplete and the dentist died before a comprehensive review by the CDC. Several of his staff did document deficiencies in basic infection control practices, however. The CDC concluded that the available evidence pointed to transmission of the virus by the dentist to each of his patients individually, rather than patient-to-patient transmission through contaminated instruments (13). The etiology of this outbreak will likely never be known, but fortunately, there have been no other recognized instances of HIV transmission from a health care worker to a patient, despite hundreds of look-back investigations testing thousands of patients who received care from an HIV-infected worker (5). Although these data are reassuring, and the risk is extremely small, great efforts to minimize the possibility of HIV transmission from health care workers to patients is warranted.

Since HBV is in general much more easily transmitted than HIV, one would predict that HBV transmission to patients from health care workers would occur with greater frequency. Transmission of HBV by hepatitis B e-antigen-positive health care workers to susceptible patients during invasive procedures is well described in over 350 instances. Although most of these HBV-infected workers were able to modify their operative technique and infection control practices with no subsequent instances of transmission, a small number of HBV-infected workers continued to transmit the virus and were subsequently restricted from doing invasive procedures (14,15).

The CDC is very concerned about the potential risk of transmitting HIV and other blood-borne pathogens to patients. During several recent studies, CDC investigators observed invasive procedures. They documented that after an accidental self-inflicted percutaneous injury of the health care worker, the contaminated sharp instrument, usually a suture needle, often recontacted the patient. This occurred 28 times after 88 percutaneous injuries sustained by surgeons in one study (16). Although the risk of transmission of a blood-borne pathogen through recontact is unknown, it is presumed to be the mechanism in some of the cases of HBV transmitted by health care workers to patients. Recontact has at least the potential risk for transmission of HIV as well (5).

E. Precautions During Routine Patient Care

Before 1987, the strategy used to protect health care workers from acquiring blood-borne pathogens, such as HBV or HIV, was the use of *blood and body fluid precautions*. Once a patient was identified as infected, health care workers were alerted to take extra steps to prevent exposure to infected materials from that patient. For example, gloves would be worn when taking the blood of a hepatitis B surface antigen-positive patient. However, early in the AIDS epidemic it was recognized that HIV testing of all patients was not likely to be accomplished and that even when consent for serological testing was obtained, delays while awaiting results would mean health care workers would continue to be at risk of exposure to infectious body fluids. Trying to guess which patients are infected, and thus applying a higher level of caution, is dangerous and foolhardy. Therefore, the CDC established *universal precautions* (UP) in 1987 (17). Under UP, health care workers are instructed to consider all patients potentially infectious.

The health care workers readily adapted UP in one form or another. Some hospitals dropped the category of *blood and body fluid precautions* altogether, while others added UP to the traditional form of CDC precautions as an added protective measure. Office-based practices embraced many of the principles of UP where appropriate during routine medical care.

The same CDC document called for extensive use of gloves and other cover-up clothing that act as a means of barrier protection. Emphasis was also placed on the use of mucous membrane protection because HBV is known to be transmitted through the mouth and eyes. Other important recommendations included the wide distribution and use of needle receptacles, a prohibition against recapping, breaking, or bending of needles, and guidelines for proper disinfection and sterilization of instruments and reusable devices.

In 1989, recognizing the risk to health care workers, the Occupational Safety and Health Administration (OSHA) set forth regulations that mandated adherence to CDC's recommendations. OSHA, using an industrial approach to prevention, required employers to develop a hierarchy of controls intended to eliminate or reduce the risk of exposure to HBV and HIV. The program required the wide use of engineering controls, modification of work practices, use of personal protective equipment, biohazard labeling of specimens and medical waste, routine hepatitis B vaccination of health care workers, and annual training in infection control practices for all such personnel (15; Table 2).

Initially, OSHA's requirements met fierce resistance from institutions (i.e., hospitals) and practitioners owing to the increased financial burden, an unscientific basis for some of the requirements, a general resistance to change, and the large burden of paperwork. However, in 1997, nearly all institutions, medical and dental offices have implemented most, if not all of the requirements, thereby avoiding the heavy financial penalties that OSHA has been known to impose.

Besides UP, another effective way to further prevent transmission of blood-borne pathogens is by improving engineering controls and work practices. Examples include intravenous tubing systems that are now manufactured with protected or plastic needles, piggy-back connectors that require no needles, self-sheathing intramuscular syringes, and many others. However caution is advised. Several extremely expensive devices, claiming to improve safety, have flooded the market. Unfortunately, many do not significantly reduce injuries, and some may, in fact, be more dangerous than the device they are intended to replace (19). Institutions and practitioners must carefully evaluate which devices or poor work practices are causing workplace injuries and substitute safer devices or work practices accord-

Table 2 Methods to Protect Health Care Workers from Blood-Borne Pathogens Based on CDC Guidelines and OSHA Regulations

Engineering controls	Personal protective equipment (PPE)
Needle receptacles	Gloves or double gloves
Protected needles	Gowns
Automatic pipettes	Safety glasses, face shields, masks
Plastic hematocrit tubes	Shoe covers or boots
Centrifuge covers	Head covering
Blunted suture needles	Plastic aprons
Instrument-passing tray	
Work practices	Employee health
Handwashing	Hepatitis B vaccine free of charge
Glove use	Postexposure follow-up with voluntary HIV testing
Voluntary HIV testing	Counseling
Clean-up of spills	AZT and other antiretroviral agents
No eating in clinical areas	Confidentiality of worker
Anticipating patient movement	Miscellaneous
Implementing safety devices	Biohazard labeling of specimens
Training	Laundering employee PPE
Annual inservice	
Basic understanding of HIV and HBV	
Transmission and epidemiology	
Use of personal protective equipment, engineering controls, safe work practices, and postexposure follow-up	

Source: Refs. 2, 15, and 17.

ingly. In many health care settings, workers continue to recap or dispose of needles improperly, accounting for the vast majority of percutaneous injuries (20).

F. Precautions During Bronchoscopy

Epidemiological evidence suggests that the risk of acquiring a blood-borne pathogen while performing bronchoscopy is very low. As discussed earlier in this chapter, HBV would pose the greatest risk, HIV the smallest, and HCV an intermediate risk. However, during certain steps of the procedure the bronchoscopist or a member of the team is at increased risk of exposure. Such times include placing an intravenous line or giving an intramuscular injection for sedation, especially in nervous or combative patients; using an exposed Wang needle for an endotracheal biopsy; attending to a postprocedure patient who develops hemoptysis or hemorrhage after a biopsy. Those physicians experienced with the procedure can likely name several other instances during which he or she unexpectedly was exposed to potentially infectious blood and secretions. To minimize the risk, the bronchoscopy team must anticipate the likelihood of an exposure, modify their work practices, and use the safest possible devices and techniques currently available.

The CDC and OSHA mandate, and common sense dictates, the use of the following precautions during any type of invasive procedure, including bronchoscopy:

1. Universal precautions apply to *all* patients. The unsuspected HIV-positive patient is potentially the most dangerous.
2. Use of personal protective equipment, including gloves, masks, eye protection, caps, shoe covers, and fluid-resistant gowns or aprons. Two pairs of gloves should be worn for procedures requiring the frequent use of needles.
3. Contaminated sharps should be disposed of immediately after use in a designated disposal container located at the site of use. Needles should never be recapped, bent, or broken. The sharps container should be exchanged by trained personnel when two-thirds full.
4. Patient movement should be anticipated when inserting an intravenous catheter or giving an injection. A second member of the team should assist when the patient is frightened or combative.
5. Sharp objects should never be left in a place that puts the operator or team member at risk. Wang needles should be handled by the bronchoscopist and disposed of immediately after use.
6. Spills of blood and blood-containing fluid should be contained and cleaned up by trained personnel as soon as possible.
7. All team members should be tested for serological evidence of immunity to HBV, and susceptible members should be vaccinated.
8. Resuscitation equipment should be on site so that the need for mouth-to-mouth resuscitation is completely eliminated.
9. Handwashing should precede and follow all patient contacts and the removal of gloves.

Some training centers have been able to minimize the risk of exposure to medical students, residents, and fellows, while maximizing education. By using video cameras and monitors mounted to the wall or ceiling, observers can safely watch at a distance of several feet away from the patient.

Pulmonologists who also serve as intensivists must apply the same principles of personal protection when they insert a peripheral or central line, or during procedures, such as suturing, intubation, thoracentesis, and whenever sharp devices are used.

G. Management of Exposure

Despite a decrease in the number of reported exposures since the implementation of UP, the fact remains that some exposure of health care workers to infectious materials from patients is unavoidable, and the workers remain at risk. Part of the problem is in breaking old habits; for example, many health care workers continue to recap needles or decline to wear gloves for venipuncture, despite adequate knowledge of the risks involved. Additionally, they face an inherent risk whenever using sharp devices. As long as there are sharp-tipped intravenous catheters, needles, cannulas, and scalpels, there will be accidental percutaneous injuries to these workers. Often these sharp devices will be contaminated with patient blood or body fluids. Postexposure management of HBV and HIV exposures is an important component of the CDC guidelines and OSHA regulations.

The need for postexposure chemoprophylaxis against HBV should be reduced considerably with the increased use of the hepatitis B vaccine in health care settings. Hepatitis B hyperimmune globulin (HBIG) and initiation of the vaccine series should be provided as soon as possible to any nonimmune exposed health care worker. Postexposure management recommendations for HCV are not uniform. Intramuscular immune globulin has been prescribed by some in the hope that it would provide passive immunity. However, recent testing and rejection of all blood products containing HCV has rendered the serum pool free of HCV, thereby removing any protective prophylactic value for needlesticks (21).

In 1990 the CDC issued guidelines for the management of occupational exposure to HIV. The protocol called for the use of zidovudine (AZT) chemoprophylaxis on an individualized basis, since the efficacy of the drug as a prophylactic agent could not be established by controlled studies. The decision to offer the drug to an exposed HCW was based on limited animal study data, a handful of human case reports, and the efficacy of AZT in treating infected individuals. The drug's manufacturer sponsored a double-blind, placebo-controlled study in an attempt to show efficacy in the prevention of seroconversion from an occupational exposure. Unfortunately, the study was terminated because HCWs did not want to take a placebo under such circumstances and the sample size needed to achieve statistical significance required thousands of exposed HCWs and was, therefore, not attainable. CDC recommendations for the voluntary use of AZT have evolved since 1990. Results from a retrospective case-control study controlling for several risk factors suggested that AZT, if taken promptly after a percutaneous injury, may decrease the risk of seroconversion. In

May of 1996, the CDC published an updated set of chemoprophylaxis guidelines that embraced combination therapy with two or three drugs, depending on the assessed risk of the exposure (22). Recipients of exposures perceived to be low risk are offered AZT and 3TC (Lamivudine), while Indinavir, a protease inhibitor, is added when the exposure has a high risk of transmission. Support for this approach comes from the exposure has a high risk of transmission. Support for this approach comes from the documented reduction of perinatal transmission of HIV with AZT, and the success of combination therapy in patients infected with HIV. Initial administration and monitoring of HCWs taking post-exposure prophylaxis should be done in consultation with an experienced clinician, keeping in mind the type of injury and the pattern of HIV drug resistance in the source patient when it is available. There are many reported side effects from those who have elected to take AZT, 3TC, and Indinavir; however, most HCWs can complete a 28-day course. The most common disturbances include fatigue, headache, nausea, and anorexia. Mild reductions in hemoglobin and neutrophils have been observed but are usually not severe enough to warrant discontinuing treatment.

Each HCW exposure to potentially infected blood and body fluids of patients requires immediate attention. The nature of the exposure, the patient source and serological testing (if consent is given), and the immune status of the HCW to HBV and HCV are determined. HBV and HBIG prophylaxis should be initiated if the HCW is susceptible. Unfortunately, there are no proven steps to prevent HCV at this time, although testing of the source patient and close follow-up of the HCW is advisable. The decision to have a baseline HIV test and subsequently take antiretroviral prophylaxis must be left up to the individual HCW after counseling from his or her physician. It is usually in the HCW's best interest to have a baseline HIV test drawn so that, should seroconversion occur, occupational acquisition of the infection can be documented for workmen's compensation and other types of insurance issues. Follow-up HIV testing should take place at 6 weeks, and then again at 3 and 6 months. For peace of mind, most HCWs will want a final follow-up test at 1 year, although the likelihood of seroconversion at this late date is small. Total elimination of HIV transmission from infected patients to HCWs will be possible only with the development of an effective HIV vaccine. Until that time, HCWs must master safe infection control techniques and avoid preventable exposures to HIV, rather than relying on chemoprophylaxis once exposure has occurred.

III. Respiratory Pathogens

A. The Occupational Risk of *Mycobacterium tuberculosis*

The recent reemergence of TB in the United States is due to the large number of foreign-born, previously infected individuals entering this country, the high prevalence of TB in HIV-infected patients, and the general disruption of public health services (especially in urban areas) that have traditionally been effective in controlling the spread of TB (i.e., surveillance, contact tracing, direct observation of treatment, ensuring of compliance with therapy, and such). Health care workers who found themselves immersed in the HIV epidemic in the 1980s decade are now facing the challenge of TB in this decade.

The common occurrence of TB in HIV-infected patients (attributable to the deleterious effect of HIV on cell-mediated immunity) has led to a large number of patients with TB who are highly contagious. For most health care workers who treat AIDS patients, the occupational risk of acquiring TB is far greater than the risk of acquiring HIV. This is due to the airborne nature of TB transmission and the difficulty in recognizing and treating TB in HIV-positive patients.

Over 20,000 new cases of TB are now reported each year in the United States. Many of these patients are hospitalized. Thus, the possibility of transmission to health care personnel and other patients remains a major concern. Although all nosocomial cases of TB in health care workers are of great concern, transmission of multidrug-resistant TB to these persons and susceptible patients is especially worrisome (23). Transmission in these cases has been primarily to HIV-infected or other immunosuppressed individuals, but the potential for spread to nonimmunocompromised health care workers is a real one.

A worker's risk of becoming infected with *M. tuberculosis* depends on the closeness of contact with infectious patients and the degree of adherence to infection control practices. For example, in one study an 11% purified protein derivative (PPD) conversion rate occurred among pulmonary fellows who frequently performed bronchoscopy on patients suspected of having TB. Infectious disease follows, who typically cared for the same TB patients, but did not perform bronchoscopy, had a 2.4% PPD conversion rate (24). Risks of acquiring TB from patients at the current time, however, are likely lower than those reported here. This study (1983–1986) as well as more recent studies that show increased rates of PPD conversion among exposed health care personnel, report data from a time prior to the use of the currently recommended precautions described in the following (25).

The CDC recommendations for prevention of TB transmission in health care settings were published in 1990 and updated in 1993 and 1994 (25). The first document provided valuable information concerning ventilation, ultraviolet light, high-efficiency particulate air (HEPA) filters, source control, risk assessment, and PPD screening of workers. The single most controversial recommendation dealt with the use of "respirators," mask-like devices worn over the face of workers to filter out infectious particles. In 1990, the CDC recommended the use of a dust mist respirator during routine care of TB patients. Although more difficult to wear and expensive, the dust mist respirator was much like a thick surgical mask with two heavy elastic straps. However, in its next revision, the CDC advocated a significantly higher level of respiratory protection, presumably at the urging of OSHA and the health care worker's unions. Although not specifying a particular type of respirator, the description of the ideal respirator required workers to don dust, mist, fume-HEPA respirators (DMF-HEPA), and in some cases powered air-purifying particulate respirators (PAPRs) or positive-pressure airline, half-mask respirators (Table 3). The later two mechanical devices require an external battery or electrical pack that connects them by a hose to the face piece that supplies air to the user. Many TB and infection control experts have argued that these recommendations have no scientific basis. There is no data showing that use of such respirators are more effective than "routine measures" to prevent transmission of TB to personnel. Additionally, they believe that use of such respirators constitutes an unreasonable burden, interferes with patient care, and is very costly. However, OSHA unilaterally mandated the implementation of the CDC guidelines, including respirator use and a respiratory protection program requiring fit testing and training of every individual with exposure to TB, in all health care facilities. Still, experts continue to object, stating

Table 3 Description of the Ideal Respirator for Routine Tuberculosis Patient Care

Standard performance criteria
Ability to filter particles 1 μm in size in the unloaded state with a filter efficiency of at least 95%.
The ability to be qualitatively or quantitatively fit tested in a reliable way to obtain a face seal leakage of less than 10%.
The ability to be checked for facepiece fit by health care workers each time they put on their respirator.
Health care workers who use a respirator should be included in a respiratory protection program.

Source: Ref. 25.

that neither TB transmission nor an unacceptably high PPD conversion rate has ever been demonstrated in an institution that followed the 1990 CDC guidelines calling for the less burdensome dust mist mask for routine patient care. Although, the respirator controversy continues and now lies within the Federal Courts, there are certain high-risk procedures for which there is no disagreement about the need for use of respirators. Bronchoscopy is one such procedure.

B. Precautions During Bronchoscopy

As with blood-borne pathogens, the prevention of TB transmission requires engineering controls, safe work practices, personal protective equipment, and an active employee health system (Table 4). The CDC standards for ventilation in rooms that are occupied by TB patients (25) focus on adequate air exchange (to dilute the number of airborne TB bacilli), and negative pressure (to keep the contaminated air in the room from escaping to adjacent hospital areas). Necessary work practices include early isolation of patients suspected to have TB, rapid diagnosis and treatment of infected

Table 4 Methods to Protect Health Care Workers from *Mycobacterium tuberculosis* Based on CDC Guidelines and OSHA Regulations

Engineering controls	Personal protective equipment (PPE)
TB isolation room:	Respirator: see discussion
Negative pressure	
Minimium 6 ACH	
HEPA filtration	
Ultraviolet light	
Work practices	Employee health
Early diagnosis and isolation	Semiannual or yearly PPD
Wearing respiratory protection	Chemoprophylaxis if positive
Closing door to isolation rooms	Follow-up on inadvertent exposures
Minimizing aerosol production	
Prompt treatment	
Postdischarge follow-up	
Training	Miscellaneous
Annual inservice	Monitoring and maintenance of engineering controls
Basic understanding of TB transmission and epidemiology	Fit testing of respirators
Use of personal protective equipment, engineering controls, safe work practices, and postexposure follow-up	Directly observed therapy (DOT)
	Risk assessment of the workplace

Source: Ref. 25.

patients, directly observed therapy, and prophylaxis of skin test-positive persons. Health workers with frequent exposure to TB patients should have PPD testing done every 6 months; all others should be tested annually.

Because of the types of patients referred to them, pulmonary specialists are at high risk for acquiring TB. The risk is even higher if he or she performs bronchoscopy, for it is a cough-producing and aerosol-generating procedure. During the procedure, a bronchoscopist is forced to position himself face-to-face with the patient, decreasing the effectiveness of environmental controls. Thus, the bronchoscopist and team members must rely on personal respiratory protection to prevent transmission of TB. In this instance, the minimal level of protection should be a DMF–HEPA respirator. The respirator should be worn until the worker leaves the room because; depending on the efficiency of the air exchange system, TB bacilli may remain airborne for several minutes following the procedure. A higher level of respiratory protection and a reevaluation of the engineering controls must be undertaken if PPD surveillance reveals occupational transmission of TB.

C. Management of PPD Conversions

Although following good infection control practices can minimize the occurrence of nosocomial TB transmission, it is probable that a small number of inadvertent exposures and subsequent PPD conversions among health care workers will be identified. No employee can or should be made to wear a respirator from the time they first enter the building until the time they leave at the end of the day. This scenario, although impossible to impose, is the only method that would theoretically ensure complete protection for a worker while working in the hospital. It is important to remember that such persons can also be exposed to TB outside the hospital; in fact, some health care workers have a higher risk of acquiring a TB infection from the community than from their work site.

When PPD testing reveals a new infection, the worker must be evaluated for chemoprophylaxis, and the worksite must be investigated for a breakdown of engineering or work practice controls. If the PPD conversion was secondary to a single or series of known exposures, the TB susceptibility pattern of the source patient should be considered in prescribing chemoprophylaxis. When the source of the exposure is unknown, then the likelihood of exposure to drug-resistant TB must be determined by the overall susceptibility patterns of the TB strains isolated at the work site during the previous 12 months.

The recommendation for chemoprophylaxis for exposure to isoniazid (INH)-sensitive strains of *M. tuberculosis* is oral INH, 300 mg daily for adults. The recommended duration of therapy is 6–12 months in an immunocompetent person and 12 months for persons with HIV infection (23). Preventative therapy guidelines for exposure to drug-resistant *M. tuberculosis* are not uniform. The American Thoracic Society (ATS) recommendations, published in 1994, suggest rifampin alone or rifampin plus ethambutol for newly infected patients exposed to cases of INH-resistant infection. Both drugs should be given in standard therapeutic doses for 6 months. For individuals exposed to multidrug-resistant TB (resistant to both INH and rifampin), the ATS recommends only observation without preventative therapy because there are no studies showing which, if any, regimen is successful in this setting. However, in an immunocompromised individual, who is at high risk for TB, therapy should be given. The ATS recommends 6 months of ethambutol and pyrazinamide if the organism is susceptible to these drugs; if the organism is resistant to ethambutol as well, pyrazinamide plus a quinoline should be given for 6 months (26).

IV. Conclusion

Pulmonary specialists, by virtue of the types of patients they care for and the types of procedures they routinely perform, are at considerable risk of contracting nosocomial infections from patients. Careful attention to safe work practices and principles of infection control represent the two most important ways to minimize acquisition of the blood-borne pathogens (HIV, HBV, or HCV) and TB.

References

1. Raucher BG. Commentary: AIDS, hepatitis, and urologic surgery. In: Whitehead E, ed. Current Operative Urology 1992. Philadelphia: JB Lippincott, 1992:344–348.
2. Centers for Disease Control and Prevention. Guidelines for prevention of transmission of HIV and HBV to healthcare and public-safety workers. MMWR 1989; 38:5–37.
3. Centers for Disease Control and Prevention. HIV/AIDS surveillance report. 1994; 6(no.1):1–27.
4. Baker JL, Kelen GD, Sivertson KT, Quinn TC. Unsuspected human immunodeficiency virus in critically ill emergency patients. JAMA 1987; 257:2609–2611.
5. Robert LM, Bell DM. HIV transmission in the health-care setting. Risks to healthcare workers and patients. Infect Dis Clin North Am 1994; 8:319–329.
6. Mangione C, Gerberding J, Cummings S. Occupational exposure to HIV: fre-

quency and rates of underreporting of percutaneous and mucocutaneous exposures by medical housestaff. Am J Med 1991; 90:85.
7. Henderson DK. HIV in the healthcare setting. In: Mandell G, Bennett J, Dolin R, eds. Principles and Practices of Infectious Diseases. New York: John Wiley & Sons, 1994; 2632–2656.
8. Cuthbert JA. Hepatitis C: progress and problems. Clin Microbiol Rev 1994; 7:505–532.
9. Seeff LB, the National Heart, Lung, and Blood Institute Study Group. Long term mortality after transfusion associated non-A, non-B hepatitis. N Engl J Med 1992; 327:1906–1911.
10. Schiff ER. Hepatitis C among health care providers—risk factors and possible prophylaxis. Hepatology 1992; 16:1300–1301.
11. Kelen CD, Green GB, Purcell RH, Chan DW, Qaquish BF, Sivertson KT, Quinn TC. Hepatitis B and hepatitis C in emergency department patients. N Engl J Med 1992; 326:1399–1404.
12. Mitsui T, Iwano K, Masuko K, Yamazaki C, Okamoto H, Tsuda F, Tanaka T, Mishiro S. Hepatitis C virus infection in medical personnel after needlestick accident. Hepatology 1992; 16:1109–1114.
13. Ciesielski C, Marianos D, Ou CY, Dumbaugh R, Witte J, Berkelman R, Gooch B, Myers G, Luo CC, Schochetman G, et al. Transmission of HIV in a dental practice. Ann Intern Med 1992; 116:798.
14. OSHA. Occupational exposure to blood-borne pathogens: proposed rule and notice of hearing. Federal Register. 1989; 54.
15. OSHA. The bloodborne pathogen standard: final rule. 1991; Federal Register. 56:1030.
16. Tokars J, Bell D, Culver D, Marcus R, Mendelson MH, Sloan EP, Farber BF, Fligner D, Chamberland ME, McKibben PS, et al. Percutaneous injuries during surgical procedures. JAMA 1992; 267:2899.
17. Centers for Disease Control. Recommendations for prevention of HIV transmission in health care settings. MMWR 1987; 32(2S):1–27.
19. Chiarello L. Summary New York State Department of Health Pilot Study of Needlestick Prevention Devices. Chicago, IL: American Hospital Association, 1992.
20. Hersey JC, Martin LS. Use of infection control guidelines by workers in healthcare facilities to prevent occupational transmission of hepatitis B virus and HIV: results from a national survey. Infect Control Hosp Epidemiol 1994; 15:243–252.
21. Mayhall CG. Postexposure immune globulin for needlestick injuries. Infect Control Hosp Epidemiol 1994; 15:564.
22. Centers for Disease Control. Note to readers update: provisional public health service recommendations for chemoprophylaxis after occupational exposure to HIV. MMWR 1996; 45:468–472.
23. Centers for Disease Control. Nosocomial transmission of multidrug-resistant tuberculosis among HIV-infected persons—Florida and New York, 1988–1991. MMWR 1991; 40:585–591.

24. Malasky C, Jordan T, Potulski F, Reichman L. Occupational tuberculosis infections among pulmonary physicians in training. Am Rev Respir Dis 1990; 142:505–507.
25. Centers for Disease Control and Prevention. Guidelines for preventing the transmission of *Mycobacterium tuberculosis* in healthcare facilities. Federal Register 1994; 28:29.
26. American Thoracic Society. Treatment of tuberculosis and tuberculosis infection in adults and children. Am Rev Respir Dis 1994; 149:1359–1374.

AUTHOR INDEX

Italic numbers give the page on which the complete reference is listed.

B

C

G

K

L

M

O

P

Q

R

S

T

U

V

W

SUBJECT INDEX

C